Applications of Mathematics in Models, Artificial Neural Networks and Arts

Vittorio Capecchi · Massimo Buscema ·
Pierluigi Contucci · Bruno D'Amore
Editors

Applications of Mathematics in Models, Artificial Neural Networks and Arts

Mathematics and Society

Springer

Editors
Vittorio Capecchi
Universita Bologna
Dipto. Scienze dell'Educazione
Via Zamboni, 34
40126 Bologna
Italy
vittorio.capecchi@unibo.it

Pierluigi Contucci
Universita Bologna
Dipto. Matematica
Piazza di Porta San Donato, 5
40126 Bologna
Italy
contucci@dm.unibo.it

Massimo Buscema
Semeion
Centro Ricerche di Scienze
della
Comunicazione
Via Sersale, 117
00128 Roma
Italy
m.buscema@semeion.it

Bruno D'Amore
Universita Bologna
Dipto. Matematica
Piazza di Porta San Donato, 5
40126 Bologna
Italy
damore@dm.unibo.it

ISBN 978-90-481-8580-1 e-ISBN 978-90-481-8581-8
DOI 10.1007/978-90-481-8581-8
Springer Dordrecht Heidelberg London New York

Library of Congress Control Number: 2010924730

Printed on acid-free paper

Springer is part of Springer Science+Business Media (www.springer.com)

Preface

The story of this book begins with the conference of 8–9 December 2007 entitled "Mathematics and Society" celebrating the 40 years of *Quality and Quantity, International Journal of Methodology* founded in 1967, under the auspices of Paul F. Lazarsfeld, by editor Vittorio Capecchi and co-editor Raymond Boudon. The journal at present is published by Springer Science & Business Media, Dordrecht. The editor is Vittorio Capecchi, the co-editors are Raymond Boudon and Massimo Buscema. It is a bimonthly publication and it is available online. In the first 10 years, *Quality and Quantity, International Journal of Methodology*published articles by authors writing from Europe and the United States, but in the last 10 years, a growing number of authors who present essays with mathematical models are living in Asia.

The conference of 8–9 December was promoted by the University of Bologna (at the conference, chancellor Pier Ugo Calzolari was present) and the AIS (Italian Association of Sociology) with Departments of Education, Mathematics and Natural and Physical Sciences and the Faculty of the Sciences of Education of the University of Bologna and with the Publishing House Springer (Myriam Poort was present). The success of the conference has produced the original project of this book edited by Vittorio Capecchi with Massimo Buscema, Pierluigi Contucci, Bruno d'Amore.

The book presents a historical introduction (by Vittorio Capecchi) followed by three parts. In the first part *Mathematics and Models* (coordinated by Pierluigi Contucci), mathematical models to study society elaborated in Department of Mathematics and Physics are compared to others that were elaborated in Department of Sociology and Economics. In the second part *Mathematics and Artificial Neural Networks* (coordinated by Massimo Buscema), the applications of ANNs to the social sciences are analysed in several directions and in the third part *Mathematics and Art* (coordinated by Bruno D'Amore), the essays explore the ways in which mathematics and arts relate each other.

In historical introduction, Capecchi analyses in what manner the relation between mathematics and sociology has changed. Three phases are presented: (1) Paul F. Lazarsfeld's choices concerning theory, methodology and mathematics as applied to sociological research; (2) the relations between mathematics and sociology from statistical methods to artificial society and social simulation models; (3) the new possibilities offered to sociology though by artificial neural networks. Then the changes in the methodological problems linked to the relation between mathematics and sociology are analysed together with the changes in the most important paradigm utilized in sociological research, namely the paradigm of objectivity; the paradigm of action research/co-research and the paradigm of feminist methodology. At the end of the introduction, some new possible synergies are presented.

The first part of the book coordinated by Pierluigi Contucci deals with models coming from the community of mathematicians and physicists as well as from scholars in sociology, economy and cognitive psychology. The leading theme of the mathematical–physical approach concerns the identifications of those model features which are responsible for the collective behaviour as derived from individual contribution for large numbers of them. The paper by P. Contucci, I. Gallo and S. Ghirlanda studies the effect of the interaction between two cultures and the possible scenarios appearing including the phase transitions. The methods used are those coming from statistical mechanics. The paper by Bolina gives a transparent introduction to the statistical mechanics general methods for those readers who are not familiar with that discipline. The paper by F. Gallo et al. applies the method introduced in the previous papers to the study of the climate change and energy virtuous behaviour especially oriented to the recommendation to public policy makers. The paper by A. Borghi et al. explains the necessity of embodied models in cognitive psychology. The paper by Robert Smith (Social Structural Research, Inc., Cambridge, MA) presents the possibility to analyse with stronger mathematical models *The Academic Mind* by Paul F. Lazarsfeld; Simone Sarti and Marco Terraneo (University of Milano-Bicocca) apply a multilevel regression technique to validate a social stratification scale; Claudio Gallo (Crs4, Cagliari) discusses the mathematical models of financial markets.

The second part of the book, coordinated by Massimo Buscema, presents essays by the Semeion Group (Massimo Buscema, Giulia Massini, Guido Maurelli, Stefano Terzi) and by Enzo Grossi (Bracco SpA, Milano), Pierluigi Sacco (IUAV, University of Venezia), Sabina Tangaro (Istituto Nazionale Fisica Nucleare, Bari). Artificial adaptive systems (AASs) are a new area of the modern applied mathematics. The main goal of AAS is to generate models from data. So, AASs are systems able to make the different models explicit, hidden in the real world. To do that, AASs present a set of specific features:

1. AASs are completely data driven or more precisely, the less the free parameters they have to presume, the better.
2. AASs generate a specific model only during their active interaction with the data. So they are bottom-up systems and they produce a data model as an end point of an iterative and a feedback loop process. This means that the final model of the data emerges automatically during the process itself. Consequently, they are dynamic systems, where the time of their learning and/or evolutionary process is part of the final model.
3. During their learning and/or evolutionary process, they process all the variables of the data in parallel. So, at the end of this process, each variable has been

defined by its global interaction with all the others (many-to-many relationships); so, theoretically, every order of variable interaction should be coded.
4. AAS has to be able to code all the consistent non-linearity hidden in the data.
5. During the learning and/or the evolutionary process, both the variables and the records (points) of the data set work as agents. This means that they interact in active way among them and with the basic parameters of the AAS equations.
6. AAS, to be validated, has to follow specific validation protocol and procedures, very similar to the procedures used in experimental physics.

In this part of the book we show new AAS algorithms, recently designed in AAS basic research, and their experimental application in real–world problems: bio-medicine and security.

These two applicative fields seem to be uncorrelated. Partially this is true. And so the application of the same algorithms to different areas is a good test to prove their capability to be really "data driven". From another point of view, bio-medicine and security are linked; both represent tough real problems, wherein the gold standard is very often grounded. Consequently, it is easy to analyse the performances of our AAS. Bio medicine and security are also very sensitive "ethic" subjects; in the first, we try to defeat the disease, in the second one, we try to cope with violence and illegality, an impressive social disease.

The third part of the book, coordinated by Bruno d'Amore, presents essays on the relation between mathematics and art. Amongst the most widespread convictions, and not only in a low cultural profile perspective, there is the following: art (in all of its aspects, but here I will focus on figurative art) is the reign of freedom and fancy, whereas mathematics is that of formalism and rigour.

This approach refers to a position according to which we are dealing with two opposite worlds, with no cultural unity. Nevertheless the aforementioned four terms (freedom and fancy, formalism and rigour) do have common deep ties and are all produced by human beings, by their need to create and communicate.

Since the Renaissance there are examples of artists–mathematicians in which such terms are indissolubly bound, reinforcing each other; it is well known that Albrecht Dürer travelled in Italy to gain knowledge of the "scientific" art, widespread in the Peninsula and not yet in Bavaria, and to take courses as a geometry student at the *Alma Mater;* without rigorous knowledge, he said, art is an empty fancy and a blindly accepted practice.

Freedom and fancy must lay on a rigorous basis that gives them *sense*; otherwise it is *ignis fatuus*, uselessness, illogical. On the other hand, today it is well known that the first gift required by any high-level mathematician is fancy. Several mathematicians stated that a person quitted mathematics and became a poet (or a painter) because he or she was not fancy enough. Furthermore, when we say that a chess player plays with fancy, we do not mean he or she does not follow the rules of that game strictly but that he or she follows them conceiving unexpected and creative strategies.

We do not want to astonish the reader with these statements; in fact, we just want to convince the few that should still be so naive to believe these trivial dichotomies.

So if it is true, as it is, that many artists in centuries (more and more often at the present time) turned to mathematics as a source of inspiration or as an object of their pictorial practice, it is also true that many mathematicians (more and more often at the present time) did not despise to look at figurative art, with very different means, instruments and objectives, as an interesting and significant field of research and cultural speculation.

We tried to reproduce here the variety of these approaches. Bruno d'Amore (his essay is about mathematics and figurative art) has invited the following colleagues to discuss them from many points of view that are perfectly entangled, but each of them following specific and distinct lines, hoping to offer a significant variety of such interests: Igino Aschieri and Paola Vighi (University of Parma), From Art to Mathematics in the Paintings of Theo van Doesburg; Giorgio Bagni (University of Udine), Mathematics, Art, and Interpretation: A Hermeneutic Perspective; Giorgio Bolondi (University of Bologna), Points, Line and Surface. Following Enriques and Kandinsky; Michele Emmer (University of Roma I), Visibili armonie: The Idea of Space from "Flatland" to Artistic Avant-garde; Franco Eugeni and Ezio Sciarra (University of Teramo), Mathematical Structures and Sense of Beauty; Monica Idà (University of Bologna), Visual Impact and Mathematical Learning; Marco Pierini (University of Siena), Art by Numbers. Mel Bochner, Roman Opalka and other Filaritmici; Aldo Spizzichino (CNR of Bologna), My Way of Playing with the Computer; Gian Marco Todesco (Digital Video SpA), Four-Dimensional Ideas.

The essays presented in these three parts are interesting not only for their contribution to mathematical methodology and to the methodology of social research but also for other two important directions of action research: (1)technological innovations regarding the quality of life (climate changes through efficient energy, mathematical models against criminality, mathematical models for medicine and so on) and (2) technological innovations for creativity (the papers of the section *Mathematics and Art* are in the direction of projects as the *Creative Cities Network* of UNESCO).

Finally this book is useful not only for those who make use of mathematics in the social sciences but also for those who are engaged in the diffusion of technological innovation to improve life quality and to spread creativity in all directions of the arts.

Bologna, Italy — Vittorio Capecchi
Roma, Italy — Massimo Buscema
Bologna, Italy — Pierluigi Contucci
Bologna, Italy — Bruno D'Amore

Contents

Contributors

Igino Aschieri Local Research Unit of Didactics of Mathematics; Mathematics Department, University of Parma, Parma, Italy, aschieri@aschig.191.it

Giorgio T. Bagni Department of Mathematics and Computer Science, University of Udine, Udine, Italy, giorgio.bagni@dimi.uniud.it

Roberto Bellotti Department of Physics, Center of Innovative Technologies for Signal Detection and Processing (Tires), National Institute of Nuclear Physics, Bari Section, Bari, Italy; University of Bari, Bari, Italy, Roberto.bellotti@ba.infn.it

Mel Bochner New York artist represented by Peter Freeman Galery, New York, USA, info@peterfreemaninc.com

Oscar Bolina Kaplan Shinyway Overseas Pathway College, HangZhou 310053, P.R. China, oscarb@kaplanshinyway.com

Giorgio Bolondi Department of Mathematics, University of Bologna, Bologna, Italy, giorgio.bolondi@unibo.it

Anna M. Borghi Department of Psychology, University of Bologna, Bologna, Italy; Institute of Cognitive Sciences and Technologies, CNR, Rome, Italy, annamaria.borghi@unibo.it

Massimo Buscema Semeion Research Center, Via Sersale, Rome, Italy, m.buscema@semeion.it

Daniele Caligiore Department of Psychology, University of Bologna, Bologna, Italy; Institute of Cognitive Sciences and Technologies, CNR, Rome, Italy, daniele.caligiore@istc.cnr.it

Vittorio Capecchi Department of Education, University of Bologna, Bologna, Italy, vittorio.capecchi@unibo.it

Pierluigi Contucci Department of Mathematics, University of Bologna, Bologna, Italy; Centre for the Study of Cultural Evolution, Stockholm University, Stockholm, Sweden, contucci@dm.unibo.it

Adam Coutts Department of Politics and International Relations, University of Oxford, Oxford, England, UK, adam.coutts@politics.ox.ac.uk

Bruno D'Amore NRD Department of Mathematics, University of Bologna, Bologna, Italy; ASP High Pedagogical School, Locarno, Switzerland; MESCUD Districtal University "Fr. José de Caldas", Bogotà, Colombia, damore@dm.unibo.it

Francesco De Carlo National Institute of Nuclear Physics, Bari Section, Bari, Italy, francesco.decarlo@ba.infn.it

Michele Emmer Department of Mathematics, University of Rome 1, Rome, Italy, emmer@mat.uniroma1.it

Franco Eugeni Department of Communication, University of Teramo, Teramo, Italy, Eugenif1@tin.it

Claudio Gallo Imaging & Numerical Geophysics, Energy & Environment Department, Center for Advanced Studies, Research and Development in Sardinia (CRS4), Pula CA, Italy, fender@crs4.it

Federico Gallo Office of Climate Change, UK Government, UK, federico.gallo@occ.gsi.gov.uk

Ignacio Gallo Department of Mathematics, University of Bologna, Bologna, Italy, gallo@dm.unibo.it

Gianfranco Gargano National Institute of Nuclear Physics, Bari Section, Bari, Italy; Department of Physics, University of Bari, Bari, Italy, g.gargano@libero.it

Stefano Ghirlanda Department of Psychology, University of Bologna, Bologna, Italy; Centre for the Study of Cultural Evolution, Stockholm, Sweden, stefano.ghirlanda@unibo.it

Enzo Grossi Medical Department, Bracco Spa, Milano, Italy; Centro Diagnostico Italiano, Milano, Italy; Semeion Research Centre, Rome, Italy, enzo.grossi@bracco.com

Monica Idà Department of Mathematics, University of Bologna, 40126 Bologna, Italy, ida@dm.unibo.it

Raffaele Mascella Department of Communication, University of Teramo, Teramo, Italy, mascella@unite.it

Giulia Massini Semeion Research Center, Via Sersale, Rome, Italy, g.massini@semeion.it

Roman Opalka Polish painter born in France, represented by Yvon Lambert Gallery, Paris, France, paris@yvon-lambert.com

Pier L. Sacco Department of Arts and Industrial Design, Iuav University, Venice, Italy, sacco@economia.unibo.it

Luca De Sanctis Department of Psychology and Mathematics, University of Bologna, Bologna, Italy, luca.desanctis2@unibo.it

Simone Sarti Department of Sociology and Social Research, University of Milan "Bicocca", Milan, Italy, simone.sarti@unimib.it

Ezio Sciarra Department of Social Sciences, University of Chieti, Pescara, Italy, esciarra@unich.it

Claudia Scorolli Department of Psychology, University of Bologna, Bologna, Italy, cscorolli@dsc.unibo.it

Robert B. Smith Social Structural Research Inc., Cambridge, MA, USA, rsmithphd@comcast.net

Aldo Spizzichino Former researcher at INAF IASF-bo, Bologna, Italy, aldo@computedart.org

Sabina Tangaro National Institute of Nuclear Physics, Bari Section, Bari, Italy, sonia.tangaro@ba.infn.it

Marco Terraneo Department of Sociology and Social Research, University of Milan "Bicocca", Milan, Italy, marco.terraneo@unimib.it

Gian M. Todesco (http://www.toonz.com/personal/todesco), Digital Video S.p.A. (http://www.toonz.com), matematita (http://www.matematita.it)

Paola Vighi Local Research Unit of Didactics of Mathematics; Mathematics Department, University of Parma, Parma, Italy, paola.vighi@unipr.it

Chapter 1
Mathematics and Sociology

From Lazarsfeld to Artificial Neural Networks

Vittorio Capecchi

Abstract In this historical introduction Capecchi analyses in what manner the relation between mathematics and sociology has changed. Three phases are presented: (a) Paul F. Lazarsfeld's choices concerning theory, methodology and mathematics as applied to sociological research; (b) the relations between mathematics and sociology from statistical methods to artificial society and social simulation models; and (c) the new possibilities offered to sociology though by artificial neural networks. Then the changes in the methodological problems linked to the relation between mathematics and sociology are analysed together with the changes in the most important paradigm utilized in sociological research namely the paradigm of objectivity; the paradigm of action research/co-research and the paradigm of feminist methodology. At the end of the introduction, some new possible synergies are presented.

The first issue of the periodical *Quality and Quantity*, edited by Vittorio Capecchi with Raymond Boudon as advisory editor, was published in English in January 1967, under the auspices of Paul F. Lazarsfeld (PFL). PFL thought that it was time that the relation between mathematics and sociology started to spread in Europe also (the periodical was in fact published with the subtitle *European Journal of Methodology*). I met PFL in 1962 in Gösing (Austria) during a seminar on *mathematics and social sciences*[1] (PFL had previously written to some Italian departments of statistics to find out whether there were young scholars trained in mathematics and sociology. At the time I had just got a degree at the Bocconi University in Milan with Francesco Brambilla and Angelo Pagani, with a dissertation entitled "Application of Markov Chains to Social Mobility"). After the seminar, I decided to edit PFL's works in Italian[2] and subsequently began to do research at the Bureau of

V. Capecchi (✉)
Department of Education, University of Bologna, Bologna, Italy
e-mail: vittorio.capecchi@unibo.it

[1]The proceedings of the seminar were published in Sternberg et al. (1965).
[2]Lazarsfeld (1967).

V. Capecchi (eds.), *Applications of Mathematics in Models, Artificial Neural Networks and Arts*, DOI 10.1007/978-90-481-8581-8_1,

Applied Social Research at the Columbia University, at the time under the direction of PFL, who used to collaborate with Robert K. Merton. In Paris, thanks to PFL, I met Raymond Boudon, who at the time was editing PFL's works in French, and together we decided to plan a periodical on the interrelation between mathematics and sociology.

The first issue of *Quality and Quantity* was published by a small Italian publishing house (Marsilio in Venice), thanks to the help of the architect Paolo Ceccarelli, who, at the time, owned some shares in Marsilio. The cover of the issue – which has always remained the same – was created by a Venetian designer. After 2 years, in 1969, the periodical started to be published by Il Mulino in Bologna, thanks to Giovanni Evangelisti, who thought that PFL's work was going to become a cornerstone of Italian sociology. Starting from 1962, the periodical was published by Dutch publishing houses (Elsevier, Kluwer and Springer). Nowadays, Springer publishes six issues a year which are also available online, with Raymond Boudon and Massimo Buscema as co-editors. In all those 40 years, *Quality and Quantity* has been very well organized by the editorial secretary Dolores Theresa Sandri.

The relation between mathematics and sociology has a long history which begins in Europe, as it is briefly illustrated by PFL (1962, p. 761) as follows:

> Sampling methods were derived as a sequence to Booth's survey of life and labour in London. Factor analysis was invented by the Englishman, Spearman. Family research, with special emphasis on quantification, come of age with the French mineralogist Le Play: Gabriel Tarde advocated attitude measurement and communication research (...) The idea of applying mathematical models to voting was elaborately worked out by Condorcet during the French Revolution. His contemporaries, Laplace and Lavoisier, conducted social surveys for the Revolutionary Government, and their student, The Belgian, Quételet, finally and firmly established empirical social research under the title, "phisique sociale" (...). In Italy, during the first part of this century, Niceforo developed clear ideas on the use of measurement in social and psychological problems brilliantly summarised in his book on the measurement of progress. The German could claim a number of founding fathers: Max Weber was periodically enthusiastic about quantification, making many computations himself; Toennies invented a correlation coefficient of his own; and during Easter vacations, von Wiese regularly took his students to villages so that they could see his concept about social relations acted out in peasant families.

In a long article dedicated to the relation between mathematics and sociology, PFL (1961) wrote that such a relationship can be divided into three phases; each phase is marked by the work of a leading scholar: (1) *government statistics* with important contribution by the German philosopher Hermann Conring (1606–1681); (2) *phisique social* with contributions by Belgium astronomer and statistician Adolphe Quételet (1796–1874) and (3) the *observation method* with contributions by the French mineralogist Frédéric le Play (1806–1882). The most representative scholar of phase that followed – the *Methodology of Sociological Research* – was certainly the sociologist and mathematician Paul F. Lazarsfeld (1901–1976). In 1954, in his introduction to *Mathematical Thinking in the Social Sciences*, PFL makes the following comments concerning the relation between mathematics and sociology:

> *Why mathematics is useful for sociology*: (i) mathematics contributes to clarity of thinking and, by permitting better organization of available knowledge, facilitates decisions as to

needed further work; (ii) how do we weave back and forth from empirical observation to the parameters of the underlying model incorporating our theoretical assumptions, in terms which are always in part probabilistic; (iii) There is little doubt that a trend toward formalization will profitably bring together a variety of pursuits in the behavioral science which, at the moment, have little contact.

Three roads seem promising; (i) We need people who are trained both in mathematics and in some sector of social sciences; (ii) At the same time, actual investigations have to be carried on; (iii) In addition to training and creative work, there is a third road. We need investigations which clarify in a more general way the possible relations between mathematics and the social sciences.

The future of relation mathematics/sociology; How the role of mathematical thinking in the social sciences will evolve is more difficult to predict, because neither mathematics not social sciences is unchangeably fixed. [3]

In this historical introduction I have tried to reconstruct the relation between mathematics and sociology, keeping in mind the last 40 years of *Quality and Quantity* and the following three phases: (a) PFL's choices concerning theory, methodology and mathematics applied to the paradigm of objectivity; (b) the relations between mathematics and sociology from statistical methods to artificial society and social simulation; (c) the new possibilities offered to sociology by artificial neural networks.

1.1 Theory, Methodology and Mathematics: the Choices of Paul F. Lazarsfeld

Paul Felix Lazarsfeld (PFL) is best known for having used in the United States (and in Europe) quantitative methods which were opposed to the qualitative methods of the Chicago School. The reception of his works in the United States, France and Italy[4] has however rightly stressed that his contribution is more complex than this. PFL's choices concerning sociological theory, methodology and mathematics can be summed up as follows:

- *Subordination of research to theory*. In order to understand PFL's choices concerning sociological theory, it should be remembered that during the 1950s and the 1960s in the United States the "grand theory" of Talcott Parsons was opposed to a "middle range theory", proposed by Robert Merton. PFL chose the method by Merton and, as noted in PFL (1953), his programme had the following goals: (a) to find the causes of individual actions and (b) to understand mutual modifications that take place as a consequence of interactions. PFL's work is in line with his theoretical objectives. He in fact was engaged, or participated, to various researches concerning individual behaviour in specific situations (unemployment

[3]Lazarsfeld (1954), pp. 3–5, 8, 10, 16. The quotations from PFL (1954) have been organized in a different way.

[4]In the United States: Merton et al. Eds. 1979; in France: Lautman and Lécuyer Eds. 1998; in Italy: Campelli Ed. 1999.

in *Die Arbeitslosen von Marienthal*, the Second World War in *The American Soldier*, the McCarthyism in *The Academic Mind*) and mechanisms subordinated to specific choices (the political vote in *The American Voter* or consumers' choices in *Personal Influence*), with the aim to evaluate the effect of interactions of the behaviour of single people. As noted by Robert Merton (1998, p. 174), "It was only the topics that varied endlessly.(...). But at their conceptual core most of those varied topics were instances of a crucial type of action: the making of choices ore, in somewhat extended sense, the arriving at decisions". In brief, research is subordinated to theoretical construction.

- *Subordination of methodology to research.* The methodology to carry out this programme is based on the paradigm of objectivity. According to PFL the Chicago School cannot be defined as a scientific one, because it proposed qualitative methods such as participating observations experimented by anthropologists, among whom was Malinowski. As noted by William Foote Whyte in his book *Street Corner Society* (1943, p. 356–357): "It would be impossible to map out at the beginning the sort of study I eventually found myself doing". His work "depended upon an intimate familiarity with people and situation" and this "intimate familiarity" was necessary "to understand the group" only through observing how it changed through time. Foote Whyte thought that there were risks in this kind of research (if the scholar at the beginning is a non-participating observer, but later on, when he has been accepted by the group, he becomes more and more participating and less and less of an observer), but these were still acceptable risks because they led to a better knowledge of people and communities that were the object of the study.

PFL prefers to run other kinds of risks and uses the paradigm of objectivity. From the point of view of the distinction between standpoint epistemology, methodology and research methods, [5] this *paradigm of objectivity* can be defined as follows:

1. *Standpoint epistemology.* Sociological research has the goal to formulate theories (explanations) on attitudes and behaviours of people who have to make choices with the most possible objectivity.
2. *Methodology.* In order to reach this objective, research is separated by actions that could derive from explanations obtained through research. The explanations are considered scientifically valid if the answers (information) given by the subjects of the research are "objective". An increased objectivity can be obtained if

[5] In this paper the term *paradigm*, in the sense attributed to it by Kuhn, has been used for the following: (a) standpoint methodology; (b) methodology; (c) research methods. The definitions are by Sandra Harding (2004, p. 44; 1987, p. 2): *standpoint epistemology* "sets the relationship between knowledge and politics"; *methodology* is "a theory and analysis of how research does or should proceed"; *research method* "is a technique for (or way of proceeding in) gathering evidence. (...) In this sense there are only three methods of social inquiry: listening to (or) interrogating informants, observing behaviour or examining historical trace and records".

the researcher does not influence the answers (information) given by the subjects of the research.
3. *Research methods*. Valid methods of research are only two: those in which there is no interaction on the part of researcher with the subject of research or those in which the interaction happens through a group of professional interviewers who use a scientific method.

The objectivity paradigm, however, is not used by PFL in a rigid and reductive way and, in *The Academic Mind*, its use in the survey leads to results that make this research closer to the one of the Chicago School. The steps of a survey, according to PFL (1958, pp. 101–104), are four:

1. *Imagery*. The flow thought and analysis and work which ends up with a measuring instrument usually begins with something which might be called imagery. Out of the analyst's immersion in all the detail of a theoretical problem, he creates a rather vague image or construct. (...).
2. *Concept specification*. The next step is to take this original imagery and divide it into components. The concept is specified by an elaborate discussion of phenomena out of which it emerged. We develop "aspects", "components", dimensions" or similar specification. (...)
3. *Selection of indicators*. After we have decided on these dimensions, there comes the third step: finding indicators for the dimensions. (...).
4. *Formation of indices*. The four steps is to put Humpty Dumpty together again (...) because we cannot operate with all those dimensions and indicators separately.

In *The Academic Mind*, one should however add a fifth step:

5. *A political use of quantitative methodology and mathematics*. Quantitative methods and the use of mathematics present results in a more "objective" way and in this way they can be used to protect the "subjectivity" of the researcher and allow her/him to express subjective evaluations that do not conform with the contemporary political climate.

This fifth step, never explicitly declared but nevertheless practised by PFL, stresses the way in which he always subordinates methodology to the goals of theory and research. As Jacques Lautman and Bernard-Pierre Lécuyer have noted (1998, p. 17), PFL's methodology is not an end to itself, because "the use of methodological innovation happened only when one encountered difficulties with theory".

- *Subordination of mathematics to methodology*. PFL's use of mathematics, within his proposed methodology for sociological research, follows two directions: (a) a direction that is subordinated to research needs and sociological theory ($S \rightarrow M \rightarrow S$, where S = sociology and M = mathematics) and (b) a direction in which mathematics has its own autonomy of elaboration, even though this is applied to sociology ($M \rightarrow S \rightarrow M$). PFL's contribution mainly follows the first direction; here the limits of mathematics are two: (i) mathematics models and methods are mainly linear with only few exceptions and (ii) it is not possible to deal with variables at the level of the nominal scale, ordinal scale or interval scale at the same time. [6]

In a sociological research, such as the survey, items at the nominal level (gender distinctions, political and geographical origins, etc.), at the ordinal level (education record), at the level of the interval scale (test result or attitude scales) and on the ratio scale (age, recurrence of behaviours, and so on) are all present at the same time. As a consequence, it is not possible to treat all items of a sociological research according to the same methods or mathematical model. Possible solutions are the following: (i) reduce part of the items in dichotomous variables and (ii) reduce part of the items in variables on the interval scale. In this way, scores between 1 and 4 are adopted in order to make items on the ordinal scale (education record) and items on the ratio scale (age) homogeneous; (iii) try to construct indices that summarize more items.

The result was that, even in PFL's most elaborated researches, mathematical applications are always realized by limited number of items and the research results are summarized in a limited number of indices. PFL's choices will be analysed with reference to three researches (*Die Arbeitslosen von Marienthal*, *Personal Influence*, *The Academic Mind*), in order to understand the ways in which sociological research can be classified.

1.1.1 Types of Sociological Research: Some Suggestions

Some suggestions concerning the classification of sociological research coordinated by PFL (or undertaken following his instructions) are illustrated in Tables 1.1, 1.2 and 1.3. Table 1.1 has been presented by Hanan Selvin (1979) to define the different study aim of a research which uses two dimensions: (a) there is a distinction between researches that take into account data already gathered (such as censuses or electoral results), which must be analysed without any possibility of modifying them, and researches that analyse data gathered on a new population of subjects that are interviewed and (b) there is a distinction between explicative researches, concerning causes, and researches that are only descriptive.

---

[6]Warren S. Torgerson (1958) gives the following definitions for the four types of scales: (i) *nominal scale*: when between the two elements A and B of the same variable, it is possible to indicate only the relation $A = B, A \neq B$; (ii) *ordinal scale*: when between two elements of the same variable, it is possible to indicate the relations $A < B, A = B, A > B$; (iii) *interval scale*: when the scale has no natural origin and operations such as A: B, $A \times B$ are possible, but the origin and units of measure are arbitrary (as in test scores); (iv) *ratio scale* when the scale has natural origin (as in the age variable) and operations such as A: $B, A \times B$ are possible.

Table 1.1 Types of sociological research: study aim

Study aim	The investigator seeks to describe an antecedent defined population	The investigator seeks to describe a new population
The investigator is interested in causality	Descriptive explanatory S. A. Stouffer (1955) *Communism, conformity and civil liberties.*	Purely explanatory studies M. Jahoda, PFL and H. Zeisel (1933) *Die Arbeitslosen von Marienthal.*
The investigator is not interested in causality	Purely descriptive P. M. Blau and O. D. Duncan (1962) *The American occupational structure.*	Nonstudy Example *: How youth feel about depression*

Source: Selvin (1979)

Table 1.2 Types of sociological research: methodological options with the paradigm of objectivity

Methodological options	No interaction	Interaction with interview
Quantitative methods	Observation of quantitative behaviours and utilization of statistics (example: *Die Arbeitslosen von Marienthal* (1933))	Survey (examples: *Personal Influence*(1955); *The Academic Mind* (1958))
Qualitative methods	Observation of qualitative behaviours and utilization of letters, diaries (examples: *Die Arbeitslosen von Marienthal* (1933); Asylums (1961))	Survey with open items (example: *The Academic Mind* (1958))

Table 1.3 Types of sociological research: sponsors and object of research

	Object of research			
Research sponsor	Towards "top"	Intermediary	Towards 'bottom' Type I	Towards "bottom" Type II
Financial research sponsor not using results	1	2	3	4
Financial research sponsor using results	5	6	7	8
Non-financial research sponsor chosen by enquiry group	9	10	11	12

Source: Capecchi (1972, 1981)

Methodological choices within the paradigm of objectivity lead to two dimensions indicated in Table 1.2: (c) a greater/smaller interaction between the researcher and the subjects of the research and (d) the greater or lesser possibility to use quantitative or qualitative methods of analysis.

Dimension (c) distinguishes between two kinds of research: (i) research with no interaction and (ii) research in which the only possible interaction is between the professional interviewer and the subjects of the research.

Among the researches in which there is no interaction with the subjects of the research are statistics, letters, diaries, etc. or cases in which people are observed without being aware of it. *Die Arbeitslosen von Marienthal* and *Asylums* (1961) by Erving Goffman are part of the latter. In *Asylums* the researcher was hired for 6 months as a masseur by a psychiatric in order to observe what was going on without influencing the interrelations among patients, nurses and doctors. It should be stressed that *Asylums*, which is realized without any interaction between the research co-ordinator and the subjects of the research, has produced very relevant changes in psychiatric practice (in Italy its translation, by Franco Basaglia, has been of major importance to start a new way to practise psychiatry). Researches without interaction as well as those based on interviews use quantitative and qualitative methods, as clearly shown by PFL's researches, which will be considered in the next section. However, it should be considered that if one chooses the paradigm of objectivity, some qualitative methodological strategies may be excluded.

In Table 1.3, shown in Capecchi (1972, 1981), researches are classified taking into account of the following: (e) the sponsor who finances the research and (f) the level (measured by the researcher) in which people and object of the research are collocated. This table was proposed in a period in which radical sociology was popular in the United States and caused worries about the possible negative role played by the sponsor and the tendency of sociological research not to take into account economic and political powers.

The research sponsor cannot be interested in using the results (this is the case of *The Fund for the Republic*, an emanation of the *Ford Foundation*, which sponsored for *The Academic Minds*) or he may be interested in using results (for example this is the case of the social democratic party in Vienna, which sponsored the *Arbeitslosen von Marienthal*, or Macfadden publications, which sponsored for *Personal Influence*). The sponsor can be a non-financial subject, when he helps the research but does not finance the research group, which therefore works for free.

Research can be different according to the kind of relation that is established between the researcher and the people, object of the research. Researchers can study power; they can study people that are, like themselves, university professors or they can study people that have less power and influence. In this latter case, two situations should be distinguished: (1) type I in which the asymmetrical relation is mainly due to social/economic variables (the unemployed in *Marienthal*, women interviewed in *Personal Influence*) and (2) type II in which the asymmetrical relation depends on other variables, such as gender, race or psychical condition (for example the patients of the psychiatric hospital studied by Goffman, etc.)

1.1.2 Die Arbeitslosen von Marienthal (1932)

In 1933, Franklin Delano Roosevelt becomes president of the United States of America; in the same year, Adolf Hitler becomes the German chancellor of the new Reichstag and begins his Nazi dictatorship. In 1932, *Die Arbeitslosen von Marienthal* is published. It belongs to PFL's Viennese period, studied by Hans Zeisel (1979), Anton Pelinka (1998), Francois Isambert (1998) and Marie Jahoda (1998). This book was published with Marie Jahoda and Hans Zeisel by the Centre of Applied Psychology, directed by PFL and financed by the Rockefeller Fund and the social democratic party of Vienna.

The objective of the research was to study the effects of unemployment on the people of Marienthal, a small industrial village in the outskirts of Vienna. The total inhabitants were 478 families, three quarters of these were fully unemployed, due to the fact that a cotton industry – Todesko, the only source of employment in the area – had closed. This is research 7 in Table 1.3. Thanks to the psychologist Marie Jahoda, the first wife of PFL, the research focused on the relationship between women and men in family life, on the way families spent their free time, the way they search employment, etc. This research was defined by its authors as an *immersion* research (sich einleben); the methodological choice of non-interaction with the people in Marienthal was taken in order to reach more objective results and was influenced, as PFL wrote (1971), by Karl Marx. Individual and contextual features were considered; analysis were mainly quantitative, based on official statistics (population statistics, complaints presented to the industrial commission, electoral results) and other kinds of data (the amount of money spent in the consumers' cooperative, the number of books borrowed from the local library, the number of subscriptions to periodicals). Another kind of survey was done; behind the window at midday sharp, the passers-by were observed to quantify the pace and the length of conversation of men and women that were going home.

It was also decided to observe the behaviour of men and women of Marienthal using qualitative methodologies. The research team organized the so-called "Clothes Project" (the team gave out 200 hundred pieces of clothes to the poorest families and in order to justify these presents they asked them to answer some questions), a "Medical Treatment Project" (the team was joined by an obstetrician and a paediatrician to give out, if necessary, free medicines), and two courses for women: one of model drawing to provide professional requalification for the less young ones and a gym course for the younger women.

The team tried to be as objective as possible, and the inhabitants of this little village started to consider it as a group of people who worked for the government to help them (by organizing courses, giving aid, etc.) and not as researchers. Even when the team used essays by school children (in exchange for Christmas presents), children thought that these were part of their routine homework.

The results led Jahoda, PFL and Zeisel to formulate a theory that was built step by step so that it was only at the end of the research that "essential ideas on the effects of unemployment emerged". The relations between the main variables were shown, and, as noted by Francoise Isambert (1998), they formed a circular interpretative model, in which unemployment represented its beginning and its end: unemployment activates a "process of degradation" which aggravates, within a negative spiral, the problems about finding a job. Families were classified into four groups: resigned (48%), apathetic (25%), actives (16%) and desperate (11%). According to this scheme by Isambert, there are therefore various levels of degradation families can find themselves in (ranging from resignation to desperation). However, there is also a "deviant minority": families defined as actives that try to find new solutions.

This research was highly valued in the Unites States by politically engaged sociologists such a Robert and Helen Lynd. The Lynds had already published *Middletown* (1929) and were influenced by PFL when later on they wrote *Middletown in Transition* (1937).

1.1.3 Personal Influence (1955)

1955 was the year of Martin Luther King. In that year in Montgomery, Alabama, Rosa Parks, a middle-aged lady, decided to rebel against black segregation, which obliged black people to sit in the back of buses, even when seats in the front were free. Rosa Parks sat in the front seats of a bus in Montgomery and for this reason she had to pay a $10 fine. This event convinced Martin Luther King, who in 1955 has just received his Ph.D. in theology from Boston University, to become the leader of a pacifist movement for the rights of blacks. He started to boycott buses and in 1956 a sentence of the US Supreme Court declared segregation on buses unconstitutional.

Personal Influence, published in 1955 by PFL in collaboration with Elihu Katz, was financed by the research office of the Macfadden publications to understand how to organize an advertisement campaign (in Table 1.3, it is number 7 research). In this case, the sponsor used the results of the research for market purposes (while in *Die Arbeitslosen von Marienthal* the socialist party intended to use the results to fight back unemployment). This research is made in the period when Lazarsfeld was active. He had arrived in the United States in 1933 with a Rockefeller fellowship and as part of a wide intellectual migration[7] from territories occupied by the Nazi [on this particular period, see essays by Christian Fleck (1998), Robert Merton (1998), Seymour Lipset (1998)]. The aim of *Personal Influence* was to analyse the influence of mass media on women consumers. PFL wanted to verify the theory of "two steps flow of communication", according to which the majority of women are not directly influenced by mass media but by a net of opinion leaders that are part of their relations. The method for such verification consisted of three surveys done between the autumn of 1944 and the spring of 1945, just before the end of the Second World War. The study focused on some consumer choices (food, household products, movies and fashion) and the opinions on social and political issues

---

[7] See the article by PFL (1969).

expressed by women of Decatur, a city of about 60,000 inhabitants in the Middle West chosen to represent "average" behaviours.

In this work, relations between men and women were not taken into account and only individual variables were considered. For mathematical elaboration of results, the analysis of the latent structure was also used, and in the appendix "On the construction of indices", the procedures that led to a summary of the main results were illustrated. These were divided into four indices: gregariousness, social status, importance and opinion leadership. When the study was published, PFL was criticized for having chosen market research in a period in which sociologists were mainly interested in fighting back what Marin Luther King called the three demons: poverty, racism and militarism. As Seymour Martin Lipset (1998, p. 264) noted:

> To Lynd and to radical students like myself, however, the fact that Paul and his Bureau of Applied Social Research (formerly the Office of Radio Research) were so involved in market research, in studies supported by the radio networks, or advertising agencies, seemed like sell-outs. We knew, or I should rather say, I knew, that I could learn much from Paul and Bureau type research, essentially survey technique. But I and others refused to be seduced by what seemed to us to be the flesh-pots of capitalism.

There were two problems in *Personal Influence*: (1) the choice of a researcher is never a neutral choice but the product of a certain historical contexts and (2) if one chooses an issue such as the influence of mass media on people, aims should be considered; studying mass media for advertisement purposes is different from studying mass media to analyse and understand power relations that focused on racists, militarist and sexiest contents.

1.1.4 The Academic Mind (1958)

The historical background of this study is McCarthyism. In the United States the "cold war" climate after the Second World War caused a fear of communism. Those who were accused of being communists – in cinema, as well as in the universities – could lose their job and be arrested. The term McCarthyism started to be used by the press in 1950 and referred to the fanatic activities during 1946 of Wisconsin Senator Joseph McCarthy. During the Truman presidency, in 1953 McCarthy accused defence secretary George Marshall, the architect of the Marshall plan and Nobel Peace Prize, of being a traitor and responsible for the spread of communism in China. During 1953, owing to his popularity, McCarthy became chairman of the Senate Committee on Government Operation, which controlled the Senate Permanent Subcommittee Investigation. During the Eisenhower presidency, this committee investigated communist influence in the "Voice of America" and also began an investigation on communist influence in the army, which ended up by considering Eisenhower himself as a threat. This obsession with communism which was supposed to have influenced the presidency also was considered excessive by the republicans and in 1954 a resolution emanated by Senator Ralph Flanders condemned Senator McCarthy. In this climate, in 1955 *The Academic Mind*, a research coordinated by PFL and Wagner Thielens, could begin. Its aim was to study the consequences of McCarthyism in American Universities and it was financed by *The Fund for the Republic*, an emanation of the *Ford Foundation*, around which progressive intellectuals, such as John Kennedy, gathered. This research received a lot of funds – one quarter of a million dollars – and had the possibility of realizing an extremely complex sample made up of 2451 university teachers, of which 11% were females, from 165 university colleges. It employed two survey firms and a team coordinated by David Riesman to control and reflect on the whole experience (in Table 1.3 it is research type 1).

This research can be analysed from a methodological point of view following three directions: (1) the use of mathematical analysis and quantitative methods to give voice to charges against McCarthyism by university teachers; (2) the analysis of surveys by David Riesman, in which the complexity of the relation between the interviewer and the subject of the research emerges and (3) the lack of attention to gender relations, which leads PFL and Thielens to keep women and men interviewed in one single group.

The first point is interesting, because *The Academic Mind* is amongst the most elaborated studies by PFL from a mathematical point of view. It has two significant characteristics: (1) the progressive reduction of items from 21 to 4 to measure two main aspects of the "apprehension" indicator: "worry" due to attitudes and behaviours that could be criticized, and "caution" for avoiding attitudes and behaviours that could be criticized for fear of sanction and (2) the use of the analysis of the latent structure to verify the non-linear relation of the four items selected concerning latent dimension "apprehension".

Such a use of mathematics and quantitative analysis, together with a neutral terminology (for example the term "permissive" instead of "liberal" or "progressive", instead of "conservative" [8]) was part of a defensive strategy that under the "pretence of objectivity" made possible to document in great details the violence of McCarthyism on American university teachers. In Chapter 2, qualitative answers given to several open items are elaborated and an accurate documentation of the violence of McCarthyism is negatively evaluated by the two authors (1958, p. 57):

> In this period an individual could be called Communist for almost any kind of behaviour, or for holding almost any kind of attitudes. In them the world "Communist" became a vague and angry label, a "dirty name" with which and individual showed his disagreement with a teacher's thinking. (...) Just as in the Salem of the 1690's good citizens were quick to see in many an act an evil intent, and in each evil intent the signs of witchcraft, so in the post war decade many detected a lurking evil in the behaviour of college teachers which must surely spring from a subtle and pervasive Communism.

[8] PFL and Thielens (1958, p. 121) explain their choice as follows: "We have used the term permissive when often the reader, quite correctly, might prefer that we speak of liberal or progressive teachers. We have avoided these two words because they have changed their meaning too often in the great debate of the last decades."

The Academic Mind marked PFL's return after market researches, to politically oriented researches similar to the one he carried out during his Viennese period. As David Riesman has noted (1979, p. 226):

> Lazarsfeld used to remark that he undertook the Teacher Apprehension Study because it gave him a chance to put to work his passion for newly discovered contextual analysis. But, as a Marxist say, it was no accident that the subject was academic freedom: he cared about that. In the post McCarthy days it seems safe to say that he had a lifelong nostalgia for socialism Vienna style.

In 1957, McCarthy died of alcoholism at the young age of 49 for not being able to bear the burden of his failure and in 1958, *The Academic Mind* was published. At the time, the Republicans were still very powerful and of the six reviews to this study, five were totally negative because PFL had dared to openly criticize McCarthy. Nowadays, however, this publication is invaluable for having given a voice to the victims of McCarthyism and for all those who wish to reconstruct the reception of McCarthyism in American universities, as Ellen W. Schrecker, who has written the most complete study on this subject (1986), has rightly noted. *The Academic Mind* is also important for a discussion concerning methods, as the long article by David Riesman (1958) notes; here he clearly illustrates the "subjective" relation between respondents and interviewers:

> an enormous variety of factors may serve to structure the expectations of both respondents and interviewers, and thus to influence what is deemed relevant- what is even conceived and thought- and what is heard and recorded.

Riesman shows that according to those who agree to paradigm of objectivity, the subjectivity that one thinks to have dispensed with by delegating the survey to a group of professional interviews is in actual fact only transferred from those who coordinate the research to the interviewers. One should also stress that the data on the sample of women interviewed has never been elaborated by Robert Smith, who shows a new way of elaborating data shown in *The Academic Mind*. This work demonstrates once again that a well-done research can always teach something.

1.1.5 Other Dimensions for the Classification of Sociological Researches

The three above-mentioned researches by PFL make it possible to integrate the six dimensions shown in Tables 1.1, 1.2 and 1.3: (a) *relations between women and men*: this can be included in the research; it can be excluded from the sample's choice; it can be excluded from the elaboration's choice; (b) *theory construction*: the theory can be constructed during the research (*Die Arbeitslosen von Marienthal*, *The Academic Mind*) or beforehand; in this case the research has the aim of verifying the theory (*Personal Influence*); (c) *individual and collective variables*: some researches consider both individual and collective variables (*Die Arbeitslosen von Marienthal*, *The Academic Mind*) and others in which almost exclusively individual variables are considered (*Personal Influence*); (d) *use of mathematics*: mathematics may be used in more than one steps of the research (*The Academic Mind*, *Personal Influence*) or not used at all (*Die Arbeitslosen von Marienthal*); (e) *radical sociology's evaluation*: this evaluation considers the political impact of the research; this can be positive (*Die Arbeitslosen von Marienthal*, *The Academic Mind*) or negative (*Personal Influence*); (f) *key word* with which a research can be summarized: immersion (*Die Arbeitslosen von Marienthal*), verification of a theory (*Personal Influence*), accusation of the power (*The Academic Mind*).

The overall result is shown in Table 1.4.

Table 1.4 Characteristics of three researches coordinated by PFL

Dimensions	Die Arbeitslosen von Marienthal (1932)	Personal Influence (1955)	The Academic Mind (1958)
Explanatory/ descriptive type	Explanatory	Explanatory	Explanatory
Antecedent/new Data	New	New	New
Quantitative/qualitative methods	Quantitative and qualitative methods	Survey for quantitative methods	Survey for quantitative and qualitative methods
Interaction with subjects	No interaction	Interaction with interview	Interaction with interview
Research sponsor	Using results	Using results	Not using results
Object of research	Towards bottom Type A	Towards bottom Type A	Towards top
Relation between women and men	Analysed	Not analysed for sample's choice	Not analysed for elaboration's choice
Theory's construction	During research	Before research	During research
Types of variables	Individual and collective variables	Individual variables	Individual and collective variables
Use of mathematics	No use	Utilization of models and indicators	Utilization of models and indicators
Radical sociology's evaluation	Positive	Negative	Positive
Key word of research	Immersion	Verification of a theory	Accusation of the power

1.2 Mathematics and Sociology from Statistical Models to Artificial Societies and Social Simulation

In this second part, the main changes in the relation between mathematics and sociology are considered after PFL. A first change has arrived from Lazarsfeld's statistical models and those published in the *Journal of Artificial Societies and*

Social Simulation. Furthermore, changes have occurred in mathematical structure of models also (due to increased possibilities offered by computer science) and in the research objectives (the passage from the paradigm of objectivity to the paradigm of action research/co-research and the paradigm of feminist methodology). The relation between mathematics and sociology($S \rightarrow M \rightarrow S$) and ($M \rightarrow S \rightarrow M$) should therefore be evaluated taking into account what occurs before the actual research begins, that is to say researchers' stance and in particular their set of values as well as methodological and political choices.

The shift from Lazarsfeld's models to simulation models and to artificial neural networks has been described in various studies. These have focused not only on the results of these researches but also on the researchers that made such shift possible, portraying the complex relationships between university research centres and laboratories both in Europe and in the United States. The studies by Jeremy Bernstein (1978, 1982), Pamela McCorduck (1979), Andrei Hodges (1983), James Gleick (1987), Steve J. Heims (1991), Morris Mitchell Waldrop (1992), Albert-Laszlo Barabasi (2002) and Linton C. Freeman (2004) are very significant in that they reconstruct the synergies and contradictions that have led to such changes.

1.2.1 The Paradigm of Action Research/Co-research

The paradigm of *action research/co-research* differs not only from the one of objectivity, which, as we have seen, characterizes PFL's researches, but also from qualitative researches such as those that have a participant observer and that are in turn criticized by PFL. Researches that use this paradigm is aimed not only at finding out explanations but also at changing attitudes and behaviours concerning people or a specific situation. Kurt Lewin (1946 republished in 1948, pp. 143–149), who is the first to utilize the term "action research", gives this definition:

> action research [is] a comparative research on the conditions and effects of various form of social action and research leading to social action. Research that produces nothing but books will not suffice. This by no means implies that the research needed is in any respect less scientific or "lower" than what would be required for pure science in the field of social events (...) [action research use] a spiral of steps, each of which is composed of a circle of planning, action, and fact finding about result of action (...) Planning starts usually with something like a general idea. For one reason or another it seems desirable to reach a certain objective. Exactly how to circumscribe this objective, and how to reach it, is frequently not clear. The first step then is to examine the idea carefully on the light of the means available. (...) The next period is devoted to executing the first step of the overall plan. (...) The next step again is composed of a circle of planning, executing, and reconnaissance or fact finding for the purpose of evaluating the results of the second step, for preparing the rational basis for planning the third step, and for perhaps modifying again the overall plan.

The action research is different from PFL's researches in which actions happen after the publication of the research results; it is also different from researches that use participant observation. The "intimate familiarity" with the subjects of the research William Foote Whyte talked about had as its objective knowledge, and in a similar fashion, Alfred Mc Clung Lee (1970, p. 7), the author of the introduction to the Reader entitled *The Participant Observer*, noted that:

> Participant observation is only a gate to the intricacies of more adequate social knowledge. What happens when one enters that gate depends upon his abilities and interrelationships as an observer. He must be able to see, to listen, and to feel sensitivity to social interactions of which he becomes a part.

The objective of the *action research/co-research* is not only knowledge but also action, and it is precisely the intertwining between research and action that characterizes this kind of research.

PFL's researches and those based on participating observation are characterized by a [hypothesis→ fieldwork→ analysis→ conclusion] sequence, and differences are in the type of field work used. In the *action research/co-research* the sequence is more complex, as it is characterized by several research steps and actions: [*Research* (hypothesis→ fieldwork→ analysis)→ *Action* (action→ outcomes→ analysis) → *New research* (hypothesis→ fieldwork→ analysis)→ *New action* (action→ outcomes→ analysis) →]. This different type of research has a spiral process, which gets interrupted only when the actors of the research have achieved the changes desired. As Kurt Lewin has noted, "[action research use] a spiral of steps, each of which is composed of a circle of planning, action, and fact finding about result of action".

This type of research functions only if close collaboration between the different types of actors in the process of research and action takes place. The relationship between those who coordinate the research and the subjects of the research is therefore very different from those researches that follow the paradigm of objectivity, in which actors and subjects are kept apart. *Action research* is also very different from the "intimate familiarity" which is based on participating observation.

In *action research/co-research*, research is characterized by an explicit agreement among three different types of actors: (1) those who coordinate the research and the research team; (2) public or private actors, who take part in the process of changing and (3) the subjects of the research. Collaboration among these three types of actors who attempt to bring about changes of attitude and people's behaviour or a certain situation allows to (i) reach the necessary knowledge to formulate new theories and (ii) individuate the necessary action to produce change.

The refusal of the paradigm of objectivity does not mean that in this kind of research, objectivity is completely absent. Objectivity is in fact pursued through an ongoing reflection concerning the various steps of the research and all actors' behaviours and attitudes involved (including those of the co-ordinator). This is therefore a self-reflective research. Kurt Lewin analyses an example of research action based in Connecticut in which actors attempt to tackle racist behaviours. He describes the work of the observers that every day transcribe what happens in the different steps of the research in order to reach self-reflection:

> The method of recording the essential events of who had attended the workshop included an evaluation session at the end of every day. Observers who had attended the various subgroup sessions reported (into a recording machine) the leadership pattern they have observed, the

progress or lack of progress in the development of the groups from a conglomeration of individuals to an integrated "we" and so on.

Remaining within the boundary of methodology, research methods change depending on the behaviour adopted by the action research and the choices of the various actors. Contrary to what happened in PFL's researches, here no method of research is precluded.

The paradigm of the *action research/co-research* can be defined through the following points:

1. *Standpoint epistemology*. The objective of the research is changing the attitudes and behaviour of people or a particular situation.
2. *Methodology*. In order to reach this objective, the research is made up of the necessary action that brings about change. Such actions are determined by the analysis of the research activity (it is an action research). The explanations reached are considered valid if the answer (information) provided by the subject of the research is obtained, thanks to the collaboration of those who do the research and the other actors (it is a co-research). A higher objectivity can be obtained if during the research all the actions by the three kinds of actors (the co-ordinator of the research, other actors and the subjects of the research. It is a self-reflective research) are observed, transcribed and evaluated;
3. *Research methods*. All methods, both quantitative and qualitative, are possible, provided that these are in line with the above-mentioned methodology.

Action research/co-research began at the end of the 1960s and the early 1970s in the United States and Europe, following the encouragement provided by the example of students' and workers' movements. In the 1980s its popularity decreased, but nowadays it is widely used once again all over the world – from Latin America to Australia – because it has proved useful in several different and significant ways.

The main applications of *action research/co-research* are the following: (a) community actions, such as the research studied by Kurt Lewin concerning integration problems of minorities in certain communities; (b) children's illiteracy and learning problems; for example the participatory action research coordinated by Paulo Freire to fight back illiteracy in Brazil, which provided the example for several action researches in education; (c) factory workers with problems connected with technological innovation and manager choices; for example the co-researches carried out in Italy and studied by Capecchi (2004); (d) groups affected by psychical problems, disabilities and old age; for example, David Epston's co-research (1999) to help people with mental problems in which a "coproduction of knowledge by sufferers and therapists" was realized; (e) interventions to help people at risk: those who have justice problems, drug addicts, etc; for example the "Sonda Project" directed by Massimo Buscema exposed in the third part of this historical introduction; (f) organization of strategies for local development in which more actors aim at tackling an economic precarious situation; for example the researches in Norway, Sweden and Denmark described by Lauge Baungaard Rasmussen (2004).

Action research/co-research has been very successful, even though its political use has been overall a downside. For example an international neo-liberalist institution, such as the World Bank, has used this type of research to try to convince the native population to take part into multinational programmes, which were aimed at exploiting them, as documented in Bill Coke and Uma Kothari (2001).

The action research/co-research has followed a trajectory similar to Bruno Latour's theories (2005, pp. 8–9). After studying innovations in the scientific field, he considers two approaches to sociology:

> *First approach:* They believed the social to be made essentially of social ties, whereas association are made of ties which are themselves non-social. They imagined that sociology is limited to a specific domain, whereas sociologists should travel wherever new heterogeneous associations are made. (...). I call the first approach "sociology of social" (...).
> *Second approach:* Whereas, in the first approach, every activity – law, science, technology, religion, organization, politics, management, etc. – could be related to and explained by the same social aggregates *behind* all of them, in the second version of sociology there exists *nothing* behind those activities even though they produce one. (...) To be social is no longer a safe and unproblematic property, it is a movement that may fail to trace any new connection and may fail to redesign any *well-formed* assemblage. (...) I call the second [approach] 'sociology of association'.

It is obvious that Latour's attention to the formation of new collective actors, such associations (which Latour calls actors-network) finds a parallel in action research, and distinguishes his approach from those using the paradigm of objectivity. Latour writes (2005, pp. 124–125):

> The question is not whether to place objective texts in opposition to subjective ones. There are texts that pretend to be objective because they claim to imitate what they believe to be the secret of the natural sciences; and there are those that try to be objectives because they track objects which are given the chance to object to what is said about them.

According to Latour, therefore, it is essential that the "objects" of the research also become "subjects" and have "the chance to *object* to what is said about them".

1.2.2 The Paradigm of Feminist Methodology

The paradigm of feminist methodology is closely related to the actions and theories of the world feminist movement. It is precisely this connection that makes this paradigm very different from the paradigm of objectivity and that of the *action research/co-research*. The feminist movement is a heterogeneous collective and political subject which, in different times and places, has realized different actions and proposed different theories. Despite such diversity, Caroline Ramazanoglu and Janet Holland (2002, pp. 138–139) write that when a researcher uses feminist methodology to realize researches for other women, we call this a "feminist epistemic community":

> An epistemic community is a notion of a socially produced collectivity, with shared rules, that authorizes the right to speak as a particular kind of knowing subject.(...) Feminist exist as an imagined epistemic community in the sense that they do not need to meet

together to exist as a collectivity and they are not simply a collection of women. It is open to investigation, however, as to what women or knowing feminists actually do have in common.

Books and articles on feminist methodology started to appear in the 1970s in English countries and have later on spread to other geographical areas and cultural settings. The following anthologies may provide an idea of the illustration and evolution of this methodology: Nona Blazer and Helen Youngelson Wachewre (1977); Helen Roberts (1981); Gloria Bowles and Renate Duelli Klein (1983); Sandra Harding and Merrill B. Hintikka (1983); Sandra Harding (1987); Joyce McCarl Nielsen (1990); Mary Margaret Fonow and Judith A. Cook (1991); Sharlene Nagy Hesse-Biber and Michelle L. Yaiser (2004).

In order to attempt to understand the directions of feminist methodology, one can begin to consider the relationship between objectivity and subjectivity. As Caroline Ramazanoglu and Janet Holland note (2002, p. 62), this relationship should be considered as part of another relation – the one between knowledge and truth. The latter considers a continuum between two polar positions that can be occupied by researchers: (1) absolute truth; this is the position of somebody who believes to be "an all-knowing observer external to and independent of what is being observed") and (2) absolute relativism; "in this position there is no way of adjudicating between different versions of *truth*".

Feminist methodology occupies a middle position between the above-mentioned extremes; on the one hand, it believes that it is always possible to find better explanations, on the other hand, it also believes that it is not possible to arrive at "an absolute truth" that is beyond the interrelations of female researchers and the subjects of the research. What are the risks that run those who do not occupy an intermediate position? Such a problem has been clearly illustrated by Sandra Harding (2004, p. 55):

> If the community of "qualified" researchers and critics systematically excludes, for example, all African Americans and women of all races and if the larger culture is stratified by race and gender and lacks powerful critiques of this stratification, it is not plausible to imagine that racist and sexist interests and values would be identified within a community of scientist composed entirely of people who benefit-intentionally or not- from institutionalised racism and sexism.

This position is similar neither to the one of PFL who, in researches such as *Die Arbeitslosen von Marienthal* and *The Academic Mind*, endorses values and who moves in the direction of Sandra Harding's theories nor to those inspired by *action research/co-research*. What emerges from Ramazanoglu and Holland (2002) as well as Harding (2004) is that all the paradigms that have been analysed here – the one of objectivity, *action research/co-research* and feminist methodology – represent intermediate positions (in between absolute truth and absolute relativism) and all differ in their different ways of pursuing "higher objectivity".

The highest objectivity pursued by feminist methodology is called by Harding (1992, p. 580) as "strong objectivity":

> Objectivism also conceptualises the desired value–neutrality of objectivity too broadly. Objectivists claim that objectivity requires the elimination of all social values and interests from the research process and the results of research. It is clear, however, that not all social value and interests have the same bed effects upon the results of research. Democracy-advancing values have systematically generated less partial and distorted beliefs than other.

This strong objectivity requires a strong reflexivity (2004, p. 55):

> Strong objectivity requires that the subjects of knowledge be placed on the same critical, causal plane as the objects of knowledge. The strong objectivity requires what we can think of as "strong reflexivity". This is because culturewide (or nearly culturewide) beliefs function as evidence at every stage in scientific inquiry: in the selection of problem, the formation of hypotheses, the design of research (including the organization of research communities), the collection of data, the interpretation and sorting of data, decision about when to stop research, the way results of research are reported and so on.

The strong reflexivity Sandra Harding speaks about is realized by "observers designated as legitimate ones"; these observers are interested not only in methods but also in political values, which should be respected during all the steps of the research. Researches informed by feminist methodology are different from PFL's researches and those conducted through the *action research/co-research.*

Researches which follow feminist methodology can dispense from *action research/co-research.* In a textbook written by Shulamit Reinharz (1992) entitled *Feminist Methods in Social Research*, the following methods are mentioned:

> Feminist Interview Research, Feminist Ethnography, Feminist Survey Research and Other Statistical Research Formats, Feminist Experimental Research, Feminist Cross-Culture Research, Feminist Oral History, Feminist Content Analysis, Feminist Case Studies, Feminist Action Research, Feminist Multiple Methods Research

Feminist action research is only one possible method of feminist methodology and action research may be feminist or not. In this regard Katheleen Weiler (1995) has criticized from the standpoint of feminist methodology a classical Freire's action research in pedagogy.

The paradigm of feminist methodology can be defined by the following points:

1. *Standpoint epistemology.* The reference point is the theories and the struggles of feminist movements. Researches confront themselves with a "feminist epistemic community".
2. *Methodology.* In order to reach this objective, the research is founded on a privileged relation between women who do research and those who are the subjects of the research. The explanations are valid if these take into account the values of feminist epistemic community. These increase and emphasize female empowerment. A higher objectivity can be obtained if the research has "observers designated as legitimate ones" who should take into account methods; these should be fair and consider feminist values in all steps of the research.
3. *Research methods.* All methods, both qualitative and quantitative, are accepted, provided that these are used as part of the above-mentioned methodology.

1.2.3 The Relation Between Mathematics and Sociology

Before beginning the analysis of the relations between mathematics and sociology, the co-ordinator of a "traditional" sociological research had to choose among several political and methodological hypotheses, which influence the research and its object. "Traditional" choices were between Marxism/conservatorism; individualism/holism; positivism/phenomenology, etc.

Nowadays, the most important political choices concern two main antagonistic economics models (the neo-liberal model and the cooperative economics and fair trade model). Nowadays, methodological choices, though different on the surface, as previously, involve (a) what kind of research and its connected methodology to be used; (b) what kind of mathematics to be used and (c) the object of research.

Choice (a) takes into consideration the following paradigms: (i) the paradigm of objectivity; (ii) the paradigm of the action research/co-research and (iii) the paradigm of the feminist methodology. Choice (b) considers some of the most significant differences of the employment of mathematics in sociology:

(i) *Linear/non-linear mathematics*. This makes a distinction between the prevalent use of linear mathematics in PFL's researches on the one hand and non-linear mathematics that characterizes several other applications on the other. Such a distinction however is not clear-cut; for example PFL has used some non-linear models to analyse the latent structure.

(ii) *Mathematics which considers dichotomic variables/fuzzy variable*. This distinction considers the possibilities offered by mathematics for the elaboration of variables. In the first part of this introduction, the different mathematical applications to variables with different levels of quantification have been illustrated (from the nominal scale to the relational one). Generally speaking, it is possible to distinguish between mathematics applied to dichotomic variables (as in the case of PFL's researches) on the one hand and mathematics in relation to artificial neural nets on the other; the latter can elaborate all types of variables, including fuzzy ones. This distinction, as the others, presents several intermediate stages.

(iii) *Mathematics in complicated/complex systems*. The history of a new way of considering complexity is illustrated in the works of James Gleick (1987) and Morris Mitchell Waldrop (1992). As it has been summed up in Enzo Grossi's contribution in Chapter 15, nowadays it is possible to make a distinction between mathematics dealing with complicated systems (linear functions, adaptation to static environment, simple casualness, deterministic, structure determines relationship, average dominate irrelevant outliers, components maintain their essence) and mathematics in complex systems (non-linear functions, interaction with dynamic environment, mutual casualness, probabilistic, structure and relationship interact, key determinant outliers, components change their essence).

As Enzo Grossi writes:

Complex systems can adapt themselves to a dynamic environment, time for them is not "noise" but rather a way to reduce potential errors. Complexity is an adaptive process; it is time sensitive, in the sense that over time, complex processes evolve and/or degenerate. Complexity is based on small elementary units working together in a small population of synchronous processes.

Intermediate cases in this case are also numerous.

Choice (c) considers the main objects of the research, which are listed below:

(i) *Main focus on explanations based on real data/main focus on experiments with simulated data.* This choice distinguishes between the employment of mathematics in order to analyse the relations between subjects/variables (as in one of PFL's researches) and the employment of mathematics to simulate an experiment whose results are based on hypotheses (as, for example, in the *Simulmatics Project*). There are also several intermediate cases; choosing the simulation model means to be more/less interested in considering real data and, therefore, is inclined to choose the first option.

(ii) *Main focus on subjects/main focus on the macro-actors and social networks.* This choice comes as a consequence of the one between individualism and holism. A cornerstone of analysis of this "traditional" choice is still the work of Bernard Valade (2001). Nowadays, the choice is between a kind of analysis more connected to individual attitudes and behaviours and one which studies groups and actors, which, however, are not viewed as a mere aggregation of individual behaviours and attitudes. Choosing the second possibility means to perform a social network analysis, whose history has been described by Linton Freeman (2004). Macro-actors are included in the actor-network theory by Callon and Latour; social formations were analysed by Harrison, White, etc. Also in this case there are several intermediate cases; for example PFL, who should be included among those who focused on subjects, has also been interested in social networks, as Linton Freeman (2004, pp. 90–98) has noted; moreover, his research *Personal Influence* can be interpreted as the analysis of individual behaviours and attitudes to obtain data that refer to social networks.

(iii) *More focus on aesthetic aspects/or on individual and collective actions.* This choice considers using fairly autonomous ways for the analysis of the fractals studied from an aesthetic point of view and the essays of this volume on the relations between mathematics and art. Also in this case, there are a few intermediate cases, because contributions to fractal studies have also been used to evaluate individual and collective actions (suffice here to mention the essays by Maldebrot on the playing the stock market).

The space created by political and methodological choices (in the three above-mentioned directions) influences the relations between mathematics and sociology. Generally these take three main directions: (1) relations of the type ($S \rightarrow M \rightarrow S$), in which mathematics is subordinated to choices of methodological research; (2) relations in which, besides the direction ($S \rightarrow M \rightarrow S$), there is also the relation ($M \rightarrow S \rightarrow M$), in which the use of mathematics is more autonomous than that of the sociological research and (3) relations in which the relation ($M \rightarrow S \rightarrow M$) is the strongest.

Taking into consideration this more general relation between mathematics and sociology, it is possible to identify five directions which show interrelation between mathematics and sociology: (1) logic for sociological theory; (2) mathematics for relation between individual and collective properties; (3) mathematics and less visible relations; (4) mathematics for the social sciences and (5) mathematical models.

These five research directions can be defined through examples that distinguish between problems and solutions; moreover, Table 1.5 gives an idea of the richness and complexity that characterize the dialogue between mathematics and sociology.

1.2.3.1 Logic for Sociological Theory

This relation is analysed through four concepts essential for the construction of a sociological theory: (1) typologies; (2) sociological explanation; (3) micro–macro relation and (d) prediction.

Typologies

Two debates are interesting as a way of formalizing the concept of typology in sociological research: (1) the debate between Tarde and Durkheim at the beginning of the twentieth century concerning the degree of fixity of possible typologies and (2) the debate between PFL and Carl G. Hempel at the beginning of the 1960s concerning the plausibility of natural sciences as a reference point for evaluating typologies proposed by sociology.

The Gabriel Tarde (1834–1904)–Emile Durkheim (1858–1917) debate ended with the prevailing of Durkheim's theories, to the point that Tarde has since then been ignored in sociological debate, and has been used again only in recent times, as the works of Gilles Deleuze (1968), Jussi Kinnunen (1996), Bruno Latour (2001) and David Toews (2003) show. Latour entitles his essay *Gabriel Tarde and the End of the Social* because Durkheim is concerned with what he calls "social sociology" and Tarde is concerned with "sociology of associations".

Tarde's attention to the sociology of associations has caused to be considered as "the founding father of innovation diffusion research", as Kinnunen has noted (1996). It is precisely this attention to phenomena that moves and comes together that has led Tarde to disagree with Durkheim, who, as Deleuze has also noted (1968), tends on the other hand to construct too rigid and immobile types (such as, for example, typologies for suicide shown in Table 1.9). As Toews has succinctly put it:

> Durkheim (...) explicitly attribute to [social types] a relative *solidity* (...) For Tarde instead of firm 'solid' types of societies, we actually think of reproduction of societies, which exhibit similar composition. Societies are not made up of an invisible, evolving, quasi-physical substance, a substance that is *indifferent*, but in the words of Tarde 'at all times

Table 1.5 Mathematics and sociology: types of problems and solutions

Types of relation	Mathematics (M)/Sociology (S)	Types of problems	Types of solutions
1. Logic for sociological theory	$S \rightarrow M \rightarrow S$	– Typologies – Sociological explanation – Micro/macro relation – Prevision	– Reduction and reconstruction of a property space – Reduction without/with mathematical models – Sociological explanation at different levels of probability – Coleman's boat – Contingent prediction
2. Mathematics for the relation between individual and collective properties	$S \rightarrow M \rightarrow S$	– Ecological fallacies and individual fallacies (selective, contextual, cross-level) – Interaction between individual level and territorial unit level	– Models to link individual level and territorial unit level – Goodman's method to analyse electoral flux with ecological data
3. Mathematics for less visible relations	$S \rightarrow M \rightarrow S$	– Less visible relations in Coleman's boat: $M \rightarrow m$ $m \rightarrow m'$ $m' \rightarrow M'$	– Analysis of cross-pressures – Analysis of deviant cases – Analysis of unexpected effects
4. Mathematics for the social sciences	$M \rightarrow S \rightarrow M$ $S \rightarrow M \rightarrow S$	– Mathematics for dichotomous variables – Mathematics for graphs – Mathematics for games and decisions – Mathematics to find order and beauty in chaos – Mathematics for fuzzy variables	– PFL's algebra of dichotomous variables – Flament's graph theory – Luce and Raiffa's theory of games and decisions – Mandelbrot's fractals – Zadeh's fuzzy logic
5. Mathematical models	$S \rightarrow M \rightarrow S$ $M \rightarrow S \rightarrow M$	– Statistical models/simulation models – Models of processes/models of structure/rational choice models, agent-based models	– Linear causal models – Latent structure analysis – Factor models – Log-linear models – System dynamics and world models – Event- or agent-based models

and places the apparent continuity of history may be decomposed into distinct and separable events, events both small and great, which consist of *questions followed by solutions*' (1903, p. 156). The problem of continuity brings to light, for Tarde, a *compositional perspective*, a perspective upon 'things' as certain repeated gatherings of elements, as particular events whose unity is no greater than that of complex, problematic compositions.(. . .) As Tarde puts it, 'repetitions and resemblances. . . are the necessary themes of the differences and variations which exists in all phenomena' (1903, p. 6). And it follows from this, in Tarde's view, that neither is 'the crude incoherence of historic facts.. proof at all against the fundamental regularity of social life or the possibility of a social science' (1903, p. 12).

The second debate on the concept of typology begins with Carl G. Hempel and Paul Oppenheim (1936). For the latter, typology is an operation of "reduction of a property space" made of different dimensions of variables, according to which a certain phenomenon can be analysed. PFL and Allen Barton (1955) were so impressed by Hempel and Oppenheim's contribution that they wrote a long essay in which they analyse the use of logical operations of reduction and reconstruction of a property space in sociology. Hempel in 1952 writes another essay on *Ideal Types and Explanation in Social Sciences*, [9] in which three kinds of types are found: (1) *classificatory types*, "in which types are concerned as classes. The logic of typological procedure is the familiar logic of classification". (2) *Extreme types*, in which types are formulated as *extreme* or *pure* types and "may serve as conceptual points of references or poles", so if a person is T is an extreme type and cannot be classified as *T* or *non-T* but more or less close to T; (3) *ideal types*. Max Weber's ideal types are described by Hempel (1965, p. 156) as follows:

> An ideal type, according to Weber, is a mental construct formed by the synthesis of many diffuse, more or less present and occasionally absent, concrete individual phenomena, which are arranged, according to certain one-sidedly accentuated points of view, into a unified analytical construct, which in its conceptual purity cannot be found in reality. (...) This characterization, and many similar accounts which Weber and others have given of the nature of ideal types, are certainly suggestive, but they lack of clarity and rigor and that call for further logical analysis.

According to Hempel, Weber's ideal types are "subjective meaningful" concepts and, from a logical point of view, are less valid of ideal types used in economic discourse such as free market. According to Hempel (1965, p. 171), ideal types in sociology "lack the clarity and prevision of the construction used in theoretical economics" and for these the formula "if P then Q" is not valid.

PFL (1962) analyses in detail this essay by Hempel (in the light of Ernest Nagel and Max Black's contributions also) and reaches the conclusion that a dialogue between philosophers of science and sociologists is fruitful only when philosophers do not merely try to understand how sociology works in order to talk about the differences between the law of natural sciences and those of sociology. As PFL writes (1947, p. 470):

> Philosophers of sciences are not interested in and do not know what the work-a-day empirical research man does. This has two consequences: either we have to become our own methodologists or we have to muddle along without benefit of the explication clergy.

PFL and Allen Barton's (1951) and Barton's (1955) contributions follow the first of these two possibilities and propose two logical operations: (1) reduction of property space in order to propose a new typology (this reduction should of course be

[9]The essay *Ideal Types and Explanation in Social Sciences* is in Hempel (1965, p. 155–171).

justified) and (2) the reconstruction of property space from a given typology in order to verify if the operation of reduction is correctly carried out.

Two examples of reconstruction of property space are useful to understand why this method is valid. The first one is the reconstruction of deviant types proposed by Robert K. Merton (1938, 1949). Merton (Table 1.6) considers the possibilities that an individual has to accept goals or institutional means offered by society to individuals.

Table 1.6 Merton's typology of deviant behaviour

Types of adaptation	Modes of adaptation to culture goals	Modes of adaptation to institutional means
I. Conformity	+	+
II. Innovation	+	−
III. Ritualism	−	+
IV. Retreatism	−	−
V. Rebellion	±	±

Source: Merton (1938, 1949)
The sign (+) indicates "acceptance", the sign (−) indicates "rejection" and the sign (±) indicates "substitution"

This theory was well received because it was related to some unusual analysis. For example under Type II "Innovation", it included the condition of Italo-American gangsters in New York. These fully accepted (+) the goals proposed by American society, but as Italians they encountered obstacles, and for this reason they rejected (−) the institutional means to reach such goals.

During the 1960s, while working for the Bureau of Applied Social Research and editing the Italian edition of PFL's collected work, I amused myself by trying to apply what I had learnt from PFL in order to challenge the typology proposed by his friend Robert King Merton. The result[10] was published in Capecchi (1963, 1966) and is summarized in Table 1.7. This adds to new elements to Table 1.6: (a) Type II Innovation was wrongly placed, because, according to Merton, this is a type that accepts (+) goals; however, he refuses legal means in order to merely substitute (±) them and (b) four new types [3], [4], [6], [8] also emerge, and they are plausible and interesting.

Another example is the reconstruction of the well-known typology of suicides by Durkheim (Table 1.8), which Hempel would have later defined as extreme types, who collocates four types of suicides in a table that analyses two separate dimensions (solidarity and laws). Of these two dimensions, the destructive effects of people who are in extreme situations (lack of/too much solidarity; lack of/too much laws) are considered. Table 1.8 is interesting because it suggests a more modern image of types of suicides, which according to Tarde were too rigid. Maintaining

[10]Capecchi's reconstruction of Merton's typology of deviance was appreciated by Blalock (1968, p. 30–31) and an analysis of this reconstruction of deviance from a sociological point of view is in Berzano and Prina (1995, p. 85).

Table 1.7 Reconstruction of Merton's types of adaptation

Adaptation to institutional means	Adaptation to culture goals +	–	±
+	I. Conformity [1]	III. Ritualism [2]	Revolution within the system [3]
–	Estrangement [4]	IV. Retreatism [5]	Inactive opposition [6]
±	II. Innovation [7]	Exasperation [8]	V. Rebellion [9]

Source: Capecchi (1963, 1966)

Table 1.8 Reconstruction of Durkheim's types of suicide

Dimensions	Danger of self-destruction for lack of	Danger of self-destruction for too much
Solidarity	*Lack of solidarity:* egoistic suicide	*Too much solidarity:* altruistic suicide
Laws	*Lack of laws:* anomic suicide	*Too much laws:* ritualistic suicide

Source: Durkheim (1897)

that single members of a society should try to avoid extreme situations means to share a view that is widespread in religion such as Taoism and Zen Buddhism, as both positions stress the importance of moving along a "fuzzy" dimension, in a continuum between two extremes.

It is important to note that Merton and Durkheim's typologies can be represented in research/action frameworks (because they are typologies that consider processes and not static types), but they do not take into account gender differences (and are therefore easily challenged by feminist methodology). A double attention to changing processes and feminist perspectives should be considered in the construction of all typologies. In Table 1.9, the logical operations of reduction of a property space are together with two different modalities: (1) with or without the results of a research and (2) with or without mathematical models. The types based on results of a research are classificatory types, while those not based on results are extreme

Table 1.9 The types of reduction of a property space in a typology

Types of reduction	Without mathematical models	With mathematical models
Without the result of a research	Pragmatic reduction	Reduction through indices
With the result of a research	Reduction according to frequencies	Reduction according to mathematical indices and models

Source: Capecchi (1966)

or ideal types. The types proposed however should be evaluated not only in relation to a correct formal method of reduction but also in relation to the values that define their content.

Sociological explanation

A possible clarification of sociological theory can be gathered from the contribution given by logic to the definition of "sociological explanation". Hempel (1965, p. 250) describes the characteristic of a causal law and a statistical law in science:

> If E [Explanandum] describe a particular event, then the antecedent circumstances [Explanans] described in the sentences C1, C2,. . .Ck may be said jointly the "cause" of the event, in the sense that there are certain empirical regularities, expressed by the laws L1, L2,. . .Lr which imply whenever conditions of the kind indicated by C1, C2,. . .Ck occur an event of this kind described in E will take place. Statements such as L1, L2,. . .Lr which assert general and unexceptional connections between specific characteristics of events, are customarily called causal, or deterministic laws. They must be distinguished from so called statistical laws which assert that in the long run, an explicitly stated percentages of all cases satisfying a given set of conditions are accompanied by an event of a certain specific kind.

As a consequence of this definition, based on sciences, such as physics, sociology has proceeded following two different trajectories: (1) it adopted as point of reference natural sciences, such as biology, that are closer to sociology than classical physics. As Stanley Lieberson and Freda B. Lynn have written (2002):

> The standard for what passes as scientific sociology is derived from classical physics, a model of natural science that is totally inappropriate for sociology. As a consequence, we pursue goals and use criteria for success that are harmful and counterproductive. (. . .) Although recognizing that no natural science can serve as an automatic template for our work, we suggest that Darwin's work on evolution provides a far more applicable model for linking theory and research since he dealt with obstacles far more similar to our own. This includes drawing rigorous conclusions based on observational data rather than true experiments; an ability to absorb enormous amounts of diverse data into a relatively simple system that not include a large number of what we think of as independent variables; the absence of prediction as a standard for evaluating the adequacy of a theory; and the ability to use a theory that is incomplete in both the evidence that supports it and in its development.

(2) It looked for a multileveled "sociological explanation" in order to propose "sociological explanations" that had weaker conditions than those shown by Hempel's "causal law". To explain this second trajectory, one can begin by considering Raymond Boudon (1995), who considers the macro-sociological explanation proposed by Max Weber: protestant religious doctrine→ capitalism. Boudon relates Weber's theory with facts that have emerged through empirical researches and obtains three situations: (1) facts that are explained by theories (for example Trevor Roper's researches. These show that several entrepreneurs in Calvinist areas, such as Holland, were not Calvinist but immigrants with other religious values); (ii) theory is not enough to explain facts (for example Scotland is from an economic point of view a depressed area, even though it is next to England and here Calvinism is as widespread as in England. In order to explain this situation a different theory is needed); (iii) facts coincide with theories (as is the case with the success

of Capitalism in the United States and England). Boudon (1999, p. 87) evaluates Weber's explanation of protestant religious doctrine→ capitalism in the following way:

> One can conclude that Weber's theory even though has not been proved right, can still be considered a valid and plausible hypothesis. It is plausible that, given certain conditions, the presence of Protestantism has encouraged economic modernisation. One could also add that if Weber did not manage to demonstrate the existence of relation of causality, it is because this relation cannot be demonstrated. The complexity of causes of economic development is such that is practically impossible to isolate one of these causes and measure its effect.

Boudon (1984) has stressed that differently from natural sciences, in sociology, a multi-levelled explanation is possible. In this regard, Charles Henry Cuin (2005, p. 43) in Table 1.10 shows four examples of sociological explanations with different degrees of probabilities and conditions.

Table 1.10 Examples of four types of sociological explanations

Absolute If *A* then *B*	All societies are stratified
Probable If *A* then probably *B* (with $pB = x$)	Individual orientation towards suicide changes inversely with the degree of integration in society
Conditional In *C* condition, if *A* then *B*	In bureaucracy, individuals' power increases if the uncertainty conditions they control become higher
Probable and conditional In *C* condition, if *A* then probably *B*	Generally in Western societies, industrialization goes hand in hand with a reduction of members of a family (a nuclear family)

Source: Cuin (2005)

Cuin (2005, p. 44) also considers "virtual laws" which include Weber's "ideal types". These virtual laws are not "considered for their value but for the role that they have in scientific imagination. They are propaedeutical for a nomological knowledge". Weber's ideal types therefore represent a weaker level of explanation that should not however be refused.

Micro/macro relation

In sociology, the micro/macro relation has been at the centre of attention of several debates, among which that quoted in Karin Knorr-Cetina and Aaron Cicourel's (1981) anthology is particularly interesting. Karin Knorr-Cetina (1981, p. 26–27, p. 40) considers three main hypothesis to analyse the micro/macro relation: (1) the aggregation of hypothesis; (2) the hypothesis of unintended consequences and (3) the representation of hypothesis.

> (a) The aggregation hypothesis: (...) *It says that macro-phenomena are made up of aggregations and repetition of many similar micro-episodes;* (b) The hypothesis of unintended

consequences, *in contrast to the aggregation hypothesis does not relate macro-phenomena to that which visibly or knowing happens in micro-situation. Rather it postulate properties of a more global systems which emerge by virtue of unintended (in addition to the intended) consequences of micro-events.* (...); (c) The representation hypothesis (...) *when ... many definitions of the situation are construed relationally by reference to other imputed, projected or reconstructed situations or events.* (...) *The main difference between the representation hypothesis and the other two hypothesis is perhaps that it conceives of the macro as actively construed and pursued within micro-social action while the aggregation hypothesis and the hypothesis of unintended consequences regard the macro-order as an emergent phenomenon composed of the sum of unintended effects of micro-events.*

The aggregation hypothesis is included in the anthology edited by Randall Collins (1981) and, as Knorr-Cetina and Cicourel (1981, p. 81) write, "admits only to time, space and number as pure macro-variable. All other variables and concepts can be translated into people's experience in micro-situation. (...) The macro consists of aggregates of micro-situation in time and space". The *hypothesis of unintended consequences* is presented by Rom Harré (1981) and Anthony Giddens (1981); according to this hypothesis, "Consequently, true macro concept like a social class must be considered as rhetorical classification which have no empirically identifiable referent other than that of the component individuals of which they form a sum" (1981, p. 139).

The *representation hypothesis* is by Aaron V. Cicourel (1981), Michel Callon and Bruno Latour (1981). It "argues that (macro) social facts are not simply given but emerge by the routine practices of everyday life" (Cicourel, 1981, p. 51); in addition it argues that "consider the macro order to consist of macro actor who have successfully translated other actors' will into a single will for which they speak" (Callon and Latour, 1981, p. 277). These macro-actors are called by Bruno Latour (2005) as "actors-network".

These three hypothesis clarify the micro/macro relation shown by James Coleman (1990) in his schema (Fig. 1.1) known as "Coleman's boat". [11] Coleman considers that an explanation at the macro-level $M \rightarrow M'$ (protestant religious doctrine→ capitalism) can be accepted only by admitting three passages:

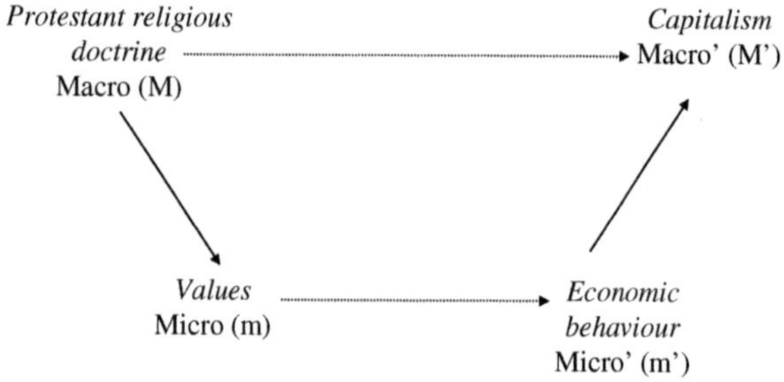

Fig. 1.1 An application of Coleman's boat to the Max Weber's explanation: protestant religious doctrine→ capitalism

[11] On this subject, see Filippo Barbera and Nicola Negri (2005).

(a) Macro–micro ($M \rightarrow m$) relation. From a macro-variable, individual characteristics are individuated. These can be explained at the macro-level (as in the example by Weber concerning the presence of Calvinism in a certain society).
(b) Micro–micro ($m \rightarrow m'$) relation. At a micro-level the relation between individuals who are Calvinist and entrepreneur's capacities is proved.
(c) Micro–macro ($m' \rightarrow M'$) relation from more individuals with entrepreneur's capacities to the variable macro-capitalism.

According to the three hypotheses in Knorr-Cetina and Cicourel's anthology, the only relation that is verifiable is ($m \rightarrow m'$).The relations ($m \rightarrow M$) and $\left(m' \rightarrow M'\right)$ are possible only if the *aggregation hypothesis* is accepted.If one accepts the *hypothesis of unintended consequences*, the macro concept of "capitalism" and "social class" must be considered as rhetorical classifications; hence the relation $M \rightarrow M'$ becomes of little significance. Further, should the *representation hypothesis* be accepted, one should take into account the formation of macro-actors (associations of Calvinist women and/or men, female/male entrepreneurs with similar values, etc.) in the social space between m/M or m'/M', which could have encouraged the relation ($M \rightarrow M'$) or made other relations possible.

Prediction

In the light of previous comments, the term "prediction" could be used but one should be careful about the way it is used and, above all, it should not be used all the time, but only when the relation ($m \rightarrow m'$) is involved. What happens however when predictions are made with a ($M \rightarrow M'$) relation? An interesting debate in this respect occurred during the *Symposium on Prediction in the Social Sciences* published in 1995 in the *American Journal of Sociology* (vol. 100, no. 6). Here Randall Collins, Timur Kuran and Charles Tilly were asked the following question: Why didn't sociologists predict the fall of the communist regime in USSR? Their answers were commented by Edgar Kiser, James Coleman and Alejandro Portes and summed by Edgar Kiser as follows:

> It may seem as though the articles by Collins, Kuran and Tilly take very different positions on the possibility of predicting revolutions, ranging from "it cannot be done" to "it already has been done". Randall Collins argue that macro-sociological prediction is possible and provides the compelling examples of his own successful prediction of the decline of the Russian empire. Timur Kuran argue that making precise prediction is not possible now and may be never possible due to empirical problems with observing preferences and the complexity of the aggregation of individual's actions in revolutionary situations. Charles Tilly claims that we have been unable to make successful prediction about revolutions because we have been using the wrong kind of theory.

Despite the differences among and the limits of these scholars (for example important gender differences are systematically ignored), a common conclusion emerges that concerns the difficulties in making macro-sociological predictions and only bland versions of such predictions are possible.

(i) *It is more correct to talk about "trends" rather than "previsions".* Randall Collins uses a geopolitical model for his predictions. As Coleman has noted (1995, p. 1618), "there is no attempt to characterise, predict, or explain the action of those who initiate a revolt or those who support the revolutionaries, despite the fact that it is their actions that constitute the revolution" (without taking into account the gender of those who begin the revolution). Despite the obvious omissions in this model, in 1980, Collins predicted that the USSR would have disappeared "within 30–50 years". Is it correct to talk about "predictions" when discussing events that are expected to happen in the next 30–50 years? According to Coleman, this is not correct, and he suggests that in such cases the term "trend" should be used instead of "prediction".

(ii) *It is more correct to talk about "explanation" rather than "prediction".* Timor Kuran deals about the micro-level of individual choices (even though he does not specify gender differences). According to him, it is impossible to make predictions in the social sciences, while it is possible to give explanation to events that have taken place. Edgar Kiser (1995, pp. 1613–1614) says that Kuran's difficulties in making predictions should be interpreted as difficulties in producing good explanations:

> Timor Kuran elaborates on the role of the micro-level on revolutions from a rational choice perspectives. (...) The main reason that revolution is so hard to predict is that the effects of structural factors vary depending on the nature of existing revolutionary thresholds are imperfectly observable due to widespread preference falsification. Kuran argues that although these factors make it almost impossible to predict revolutions they do not hinder our ability to explain them after the fact. Although his sharp distinction between prediction and explanation is useful, Kuran's arguments understates the difficulty of producing good explanation.

(iii) *It is more correct to make "contingent prediction" rather than "invariant prediction".* Charles Tilly (1995, pp. 1605–1606) writes that "The construction of invariant models of revolution is a waste of time", while "contingent predictions" are useful (despite the fact that these are not easy for lack of theory); by these he means predictions on specific situations (in this case, revolutions) and contexts. It is however important to remember that Charles Tilly is a historian and for this reason his explanations are wide and articulated.

1.2.3.2 Mathematics for the Relation Between Individual and Collective Properties

In PFL essay (1958, p. 111, 114) and PFL and Herbert Menzel (1961), a distinction is made between individual properties (those which pertain to single members of a certain community) and collective properties (those which pertain to properties of collectives).

I. Properties of individual members of collectives: (a) *absolute properties* (characteristics of members as sex); (b) *relational properties* (information about the substantive relationships between the member described and other members);

(c) *comparative properties* (characteristics of members as their IQ); (d) *contextual properties* (these describe a member by a property of his collective). II. Properties of collectives: (a) *analytical properties*: obtained by performing some mathematical operation upon some properties of each single member (average income of a city); (b) *structural properties*: properties of collectives obtained by performing some mathematical operation upon the relations of each member to some or all the others (results of a socio metric test, etc.); (c) *global properties:* properties which are not based on information about the properties of individual members (populations size, etc.).

Boudon (1963) suggests that two types of relation should be distinguished: (1) *type I* when these occur in analytical properties and (2) *type II* when these occur between structural and global properties. Complex mathematical problems arise when *type I* correlations are considered and, in order to understand what mistakes may occur, three examples related to *Le suicide* by Emile Durkheim should be quoted.

The first kind of mistake occurs when the researcher does not take into account the procedures through which statistics is constructed. John Maxwell Atkinson (1971, 1978) talking about suicidal statistics analysed by Durkheim stresses that these are not "facts", as Durkheim thought, but merely "definitions of the situation" constructed by social actors such as police, doctors and coroners. For example, as stated in Capecchi and Pesce (1993, p. 112), Durkheim statistics (1897, p. 165) showed that in 1846/1847 the Italian region with the highest number of suicides was Emilia Romagna (62.9 for millions of inhabitants, while the national average was about 30). However, as stressed by Atkinson, the number of suicides also depends on the presence of Catholics in the region. For Catholics, in fact suicide is a sin and therefore the families of the person who committed suicide are likely to hide it. The higher presence of suicides in Emilia Romagna therefore should be interpreted as an indicator of religious habits, and not as an indicator of feelings of desperation amongst the population. When one deals with "official statistics", it is important to consider "how the statistics has been built", as Maxwell Atkinson notes.

A second kind of mistake occurs when the researcher considers correlations between variables at the level of territorial units which are then interpreted at the level of individual behaviour. This mistake is commented by Robison (1950) and Hanan Selvin (1958, p. 615) in relation to Durkheim's correlation, according to which higher suicide rates are related to higher number of "persons with independent means" (1987, p. 271). This allowed Durkheim to conclude that "poverty protects from suicide". Robinson and Selvin rightly comment that:

> This result is consistent with either of the following hypothesis: none of the people who commit suicide has independent means, or all of them have independent means. The ecological association between characteristics of department reveals nothing about the individual association between a person's wealth and whether or not he commits suicide.

Not all cases of "ecological associations" lead to "ecological fallacies", but the possibilities for mistakes are very high and Hayward R. Alker (1969) identifies three types of ecological fallacies (selective, contextual and cross-level).

A third kind of mistake occurs when the researcher based his interpretation on his prejudices. Durkheim (1897, p. 183), for example, notes that in France, between 1889 and 1891, suicide rates among female widowers were lower than those among male widowers. Notwithstanding the mistake that he makes when he interprets data on the ecological level as data on the individual level, the explanation that Durkheim provides of this is telling. Durkheim could have provided a straightforward and easy explanation based on his assumption that for women it is easier to build a network of social relation than is for men. However, this is not considered as a possible explanation. Durkheim's prejudices against women led him to explain the lower suicide rate by invoking women's lower sensitivity and their propensity to be satisfied with their lot.

Durkheim (1897, pp. 231–2) has written:

> For women it is easier to live in isolation than for men (...) Women's privilege in this respect is due to the fact that their sensitivity is more primitive and not very developed (...) She has less needs and is happy with what she has. Provide an old woman with a devotional practice, a pet to take care of and she is happy. If a woman remains attach to religious values is because these are a defence against suicide, and precisely these simple social norms are enough for her. On the contrary, for men, these social norms are not enough because he is a more complex being.

These mistakes should be taken into consideration when one tries to use mathematics to analyse two main levels of variation: (1) *variations among individuals* (on variables such as sex, age, education, party preference) and (b) *variations among proximal territorial units* (quarters, villages, rural communes, etc.).

Mattei Dogan and Stein Rokkan (1969) have reflected on the possibility of using mathematics for these two levels (which can be considered separately or together). They are the authors of Table 1.11, in which they consider four types of possible analyses: I. The main goal is to explain individual choices (for example how

Table 1.11 Level of dependent variable and focus of analysis

Focus of analysis→ level of dependent variable	One level	Interaction of two level
Individual	I. Either individual data (e.g. from surveys) treated without reference to territorial context *or* territorial aggregate data used to analyse individual variations	III. Either individual data used jointly with contextual data for territorial units or :aggregate/global data to test interaction between levels
Territorial unit	II. Aggregate/global data for territorial units used to describe and account for variation at territorial level	IV. Either joint use of individual/aggregate/global data to test *sources of change* in territorial structure or aggregate/global data to test Interaction between levels

Source: Dogan and Rokkan (1969)

a wealth variable – to own or not your own house – can influence the political vote). If one does not have individual data but only territorial unit data (as it is the case for electoral data or census data), one can make hypotheses on individual behaviour starting from ecological correlations. II. The primary interest consists in mapping the characteristics of different territorial units (for example to verify male and female religious behaviour in different areas of the same territory, from the city centre, to boroughs in the outskirts, to small rural villages far away from the city). III. The main interest is focused on an individual level (for example to explain female and male electoral or religious choices); at the same time, the analysis of such behaviours can be put in relation to their spatial and territorial context. For example Boudon (1958) considers individual behaviour and formulates two hypotheses: (a) individual behaviour is influenced by the frequency of a certain behaviour in a certain context and (b) individual behaviour is influenced by the characteristics of a certain context. IV. Dependent variables occur at the level of territorial units, while explicative variables occur both at the territorial and the individual level because in this case one is interested in understanding variations at territorial level through a micro/macro interaction. For example conflicts between centre and outskirts of a city can be explained by considering the characteristics of these two areas as well as individual aggregate behaviours that occur there.

A very important contribution in the field of mathematics has been given by Leo A. Goodman (1959). He has demonstrated that, provided certain conditions and certain hypotheses, it is possible to interpret individual behaviour based on ecological data. For example if one knows electoral behaviour pertaining to two different elections in two different polling stations (and the results of the smallest unit), it is possible to estimate electoral mobility. Piergiorgio Corbetta, Arturo Parisi and Hans Shadee (1988) have applied the "ecological regression" technique to calculate electoral fluxes in two consecutive elections in eight Italian cities. On this, see the methodological discussion that appeared in AAVV (1993).

1.2.3.3 Mathematics for Less Visible Relations

PFL (1949, p. 379) wrote: "Finding regularities and determining criteria of significance are concerns the social sciences have in common with the natural sciences. But there are crucial differences between the two fields of enquiry. The world of social events is much less *visible* than the realm of nature". In this section, some examples of mathematical applications in less visible situations that may occur in micro/macro relations pertaining to Coleman's boat: $(M \rightarrow m)$, $(m \rightarrow m')$, $(m' \rightarrow M')$ are considered:

$$(M \rightarrow m)\,\text{relation}$$

If one wishes to find explanations on the micro-level starting from analyses at the macro-level, it is necessary to individuate mechanisms that are less visible than the macro-level. A good example of this is the cross-pressures shown in *People's Choice* by PFL, Bernard Berelson and Hazel Gaudet (1944). At the macro-level, this research showed that some groups of people, three months before the elections, knew with certainty who they would have voted for, while other people were uncertain about their vote and took a decision few days or hours before the elections. According to the authors, the explanation for this kind of behaviour is to be found in degree of cross-pressures. Studies on electoral behaviour in the United States showed that catholic, poor and black men and women tended to vote for the Democratic Party, while protestants, rich and white men and women voted for the Republican Party. What happens however in the case of a rich and catholic man? And in the case of a protestant black woman? The study showed that the more the cross-pressures in an individual, the longer the person takes to decide about his/her vote.

Another example is provided by PFL (1949, p. 380), who in *The American Soldier* presents a list of six statements:

1. Better educated men showed more psycho-neurotic symptoms than did those with less education (the mental instability of the intellectual as compared to the more impassive psychology of the man in the street has often been commented on).
2. Men from rural backgrounds were usually in better spirits during their army life than were soldiers from city backgrounds (after all, they are more accustomed to hardships).
3. Southern soldiers were better able to stand the climate in the hot South Sea Island than northern soldiers (of course, southerners are more accustomed to hot weather).
4. White privates were more eager to become non-coms than were Negroes (the lack of ambition among Negroes is almost proverbial).
5. Southern Negroes preferred Southern to Northern white (isn't it well known that southern whites have a more fatherly attitude towards their "darkies"?).
6. As long as fighting continued, men were more eager to be returned to the States than they were after the German surrender (you cannot blame people for not wanting to be killed).

After this, PFL, however, adds:

> Every one of these statements is the direct opposite of what actually was found. Poorly educated soldiers were more neurotic that those with high education; Southern showed no greater ability than Northerners to adjust to a tropical climate; Negroes were more eager for promotion than white; and so on.

$(m \to m')$relation

In this kind of relation there are two possible sources of invisibility: (1) in the choice of variables whose analysis can produce relations such as $(m \to m')$ and (ii) in the higher or lower attention to cases that deviate from the $(m \to m')$ relation.

The first case occurs when, as in *The Academic Mind*, one gives up analysing the gender differences when investigating their reactions of fears of McCarthyism.

The mathematical analysis tends to make the presence of 13% of female university teachers even more invisible, while an analysis based on gender distinction would have produced new $(m \rightarrow m')$ relations.

The second case has been stressed by PFL, who, when faced with a $(m \rightarrow m')$ relation that involves the majority of people interviewed, wonders why a minority always "deviates" and chooses a ($m \leftarrow m$') relation. Such an attention towards deviant cases leads PFL (1962, p. 766) to indicate in his presidential address two possible development in sociological research:

> One type can be called the investigation of "positive deviant cases". We take it for granted that certain types of situation usually take unfavourable turns. And yet sometimes exceptions occur: local or regional elections in which a good candidate wins in spite of the fact that his adversary has the power of the machine on his side (...). Another type of study can be called the pretesting of new social ideas. A new notion of creative reform-especially if it has just check on its assumptions and to prefect its design, partly to improve its feasibility and partly to facilitate its public acceptance.

Also in this case it is possible to use mathematical methods to ascertain the distance between more frequent and deviant types and attempt to provide an explanation for less frequent situations:

$$(m' \rightarrow M')\text{relation}$$

In this kind of relation, the non-aggregative explanations found in the essay by Karin Knorr-Cetina (1981) are less visible: the hypothesis of unintended consequences and the representation hypothesis.

Concerning the hypothesis of unintended consequences, Raymond Boudon (1977, pp. 61–132) has used mathematics to clarify some of these unexpected results. By way of a mathematical simulation, he demonstrates, for example, that a reduction of differences in the education does not imply that social mobility increases (which is the expected result), that is to say the possibility of having a better job. Unexpected and undesired results are therefore possible and mathematics can be useful to better understand how these results can occur. Concerning the representation hypothesis, a research base on a survey cannot identify the associations (that is to say the macro-actors) in a certain area and that can contribute to find a $(m' \rightarrow M')$ explanation, despite the fact that a certain kind of research can make them invisible.

1.2.3.4 Mathematics for the Social Sciences

These contributions precede and/or accompany the mathematical models which will be described in the next part. These are of the ($M \rightarrow S \rightarrow M$) kind, and, as a consequence, here mathematics is more prominent than sociological applications. Despite this, relations of the ($S \rightarrow M \rightarrow S$) kind are achieved. Let us consider PFL's contribution (1961) to algebra in dichotomic variables. PFL has written several essays on this subject (some have not been published yet). These kinds of essays are clearly very strictly related to the latent structural models.

Another kind of mathematics that is very important for the social sciences is the theory of graphs that has been systematically illustrated by Claude Flament (1965) and Claude Berge (1965) (under the direction of PFL) during seminars on mathematics for the social sciences organized by the UNESCO. From this perspective, the contributions of R. Duncan Luce and Howard Raiffa (1957) to the theory of games and decision making are also important to understand another kind of mathematical models. Fractal geometry can be considered a mathematics for the social sciences. Benoit Mandelbrot (1965) participated in the UNESCO seminars organized by PFL. Despite this, he is best known for his theories on fractal theory in Mandelbrot (1975, 1977, 1982). These have led to studies such as Heinz-Otto Peitgen and Peter H. Richter's (1986) *The Beauty of Fractals: Images of Complex Dynamical Systems*. Also significant are the contributions of fuzzy logic, which have been systematically illustrated by Lotfi A. Zadeh (1965) and carried forward by Bart Kosko (1993). Kosko has declared that accepting *fuzzy thinking* means to leave Aristotelian philosophy behind in order to embrace Buddhist philosophy.

1.2.3.5 Mathematical Models

Denis Howe, in his *Free Online Dictionary*, defines "model" as follows:

> Model is a description of observed behaviour simplified ignoring certain details. Models allow complex (systems) to be understood and their behaviour predicted within the scope of the model, but may give incorrect description and prediction for situations outside the realm of intended use.

Mathematical models used in sociology have the following three characteristics: (a) simplification; (b) explanation; (c) prediction. The results of the model can be compared with the collected data from reality obtained through research. A model is not invalidated because it is too simplified (and therefore too far away from reality); a model is valid if it is "useful" and asks interesting questions, creates new explanations and theories and fulfils interesting expectations.

The classification of mathematical models takes into consideration two main distinctions. The first one used, for example, by Nigel Gilbert and Klaus Troitzsch (2005) is between (Ia) *statistical models* of a general type that are articulated in *model of classification* and *models of relation between variables* and (Ib) *models of simulation*. A second distinction used, for example, by Aage B. Sorensen (1978) and Christofer Edling (2002) is between (IIa) *models of processes;* (IIb) *models of structure*; (IIc) *rational choice models, agent-based models and artificial society models*. Despite the fact that these two distinctions overlap, it is still useful to consider them separately, because they represent different methodological problems and cause different contributions to emerge.

1.2.3.6 (Ia) Statistical Models

This first group considers general statistical models whose characteristics are summed up by Nigel Gilbert and Klaus Troitzsch (2005, p. 16) in the following passage:

> With statistical models (...) the researcher develop a model (for example a set of equations) through abstraction from the presumed social processes in the target. These equations will include parameters (for example beta coefficients) whose magnitudes are determined in the course of estimating the equations (this is the step where a statistical package would normally be used). As well as developing a model, the researcher will have collected some data with which to perform the estimation (for example survey data on the variable included in the equations). The analysis consists of two steps: first, the researcher ask whether the model generates prediction that have some similarity to the data that have actually been collected (this is typically assessed by means of statistical hypotheses) and second, the researcher measures the magnitude of parameters (and perhaps compares their relative size, in order to identify the most important).

The general logic of these models is expressed in Fig. 1.2.

Fig. 1.2 The logic of statistical modelling as a method. Source: Gilbert and Troitzsch (2005)

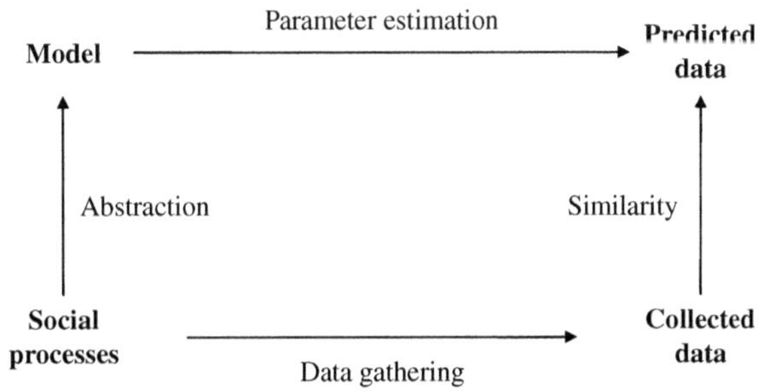

PFL's researches have focused on the importance of *linear causal models* and the *latent structure analysis*. These strategies have been compared with the models of multiple regression (more frequently used in economics) or models of *factor analysis* and *principal component analysis* (more frequently used in psychology). A few examples are sufficient to point to some problems related to these models. Let us consider, for example, the category of *linear causal models*. During the 1960s, these raised a lot of interest for four reasons:

(1) They allowed to clarify the causal relations among variables in a sociological research.
(2) They allowed a comparison with mathematical methods of linear multiple regression used in economics.
(3) They allowed to easily explore the relations among variables.
(4) They allowed the use of data analyses on panel.

The first instance of a formulation of *linear casual models* can be traced back to PFL's research *The People's Choice*, which he wrote together with Berelson and Gaudet (1944). In this research, three variables were considered: X_1 (degree of education of the electorate), X_2 (interest for the electoral campaign) and X_3 (participation in the election). PFL showed that the three variables were related; however, if one considered the relation between X_1 (education) and X_3 (vote) with X_2 constant, this relation tended to zero. That is to say that if a person was very interested in the electoral campaign, he/she would go to vote independently from his/her education, while if a person was not interested in the electoral campaign, he/she would not vote (independently from his/her education).

What PFL showed was a very simple linear casual model of the kind $X_1 \to X_2 \to X_3$ is the independent variable, X_2 the intervening variable and X_3 the dependent variable. Herbert A. Simon (1954) and Hubert M. Blalock (1962) showed that this casual scheme can be indicated by the following equations:

$$X_1 = e_1$$

$$X_2 = b_{21}X_1 + e_2$$

$$X_3 = b_{32}X_2 + e_3$$

It is easy to demonstrate that $b_{21} = \sigma_2/\sigma_1 r_{12}$ and that $b_{32} = \sigma_3/\sigma_2 r_{23}$; hence, considering the relation between coefficient b_{ij} and the linear correlation coefficient r_{ij}, the system $X_1 \to X_2 \to X_3$ can be verified when $r_{12} \neq 0$, $r_{13} \neq 0$, $r_{23} \neq 0$, $r_{23.1} = 0$. Moreover, as the numerator of $r_{23.1}$ results from r_{13} to $r_{12}r_{13}$, if $r_{23.1} = 0$, it means that $r_{13} = r_{12}r_{23}$ is also true.

The debate that ensued this formulation by Simon and Blalock was followed up by Sewall Wright (1960), Raymond Boudon (1965, 1967) and Otis Dudley Duncan (1966); a summary of this debate is in Capecchi (1967, 1967b), and Blalock (1985) contains a more recent analysis. From this debate two main possibilities for casual models emerge: (1) the possibility to evaluate the coefficients b_{ij} using the statistical contribution of the multiple regression, keeping the possibility of standard or nonstandard *path coefficient* open and (2) a very simple method to understand immediately, given an exact coefficient matrix, which kind of possible casual configuration is possible among different variables.

Drawing on my experience with two applications of linear casual models, [12] I can point out three kinds of problems.

First, in order to define the asymmetric direction $X_1 \to X_2$ instead of $X_1 \leftarrow X_2$, the researcher uses three criteria: (1) the asymmetric relation *Milieu characteristics→ Individual characteristics→ Attitudes→ Behaviours*; (2) the asymmetric relation *General →Specific* and (iii) the asymmetric

[12]The two applications of linear casual models I am referring to here are (a) an application to classify the differences between active members of the Communist Party and Christian Democrats, which appeared in English in Capecchi (1973) and (b) an application on the behaviour of voters in Italy, which appeared in English in Capecchi and Galli (1969).

relation *Preceding*→ *Following*. The problem is that only the asymmetric relation *Preceding*→ *Following* is always valid, for example *Parents' education*→ *Children's education*; in the two other kinds of asymmetric relations the choice between $X_1 \rightarrow X_2$ and $X_1 \leftarrow X_2$ often depends on the academic community, which tends to consider certain variables as independent, dependent or intervening. *Second*, in some cases, we can have the presence of both $X_1 \rightarrow X_2$ and $X_1 \leftarrow X_2$ at the same time even if the influence of these two is different and one has a main direction (for example $X_1 \rightarrow X_2$) while the other a less consistent feedback ($X_1 \leftarrow X_2$). *Third, problem* arises when in area A (or in relation to the characteristic A of the variable X_4) the relation $X_1 \rightarrow X_2 \rightarrow_3$ can be realized, while in area B (or in relation to characteristic B of the variable X_4) the relation $X_1 \rightarrow X_3 \leftarrow X_2$ can be realized.

These limits were the object of many essays, such as that by John A. Sonquist (1969), who, as a preliminary operation, proposes to choose accurately among the possible variables, taking into account the different plausibility of the casual relations which can be suggested. Owing to these difficulties, in many cases, researches on asymmetric relations [($X_1 \rightarrow X_2$) or ($X_1 \leftarrow X_2$)] have been abandoned in favour of relations of contiguity [relations of the kind ($X_1 \leftrightarrow X_2$)]

The analysis of the latent structure presented by PFL (1954) and by PFL and Neal Henry (1968) is based on dichotomic data and allows to individuate (a) the number of the homogeneous classes in which the subjects can be classified and (b) the "trace lines" that allow to individuate the probability that a subject answers positively to an item in relation to a latent dimension based on items of the same type.

An interesting application of this model can be found in PFL and Wagner Thielens (1958, p. 82). There is a clear difference between latent structure analysis and principal components method or factor analysis; in the latter the items are not related to a latent dimension but rather to "factors" or "principal components" individuated by orthogonal axes, which have to be named. A comparison between these two models was made by David J. Bartholomew (1987).

In this area, other models have also been illustrated; some of them can however be used only for specific kinds of variables: the models of classification based on entropy by Capecchi and Moller for dichotomic variables, the unfolding models by Coombs for data on the ordinal scale level, the radex by Guttman, the log-linear models, the models by Leo A. Goodman for categorical data, the correspondence analysis by Jean Paul Benzécri, the models based on the LISREL technique, etc.

All these models are variants of the statistical model previously defined and are different for (a) the mathematical characteristics of the used variables; (b) the measures of connection/correlation; (c) the hypotheses based on the model; (d) the greater/smaller attention given to models of classification or models of relations among variables and (e) the tendency to consider or fail to consider the time changes within the model.

For example the model proposed by Capecchi (1965) and by Capecchi and Frank Moeller (1968, 1975) is a classification model based on dichotomic data and uses as connecting measures the part shared by the entropies of the variables. It does not consider time changes and, in order to identify homogeneous classes, uses the second theorem by Shannon.[13]

In this area it is possible to make a comparison among different models based on the same kind of data. For example Leo A. Goodman (2007) considers different models of nominal (categorical) data. He illustrates the concepts of *independence*, *quasi-independence, symmetry, quasi-symmetry* and *symmetric association*, and makes a comparison among log-linear models, recursive models, latent structure analysis and latent class models. His conclusions (2007, pp. 16–17), wisely written, are interesting because they speak of the pleasure one can experience in playing with mathematical models; it is a pleasure that can be compared with magic and serendipity:

> The results obtained by applying the concept described in this essay to substantive data of interest sometimes seem magical – the sudden release of form formerly hidden, embedded in a block of dense data – but perhaps "serendipity" better describe the way in which these concepts were developed. In this essay, I have noted that the information to which I was exposed in my work on one statistical problem, in one substantive area of interest, that led me able to look at a second substantive area of interest, and than be able to see what was the statistical problem that needed to be dealt with there and how to proceed with work on it (...) and so on. By a serendipitous result I do not mean here a result obtained by accident or chance, but rather a result obtained by an accidental exposure to information and a prepared mind.

1.2.3.7 (Ib) Models of Simulation

As Gilbert and Troitzsch (2005, p. 17) write, models of simulation show differences and similarities with previous models. The relation between model and simulation of data is shown in Fig. 1.3.

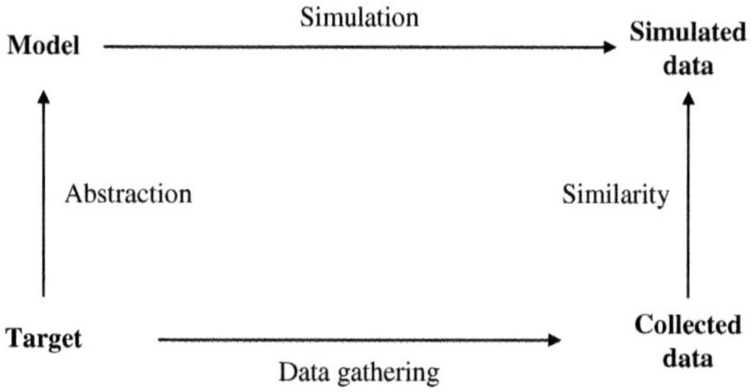

Fig. 1.3 The logic of simulation as a method

The evaluation of a simulation model given by Gilbert and Troitzsch (2005, p. 17) is as follows:

[13]The models presented by Capecchi and Moeller in a wider social entropy theory is in Kenneth D. Bailey (1990).

> Once again, the researcher develops a model based on presumed social processes. But this time, the model might be in the form of a computer program rather than a statistical equation. The model is run and its behaviour measured. In effect, the model is used to generate the simulated data. These simulated data can then be compared with data collected in the usual ways to check whether the model generates outcomes which are similar to those produced by the actual processes operating in the social world.

One of the first simulation models realized in sociology is the one known as "The Simulmatics Project" described by Ithiel de Sola Pool and Robert Abelson (1961). With this model one aimed at understanding the reaction of voters to John F. Kennedy's political campaign, though later on this model was also used to understand how the referendum about the fluoridation of drinking water took place. One of the first comments concerning simulation models in sociology dates back to 1965 and appeared in a special issue of *Archives Europèennes de Sociologie* entitled "Simulation in Sociology". Raymond Boudon (1965) wrote the introduction of this issue and analysed the differences between applications by James Coleman, Elihu Katz and Herbert Menzel (1957) [14] on the one hand and applications of simulation models on the other. Coleman, Katz and Menzel's research was very interesting as it dealt with issues of the diffusion of a new drug among doctors and patients, a typical issue as long as simulation models are concerned. Coleman, Katz and Menzel carried out a complex survey. As the three authors wrote (1957, p. 254):

> The research is thus based on three kinds of data: the month of each doctor's first prescription of the new drug obtained through a search of pharmacists' files; data about the informal social structure of the medical community derived from doctors' replies to sociometric questions in an interview; and many individual attributes for each doctor, likewise obtained by interview.

The data that were obtained were useful to identify the way in which the new drug was marketed; it was found that this changed according to doctors' position in the community. The authors were in this way able to trace different curves for the marketing of the drug.

This kind of research can also be carried out with a simulation model; the issue of *Archives Europèennes de Sociologie* introduced the model by Torsten Hägerstrand (1965). This dealt with innovations promoted by the Swedish government – subsidies to improve pasture and a systematic control of bovine tuberculosis – in small rural farms in southern Sweden. As Boudon has noted, in order to study the way these innovations spread, Hägerstrand does not focus on "relational properties" between farms (equivalent to sociometric equivalents used in Coleman, Katz and Menzel's research), instead he looks for "structural properties" related to that particular territory. According to Hägerstrand, an indicator is represented by telephone calls from and to agricultural farms. The further the distance between farms, the smaller the amount of telephone calls. A second indicator is "local migration" that in rural areas depends on marriage, exchange of farm labourers between farms, exchange of farms between farmers. Also in these cases, the further the distance

[14] For a more complete analysis, see Coleman et al. (1966).

between farms, the smaller the amount of migration. As Boudon writes (1965, p. 10):

> Hägerstrand's model introduces two hypotheses with a typically sociological dimension: the hypothesis of non-isotropy in space and the hypothesis of a social distance that, according to an empirical law, increases more rapidly than geographical distance.

Hägerstrand presents rules that can be applied to the diffusion of information among rural farms and employs the Monte Carlo technique to obtain random numbers in order to begin a process of simulation within a matrix in which spatial probabilities of contact are different. As Hägerstrand (1965, p. 50) sums up:

> We are going to simulate diffusion of an innovation within a population by the aid of the Monte Carlo technique. In this connection the Monte Carlo approach may be said to imply that a society of "robots" is created in which "life" goes on according to certain probability rules given from the start. The technique can best be described as a game of dice in which the gaming table represent a part of the Earth surface, the piece represent individual living in the area and the rules of the game constitute the particular factors which we want to study in operation. The dice produces step by step new situation within the range of variation which is implicit in the rules. The dice is the motive power of life in the model.

As noted by Jean-Philippe Cointet and Camille Roth (2007), the model proposed by Hägerstrand is included in *knowledge diffusion models*; their structure consists of (a) an underlying social network topology and (b) a particular design of interaction rules driving knowledge transmission. Furthermore, this kind of model (in a similar way to all models of simulation) poses the problem of how close to reality the model is. Hägerstrand found consistent convergences between data obtained with the simulation model and empirical data obtained in rural areas of southern Sweden.

The history of simulation models in the social sciences has been written by Klaus Troitzsch (1997) and Fig. 1.4 shows a summary of such a history.

Troitzsch distinguishes between (a) models which derive from differential equations and stochastic processes and (b) models that can be defined as object-, event- or agent-based models.

The first category includes *system dynamics and world models* which use software such as DYNAMO, STELLA and WORLD 1, 2 and 3. The best known scholar using these models is Jay Wright Forrester, the founder of systems dynamics, whose theory, methodology and philosophy have been applied to industrial dynamics, environmental changes, politics, economics, as well as medicine and engineering. As Forrester (1971, p. 4) has written:

> People would never send a space ship to the moon without first testing prototype models and making computer simulations of anticipated trajectories. (...) Such models and laboratory tests do not guarantee against failure, but they do identify many weaknesses which can be corrected before they cause full-scale disasters. Social systems are far more complex and harder to understand than technological systems. (...) But what justification can there be for assuming that we do not know enough to construct models of social system but believe we do know enough to directly redesign social systems by passing laws and starting news programs? I suggest that we know enough to make useful models of social systems.

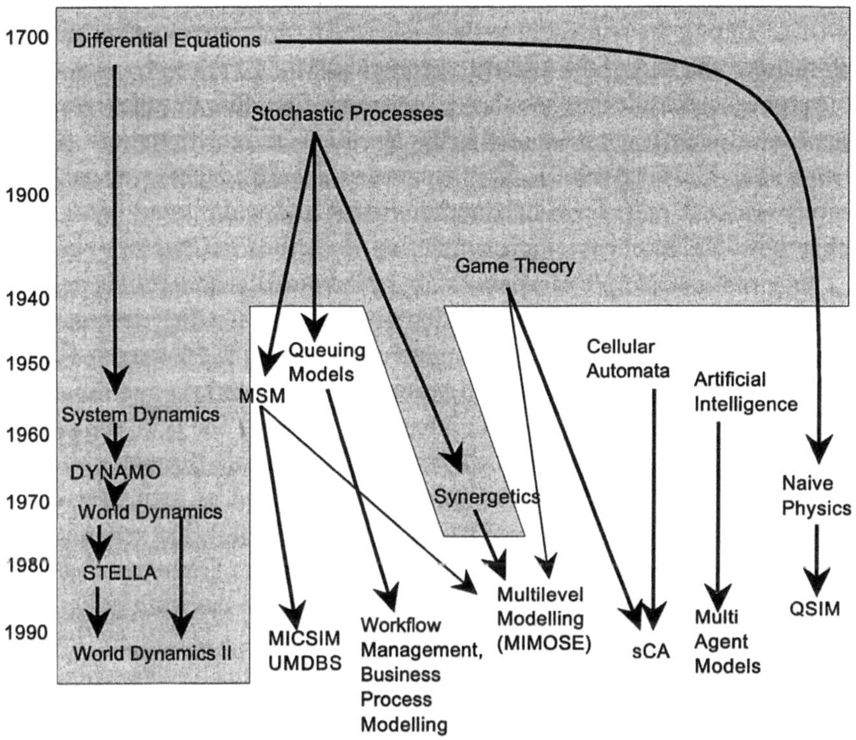

Fig. 1.4 The development of contemporary approaches to simulation in the social sciences. Source: Troitzsch (1997). Grey shaded area, equation-based models; white area, object-, event- or agent-based models

The first model of society illustrated by Forrester (1969) was about urban dynamics and consisted of an early demonstration of how social systems can have a counterintuitive nature. Forrester (1971, p. 7) writes:

> We examined four common programs for improving the depressed nature of central cities. One program was creation of jobs by busing the unemployed to suburban jobs or through governmental jobs as employer of last resort. Second was a training program to increase skills of the lowest-income group. Third was financial aid to depressed cities from federal subsides. Fourth was construction of low cost housing. All of these were shown to lie between neutral and highly detrimental regardless of the criteria used for judgment. The four program range from ineffective to harmful judged either by their effect on the en the economic health of a city or by their long-range effect on the low-income population. The results both confirm and explain much of what has been happening over the last several decades in cities.

Politicians found it difficult to accept the results of Forrester's model; such difficulties were connected with their incapacity to predict the consequences of single partial actions and their lack of an interrelated vision that includes all components of the population. As summed up by Forrester (1971, p. 9) "Programs aimed at improving a city can succeed only if they result in eventually raising the average quality of life for the country as a whole" because "any proposed program should deal with both the quality of life and the factors affecting the population".

Such an attention to consequences and interactions can also be found in the most famous model by Forrester written for *Il Club di Roma* founded by Aurelio Peccei, whose analyses are summed in his volume *World Dynamics* (1971) and his project *The Limits to Growth* edited by Donella Meadows et al. (1972). Forrester (1971, p. 12) writes:

> The model of world interaction showed different alternative futures depending on whether social policies are adopted to limit population growth while a high standard of living is still possible or whether the future is ignored until population is suppressed by pollution, crowding, disease, water and resource shortage, social strife, hunger. (...) Unless we choose favourable processes to limit growth, the social and environmental systems by their internal processes will choose for us.

The only prediction that was incorrect was the success of the book. As Forrester (1989, p. 11) writes:

> In 1971 World Dynamics seemed to have everything necessary to guarantee no public notice. First it had forty pages of equations in the middle of the book that should be sufficient to squelch public interest. Second the interesting messages were in the form of computer output graphs, and most of the public do not understand such presentations. Third the book was brought out by a publisher that had published only one previous book and I doubted that it would have the commercial status to even get reviewed. I thought I was writing for may be 200 people who would like to try and interesting model on their computer. But, as you know, I was wrong.

In the second category (b) Gilbert and Troitzsch (2005) include six kinds of models: (b1) *micro-analytical simulation models* (MSMs); the model is based on characteristics belonging to a single person (sex, age, marital status etc.) and a set number of transiting probabilities due to the fact that these models use software such as MICSIM and UMDBS. (b2) *Queuing models or discrete event models*. In these models, time is neither continuous nor formed by equidistant discrete steps, rather it proceeds from event to event. Gilbert and Troitzsch (2005, p. 80) choose as an example the simulation of an airport:

> In terms of queuing metaphor of discrete event models, there are at least three different kinds of objects, namely servers, customers and queues. Technically speaking, there is one additional object, the agenda, which keeps track of the events and schedules them. Queuing models are stochastic. In the queuing models are stochastic. In the queuing metaphor the time between customers' arrivals as well as the time needed to serve a customer are random, following a certain random distribution. Discrete event models are dynamic: states of serves, queues and customers depend on past states.

(b3) *Multilevel simulation models*. Models of this kind are exemplified by the MIMOSE software used to simulate the interaction among members of a population. An interesting example is represented by the simulation of gender segregation in German high schools. (b4) *Cellular automata*. These models have been used in physics but are also useful for simulation in the social sciences (sCA means cellular automata and is used for simulation in the social sciences) when the focus is on the emergence of properties from local interaction. Among the examples quoted by the authors are studies by Robert Axelrod (1970) on the formation of new alliances among political actors and about migrations. (b5) *Multiagent models*. These models derive from studies on artificial intelligence (AI) and simulate agents that interact "intelligently" with their environment. Examples of these include the artificial society *Sugarshape* by Epstein and Axtell, the MANTA Project (modelling an anthill activity) and the EOS Project (evolution of organized society). (b6) *Models from physics*. Applications of this kind of models by Pierluigi Contucci and Stefano Ghirlanda (2007) are included in *Quality and Quantity*. Contucci and Ghirlanda have applied statistical mechanics methods – a branch of theoretical physics – to social problems (for example intercultural contacts as a consequence of immigration). Other researches by Fabio Bagarello (2007) and Nicola Bellomo, Maria Letizia Bertotti, and Marcello Delitala (2007) have applied principles from quantum mechanics and kinetic theory of active particles to sociological problems.

1.2.3.8 (IIa) Models of Process

PFL (1955, 1965) wrote several essays on models of process taking into account recurring information (panels) concerning attitudes and behaviours as one of the main fields of application of mathematics to sociology (?). In this area, James Coleman's contributions (1964, 1964b, 1973) are very significant. In 1964 he wrote two studies in which he illustrated continuous-time models and discrete space stochastic process models for studying transition. Here he analysed phenomena such as attitudinal changes, unemployment amongst students of vocational institutes, consumer behaviour, voting behaviour and group contagion. In his study published in 1973, models of processes became less prominent, and models of rational choice theory started to be developed. His most important applications of process models were analyses of changes (shown through panels) in attitudes and behaviours (consumers' behaviour, political behaviour) of social mobility. The following annotations on models of process are possible, thanks to essays by Capecchi (1967) and Boudon (1973) and historical quantitative research by Barbagli, Capecchi and Cobalti (1987) on social mobility in an Italian region.

James Coleman (1946, 1973) is considered one of the most important scholars of mathematical models of process. In a study dated 1946, Coleman develops continuous-time, discrete space stochastic process models for studying transition and analysing phenomena such as behavioural changes, diffusion processes, electorate behaviour and group contagion. In 1973, a study on the employment of mathematics for social action was followed by the definition of models of multistage decision processes, which are applied to an analysis of the behaviour of an electorate.

As Aage B. Sorensen writes (1978, p. 349), all mathematical models of processes share "change in variables characterizing individuals, social groups and social structures", and for this reason it is important to define what change means, what are the aims of this analysis of processes and which are the criteria of evaluation:

> Change is seen as a result of other variables (possibly including time) operating on the variable of interest in a certain way-that is the process is conceived of as causal. (...) The analysis of causal processes involves two main tasks. The first is to specify the mechanism of change, i.e. to model how change occurs. The second is to assess the causal influences transmitted by the mechanism of change. (...) A mathematical model of social process may be evaluated by two main criteria: the empirical adequacy of the model (the model's ability to account for the observed course of a process) and the theoretical adequacy of the model (whether the model represents an adequate sociological conception of a process that advances our knowledge and understanding of the process).

The most important distinction, as long as models of process are concerned, is between (i) stochastic models and (ii) deterministic models. As Christofer Endling (2002, p. 202) writes:

> In a deterministic process we can fully determine its future state if we know the current state of the process. If we are dealing with a stochastic process, on the other hand, its future state can only be predicted from the present with some probability. Deterministic processes are described by differential (or difference) equations. The main tool for describing stochastic processes is the stationary Markov process, of which the Poison process and the Brownian motion are variants (differential equations are used in constructing stochastic models as well as to model change in probability distributions. (...) A deterministic model deals with change in variables, and a stochastic model deals with change in probabilistic distribution.

Endling quotes the study by David Bartholomew (1982) as an example of stochastic processes and the one by Joshua Epstein (1997) as an example of deterministic processes. The models of process have been applied to different problems. Several models have been used to analyse social mobility and changes in electoral behaviour; other models have been used to tackle social integration and diffusion of innovations.

1.2.3.9 (IIb) Models of Structure

Mathematical Thinking in the Social Sciences edited by PFL (1954) contains an essay by Nicolas Rashevsky, a mathematician and biologist. Besides analysing imitative behaviour, Rashevsky shows mathematical models of structure applied to the distribution of wealth in selfish and altruistic societies. In this area of models, one of the most important fields of study leads to the identification of social networks characterized by the convergence of disciplines such as sociology, economy, psychology, physics and mathematics (cf. Barabasi 2002; Freeman 2004). These models are characterized by four features:

(1) Social network analysis is motivated by a structural intuition based on ties linking social actors.
(2) It is grounded in systematic empirical data.
(3) It draws heavily in graphic imagery.
(4) It relies on the use of mathematical and/or computational models

Among the first applications are those by PFL and Merton (1954) about friendship. It is also important to remember that PFL has formulated the two-step flow of communication theory which has been applied to voters' behaviour in *The people's Choice* (1944) and consumer's behaviour in *Personal Influence*.

Noteworthy is a theoretical trajectory illustrated in Barabasi (2002) that connects the work of the Hungarian writer Frigyes Karinthy to the American sociologists Stanley Milgram and Mark Granovetter. A short story by Frigyes Karinthy published in 1929 and entitled *Lancszemek (chains)* illustrates an experiment; the hypothesis is that any person in this world can come into contact with another person in any other part of the world only through five stages. In this short story the protagonist plans to contact a Nobel Prize. What should one do? First this Nobel Prize must have met the Sweden King. He is obsessed with chess games and he is a good friend of a tennis player who knows very well the character in Karinthy's short story. Milgram is well known for the "Milgram experiment" in which he shows that subservience to authority can lead to the killing of another person. Milgram (1967) formalized the literary experiment by Karinthy. By showing that two people that had never met each other could find a way to come into contact with one another, he showed that the world on interconnections is very small. Granovetter (1973) illustrates this theory further. He shows that interpersonal relations have both strong clusters with very tight interpersonal connections and "weak connections" among strong clusters. It is important to have not only strong connections with a few clusters but also weak connections with clusters that are remote.

In this way, an important interpretative hypothesis on social networks starts to be illustrated. These in turn produce expressions such as social capital (used by Pierre Bourdieu with economic cultural and symbolic capital) in studies such as those by Gugliotta et al. (2007) or by Currarini et al. (2008), which propose an updated analysis of two issues previously analysed by PFL: friendship and opinion leaders.

Finally it is important to remember that the most important theoretical contribution in this category of models is that of Harrison White. Harrison White is a significant figure because his work exemplifies the shift from models of process to models of structure. Mathematical models of structure introduced by White (1963, 1970) consider two situations: structure of kinship in different groups of people and structure of career in firms. The analysis of the structure of kinship was not evaluated positively by the *American Journal of Sociology*, where it was reviewed by Raoul Naroll (1965), because it was considered a contribution to mathematical models rather than a contribution to the problems analysed (a classical example of $M \rightarrow S \rightarrow M$). Much more appreciated was White's study which appeared in 1970, which analyses the mobility of organizations. Instead of studying mobility from the point of view of people, this study uses a vacancy chain model (as in the above-mentioned research by Hägerstrand, this research also prefers to act on "structural properties" in work places rather than on "relation properties" of people). This research has been undertaken by Ivan Chase (1991, p. 152), who, while positively evaluating White's contributions, mentions three of the structural models that he himself uses:

> First, the present Markov models do not treat the actual, detailed influences at work in selecting particular individuals for particular vacant openings. (...) Second the Markov models presently used are quite crude. Positions are roughly grouped into a few broad strata, probability of a vacancy moving between the various states have to be measured empirically and cannot be predicted from first principles. (...) Third, vacancy chain theory, in its present formulation, does not lend itself to answering questions about the equality of access of various groups to mobility opportunities and this question motivate, in part, some of the more traditional approaches to mobility.

The importance given by White to models of structures transpires in his theoretical position in his volume *Identity and Control* (1992), who was reprinted and revised in 2008. As White writes (2008, p. xvii, xxi):

> The principal question for this book is How? My colleague Charles Tilly recently published an enticing book simply entitled Why? It seem to me that Why? is becoming the easy question for social analyst. An analyst can drown in thousand of answers, sought and unsought, since all studies are geared, trained, socialized to say why, to give reasons. These can just cancel out, leaving the play with How? which is to insist on setting context. (...) Sociocultural context is active, not passive; it gets negotiated rather than uncovered or invoked. This book construes context of a process seen from instances of a process seen from one view as drawing from instances of context found in various other view besides itself.

White's theoretical position is innovative and contrasts with the theory of rational choice by James Coleman. In one of his interviews to Alair MacLean and Andy Olds, White writes (2001):

> Identity and Control is at least an effort to show what's really going on when you are trying to get action, when you are trying to get control. (...) Of course you're doing rational choice, but that's the boring stuff. You have to do rational choice. You have to do something. You have to have some infrastructure. That's not where the action is. The action is what's generation the constraints. How is it all fitting together? Or in a more simpleminded way, where are the utilities coming from?

As summed up by Reza Azarian (2005, p. 35), in order to answer these questions, White presents a theory based on four tenets:

> (i) actors and their actions are viewed as interdependent rather than independent, autonomous units; (ii) ties between actors are channels for transfer of resources of various kinds; (iii) social structures are conceptualized as lasting patterns of relations among actors; and finally (iv) the structural location of a node has important perceptual, attitudinal and behavioural implications and has significant enabling, as well as constraining, bearings on its social actions.

White delineates a new conceptual network in which terms such as "identity", "control", "values", "story", "reference group", "networks", "interface" have new meanings and in which new concepts, such as "disciplines", "styles", "rhetoric" or "regimes", are also introduced. The result is a *structural theory of action* and, as stressed by Michel Grossetti and Fréderic Godart (2007), one can say that:

> Identity and Control goes beyond traditional sociological dichotomies such as micro/macro, individualism/holism, experience/structure, static/dynamic by relying on an approach based on social network and network of meaning.

White's approach, as stressed by Reza Azarian (2005), Michel Grossetti and Fréderic Godart (2007), takes some distance from the traditional individualism, holism and interactionist approach, and is similar to theory of *fields* (various relatively autonomous social spaces) by Pierre Bourdieu (1979); social network analysis, illustrated in studies by Alain Degenne and Michel Forsé (1994), whose history has been written by Linton Freeman (2004); social capital theory analysed by Nan Lin (2001) and the actor-network theory by Bruno Latour (2005).

A good anthology of the applications of this kind of models is the book of Mark Newman et al. (2006). This anthology starts first with applications (Frigyes Karinthy, Paul Erdos and Alfred Renyi, Anatol Rapoport, Ithiel de Sola Pool, Stanley Milgram) and describes three kinds of models: random graph models, the small world models and model of scale-free networks.

1.2.3.10 (IIc) Rational Choice Models, Agent-Based Models, Artificial Society Models

These models derive from *rational choice theory* (RCT), according to which all social phenomena are the result of individual rational choices. Between 1946 and 1973, Coleman started to support the rational choice theory in sociology, a new position which he theorized in his *Foundations of Social Theory* (1990). As Peter Marsden (2005, p. 11, 15) writes:

> Foundation of social Theory (FST) was Coleman's main theoretical project and the one that that he regarded as his most significant. It aspires toward a transdisciplinary theory of social systems that allows social science to aid in designing improved forms of social organisation. (...) Proceeding under methodological individualism, Coleman assumed simple microfoundation: interrelated purposive actors using resource to pursue interests. From such assumption, FST worked towards accounts for such social phenomena and authority systems, structure of trust, social norms, collective behaviour, corporate actors and revolution. Coleman begins FST by highlighting the micro–macro transition as the foremost theoretical problem for social science, arguing that explanation of system behaviour in term of lower-level constituent elements are apt to be more general and more useful for interventions than those that do not probe beneath the system level (...) FST was reviewed very widely after its publication in 1990. At least four review symposia were devoted to it. Although the tone and the content of review varied and most acknowledged FST as a major theoretical work, on balance tended to be critical. Many commentators were dubious of the rational micro model and sceptical that sociology can be constructed on individualist postulates, observing, among other things, that choice take place within existing institutional complexes.

In this chapter, Coleman's position has been quoted in relation to the Coleman's boat: $(m - m')$, $(M{-}m)$ and $(m' - M')$ strategies. Coleman's position therefore is related to a form of methodological individualism, however, as Udehn (2002) writes, Coleman's position is so innovative with respect to traditional approaches such as those of PFL that it is possible to speak of "structural individualism".

RCT was at the beginning applied only to economics; the shift from economics to sociology raises some problems. James Coleman (1986, pp. 1–2) illustrates this shift as follows:

> Rational action of individuals has a unique attractiveness as the basis for social theory. In an institution or a social process can be accounted for in terms of the rational actions of individuals, then and only then can we say that it has been "explained". (...) Certain phenomena derive rather directly from the conception of rational actions of individuals. (...) The simplest and the most direct of those arise from voluntary action of two people engaging in a social exchange. It is this structure of action that forms the basis for all of classical and neoclassical economic theory. (...) All political process, must social institutions, collective behaviour such as fads and panic, organizational functioning, status systems, system of norms and a host of other phenomena cannot be treated merely as extensions of economic systems involving exchange of private goods. In fact, every day language points to a phenomenon wholly outside that domain: the emergence of another class of "actors" which cannot be identified with any single physical person. Whenever we speak of "a family" moving from one city to another, a "firm" lowering its process, "a union" going on strike, 2a nation" going to war, we are speaking of a class of actors other than individual persons, but speaking of them "acting" just as we would speak of an individual person.

According to Coleman, in RCT applied to sociology, two changes occur: (1) there are more phenomena analysed (collective behaviour, organizational functioning, status systems, system of norms, etc.) and (b) there are more kinds of actors involved (individual persons and "corporate actors" such as families and firms).

RCT can be described, as Raymond Boudon does (2003, p. 3), by six postulates:

> RCT can be described by a set of postulates. (...) The first postulate, P1, states that any social phenomenon is the effect of individual decisions, actions, attitudes, etc. (individualism). A second postulate, P2, states that, in principle at least, an action can be understood (understanding). As some action can be understood (understanding). As some actions can be understood without being rational, a third postulate, P2, states that any actions caused by reasons in the mind of individuals (rationality). A fourth postulate, P4, assumes these reasons derive from consideration by the actor of the consequence of his or her actions as he or she sees them (consequentialism, instrumentalism). A fifth postulate, P5, states that actors are concerned mainly with the consequences to themselves of their own action (egoism). A sixth postulate, P6, maintains that actors are able to distinguish that costs and benefits of alternative lines of action and that they choose the line of action with the most favourable balance (maximisation, optimization).

Boudon (2003, p. 10) notes that the first three postulates are more general than the others; he calls this set cognitivist theory of action (CTA) and concludes by noting that CTA has more advantages than does RCT:

> It is essential for sociology as a discipline to be aware that many traditional and modern sociological studies owe their explanatory strength to the use of a cognitive version of methodological individualism, as opposed to an instrumental one, mainly represented by RCT.

This does not imply that there are no applications of RCT, which are on the contrary very useful. A series of examples (ranging from the easy to the more complex one) are useful to understand the methodological problems involved.

A very simple example is represented by the application of the "prisoner's dilemma" (PD), which is quoted at the beginning of all studies on game theories and considers the possible answers (and their consequences) provided by two prisoners. The best solution for them is silence (that is to say cooperation and a 6-month period in jail); however, the search for the best possible option (the possibility to be free) and the fear for the worst punishment (10 years in jail) lead to defection (5 years in prison) as the best solution possible (known as "pareto-suboptimal solution).

	Prisoner B stays silent (*cooperate*)	Prisoner B betrays (*defect*)
Prisoner A stays silent (*cooperate*)	Each serves 6 months	Prisoner A: 10 years; prisoner B: goes free
Prisoner A betrays (*defect*)	Prisoner A: goes free; prisoner B: 10 years	Each serves 5 years

This example is used by Raymond Boudon (2003, p. 4) and is related to questions such as "Why did the Soviet Empire collapse suddenly in the early 1990s?" that he attempts to answer and which has already been mentioned in the section on prediction. Boudon considers that, even if cooperation through bilateral disarmament would be better for the two actors (the US government and the USSR government), the search for power and the fear for punishment lead both actors to acquire more armaments (a pareto-suboptimal solution):

> If I (the US government) do not increase my military potential while the other party (the government of USSR) does, I run a deadly risk. Thus, I have to increase military spending, even though, as a government, I would prefer to spend less money on weapons and more on, say. Schools, hospitals, or welfare because they would be more appreciated by the voters. In this situation, increasing one's arsenal is a dominant strategy, although its outcome is not optimal. (...) The "foolish" outcome was the product of "rational" strategies.

In what way does this analysis explain the collapse of the Soviet Empire? As Boudon writes (2003, p. 4), in this game the winner is the US government, because he has more economic power and can invest on armaments, while the USSR has not got these possibilities and is for this reason out of the game:

> The game stopped when the PD structure that had characterized the decades long interaction between the two powers was suddenly destroyed. It was destroyed by the threat developed by then U.S. President Reagan of reaching a new threshold in the arms race by developing the SDI project, the so called Star Wars (...). Economically, the project was too expensive the Soviet government saw that there was no way to follow without generating serious internal economic problems. Hence, it did not follow and by not so doing, lost its status of superpower, which had been uniquely grounded in its military strength.

Boudon writes that "of course there are other causes underlying the collapse of the Soviet Union", but this does not stop RCT from explaining what has happened, at least in part. Another example of an application of game theory to military events is included in the essay by Philippe Mongin (2008), which analyses the last controversial decisions of Napoleon at Waterloo. Also in this case, this analysis reaches evaluations that are innovative with respect to more traditional historical analysis.

One of the most interesting uses of game theory is by Robert Axelrod, who has written an important theory in praise of cooperation. The game of the dilemma of the prisoners is reorganized according to the following schema:

	B cooperate	*B defect*
A cooperate	$A = 3, B = 3$ Reward for mutual cooperation	$A = 0, B = 5$ Temptation to defect
A defect	$A = 5, B = 0$ Temptation to defect	$A = 1, B = 1$ Punishment for mutual defection

It is interesting to note that the game between the two actors based on a reward/payment logic leads to a situation in which both actors move towards the defect strategy. However, if the game carries on, the situation evolves towards cooperation. Axelrod shows that, if one repeats the game and considers the different strategies, the TIT-FOR-TAT strategy is the winning option; here the first move of A always tends towards cooperation and the moves change only if B chooses a different move. The TIT-FOR-TAT winning strategy in this simulation tends towards mutual cooperation and can also be noted in real societies. Axelrod (1981, 1984, 1997) shows examples of cooperation taken from events in different points in time, such as the First World War and the contemporary period. To understand the interest raised by these analyses, some comments by John Barrie (2006) in *Disarmament Diplomacy*, in which he considers three important elements in Axelrod's analysis and the TIT-FOR-TAT model in favour of unilateral disarmament, are quoted:

> An important discovery was that the length of the game is a key aspect of his success. (...) A second insight Axelrod observed that " a world of meanies can resist invasion by anyone using any other strategy-provided that the newcomers arrive one at time. The problem of course, is that a single newcomer in such a mean world has no one who will reciprocate any cooperation. If the newcomers arrive in small clusters, however, they will have a chance to thrive". Third, Axelrod showed that players using nice tit-for-tat strategies that never defect first are better than others at protecting themselves from invasion by competing strategies. They do this by only defecting against those that defect against them. It may be recalled that a population of individuals that always defects can withstand invasion by any strategy provided players using other strategies come one at time. By comparison, Axelrod notes "With nice rules the situation is different. If a nice rule can resist invasion by other rules coming one at time, then it can resist invasion by clusters, no matter how large. So nice rules can protect themselves in a way that always defecting cannot." The cooperation can evolve in a broader world of defectors is an important theoretical insight reflecting both common sense and historical experiences, and can be observed in a wide range of phenomena studied by many disciplines. [15]

It is important to observe that the experiments made by Axelrod are useful to answer important questions from a sociological viewpoint and lead to unexpected results and complex reflections. For example in Axelrod (1997), there are two very important contributions. In *A Model for the Emergence of New Political Actors*, Axelrod's question is "How can new political actors emerge from an aggregation of

[15] Axelrod's quotations in this article by John Barrie are from Axelrod (1981, pp. 315–316).

smaller political actors?" Axelrod's answer (1997, p. 124) shows how new levels of organization can be reached:

> This essay presents a simulation model that provides one answer. In its broader perspective, the work can be seen as a part if the study of emergent organization through "bottom up" processes. In such "bottom up" process small units interact according to locally defined rules, and the result is emergent properties of the system such as the formation of new level of organization.

In his essay *The Dissemination of Culture: A Model with Local Convergence and Global Polarization*, Axelrod's question is "If people tend to become more alike in their beliefs, attitudes and behaviour, why don't all their differences eventually disappear? His answer is equally interesting (1997, p. 171):

> The proposed model shows how individual or group differences can be durable despite tendencies toward convergence. It treats culture as the attributes that social tendencies toward convergence. It treats as the attributes that social influence can influence. Unlike previous models of cultural change or social influence, this one is based on the interplay between different dimensions or features that characterize people. The basic assumption is that the opportunity for interaction and convergence is proportional to the number of features that two neighbors already share. Stable cultural difference emerge as regions develop in which everyone shares the same culture, but have nothing in common with the culture of neighboring regions. The degree of polarization is measured by the number of different cultural regions that exist when no further change is possible.(...) The social influence model illustrates three fundamental points: 1. Local convergence can lead to global polarization. 2. The interplay between different features of culture can shape the process of social influence. 3. Even simple mechanism of change can give counterintuitive results, as shown by the present model, in which large territories generate surprisingly little polarization.

As summed up by Axelrod (1997, p. 148), the simulation shows "that the number of stable homogeneous regions decreases with the number of features, increases with the number of alternative traits per feature, decreases with the range of interaction, and (most surprisingly) decreases when the geographic territory grows beyond a certain size".

As stressed by Michael W. Macy and Robert Willer (2002, p. 151), the results are surprising and make a case for the "paradox of mimetic divergence":

> Axelrod's models couple local influence (the tendency for people who interact frequently to become more similar over time) and homophily (the tendency to interact more frequently with similar agents). (...) He found that "local convergence can lead to global polarization" and that unique subcultures can survive in the face of a seemingly relentless march toward cultural conformity. Stable minority subcultures persist because of the protection of structural holes created by cultural differences that preclude interaction, thereby insulating agents from homogenizing tendencies. Axelrod's models also reveal a surprising effect of population size. Intuitively, one might expect larger numbers of stable subcultures to emerge in larger population. However Axelrod found a non linear effect, in which the number of minority cultures first increases with population size but then decrease. The counter-intuitive result illustrates the principle of "gambler's ruin". Large populations allow for larger cultural movements that can survive random fluctuations in membership better than smaller competitors. As the big get bigger, the number of minority subcultures diminishes.

Axelrod's models of simulation are included in the agent-based models; an introduction to these kinds of models has been written by Nigel Gilbert (2008, p. 2), who defines them as follows:

> Formally, agent based modelling is a computational method that enables a researcher to create, analyse and experiment with models composed of agents that interact with an environment. (...) Computational models are formulated as computer programs in which there are some inputs (independent variables) and some outputs (like dependent variable) and an experiment consists of applying some treatment to an isolated system and observing what happens.

The characteristic of these models have been defined in Fig. 1.3; Gilbert takes into account the target of the model and finds three main types of agent-based models:

> (i) *Scale models* are smaller versions of the target. Together with the reduction in size is a systematic reduction in the level of detail or complexity of the model; (...) (ii) An *ideal type model* is one in which some characteristics of the target are exaggerated in order to simplify the model; (...) (iii) *Analogical models* are based on drawing an analogy between some better understood phenomenon and the target.

Gilbert shows that applications of these models have been made in more directions (urban models, opinion dynamics, consumer behaviour, industrial network, supply chain management, electricity market, etc.): from the analysis of youth subcultures to the study of terrorist groups and from the diffusion of certain industrial activities to geographical information systems.

Some studies, such as the Sugarshape model described by Joshua M. Epstein and Robert Axtell (1996, p. 4), can be mentioned. This defines artificial society models as follows:

> In this approach fundamental social structures and group behaviours emerge from the interaction of individuals operating in artificial environments under rules that place only bounded demands on each agent's information and computational capacity. We view artificial societies as laboratories, where we attempt to "grow" certain social structure in the computer -or in silico- the aim being to discover fundamental local or micro mechanism that are sufficient to generate the macroscopic social structure and collective behaviours of interest.

Within this category of models, particularly important are the simulations of cities realized by Michael Batty (2005, p. 317). He describes his models as follows:

> The model we have developed is composed of an individual behaviour dynamics for agent that are largely conditioned by autonomous responses to highly localized spatial conditions. We have assumed that the model is calibrated in a traditional manner by scaling up the actions of individual agents into some global pattern, which is then matched against some set of observed data. Our assumption is that such global behavior can be predicted and possible controlled through intervention that change the spatial geometry of the system with consequent impact on individual behavior.

If one considers the articles in *Journal of Artificial Society and Social Simulation*, there are different areas of application for these models: from the simulation of everyday life in a coffee place to the spread of new religious movements and the formation of leadership, from the spread of xenophobia to the diffusion of altruistic feelings. The Italian scientific contribution to this periodical has strong connections with psychology experts, who in turn gather around the periodical entitled *Sistemi intelligenti* founded and edited by Domenico Parisi. One could think, for example, of the article by Gigliotta et al. (2007). Other scientific contributions that analyse the dynamics of industrial innovation are Fioretti (2001); Squazzoni and Boero (2002); Albino et al. (2003); Boero et al. (2004); Borrelli et al. (2005). In these articles both traditional industrial areas (such as Prato for textiles) and more innovative clusters of small and medium firms are analysed.

1.3 Possibilities for Sociology of Artificial Neural Networks

The history of the ANNs can be summed up in four phases: (i) preliminaries; (ii) expansion within studies on artificial intelligence; (iii) delusion; (iv) expansion with ANN applications in all directions.

The reconstruction of the preliminaries can be partly subjective. As we are talking about AI, I would like to include among preliminary contributions the work of Edgar Allan Poe (1836), who analysed a fake automaton (the chess player Kempelen), pointing out the differences between human and artificial intelligence. Less creative and subjective preliminary contributions are those by Alan Turing and Norbert Wiener. Steve Heims (1991) noted that when Wiener organized the first conferences in cybernetics and the social sciences in New York in 1946 under the auspices of The Macy Foundation, he invited PFL also. He participated in one of the meetings, but, unlike Gregory Bateson, showed little interest for analyses which anticipated ANN. This showed that a rift opened between PFL's social sciences and a mathematical analysis that anticipates the ANN. Among the most specific preliminaries are those of the neurophysiologist Warren McCulloch and of the mathematician Walter Pitts, who in 1943 wrote a paper on how neurons might work showing a model of ANN with electric circuits. In 1948 W. Ross Ashby published the article *Design for a Brain* and in 1949 Donald Hebb's *The Organisation of Behavior* was also published. Here a law for synaptic neuron learning (The Hebbian learning law) was illustrated for the first time.

The phase of expansion of the ANNs starts in 1951 with the publication of *Foundation* by Isaac Asimov, in which psychohistorian Hari Seldon presents a new theory: the evolution of human society through a number of complex mathematical laws, and in the same year, Marvin Minsky created the first ANN while working at Princeton. In 1957, Frank Rosenblatt at the Aeronautical Laboratory of Cornell University created *Perceptron*; in 1959, Bernard Widrow and Marcian Hoff at Stanford developed two models called ADELINE and MADALINE (from multiple adaptive linear elements); in 1960, Rosenblatt published his book *Principles of Neurodynamics* about modelling the brain.

This enthusiasm for ANN was followed by a period of disillusion, which reached its peak in 1969, with the publication of *Perceptrons* by Marvin Minsky and Seymour Papert. This study illustrated the limits of an ANN built by Rosenblatt. In the 1970s, ANN continued to be studied by single researchers (in 1971, Crossberg started to publish his studies on non-linear ANN, in 1972, Kahonen discovered the *Learning Vector Quantization*, in 1974, Werbos started the *Back-propagation*

Algorithm, etc) but it was only in the 1980s that ANN became a powerful kind of algorithm, whose application was no longer limited to psychological research but was applied to all the social sciences. Among those responsible for this renewed interest for ANN was John Hopfield, who, in 1982, read to the National Academy of Science his essay *Neural Networks and Physical Systems with Emergent Collective Computational Abilities*"; Kahonen, who in 1982 published his *Self Organizing Map* (SOM); Carpenter and Grossberg, who in 1983 introduced the *Adaptive Resonance Theory* (ART). Further, in 1984, the Boltzmann machine was introduced; in 1986, Rumelhart and McClelland edited the volume *Parallel Distributed Processing: Explorations in the Microstructure of Cognition* and in 1988, Broomhead and Lowe introduced the radial basis function (RBF), etc.

Today ANN represents a mathematical instrument that allows to solve problems in different disciplines. For this reason, it is important to consider ANN relation with sociology, especially with respect to the models illustrated in the first and the second part of this introduction and understand its possible applications.

1.3.1 Sociology and Artificial Neural Networks

What are the differences between ANN and the statistical and simulation models applied in sociology and analysed in the previous part? We can start by considering the schemes in Figs. 1.2 and 1.3 and then proceed by comparing them with the equivalent scheme in Fig. 1.5, in order to highlight some differences.

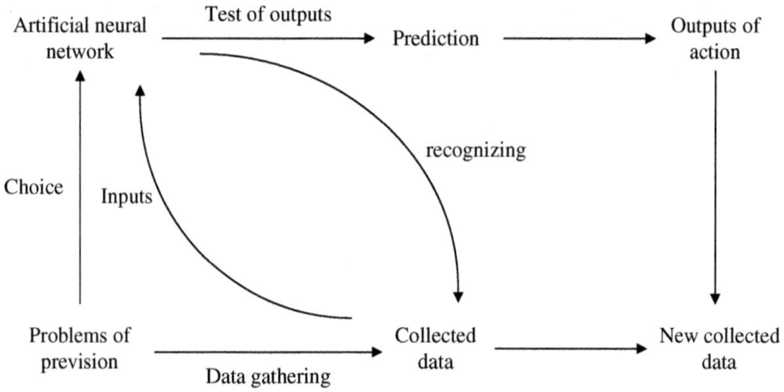

Fig. 1.5 The logic of prevision of artificial neural network

In statistical and simulation models applied to sociology, the starting point is the real world named "social processes" and "target". This starting point applies also to the net of relations centred around ANNs. In this case, however, the most proper term to indicate the main features of the real world is "problems of prediction". ANNs, in fact, can be distinguished from other mathematical models applied to sociology because they offer the possibility to make predictions.

Depending on the "problem of prediction" that the research wants to focus on, a family of ANNs is individuated, but the choice of ANN is made taking into account the relation *collected data→ ANN and ANN→ collected data.* The collected data are in fact the input of ANN (similar to the collected data in a traditional statistical model). However, differently from what happens in Figs. 1.2 and 1.3, ANN *learns* from the interaction of these data and forms its own rules.

As Massimo Buscema clarifies in Chapter 10, depending on the problem to solve, there are three main families of ANNs (supervised ANN, associative memories, autopoietic ANN); the architecture of the ANNs is formed by *nodes* and *connections*. What differentiates ANNs from the mathematical models illustrated in the second part of this introduction is the fact that ANNs are "mechanisms of elaboration of data", which produce their own rules and which are in turn characterized by iterative exploration of the collected data. ANNs are *adaptive*. As Buscema stresses, they are part of the *artificial adaptive systems*. It is for this reason that Fig. 1.5 shows a circular relation connecting *ANN/collected data.*

After this interaction, results are tested in different ways depending on the prediction problem in order to find the best prediction possible at the level of a single person – unlike what happened in relation to the prediction problems previously noted in sociological research. In sociological research which uses statistical models, one can make prediction at micro-levels ($m \rightarrow m'$) and also at macro-levels ($M \rightarrow M'$), though these predictions are different. At micro-levels, predictions concern relations among variables with probability (defined by frequencies); at macro-levels these predictions are vaguer and more difficult to attain. In both cases, explanations (see the examples in the table) coincide with predictions. The shift from variables to individuals occurs in models of simulation in which hypotheses (of explanation) on the behaviour of a group of individuals are made. Simulated data (prediction) are then compared with the collected ones. In the ANNs the concept of prediction is on the contrary collocated in a different phase and has a different meaning. The interaction between collected data and ANN gives rise to a model that can be interrogated and allows predictions. As it is well illustrated in Massimo Buscema and the Semeion Group's work shown in the next paragraph, once the interaction between collected data and ANN has been tested, this model can be interrogated and predictions on single individuals or ideal types can be made. For example answers to questionnaire are indicative to make predictions on drug addictions and failures at school for young people; these are also useful to understand the incidence of Alzheimer in old age and other risks. This prediction is not compared with the collected data but is compared with the new *collected data* (the results concerning marks of students in new classes, concerning aging people, etc) that are influenced by action. If risks of contracting Alzheimer are high, one has got time to intervene; if risks of getting bad marks are high, one can intervene with special classes. It is for these reasons that in Fig. 1.5 we have a trajectory from prediction to action and then the results of this action are compared with the new collected data.

In order to explain the characteristics of ANNs, some reference should be made to the applications of ANNs to sociology carried out by the Semeion Research Institute (illustrated in the following paragraph). In this respect, four kinds of relations can be considered: ANNs/collected data; ANNs/methodology; ANNs /kind of research; ANNs/theory.

(a) *ANNs/collected data.* As it is shown in the application which will be illustrated in the following paragraph, the input data of ANN can have different provenances and forms (a survey, a census data, an image, a temporal sequence of data, a transition matrix, data based on territorial units, etc.). ANNs can define strategies of connection and predictions with variables that are not limited to the four levels indicated by Torgerson (nominal, ordinal, interval scales or relations) but also extend to fuzzy variables or variables represented by a pixel in an image.
(b) *ANNs/methodology* The four themes dealt by logic in traditional sociology (typologies, explanation, micro/macro, prevision) provide a hint to understand how different ANNs are from the mathematical models presented in the first and second part of this introduction. Concerning the individuation of *typologies*, ANNs also allow to reach "typical profiles", "ideal types", "typologies" [see researches (d), (e) in the following paragraph]. However, the way in which these typologies are defined and the possibilities to challenge them are different from the typologies introduced by PFL. Similarly, the concept of *explanation* is also different, because ANNs do not present hypothesis of explanation about collected data as in statistical or simulation models. The prevision may be realized also if data present only a situation of "synchronicity" [16] without hypothesis of causal relations between variables.
Moreover, in ANNs, the micro–macro relation is also different, because there is a shift from a macro-analysis that takes into account the relations of a set of variables and subjects to micro-predictions on a single subject (these differences are even more marked when the starting point is represented by an image analysed using the dynamics of its pixel). In ANNs the prediction is different from the one found in models of simulation, because it is constructed through real subjects as well as ideal typologies.
(c) *ANNs/kind of research.* One can easily find out that among the three paradigms that are most often used in sociological research (paradigm of objectivity, action research/co-research paradigm and feminist research paradigm), the one that is most used by the Semeion Research Institute is the *action research–co-research paradigm* because ANNs are utilized for change (the reduction of drug abuse, aid to people with diseases, etc.). In some cases there is a possibility of using ANNs in conjunction with a *feminist paradigm* (this is the case of differences between female and male mobility).
(d) *ANNs/theory*. Concerning this issue, it is important to answer a question posed by some Italian sociologists who gathered for a seminar on sociology organized by Enzo Campelli in Rome in 2007 (I participated in that seminar with a paper

[16] About "synchronicity" linked to the discussion between Jung and Wolfgang Pauli, the book edited by Lance Storm (2008) is suggested.

co-written with Buscema). To understand the whole issue however the context should be clarified. According to scholars, ANNs are different from the models showed in Figs. 1.2 and 1.3 because they do not formulate hypothesis on the relations that exist among independent, intervening and dependent variables (that is to say among input and output data). If the term "model" is identified with "hypotheses on reality", ANNs, then, *are* not "models".

Beginning from this assumption, some sociologists present in the above-mentioned seminar asked the following question: if ANNs are "mechanisms of elaboration of data" that do not make hypothesis on the relations between input and output, does it follow that these are a kind of UFO (a black box) not concerned with the search for new theories antagonist to the choices made by PFL (subordination of research to theory, subordination of methodology to research, subordination of mathematics to sociology)? The answer is "no" for two reasons. First of all, ANNs are not UFOs that transform input into output, but IFOs (identified flying objects) because each ANN has its specific and well-defined characteristics. Besides, as shown in the research by Massimo Buscema and the Semeion Research Group, the relation *ANN/collected data* is complex and points research in two directions: (1) towards a search for the best ANN which should then be improved mathematically and (2) towards the proposal of new theoretical contributions in order to improve the quality of collected data.

Let us consider the *Sonda Project*, illustrated in volumes by Massimo Buscema and the Semeion Group (1992, 1994) [discussed in point (a) of the following paragraph]. In this research concerning the possibility to predict if a person will become a drug addict, it is the *ANN/collected data* relation that leads the Semeion Research Institute not only to elaborate a new ANN but also to propose a more complex "theory" concerning drug addiction. The results of *ANN/collected data* relation lead to very good predictions (more than 90% probabilities) because (i) a mathematically improved ANN has been used and (ii) a more complex theory on the causes of drug addiction has also been used. In other words, a more complex theory on the causes of drug addiction has been used. Therefore, if one uses "good" ANNs in order for the applications to work, one also needs a "good" sociological theory.

One should take into account the research of the Semeion Research Institute and note that in several cases, "theoretical" contributions come from the inside history of ANNs, a history that is at the crossroads of different disciplines and different *theoretical* contributions. Studies such as those by Gleick and Waldrop already mentioned show that mathematical analysis of "complexity" can be achieved by way of several theoretical contributions, as it is interestingly shown by Buscema (2002). In this study on professional behaviour, theoretical contributions derive from Algirdas-Julien Greimas' work, which has enabled Buscema to explore ANNs and to connect mathematical and theoretical contributions in his *squashing theory*. An illustration of the *squashing theory* is the famous novel *Flatland: A Romance of Many Dimensions* by Edwin Abbott. This employs geometrical figures in place of characters in order to show how a two-dimensional world derives from a three-dimensional world and so on. According to "squashing theory" of Buscema, the inferior dimensions are the result of a "squash "of superior dimensions. As Buscema writes, there are three principles that characterize squashing theory (1994, pp. 195–197):

> *Principle of totality*. In order to obtain the map of a subject, one has to obtain vital information on all his/her properties that are stable in time without consideration for hierarchy and isotropy. (...) The system of calculus should be used to include in the same unity these heterogeneous constellations of information, and establish which of these are in a relation of indifference, solidarity or antagonism with the subject or group of subjects. This is because all subjects are characterized by a heterogeneity of aspects and their personalities depend on the way in which such co-existence has or has not been structured. (...); (ii) *Principle of variety*. When the amount of the kinds of information must be reduced drastically, it is necessary to collect information that are as different as possible the one from the other. (...) Each subject should be considered as a society with a variety of characteristics, attitudes and behaviours, their models of reciprocal interaction should represent the objective of the analysis and not a pre-ordered constraint. From this, one can obtain three sub-principles: (1) *fuzzy participation*: the possibility of a stable human behaviour implies the negative or positive fuzzy participation of all those characteristics that form the unity of that subject; (2) *amplified indifference:* those characteristics that are indifferent to human behaviour contribute with their indifference to make other characteristics significant either positively or negatively. (...) The relations of indifference are the result of a process that the system executes in order to maintain its own internal unity, amplifying the relations of solidarity and exclusion. (3) *Equi-finality*: different subjects can manifest their behaviour through fuzzy participations that are different from the various properties they mitigate. There is always a function able to distinguish different subjects who have – albeit in a variety of different ways – the same behaviour from subjects who, on the contrary, use various strategies to hide the fact that they have the same behaviour; (...) (iii) *Principle of automatization* The kind of information available on a subject and/or a group of subjects must be as brief as possible. It is therefore necessary to proceed towards a figurative automatization through which a map for the subject is drawn.

ANNs' challenge to sociology does not therefore involve merely mathematics but it has a theoretical and methodological nature.

1.3.2 Semeion Research Institute's Applications to Sociology

In order to reflect on the possibilities of applications of ANNs, it is useful to quote some of the applications by Massimo Buscema and the Semeion Research Group (Table 1.12).

(a) *How to predict for strategies of prevention?* Sociological research attempts to individuate which characteristics of a subject are significant to predict whether, given a certain environment, he/she will become a drug addict, a heroin addict or will fail exams at school. Such a search is problematic. From a technical point of view, this prediction makes use of only an output. Particularly interesting in this respect has been the *Sonda Project*, illustrated in books by Massimo Buscema and the Semeion Group (1992, 1994), which considers the possibility of predicting if a person will become a drug addict.

In this project, the choice of the relation *collected data/ANN* is the following. The survey has led to a general questionnaire of 112 items that focuses on aspects that

Table 1.12 Examples of application of ANNs of the Semeion Research Institute

Sociological problem	Type of collected data	Type of ANN	Applications of the Semeion Research Group
(a) How to predict for strategies of prevention	– Survey based on subjects who take and do not take drugs	– Feedforward with supervision	– Drug addiction – Heroin abuse – Dropout students – Depression
(b) How to predict connection among data	– Survey on different samples – Census data	– Backpropagation – SOM (self-organizing map) – P-I function (pseudo-inverse function)	– Less variables with the same content of information – Vocational training – Artificial increase of a dimension of a sample
(c) How to predict from images	– Radiological images– satellite images	– ACM (active connession matrix) -J-Net System	– Medical diagnostic – Pollutions – Analysis of a work of art
(d) How to predict historical series of data	– Electroence-phalographic data (EEG) – Stock exchange data	– IFAST (implicit function as squashing time)	– Alzheimer disease – Stock exchange
(e) How to predict social networks	– Social networks of individuals	– Self-organizing maps (SOMs) and auto-contractive maps (AutoCMs)	– Criminal networks – Power networks
(f) How to predict about individuals in process models	– Social mobility data in different generations	– Backpropagation	– Male and female – Social mobility
(g) How to predict from ecological data	– Information about cities	– Backpropagation with constraint satisfaction – Internal recirculation net	– Classification and typologies of cities

are essential to understand how one becomes (or does not become) a drug addict; these include education, abode, employment, religion, economics, his/her relation with justice, alcohol and smoke, health conditions, micro-vulnerability and family condition, his/her perception of people that entertains a close relationship with the subject, spare time and friendship. To this basic questionnaire, 98 items have been added only for drug addicts only, and 7 items only for those who are not explicitly connected to drug abuse. We have therefore two questionnaires: (1) a 210–items questionnaire named *Very*. This questionnaire has been used with drug addicts in a community and those who have left the community in the last 5 years and (2) a

119-items questionnaire named *Net*. This has been used for subjects who do not take drugs. The basic questionnaire focuses around these issues.

The artificial neural network employed is a *feedforward* supervised and produced by the Semeion Group, which employs *squashing theory*, whose main principles and characteristics have been illustrated above. The application of this network (141 input units, 2 hidden units and 1 output unit) to analyse the answers given by groups or subsamples of subjects has defined two phases of *testing* and *prediction*. The *testing* phase consists of 10 experimentations on samples of drug addicts and non-drug addicts, while the *prediction* phase calculates the different percentage of drug addiction in a sample of non-drug addicts, depending on the number of items and the kind of network considered. The most important result of this experimentation is the fact that with a net based on *squashing theory* and taking into consideration all the items, the prediction probabilities are over 90%. Concerning this experimentation, one can state (i) that the net chosen is superior to all other nets and (ii) the importance of all directions pointed by the questionnaire, rather than mere hypotheses of explanation – intervention which considers only psychological, familiar and social factors.

As the research is a research-action type, the operative and theoretical choices used to face the problem of drug addiction are also important. The theoretical choice consists in positively evaluating the intervention and considering people at risk according to their potentials. A permanent observatory to observe signs of hardship in its first stages is being proposed. This is articulated in (i) a "shop" with an entrance on the street in which young people are encouraged to participate in audio visual and computerized activities on the city; (ii) a mobile unit to contact subjects in their own spaces and (iii) an "idea bank" to encourage the realization of projects. All these can play a key role in transforming subjects from passive and easily manipulated individuals to subjects of change. Subjects are encouraged to gather in "gangs" and small groups, and try to find ideas and solutions for their projects.

This project has been experimented in the military hospital for legal medicine in Verona in order to verify people's vulnerability to heroine abuse while doing their military service. The illustration of this experiment is in Buscema (1999, pp. 15–94). In an essay by Guido Maurelli and Stefano Terzi (1999), the application of ANNs to predict the emergence of depression among inhabitants of isles that are isolated from the mainland is illustrated. The same ANN as the one used in the *Sonda Project* was also used to predict school behaviour.

This research has been carried out by Vincenzo Carbone and Giuseppino Piras (1999) in collaboration with the Semeion Research Group using an interview plan consisting of 224 items. Thanks to this research, some differences between the best students and dropouts have been individuated. If this kind of research had been repeated each year, it could have provided teachers useful information concerning their new pupils. It should be stressed that ANNs allow to make predictions at individual levels, so teachers of new classes who use predictions could in theory predict the student's overall or partial success (for example the probabilities of succeeding in mathematics). Providing teachers with this kind of information raises ethical problems. One wonders, for example, about the behaviour of a teacher who knows from the start who the best and worst students are. Would he/she try to challenge this tendency (dedicating more attention to dropout subjects) or would he/she try to re-confirm the negative evaluation (because "ANN says so")? And what if we knew in advance that a subject was going to develop a "deviant" behaviour? The famous novel *Minority Report* by Philip Dick, which describes a future society in which people are arrested for deviant behaviours, not yet manifested but merely predicted (a prediction that might be based on RNNs?), contributes to challenge and questions the validity and diffusion of these methods.

(b) *How to predict connections among data in the same or different samples*? In this area are included three kinds of problems typically encountered in sociological research: (1) How to move from a high number of items to a smaller number of variables without losing useful information (PFL has referred to this problem as the shift from items to variables and from variables to indicators)? (2) How to related characteristics belonging to a group of subjects to characteristics required by a set of social roles? (iii) How is it possible to use a restricted sample of subjects to obtain information for an artificially enlarged sample of subjects?

The first two problems have been in Massimo Buscema and the Semeion Research Group's research (2002). The first one is concerned with the shift from a *tactical questionnaire* (made up of 806 variables in order to map "generic" competences of people of working age) to a questionnaire of 61 generic competences (for subjects considered the best professionals in 1 of the 30 macro-professions, plus a class of subjects defined as "not the best ones"). This shift has been realized by using the ANN backpropagation characterized by self-momentum (Buscema and Semeion Group 1999a, pp. 189–222): a network of 806 input variables and 61 output variables with two strata of hidden units (80 units for each stratum).The second problem, the one that concerns the attempt to project 61 generic competences in 30 jobs (plus one), has been solved by using an ANN of the SOM (self-organizing map) kind, which classifies subjects on the basis of their generic competences and then projects them on a two-dimensional map. The solution to these two problems has been illustrated in a research characterized by interesting theories and practical solutions. The theories illustrated by Buscema (2002, pp. 21–37), which consider competences regarding action, recognition (that is to say "to be and to appear") and manipulation (passions), have been inspired by the work of Algirdas-Julien Greimas. As Buscema (2002, p. 32) writes, "if manipulation is action performed by a subject on another subject in order to make him/her perform such action, passion is the attempt on the part of a manipulating subject to convince the manipulated subject to perform an action". Practical solutions have led to the "Loop" project (also available on line) which allows one person to make an auto-evaluation in order to be included in the professional space.

The solutions to the third problem have been illustrated in an essay by Cinzia Meraviglia, Giulia Massini, Daria Croce and Massimo Buscema (2006). The objective of this essay is to "artificially" increase the dimension of a sample in order to be able to perform complex hypothesis of testing. This sometimes proves very hard, especially when small-sized samples are involved. The method used to generate new (virtual) data from a small observed data set consists of a pseudo-inverse function

(P-I function) elaborated by Buscema and the Semeion Research Group. This is based on three principles (2006, p. 826):

> (i) Every sample of data pointes can be interpolated by an unlimited number of non linear continuous functions; (ii) Each one of those functions has a different probability to represent accurately the real universe from which a given sample is taken; (iii) An Artificial Neural Network (ANN), provided that it has hidden units, is a universal continuous function (or model).

(c) *How to predict from images?* This area of application of ANN has been successfully experimented in medicine through radiological images. In order to understand how radiological images can be used to make predictions (see the essay by Massimo Buscema and Enzo Grossi published in Chapter 16). This uses the J-Net System, a new paradigm developed by the Semeion Research Institute, for ANNs which are applied to diagnostic imaging. The strategy adopted considers the initial image as a *matrix of pixel* analysed as a dynamic system. The move is explained by the two authors as follows:

> The phenomenon to we refer in general, in our research concern the image which is perceived by our senses when a light-shrouded subject appears to us precisely as a phenomenon, can be represented for its analytic treatment by a matrix of points corresponding to the pixels the assumed initial images. Trying to extract from this image – from this phenomenon – other information about the subject producing it, which is not visible in the initial image's, which is not visible in the initial image which has being considered, allows us to consider the initial image's matrix of pixel as a dynamic system which develops in its phase space until it creates a final configuration matrix of the pixel. It is important not to mistake the space phase with the two dimensional or three dimensional space of the initial image. In fact, it is the other dimension which is derived by the intensity of connection forces of the pixels to each other which is added to the latter space's dimension.

In the research published in this volume is shown how the image of a tumour, analysed with the J-Net System, predicts its evolution providing information hidden to the gaze of the doctor (this prediction image can be compared with the real image of the tumour a year later).

As stressed by Guido Maurelli and Stefano Terzi (1999), the field of application of ANN to images is very wide; one can think, for example, of satellite images used to understand and monitor how pollution evolves in a certain area. There is another area of application of the ANN images that is worth mentioning. In his article on Magritte, the psychologist Nicola Colecchia (2004) puts forward the possibility to apply an ANN to a picture by Magritte entitled *Meditazione* (1937), which shows three lit candles that move towards an unknown destiny in a fashion that recalls the movement of worms. The question is: could the application of an ANN to this image give interesting results? Is it possible to make predictions on a work of art?

(d) *How to make prediction moving from a historical series of data?* In a study by Massimo Buscema et al. (1997), prediction-based ANNs applied to historical series concerning the rate of exchange are illustrated. These are based on an internal reconciliation network (RC) and show predictions based on the market using squash networks together with self-momentum and backpropagation networks. Historical series of different data are those based on electroencephalographic data (EEG).

Works by Grossi and Buscema (2005) and Buscema et al. (2007) have shown that an ANN assembled in a new methodology named IFAST (implicit function as squashing time) capable of compressing the temporal sequence of electroencephalographic (EEG) data into spatial invariants is very useful to predict Alzheimer disease. In this direction is the study of Benoit Mandelbrot and Richard L. Hudson (2004) about the (mis)behaviour of markets.

(e) *How to make predictions about social networks?* A first example of this kind of analysis is offered by Massimo Buscema in Chapter 14. In this essay, a data set is used; this is made up of 28 variables (which can be divided into more micro-variables), concerning 1.117 persons arrested in London for selling drug during a 4-month period. Two different autopoietic ANNs have been used: the self-organizing maps (SOMs) and the auto-contractive maps (AutoCMs). The results obtained from the SOM are very interesting, because they allow to define both a map and different profile types (divided into gender, ethnic group, kind of drug they used). Here a variable (for example the variable "woman") is used to define a "profile" based on major or minor associations that the variable "woman" shares with all the other variables. The results of the AutoCM lead to other tables and profiles, which can be compared with the previous ones and a particular methodology: the model fusion methodology (MFM). This is useful to see which algorithm is more consistent than the others. In order to achieve a fusion among these different algorithms, Buscema opts for the following method:

> a. Every of the presented algorithm proposes a specific tree of dependencies among the variable of the same data set. b. We need to extract from all these trees only one graph whose links among the variables are the most robust and believable. c. So we overlap all the trees and we conserve only the connections selected at least by two different algorithms; in other words if two different algorithms, using a different mathematics, outline the same link between two variables, then it is more probable that between these two variables this link is "real".

A second example is offered in the essay written by Cinzia Meraviglia (1999), in collaboration with the Semeion Research Institute. This poses a "typical" problem in the sociological research: in which way is it possible to predict the different "male" and "female" profiles, taking into account the main variables that more frequently individuate occupational mobility (education of both father and mother, education of the interviewed person, education of the partner, job of the father, job of the interviewed person when he/she started working, last job of the interviewed person)? In order to obtain these profiles, an ANN with a backpropagation algorithm has been used, elaborated by the Semeion Research Group. Its results were interesting and offered a way to measure the different weight of the variables in relation to the two profiles.

(f) *How to predict from ecological data?* The essay by Buscema and Lidia Diappi (1999) presents two examples of application of ANN, starting from ecological data. In the first example, 129 variables are the input, referring to five European cities (Barcelona, Lion, Milan, Munich, Stuttgart). Two methods have been used: (1) learning with backpropagation (BO) and enquiry with constraint satisfaction (CS) and (ii) internal recirculation (RC) net and return enquiry.

Inquiries are of two different kinds. The network was asked to reproduce the "Lion model" and, while the RC net has easily recognized the "model" of this city, the BC-CS has pointed out the differences between Lion and other cities. A different enquiry was also carried out. It began by defining "ideal cities" (the "ecological city", the "technological city"). Then, a second application was made, taking into account 95 Italian cities, characterized by 43 variables; this analysis has allowed to individuate some typologies: cities with the highest socio-environmental benefits or with the highest socio-economic benefits and cities with the lowest socio-environmental costs or with the lowest socio-economic costs.

1.3.3 Possibilities of ANNs to the Relation Between Mathematics and Society

With respect to PFL analysis and statistical models of simulation mentioned in the second part, ANNs show elements of continuity and also of radical change. The elements that show continuity are those mentioned by Leo Goodman (2007) when he talks about mathematics applied to sociology as a method endowed with "magic" (because it reveals what is hidden) and/or "serendipity" (because it brings to light unexpected relations). It is certain that "magic and/or serendipity" can be found both in PFL's models and in ANNs. Moreover, several elements of continuity can be found in the three choices proposed by PFL. In the essays in this volume, three main possibilities of application of ANNs can be found.

The first possibility consists in using ANNs together with statistical models of simulation to understand how different methods can contribute to the explanation of data concerning a single research. For example applications of models of simulation to climatic changes and problems of conflict/integration in different cultural backgrounds illustrated in this volume by Pierluigi Contucci could be compared, using the same data with ANN application on the same issues. Moreover, different methodologies could also be compared as Robert Smith shows in this volume with reference to data concerning "classic" researches such as PFL's.

The second possibility consists in widening applications of ANNs to areas that are significant from a sociological point of view and that have not been analysed with ANNs. For the most part, applications of ANNs by the Semeion Research Institute have used ANNs to improve the quality of life (in order to prevent deviant behaviours, life-threatening illnesses, to find out criminal connections, etc.). Three areas of application of ANNs that could prove very interesting for sociological research could be (1) economic and financial power, both as far as organized criminality is concerned and relationship between criminality and politics. These ANNs could be used to unveil hidden relationships and could be applied to local, national and international data banks. In the present international situation characterized by neo-liberal politics and organized criminality, this could prove very useful. (2) Researches connected with feminist methodology. ANNs' connection with action research/co-research would prove in this case particularly useful and (3) creativity and the arts. As shown in the third part of this volume, ANNs could enter a dialogue with the above areas, also with music and all visual arts.

A third possibility consists in getting a better understanding on the way in which ANNs can contribute to the theory/explanation of sociological research. This part is very interesting because ANNs illustrate the concepts of explanation, prediction, etc. from a different perspective. As shown in the squashing theory" by Massimo Buscema, important considerations concerning applications of ANNs or their structure still remain to be explored.

Bibliography

AAVV (1993). Quale mobilità intellettuale? Tendenze e modelli. La discussione metodologica sui flussi elettorali. *Quaderni Fondazione Giangiacomo Feltrinelli.* 33, 1–330.

Albino, V., Carbonara, N., and Giannoccaro, I. (2003). Coordination mechanism based on cooperation and competition within industrial districts: an agent based computational approach. *J. Artificial Soc. Social Simulation* 6(4), online.

Alker, H. R. Jr. (1969). A typology of ecological fallacies. In M. Dogan and S. Rokkan (Eds.), *Quantitative ecological analysis in the social sciences* (pp. 69–86). Cambridge, MA: The MIT Press.

Atkinson Maxwell, J. (1971). Social reaction to suicide. In S. Cohen (Ed.), *Images of deviance.* Harmondsworth: Penguin books.

Atkinson Maxwell, J. (1978). *Discovering suicide. Studies in the social organization of sudden death.* London: Macmillan.

Axelrod, R. (1970). Conflict of interest. *A theory of divergent goals with applications to politics*, Chicago, IL: Markam

Axelrod, (1981). The emergence of cooperation among egoists, *Am. Pol. Sc. Rev.* 75, 306–18

Axelrod, R. (1984). *The evolution of cooperation.* New York: Basic Books.

Axelrod, R. (1997). *The complexity of cooperation. Agent–based models of competition and collaboration.* Princeton, NJ: Princeton University Press.

Azarian, G. R. (2005). *The general sociology of Harrison C. White. Chaos and order in networks.* London: Palgrave MacMillan.

Bagarello, F. (2007). The Heisenberg picture in the analysis of stock markets and in other sociological context. *Quality and Quantity*, IV, 41, 533–555

Bailey, K. D. (1990). *Social entropy theory.* Albany, NY: State University of New York Press.

Barabasi, A.-L. (2002). *Linked. The new science of networks.* Cambridge, UK: Perseus; tr. it. *Links, La nuova scienza delle reti*, Torino: Einaudi 2004.

Barbera, F, and Negri N. (2005). La connessione micro – macro. Azione – aggregazione – emersione. In M. Borlandi and L. Sciolla (Eds.), *La spiegazione sociologica. Metodi, tendenze, problemi* (pp. 93–112). Bologna: Il Mulino.

Bartholomew, D. J (1982). *Stochastic models for social processes.* New York: Wiley.

Bartholomew, D. J. (1987). *Latent variable models and factor analysis.* New York: Oxford University Press.

Barton, A. H. (1955). The concept of property space in social research. In P. F. Lazarsfeld and M. Rosemberg (Eds.), *The language of social research* (pp. 40–53). Glencoe: The Free Press.

Batty, M. (2005). *Cities and complexity. Understanding cities with cellular automata, agent- based models and fractals.* Cambridge, MS: The MIT Press

Baungaard Rasmussen, L. (2004). Action research. Scandinavian experiences. *Artificial Intelligence Soc.* 18, 21–43.

Bellomo, N., Bellotti L. L, and Delitala M. (2007). From the kinetic theory of active practice in the modelling of social behaviours and politics. *Quality and Quantity*, IV, 41, 345–555.

Berge, C. (1965). Graph theory and application. In S. Sternberg, V. Capecchi, T. Kloek and C. T. Lenders (Eds.), *Mathematics and social sciences* (pp. 83–98). Paris: Mouton/Unesco.

Bernstein, J. (1978, 1982). *Science observed, experiencing science*. New York: Basic Books, tr. it, *Uomini e macchine intelligenti*, Milano, Italy: Adelphi 1990.

Berzano, L. and Prina, F. (1995). *Sociologia della devianza*. Firenze: La Nuova Italia Scientifica.

Birke, L. (1986). *Women, feminism and biology*. New York: Methuen.

Blalock, H. M. (1962). Four variable causal models and partial correlation. *Am. Sociol. Rev*. 69, 182–194.

Blalock, H. M. (1968). *Theory construction. From verbal to mathematical formulation*. Englewood Cliffs, NJ: Prentice Hall.

Blalock, H. M, Aganbegian, A., Borodkin, F. M., Boudon, R., and Capecchi, V. (Eds.) (1975). *Quantitative sociology. International perspectives on mathematical statistical modelling*. New York: Academic Press.

Blalock, H. M. (Ed.) (1985). *Causal models in the social sciences*. New York: Aldine Publishing Company.

Blazer, N. and Youngelson, W. (Eds.) (1977). *Women in a man-made world*. Chicago, IL: Rand McNally.

Boero, R., Castellani, M., and Squazzoni, F. (2004). Micro behavioral attitudes and macro technological adaptation in industrial districts: an agent – based prototype. *J. Artificial Soc. Social Simulation* 8(4), online.

Borlandi, M. and Sciolla, L. (Eds.) (2005). *La spiegazione sociologica. Metodi, tendenze, problemi*. Bologna, Italy: Il Mulino.

Borrelli, F., Ponsiglione, C., Iandoli, L., and Zollo, G. (2005). Inter organizational learning and collective memory in small firms clusters: An agent based approach. *J. Artificial Soc. Social Simulation* 8(3), online.

Borrie, J. (2006). Cooperation and defection in the conference of disarmament. *Disarmament Diplomacy* 82, Spring.

Boudon, R. (1963). Propriétés individuelles et propriétés collectives: un problème d'analyse écologique. *Revue française de sociologie* IV(3), 275–299.

Boudon, R. (1965). Réflexion sur la logique des modèles simulés. *Archives Européennes de Sociologie* VI(1), 3–20.

Boudon, R. (1967). *L'analyse mathématique des faits sociaux*. Paris: Plon.

Boudon, R. (1977). *Mathematical Structures of Social Mobility*. Amsterdam, The Netherlands: Elsevier Scientific Publishing Company.

Boudon, R. (1977). *Effets perverse et ordre social*. Paris, France: Presse Universitaire de France.

Boudon, R. (1984). *La place du desordre. Critique de theorie de changement social*. Paris, France: Presse Universitaires de France.

Boudon, R. (1987). The individualistic tradition in sociology. In J. C. Alexander et al. (Eds.), *The micro–macro link* (pp. 33–45). Berkeley, CA: University of California Press.

Boudon, R. (1999). L'Ethique protestante de Max Weber: le bilan de la discussion. In R. Boudon (Ed.), *Etudes sur les sociologues classiques* (pp. 55–92). Paris, Quadrige/Presse Universitaire de France.

Boudon, R. (2003). Beyond rational choice theory. *Ann. Rev. Sociol*. 29, 1–21

Bourdieu, P. (1979). *La distinction, critique sociale du jugement*. Paris, France: Les Editions de Minuit.

Bowles, G. and Duelli Klein, R. (Eds.) (1983). *Theories of women's studies*. Boston, MA: Routledge and Kegan Paul.

Briggs, J. (1992). *Fractals. The pattern of chaos*. New York: Simon & Schuster.

Buscema, M. and Semeion Group (1992). *Il Progetto Sonda. La prevenzione dai comportamenti auto ed eterodistruttivi*. Roma: Edizioni Semeion.

Buscema, M. and Massini, G. (1993). *Il Modello MQ. Reti neurali e percezione interpersonale*. Roma: Armando Editore.

Buscema, M. (1994). *Squashing theory. Modello a reti neurali per la previsione di sistemi complessi.* Roma: Armando Editore.
Buscema, M., Matera, F., Nocentini, T., and Sacco, P. L. (1997), *Reti neurali e finanza.* Roma: Armando Editore
Buscema, M. (Ed.) (2006). *Sistemi ACM e imaging diagnostico.* Milano, Italy: Springer Verlag Italia.
Buscema, M. and Semeion Group (1999a). *Reti neurali artificiali e sistemi sociali complessi, Teoria-modelli applicazioni. Vol I Teoria e modelli.* Milano, Italy: Franco Angeli.
Buscema, M. and Semeion Group (1999b). *Reti neurali artificiali e sistemi sociali complessi, Teoria-modelli applicazioni. Vol II Applicazioni.* Milano, Italy: Franco Angeli.
Buscema, M. and Drappi, L. (1999). La struttura complessa delle città. Reti neurali per un sistema cognitivo. In M. Buscema and Semeion Group (Eds.), *Reti neurali artificiali e sistemi sociali complessi. Teoria-modelli- applicazioni.* Vol II Applicazioni (pp. 228–260). Milano: Franco Angeli.
Buscema, M. and Intraligi, M. (1999). Reti Neurali Artificiali per il riconoscimento della vulnerabilità da eroina e simulazione di scenari dinamici. In Buscema M. and Semeion Group (Eds.), *Reti neurali artificiali e sistemi sociali complessi. Teoria-modelli- applicazioni.* Vol II Applicazioni (pp. 40–95). Milano: Franco Angeli.
Buscema, M. and Semeion Group (2002). *Reti neurali artificiali per l'orientamento professionale. Progetto Loop.* Milano, Italy: Franco Angeli.
Buscema, M., Rossigni, P., Babiloni, C., and Grossi, E. (2007). The IFAST model, a novel parallel nonlinear EEG analysis technique distinguishes mild cognitive impairment and Alzheimer's disease patients with high degree of accuracy. *Artificial Intelligence in Med.* 40, 127–143.
Callon, M. and Latour, B. (1981). Unscrewing the big Leviathan: how actors macro-structure reality and how sociologist help them to do so. In K. Knorr-Cetina and A. V. Cicorel (Eds.), *Advances in social theory and methodology. Toward an integration of micro and macro sociologies* (pp. 277–303). Boston, MA: Routledge & Kegan Paul.
Campelli, E. (Ed.) (1999). Paul Felix Lazarsfeld: un classico "marginale". *Special Number of Sociologia e ricerca sociale*, n. 58/59.
Capecchi, V. (1963). Analisi qualitativa e quantitativa in sociologia. *Quaderni di Sociologia* XII(4), 171–200.
Capecchi V. (1964). Une methode de classification fondée sur l'entropie. *Revue Française de Sociologie* V, 290–306.
Capecchi, V. (1965). L'analisi delle preferenze politiche. *Rassegna italiana di sociologia* 6(2), 199–261.
Capecchi, V. (1966). Typologies in relation to mathematical models. *Ikon* 58, 1–62.
Capecchi, V. (1967). Metodologia e ricerca nell'opera di Paul F. Lazarsfeld. Introduzione a P. F. Lazarsfeld. op.cit. VII-CLXXXIV.
Capecchi, V. (1967b). Problèmes méthodologiques dans la mesure de la mobilité sociale. *Archives Européennes de Sociologie* (12), 285–318.
Capecchi, V. and Moeller, F. (1968). Some application of entropy to the problems of classifications. *Quality and Quantity* 2, 63–84.
Capecchi, V. and Galli, G. (1969). Determinants of voting behaviour in italy: a linear causal model of analysis. In M. Dogan and S. Rokkan (Eds.), *Quantitative ecological analysis in the social sciences* (pp. 233–283). Cambridge MA: The MIT Press.
Capecchi, V. (1972). Struttura e tecniche della ricerca. In Rossi P. (Ed.), *Ricerca sociologica e ruolo del sociologo.* Bologna, Italy: Il Mulino, 23–129.
Capecchi, V. (1973). Some examples of classification and causal analysis. *Quality and Quantity* 7, 131–156.
Capecchi, V. and Moeller, F. (1975). The role of entropy in nominal classification. In H. M. Blalock, Aganbegian, F.M. Borodkin, R. Boudon and V. Capecchi (Eds.), *Quantitative sociology. International perspectives on mathematical statistical modelling* (pp. 381–428). New York: Academic Press.

Capecchi, V. (1981). From sociological research to the inquiry. In D. Pinto (Ed.), *Contemporary Italian sociology. A reader* (pp. 223–230). Cambridge, UK: Cambridge University Press.
Capecchi, V. (1985). Appunti per una riflessione sulla metodologia della ricerca sociologica. *Quaderni di sociologia* 4–5, 112–169.
Capecchi, V. and A. Pesce (1993). L'Émilie – Romagne. In V. Scardigli (Ed.), *L'Europe de la diversité. La dynamique des identit és régionales* (pp. 89–123). Paris: Ceres.
Capecchi, V. (1996). Tre Castelli, una Casa e la Città inquieta. In C. Cipolla and A. De Lillo (Eds.), *Il sociologo e le sirene* (pp. 37–99). Milano, Italy: Franco Angeli.
Capecchi, V. (2004). A changing society and problems of method: a politically committed research type. *Artificial Intelligence Soc.* 1, 149–174.
Carbone, V. and Piras, G. (1999). Orientamento e dispersione scolastica: le Reti Neurali Artificiali come support dell'azione formativa. In M. Buscema Semeion Group (Eds.), *Reti neurali artificiali e sistemi sociali complessi. Teoria-modelli- applicazioni.* Vol II Applicazioni (pp. 170–200). Milano: Franco Angeli.
Chase, I. D. (1991). Vacancy chains. *Ann. Rev. Sociol.* 17, 133–154.
Cicourel, A. V. (1981). Notes non the integration of micro- and macro- levels of analysis. In K. Knorr-Cetina and A.V. Cicourel (Eds.), *Advances in social theory and methodology. Toward an integration of micro and macro sociologies* (pp. 51–79). Boston: Routledge & Kegan Paul.
Colecchia, N. (2004). *Magritte nella rete. Approccio neurale al linguaggio pittorico.* Milano, Italy: Franco Angeli.
Coleman, J. (1946). Some sociological models. In S. Sternberg, V. Capecchi, T. Kloek, and C. T. Lenders (Eds.), *Mathematics and social sciences* (pp. 175–212). Paris: Mouton/Unesco.
Coleman, J. S., Katz, E., and Menzel, H. (1957). The diffusion of an innovation among physicians. *Sociometry* XX, 253–270.
Coleman, J. S. (1964). *Introduction to mathematical sociology.* New York: Free Press.
Coleman, J. S (1964b). *Models of change and response uncertainty.* Englewood Cliffs, NJ: Prentice Hall inc.
Coleman, J. S., Katz, E., and Menzel, H. (1966). *Medical innovation: a diffusion study.* Indianapolis, IN: Bobbs–Merrill.
Coleman, J. S. (1973). *The mathematics of collective action.* London: Heinemann Educational Books.
Coleman, J. S. (1979). Purposive Actors and Mutual Effects. In R. K. Merton, J. S. Coleman, P. H. Rossi (Eds.), *Qualitative and quantitative social research*, Papers in Honour of Paul F. Lazarsfeld (pp. 98–118). New York, NY: The Free Press.
Coleman, J. S. (1986). *Individual interests and collective action. Selected essays.* Cambridge, UK: Cambridge University Press.
Coleman, J. S. (1990). *Foundation of social theory.* Cambridge, MA: The Belknap Press of Harvard University Press.
Coleman, J. S. (1995). Comment on Kuran and Collins. *Am. J. Sociol.* 100(6), 1616–1619.
Collins, R. (1981). Micro-translation as a theory-building strategy. In K. Knorr-Cetina and A. V. Cicourel (Eds.), *Advances in social theory and methodology. Toward an integration of micro and macro sociologies* (pp. 61–107). Boston: Routledge & Kegan Paul.
Coke, B. and Kothari, U. (Eds.) (2001). *Participation: The new tyranny?.* London: Zed.
Cointet, J.-P. and Roth, C. (2007). How realistic should knowledge diffusion models be?. *J. Artificial Soc. Social Simulation* 10, 1–18.
Contucci, P. and Ghirlanda, S. (Eds.) (2007). How can mathematics contribute to social sciences. *Special Number of Quality and Quantity*, IV, 41.
Corbetta, P., Parisi, A., and Shadee H. M. A. (1988). *Elezioni in Italia*, Bologna: Il Mulino.
Cuin, C. H. (2005). Esistono leggi sociologiche?. In M. Borlandi and L. Sciolla (Eds.), *La spiegazione sociologica. Metodi, tendenze, problemi* (pp. 33–44). Bologna, Italy: Il Mulino.
Currarini, S., Jackson, M. O., and Pin, P. (2008). An Economic Model of Friendship: Homophily, Minorities and Segregation. Paper presented at the 2007 European Meetings of the Econometric Society in Budapest.

Degenne, A. and Forsé, M. (1994). Les réseaux sociaux, Paris: Armand Colin.
Deleuze, G. (1968). *Différences et répétition*. Paris, France: PUF.
De, S. P. and Abelson, R. (1961). The simulmatics project. *Pub. Opin. Quart.* 25, 167–183.
Dogan, M. and Rokkan, S. (Eds.) (1969). *Quantitative ecological analysis in the social sciences*. Cambridge, MA: The MIT Press.
Duncan, O. D. (1966). Path analysis: sociological examples. *Am. J. Sociol.* 72, 1–16.
Durkheim, E. (1987). *Le suicide Reprint*. Paris: Presses Universitaires de France, 1960.
Edling, C. R. (2002). Mathematics in sociology. *Ann. Rev. Sociol.* 28, 197–220.
Epstein, J. M. (1997). *Nonlinear dynamics, mathematical biology, and social science*. New York, NY: Addison-Wesley Publishing Company.
Epston, D. (1999). Co-research: the making of an alternative knowledge. Chapter 16 in *Narrative therapy and community work: A conference collection*. Adelaide, SA: Dulwich Centre Publications.
Flament, C. (1965). *Theorie des graphes et structures sociales*. Paris, France: Gauthier Villars.
Fleck, C. (1998). The choice between market research and sociography, Or: What happened to Lazarsfeld in the United States? In J. Lautman and B. P. Lécuyer (Eds.), Paul Lazarsfeld (1901–1976), *La sociologie de Vienne à* New York, NY (pp. 83–119). Paris: L'Harmattan.
Fioretti, G. (2001). Information structure and behavior of a textile industrial district. *J. Artificial Soc. Social Simulat.* 4(4), online.
Fondazione Giangiacomo Feltrinelli (1993). Quale mobilità elettorale? Tendenze e modelli. La discussione metodologica sui flussi elettorali. *Quaderni Fondazione Giangiacomo Feltrinelli* 33, 1–330.
Fonow, M. M. and Cook, R. A. (Eds.) (1991). *Beyond methodology, feminist scholarship as lived research*. Bloomington, IN: Indiana University Press.
Foote White, W. (1943). *Street corner society*. Chicago, IL: University of Chicago Press.
Forrester, J. W. (1969). *Urban dynamics*, Waltham MA. Pegasus Communications.
Forrester, J. W. (1971). Counterintuitive behaviour of Social systems. *Technol. Rev.* 73, 53–68.
Forrester, J. W. (1989). The beginning of social dynamics. *Paper for the International Meeting of the System Dynamic Society*, Stuttgart, Germany, July 13
Freeman, L. C. (2004). *The development of social network analysis: a study in the sociology of science*. Vancouver, BC: Empirical Press, tr. it. *Lo sviluppo dell'analisi delle reti sociali* a cura di Memoli R.
Garfinkel, S. L. (1987). *Radio Research. McCarthyism and Paul F. Lazarsfeld*. Thesis of Ph.D., Columbia University.
Giddens, A. (1981). Agency, institution and time space analysis. In K. Knor-Cetina and A. V. Cicourel (Eds.), *Advances in soical theory and methodology. Toward an integration of micro and macro sociologies* (pp. 161–174). Boston: Routledge & Kegan Paul.
Gigliotta, O., Miglino, G. and Parisi, D. (2007). Group of agents with a leader. J. Art. Soc. Soc. Simul. 10(41) 1
Gilbert, N. and Troitzsch, K. G. (2005). *Simulation for the social scientist*. 2nd edition. New York: Open University Press.
Gilbert, N. (2008). *Aged based models*. Thousand Oaks (Ca): Sage.
Gleick, J. (1987). *Chaos*. New York: Viking Penguin Inc. tr. it., *Caos. La nascita di una nuova scienza*, Milano, Italy: Rizzoli 1989.
Goodman, L. A. (1959). Some alternatives to ecological correlations. *Am. J. Sociol.* LXIV, 610–624.
Goodman, L. A. (2007). Statistical magic and/or statistical serendipity: an age of progress in the analysis of categorical data. *Ann. Rev. Sociol.* 33, 1–19.
Granovetter, M. S. (1973). The strength of weak ties. *Am. J. Soc.* 78, 1360–1380.
Grossetti, M. and Godart, F. (2007). Harrison white: des réseaux sociaux à une theorie structurale de l'action. *SociologieS, Revue scientifique internationale*, Octobre
Grossi, E. and Buscema, M. (2005). The potential role played by artificial adaptive systrems enhancing our Understeanding of Alzheimer disease. *Neurosci. Res. Commun.* 35 (3), 246–263

Hägerstrand, T. (1965). A Monte Carlo approach to diffusion. *Archives Européennes de Sociologie* VI(1), 43–67.

Harding, S. and Hintikka, M. B. (Eds.) (1983). *Discovering reality. Feminist perspectives on epistemology, metaphysics, methodology and philosophy of science*. Dordrecht, The Netherlands: Reidel Publishing Company.

Harding, S. (Ed.) (1987). *Feminism and methodology*. Bloomington, IN: Indiana University Press.

Harding, S. (1991). *Whose science, whose knowledge? Thinking from women's lives*. Ithaca, NY: Cornell University Press.

Harding, S. (1992). After the neutrality ideal: science, politics and strong objectivity. *Soc. Res.* 59(3), 567–588.

Harding, S. (2004). Rethinking standpoint epistemology. What is strong objectivity? In S. Nagy Hesse-Biber and M. L. Yaiser (Eds.), *Feminist perspectives on social research* (pp. 39–64). New York, NY: Oxford University Press.

Harré, R. (1981). Philosophical aspects of the macro- micro problem. In K. Knor-Cetina and A. V. Cicourel (Eds.), *Advances in social theory and methodology. Toward an integration of micro and macro sociologies* (pp. 139–160). Boston: Routledge & Kegan Paul.

Heims, S. J. (1991). *The cybernetics group*. Boston, MA: The Massachusetts Institute of Technology, tr. it., *I cibernetici. Un gruppo e un'idea*, Editori Riuniti, Roma 1994.

Hempel, C. G. and Oppenheim, P. (1936). *Der Typusbegriff im Lichte der Newen Logik*. Leiden: Sijthoff.

Hempel, C. G. (1965a). *Aspects of scientific explanation and other essays in the philosophy of science*. New York: The Free Press.

Hempel, C. G. (1965b). Typological methods in the natural and the social sciences. In C. G. Hempel (Ed.), *Aspects of scientific explanation and other essays in the philosophy of science* (pp. 155–171). New York, NY: The Free Press.

Hodges, A. (1983). *Alan Turing. The Enigma*. New York: Burning Books, tr. it. *Storia di un enigma. Vita di Alan Turing 1912–1954*. Torino, Italy: Bollati Boringhieri 1991.

Isambert, F. (1998). La méthodologie de Marienthal. In J. Lautman and B. P. Lécuyer (Eds.), *Paul Lazarsfeld* (1901–1976). La sociologie de Vienne à New York (pp. 49–64). Paris: L'Harmattan.

Jacobs, G. (Ed.) (1970). *The participant observer. Encounters with social reality*. New York: George Braziller.

Jahoda, M., Lazarsfeld, P. F. and Zeisel, H. (1932). *Die Arbeitslosen von Marienthal*. Leipzig: Hitzel, tr. it. *I disoccupati di Marienthal*, Edizioni Lavoro, Roma 1986.

Jahoda, M. (1998). Paul Felix Lazarsfeld in Vienna. In J. Lautman and B. P. Lécuyer (Eds.), *Paul Lazarsfeld* (1901–1976), La sociologie de Vienne à New York (pp. 135–146). Paris: L'Harmattan.

Katz, E. and P. F. Lazarsfeld (1955). *Personal influence. The part played by people in the flow of mass communication*. Glencoe: The Free Press.

Kinnunen, J. (1996). Gabriel Tarde as a founding father of innovation diffusion research. *Acta Sociologica* 39(4), 431–442.

Kiser, E. (1995). What can sociological theories predict? comment on collins, Kuran and Tilly. *Am. J. Sociol.* 100(6), 1611–1615.

Knorr-Cetina, K. and Cicorel, A. V. (Eds.) (1981). *Advances in social theory and methodology. Toward an integration of micro and macro sociologies*. Boston, MA: Routledge & Kegan Paul.

Knorr-Cetina, K. (1981). Introduction: The micro-sociological challenge of macro-sociology: towards a reconstruction of social theory and methodology. In K. Knorr-Cetina and A. V. Cicorel (Eds.), *Advances in social theory and methodology. Toward an integration of micro and macro sociologies* (pp. 2–47). Boston, MA: Routledge & Kegan Paul.

Kosko, B. (1993). Fuzzy thinking. *The New Science of Fuzzy Logic*. New York, NY: Hyperion.

Latour, B. (2001). Gabriel tarde and the end of the social. In P. Joyce (Ed.), *The social in question. New bearings in history and the social sciences* (pp. 117–132). London: Routledge

Latour, B. (2005). *Reassembling the social. An introduction to actor-network-theory*. Oxford: Oxford University Press.

Luce, R. D and Raiffa H. (1957). *Games and decisions: Introduction and critical survey*. New York: John Wiley and Sons.
Lautman, J. and Lécuyer B. P. (Eds.) (1998). *Paul Lazarsfeld (1901–1976), La sociologie de Vienne à New York*. Paris, France: L'Harmattan.
Lautman, J. and Lécuyer B. P. (1998). Presentation. In J. Lautman and B. P. Lécuyer (Eds.), *Paul Lazarsfeld (1901–1976), La sociologie de Vienne à New York* (pp. 9–19). Paris, France: L'Harmattan.
Lazarsfeld, P. F., Berelson, B. and Gaudet, H. (1944). *The people's choice*. New York: Duell, Sloan & Pearce.
Lazarsfeld, P. F. (1949). The American soldier. An expository review. *Pub. Opin. Quart.* XIII, 377–404.
Lazarsfeld, P. F. and Barton A. H. (1951). Classification, Typologies and Indices. In D. Lerner and H. D. Laswell (Eds.), *The policy sciences*. Stanford: Stanford University Press.
Lazarsfeld, P. F. (1953). Some historical notes on the empirical study of action, Upublished Report, tr. it. Lo sviluppo storico dello studio empirico dell'azione". In P. F. Lazarsfeld (1967) *Metodologia e ricerca sociologica* (Italian Anthology edited by V. Capecchi) (pp.109–175). Bologna: Il Mulino.
Lazarsfeld, P. F. (1954). Introduction: mathematical thinking in the social sciences. In P. F. Lazarsfeld (Ed.), *Mathematical thinking in the social sciences* (pp. 3–16). Glencoe: The Free Press.
Lazarsfeld, P. F. and Merton, R. K. (1954). Friendship as a social process: a substantive and methodological analysis. In M. Berger (Ed.), *Freedom and control in modern society* (pp. 18–66). New York: Van Nostrand.
Lazarsfeld, P. F. (1955). Mutual effects of statistical variables, Bureau of applied social research. Unpublished paper, Lazarsfeld P. F. *Metodologia e ricerca sociologica* (pp. 557–592), Bologna, Italy: Il Mulino, 1967.
Lazarsfeld, P. F. (1958). Problems in methodology. In R. K. Merton, L. Broom, and L. S. Cottrell jr. (Eds.), *Sociology today* (pp. 39–78). New York: Basic Books.
Lazarsfeld, P. F. and Thielens, W. jr. (1958). *The academic mind*. Glencoe: The Free Press.
Lazarsfeld, P. F. (1961). Notes on the history of quantification in sociology: trends, sources and problems. *Isis* 52, 277–333.
Lazarsfeld, P. F. and Menzel, H. (1961). On the relation between individual and collective properties. In A. Etzioni (Ed.), *Complex organization, a sociological reader* (pp. 422–440). New York: Holt Rinehart and Winston.
Lazarsfeld, P. F. (1962). The sociology of empirical social research. *Am. Sociol. Rev.* 17(6), 757–767.
Lazarsfeld P. F. (1965). Repeated observation on attitude and behaviour items. In S. Sternberg, V. Capecchi, T. Kloek and C. T. Lenders (Eds.), *Mathematics and social sciences* (pp. 121–142). Paris: Mouton/Unesco.
Lazarsfeld, P. F. (1967). *Metodologia e ricerca sociologica*. Bologna, Italy: Il Mulino – a cura di V. Capecchi.
Lazarsfeld, P. F. (1971). Foreword – forty years later. *Prefazione alla edizione inglese*, tr. it., Jahoda, M., Lazarsfeld, P. F., Zeisel, H., *I disoccupati di Marienthal* (pp. 43–51). Roma: Edizioni Lavoro, 1986.
Lewin, K. (1946). Action research and minority problems. *J. Soc. Issues* 2, 34–46. Published in K. Lewin (Ed.) (1948). *Resolving social conflict: selected papers on group dynamics*. New York: Harper.
Lieberson, S. and Lynn, F. B. (2002). Barking up the wrong branch: scientific alternatives to the current model of sociological science. *Ann. Rev. Sociol.* 28, 1–19.
Lin, N. (2001). *Social capital: A theory of social structure and action*. New York, NY: Cambridge University Press.
Lipset, S. M. (1998). Paul F. Lazarsfeld of Columbia: A Great Methodologist and Teacher. In J. Lautman and B. P. Lécuyer (Eds.), *Paul Lazarsfeld (1901–1976), La sociologie de Vienne à New York* (pp. 255–270). Paris, France: L'Harmattan.

Lynd, R. S. (1939). *Knowledge for what? The place of social science in American culture.* Princeton University Press, Princeton, trad. it. *Conoscenza perché fare. Le scienze sociali nella cultura americana*, Guaraldi, Firenze 1976.
Macy, W. M. and Willer, R. (2002). From factors to actors: computational sociology and agent-based modelling. *Ann. Rev. Sociol.* 28, 143–166.
Mandelbrot, B. (1965). Macro-statistical models and aggregative laws of behavior. In S. Sternberg, V. Capecchi, T. Kloek, and C. T. Lenders (Eds.), *Mathematics and social sciences* (pp. 213–239). Paris: Mouton/Unesco.
Mandelbrot, B. B. (1975). *Les objects fractals*. Paris, France: Flammarion.
Mandelbrot, B. B. (1977). *Fractals: form, chance and dimension*. San Francisco, CA: Freeman.
Mandelbrot, B. B. (1982). *The fractal geometry of nature*. San Francisco, CA: Freeman.
Mandelbrot, B. B and Hudson, R. L. (2004). *The (Mis)behaviour of market. a fractal view to risk, ruin and reward*, tr. it. *Il disordine dei mercati. Una visione frattale di rischio, rovina e redditività*, Torino: Giulio Einaudi Editore.
Marsden, P.V. (2005). *The sociology of James Coleman*. Ann. Rev. Soc. 31, 1–24
Marsed, P. V. (2005). *The sociology of James Coleman*. Ann. Rev. Sociol. 31, 1–24.
Maurelli, G. and Terzi, S. (1999), Panoramica di sperimentazioni effettuate con Reti Neurali Artificiali. In M. Buscema and Semeion Group (Eds.), *Reti neurali artificiali e sistemi sociali complessi. Teoria-modelli- applicazioni*. Vol II Applicazioni (pp. 284–312). Milano: Franco Angeli.
McClung, L. A. (1970). On context and relevance. In G. Jacobs (Ed.), *The participant observer. Encounters with social reality* (pp. 3–16). New York: George Braziller.
McCorduck, P. (1979). *Machines who think*. New York: Freeman, tr. it. *Storia dell'intelligenza artificiale*, Padova: Franco Muzzio Editore 1987.
Meadows, D. H. et al. (1972). *Limits to growth*. New York, NY: Universe Books.
Meraviglia, C. (1999). Questioni di mobilità maschie e femminile: tecniche a confronto. In M. Buscema & Semeion Group (Eds.), *Reti neurali artificiali e sistemi sociali complessi. Teoria-modelli- applicazioni*. Vol II Applicazioni, (pp. 201–213). Milano: Franco Angeli.
Meraviglia, C. (2001). *Le reti neurali nella ricerca sociale*. Milano, Italy: Franco Angeli.
Meraviglia, M., Massini, G., Croce, D., and Buscema, M. (2006). GenD an evolutionary system for resampling in survey research. *Quality and Quantity* 40(5), 825–859.
Merton, R. K. (1938). Social structure and anomie. *Am. Sociol. Rev.* 2, 672–682.
Merton, R. K. (1949). *Social theory and social structure*. Glencoe: The Free Press, trad. it. *Teoria e struttura sociale*, Il Mulino, Bologna, 1959.
Merton, R. K., Coleman, J. S., and Rossi, P. H. (Eds.) (1979). *Qualitative and quantitative social research, papers in honour of Paul F. Lazarsfeld*. New York: The Free Press.
Merton, R. K. and Barber, E. G. (1992) *The travels and adventures of serendipity. A study in historical semantics and the sociology of science*. tr. it. *Viaggi e avventure della Serendipity*, Bologna, Italy: Il Mulino, 2002.
Merton, R. K. (1998). Working with Lazarsfeld: Notes and context. In J. Lautman and B. P. Lécuyer (Eds.), *Paul Lazarsfeld (1901–1976), La sociologie de Vienne à New York* (pp. 163–211). Paris, France: L'Harmattan.
Milgram, S. (1967). The small world problem. *Psychol. Today* 2, 60–67.
Mongin, P. (2008). Retour à Waterloo: histoire militaire et théorie des jeux. *Annales*, I, 63, 39–69.
Nagy, H., Biber, S. and Yaiser, M. L. (Eds.) (2004). *Feminist perspectives on social research*. New York: Oxford University Press.
Naroll, R. (1965). Book review of Harrison White. *Am. J. Soc.* II, 71, 217–8.
Newman, M., Barabasi, A.-L., and Watts, D. J. (Eds.) (2006). *The structure and dynamics of networks*. Princeton, NJ: Princeton University Press.
Nielsen, J. McC. (Ed.) (1990). *Feminist research methods*. Boulder, CO: Westview Press.
Nin, N. (2001). *Social capital. A theory of social structure and actions*. Cambridge, UK: Cambridge University Press.
Peitgen, H.-O. (1986). *The beauty of fractals. Images of complex dynamical systems*. Berlin, Germany: Springer Verlag.

Pelinka, A. (1998). Paul F. Lazarsfeld as a pioneer of social sciences in Austria. In J. Lautman and B. P. Lécuyer (Eds.), *Paul Lazarsfeld (1901–1976), La sociologie de Vienne à New York* (pp. 23–32). Paris, France: L'Harmattan.

Poe, E. A. (1836). *Maelzel's chess player, Southern literary messenger*. tr. it *Il giocatore di scacchi di Maelzel*. Milano, Italy: SE , 2000.

Ramazanoglu, C. (1989). *Feminism and the contradictions of oppression*. London: Routledge & Kegan Paul.

Ramazanoglu, C. and Holland, J. (2002). *Feminist methodology: Challenges and choices*. Thousand Oaks: Sage.

Riesman, D. (1958). Some observations on the interviewing in the teacher apprehension study. In P. F. Lazarsfeld and W. Thielens Jr. (Ed.), *The academic mind* (pp. 266–377). Glencoe: The Free Press.

Riesman, D. (1979). Ethical and practical dilemmas of fieldwork in academic settings: a personal memoir. In R. K. Merton, J. S. Coleman, and P. H. Rossi (Eds.), *Qualitative and quantitative social research, papers in honour of Paul F. Lazarsfeld* (pp. 210–231). New York: The Free Press.

Roberts, H. (Ed.) (1981). *Doing feminist research*. London: Routledge & Kegan Paul.

Robinson, W. S. (1950). Ecological correlation and the behaviour of individuals. *Am. Sociol. Rev.* XV, 351–357.

Selvin, H. C. (1958). Durkheim's suicide and problems of empirical research. *Am. J. Sociol.* 63, 607–619.

Selvin, H. C. (1979). On following in someone's footsteps: two examples of Lazarsfeldian methodology. In R. K.Merton, J. S. Coleman, and P. H. Rossi (Eds.), *Qualitative and quantitative social research* (pp. 232–244). New York: The Free Press.

Simon, H. M. (1954). Spurious correlation: a causal interpretation. *J. Am. Stat. Assoc.* 49, 467–479.

Sonquist, J. A. (1969). Finding variables that work. *Pub. Opin. Quart.* 33, 83–95.

Sorensen, A. B. (1978). Mathematical models in sociology. *Ann. Rev. Sociol.* 4, 345–371.

Squazzoni, F. and Boero, R. (2002). At the edge of a variety and coordination. An agent –based computational model of industrial districts. *J. Artificial Soc. Social Simulat.* 6(4), online.

Sternberg, S. with Capecchi, V., Kloek, T., and Laenders, C. T. (Eds.) (1965). *Mathematics and social sciences*. Paris, France: Mouton /Unesco.

Storm, L. (Ed.) (2008). *Synchronicity. multiple perspectives on meaningful coincidence*. Grosseto, GR: Pari Publishing.

Taschwer, K. (1998). Discourses on society in *Red Vienna*: some contexts of the early Paul F. Lazarsfeld. In J. Lautman and B. P.Lécuyer (Eds.), *Paul Lazarsfeld (1901–1976), La sociologie de Vienne à New York* (pp. 33–48). Paris, France: L'Harmattan.

Tilly, C. (1995). To explain political processes. *Am. J. Sociol.* 100(6), 1394–1610.

Toews, D. (2003). The new tarde. sociology after the end of the social. *Theory, Cult. Soc.* 20(5), 81–98.

Torgerson, W. S. (1958). *Theory and methods of scaling*. New York: John Wiley and Sons inc.

Troitzsch, K. G. (1997). Social simulation: Origins, prospects, purposes. In R. Conte, R. Hegslemann, and P. Terna (Eds.), *Simulating social phenomena* (pp. 41–54). Berlin: Springer.

Udehn, L. (2002). *The changing fase of methodological individualism. Ann. Rev. Soc.* 28, 479–507.

Valade, B. (2001). De l'explication dans les sciences sociales: holisme et individualisme. In J. -M. Berthelot (Ed.), *Epistémologie des sciences sociales* (pp. 357–405). Paris: Presse Universitaire de France.

Waldrop, M. M. (1992). Complexity. *The emerging science at the edge of the order and chase.* New York, NY: Simon and Schuster.

Weiler, K. (1995). Freire and a feminist pedagogy of difference. In J. Holland, M. Blair, and S. Sheldon (Eds.), *Debates and issues in feminist research and pedagogy* (pp. 23–44). Clevedon, UK: Multilingual Matters Ltd.

White, H. C. (1963). *An anatomy of kinship*. Englewood Cliffs, NJ: Prentice Hall.

White, H. C. (1970). *Chains of Opportunity*. Cambridge, MA: Harvard University Press.

White, H. C. (1992). *Identity and control: a structural theory of social action*. Princeton, NJ: Princeton University Press.

White, H. C. (2001). *Interview*. In A. McLean and A. Olds, online.

White, H. C. (2008). *Identity and control: how social formation*. Princeton, NJ: Princeton University Press.

Wright, S. (1960). Path coefficients and path regression: alternative or complementary concepts. *Biometrics* 16, 189–202.

Zadek, L. A. (1965). Fuzzy sets. *Inf. Control*, 8, 338–53.

Zeisel, H. (1979). The Vienna years. In R. K. Merton, J. S. Coleman, P. H. Rossi (Eds.), *Qualitative and quantitative social research, papers in honour of Paul F. Lazarsfeld* (pp. 10–15). New York: The Free Press.

Part I
Mathematics and Models

Chapter 2
Equilibria of Culture Contact Derived from In-Group and Out-Group Attitudes

Pierluigi Contucci, Ignacio Gallo, and Stefano Ghirlanda

Abstract Modern societies feature an increasing contact between cultures, yet we have a poor understanding of what the outcomes might be. Here we consider a mathematical model of contact between social groups, grounded in social psychology and analyzed using tools from statistical physics. We use the model to study how a culture might be affected by immigration. We find that in some cases, residents' culture is relatively unchanged, but in other cases, residents may adopt the opinions and beliefs of immigrants. The decisive factors are each group's cultural legacy and its attitudes toward in- and out-groups. The model can also predict how social policies may influence the outcome of culture contact.

2.1 Introduction

Contact between cultures is a prominent feature of modern society, driven by large-scale migration, global media, communication networks, and other socio-economic forces (Lull 2000). Understanding how human cultures interact is crucial to such issues as immigration management and the survival of national and minority cultures (Cornelius et al. 1994, Givens and Luedtke 2005), yet the dynamics of culture contact is poorly known. Here we explore the problem considering a single cultural trait that can take two forms, such as being in favor or against the death penalty, or whether to wear a particular piece of clothing or not. We are interested in (1) how the two trait forms are distributed among subgroups in a population, e.g., residents and immigrants, males and females, social classes and (2) how different subgroups influence each other's traits.

P. Contucci (✉)
Department of Mathematics, University of Bologna, Bologna, Italy; Centre for the Study of Cultural Evolution, Stockholm University, Stockholm, Sweden
e-mail: contucci@dm.unibo.it

V. Capecchi (eds.), *Applications of Mathematics in Models, Artificial Neural Networks and Arts*, DOI 10.1007/978-90-481-8581-8_2,

We start with assumptions about how individuals may change their opinions and behaviors as a consequence of social interactions and then derive the population-level consequences of such assumptions using tools from statistical physics. We study the case of immigration in detail and conclude that culture contact may sometime result in residents taking on the opinions and beliefs of immigrants, depending on each group's cultural legacy, its attitudes toward in- and out-groups, and social policies.

Our main assumption about how individuals may change their traits is the so-called similarity-attraction hypothesis of social psychology: an individual tends to agree with those who are perceived as similar to oneself and to disagree with those who are perceived as different (Byrne 1971, Grant 1993, Byrne 1997, Michinov and Monteil 2002). Additionally, individuals can be influenced by other forces favoring one form of a trait over the other. For instance, a media campaign may advertise in favor or against a given idea or behavior. To determine the distribution of opinions among subgroups of a population (after they have been in contact for some time), we apply statistical mechanics, a branch of theoretical physics that studies the collective properties of systems composed of many parts that interact according to given rules. These techniques were originally developed to derive the laws of thermodynamics from molecular dynamics (Thompson 1979) but have also been applied to biological (Amit 1989, Arbib 2003) and social systems, including models of social choice (Schelling 1973, Granovetter 1978, Durlauf 1999, Watts 2002, Nancy 2003).

The latter considers how collective opinions or choices emerge within a homogeneous social group. The model we discuss here is, to our knowledge, the first one to consider populations consisting of different social groups in interaction.

2.2 General Framework

We now outline a general framework for modeling group-level consequences of interactions among individuals (Contucci and Ghirlanda). Individual i is described by a binary variable $s_i = \pm 1$, representing the two possible forms of the considered trait ($i = 1,\ldots, N$). A group is characterized by the mean value $m = \frac{1}{N}\sum_i s_i$, which can be measured by, say, a referendum vote or a survey. To apply statistical mechanics we formalize the interaction between individuals as follows. Let L_{ik} be the similarity that individual i perceives with k and assume that L_0 is the level of similarity above which individuals tend to agree and below which they tend to disagree. We can then recast the similarity-attraction hypothesis in the form of a minimization rule, assuming that i, when interacting with k, tends to assume the trait value that minimizes the quantity

$$H_{ik}(s_i, s_k) = -(L_{ik} - L_0)s_i s_k \qquad (2.1)$$

This assumption agrees with the similarity-attraction hypothesis because when $L_{ik} > L_0$, the expression is minimized by agreement ($s_i s_k = 1$) and when $L_{ik} < L_0$, the expression is minimized by disagreement ($s_i s_k = -1$). For simplicity we let

$L_{ik} - L_0 = J_{ik}$ in the following. Then $J_{ik} > 0$ favors agreement and $J_{ik} < 0$ favors disagreement. We say "favor" because we do not assume strict minimization. Rather, we assume that a trait value yielding a lower value of (2.1) occurs with a higher probability, but not with certainty (see Appendix). The rationale for this assumption is that similarity to others is not the sole determinant of an individual's trait (Byrne 1997, Michinov 1992).

When an individual interacts with many others, we assume that she tends to minimize the sum H_i of all functions (2.1) relative to each interaction:

$$H_i(s_i) = \sum_k H_{ik}(s_i,s_k) = -\sum_k J_{ik}s_is_k \tag{2.2}$$

where the sum extends over all individuals with whom i interacts. In summary, the effect of changing one's trait is gauged depending on whether it makes an individual agree or disagree with others.

The effect of factors such as the media or social norms is, for each individual, to favor a particular trait value. This can be included in our minimization scheme by adding a term to equation (2.2):

$$H_i(s_i) = -\sum_k J_{ik}s_is_k - h_is_i \tag{2.3}$$

The added term means that $S_i = 1$ is favored if $h_i > 0$, while $s_i = -1$ is favored if $h_i < 0$. We now define a group-level function$H$ as the sum of individual functions:

$$H(s) = \sum_i H_i(s_i) = -\sum_{i,k} J_{ik}s_is_k - \sum_i h_is_i \tag{2.4}$$

where $s = \{s_1,\ldots,s_N\}$ is the set of all individual traits. The function H is referred to as the system *Hamiltonian* in statistical mechanics, where it usually arises from consideration of a system's physical properties. Here, on the other hand, we have designed the function H so that lower values of H correspond to group states that, given our assumptions about individual psychology, are more likely to occur. It is this property that allows us to use statistical mechanics (Thompson 1979). Note that we do not assume that individuals explicitly carry out, or are aware of, the computations in equation (2.4).

2.3 Culture Contact in Immigration

We consider a large and a small group, referred to, respectively, as *residents* (R) and *immigrants* (I). We are interested in the effect of one group upon the other, i.e., how culture contact changes the mean trait values in the two groups. If residents and immigrants have markedly different culture, the similarity-attraction hypothesis implies that J_{ik} should be positive for interactions within a group and negative for interactions between groups. A simple assumption (called *mean field* in statistical mechanics) is that J_{ik} depends only on group membership. This corresponds to the in-group and out-group concepts of social psychology (Brown 2000) and can be formalized as follows:

$$J_{ik} = \begin{cases} \frac{J_{res}}{2N} > 0, \quad i,k \in R \\ \frac{J_{\text{int}}}{2N} < 0, \quad i \in R, k \in I \text{ or } i \in I, k \in R \\ \frac{J_{\text{imm}}}{2N} > 0, \; i,k \in I \end{cases} \tag{2.5}$$

where the factor 1/2*N* guarantees that the group function, equation (2.4), grows proportionally to the number of individuals. Before the two groups interact, residents and immigrants are each characterized by a cultural legacy that includes given mean values of the considered trait, say $m^*_{\text{res}}$and m^*_{imm}. Our goal is to predict the values $m^*_{\text{res}}$and m^*_{imm} after the interaction has taken place. To describe the effect of cultural legacies, we reason as follows. Within a group, a mean trait $m^* \neq 0$ means that the two forms of the trait are not equally common. Thus preexisting culture can be seen as a force that favors one trait value over the other and can be modeled by a force term as in equation (2.3). In other words, a model in which individuals are biased so that the mean trait is m^* is equivalent to a model with unbiased individuals subject to a force h^* of appropriate intensity. The latter can be calculated by standard methods of statistical mechanics as

$$h^* = \text{atanh}(m^*) - Jm^* \tag{2.6}$$

where atanh(·) is the inverse hyperbolic tangent and *J* is the in-group attitude (Thompson 1979, Contucci & Ghirlanda). Statistical mechanics also allows to calculate the values of $m_{\text{res}}$and m_{imm} after culture contact as the solution of a system of equations (see Appendix):

$$\begin{cases} m_{\text{res}} = \tanh\left((1-\alpha)J_{res}m_{res} + \alpha J_{\text{int}}m_{\text{imm}} + h^*_{\text{res}}\right) \\ m_{\text{imm}} = \tanh\left((1-\alpha)J_{\text{int}}m_{res} + \alpha J_{imm}m_{\text{imm}} + h^*_{\text{imm}}\right) \end{cases} \tag{2.7}$$

where tanh(·) is the hyperbolic tangent,α is the fraction of immigrants in the compound group, and h^*_{res} and h^*_{imm} are calculated for each group according to equation (2.6). Numerical analysis of these equations reveals two main patterns of behavior depending on the sign of the product $m^*_{\text{res}}m^*_{\text{imm}}J_{\text{int}}$ (Fig. 2.1). When $m^*_{\text{res}}m^*_{\text{imm}}J_{\text{int}} > 0$, a small fraction of immigrants cause only small changes in residents' trait, as intuition would suggest. This includes two distinct cases: either the two groups agree before the interaction ($m^*_{\text{res}}m^*_{\text{imm}} > 0$) and have similar culture ($J_{\text{int}} > 0$, Fig. 2.1a) or they disagree and have dissimilar cultures ($m^*_{\text{res}}m^*_{\text{imm}} < 0$ and $J_{\text{int}} < 0$, Fig. 2.1d). The second pattern of results occurs when $m^*_{\text{res}}m^*_{\text{imm}}J_{\text{int}} < 0$, in which case there exists a critical fraction of immigrants α_c, above which residents suddenly change to a nearly opposite mean trait value. This can happen either when

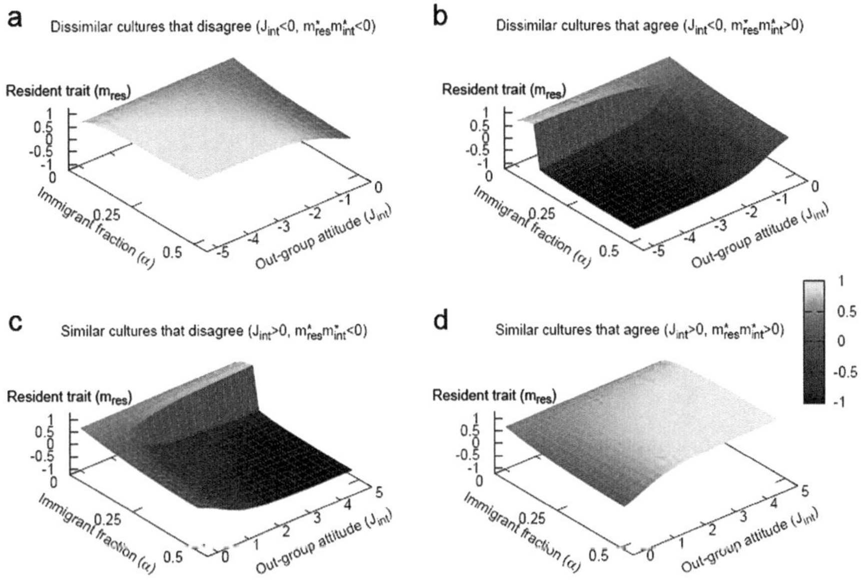

Fig. 2.1 Influence of immigration on resident culture. Each panel portraits the mean resident trait after cultural contact m_{res} as a function of the fraction of immigrants α and the strength and sign of out-group attitude J_{int}. Dramatic shifts in resident trait occur only when $J_{int}m^*_{res}m^*_{imm} < 0$ **(b,d)**, but not when $J_{int}m^*_{res}m^*_{imm}$ **(a,c)**, where m^*_{res} and m^*_{imm} are residents' and immigrants' mean traits before cultural interaction, respectively. Parameter values: $J_{res} = 1, J_{imm} = 0.7, m^*_{res} = 0.7, m^*_{imm} = -0.5$ **(a,c)** or $m^*_{imm} = 0.5$ **(b,d)**

the two groups agree and have dissimilar culture ($m^*_{res}m^*_{imm} > 0$ and, Fig. 2.1b) or when the groups disagree and have similar culture ($m^*_{res}m^*_{imm} > 0$ and $J_{int} > 0$, Fig. 2.1c). This dramatic phenomenon only exists when attitudes toward the out-group (either positive, Fig. 2.1b, or negative, Fig. 2.1c) are strong enough. The shift can thus be inhibited by decreasing the magnitude of J_{int}. According to our assumptions, this amounts to making the groups less similar when they are similar and less different when they are different.

There are other ways in which dramatic shifts in residents' trait may be prevented. It is possible, for instance, to reduce the strength of residents' in-group attitude J_{res} (Fig. 2.2). According to the similarity-attraction hypothesis, a higher value of J_{res} corresponds to higher in-group similarity. Hence our model suggests that a more culturally homogeneous group has a greater risk of undergoing a dramatic transition when confronted with an immigrant culture. That is, encouraging cultural diversity among residents may make their culture more robust. One may also try to influence individuals directly, introducing, e.g., social incentives that encourage a given trait [modeled by h terms as in equation (2.3)]. Consider a situation in which residents are predicted to change trait when the fraction of immigrants passes a critical value α_c (Fig. 2.1b). In such a case, α_c can be increased subjecting individuals to an incentive h that favors the residents' original trait (Fig. 2.3a). An incentive in the opposite direction, on the other hand, decreases α_c, suggesting that

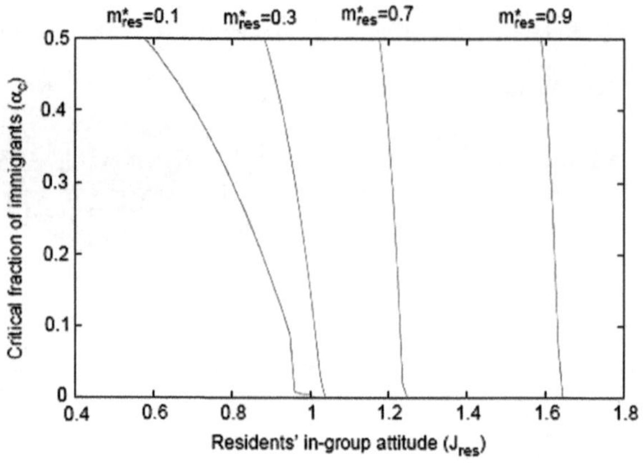

Fig. 2.2 In-group attitudes and shifts in cultural traits. Each line shows the critical fraction of immigrants α_c, above which a sudden shift in residents' trait is observed, as a function of the strength of residents' in-group attitude J_{res}. The *curves* are identical for the cases in Fig. 2.1b and c, i.e., for positive or negative J_{int}. For each value of m^*_{res} (*different lines*), lowering J_{res} sharply increases the fraction of immigrants that can be sustained before residents significantly change trait

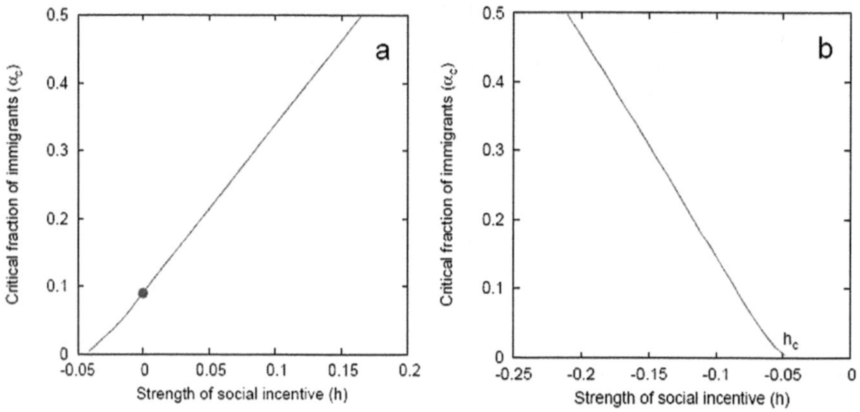

Fig. 2.3 Social incentives and shifts in cultural traits. Both panels plot the critical fraction of immigrants α_c, above which a sudden shift in residents' trait is observed, as a function of the strength of a social incentive capable of affecting individual traits, modeled as an external force h [equation (2.3)]. (**a**) A social incentive is added to the situation in Fig. 2.1b ($h = 0$, *red dot in this figure*). If h favors (opposes) the residents' original trait value, the critical fraction of immigrants is raised (lowered).(**b**) A social incentive is added to the situation in Fig. 2.1d, in which no dramatic change is predicted. When h is decreased from 0 toward negative values, residents' trait changes very slightly (not shown), until a critical value h_c is reached when a sudden shift in residents' trait is predicted with a very small fraction of immigrants. Parameter values as in Fig. 2.1

the impact of social policies can be dramatic. Indeed, we show in Fig. 2.3 that an incentive h can trigger dramatic changes even when these are impossible with $h = 0$, as, for instance, in Fig. 2.1d.

2.4 Discussion

Clearly, our model is only an approximation to the complexities of culture contact. Yet it exhibits a rich set of behaviors that, we hope, may help to understand this complex phenomenon and promote the development of more refined models. Our approach can be developed by considering more individual traits (so that changes in culture as a whole can be assessed), more realistic patterns of interactions among individuals (social networks), individual variability in in-group and out-group attitudes, and more complex rules of individual interaction. Our basic hypothesis (similar individuals imitate each other more strongly than dissimilar ones), however, is well rooted in social psychology (Byrne 1971, 1997), including studies of intergroup behavior (Grant 1993, Michinov and Monteil 2002), and we expect it to remain an important feature of future models.

Acknowledgments We thank Francesco Guerra, Giannino Melotti, and Magnus Enquist for discussion. Research supported by the CULTAPTATION project of the European Commission (FP6-2004-NEST-PATH-043434).

Appendix

Statistical mechanics assigns to each system configuration s a probability that is inversely related to the value of $H(s)$ through an exponential function (Thompson 1979):

$$\Pr(s) = \frac{e^{-H(s)}}{\sum_s e^{-H(s)}} \tag{2.8}$$

where the denominator is a normalization factor ensuring $\sum_s \Pr(s) = 1$. Equation (2.8) can be proved in a number of important cases (Thompson 1979) but is also used heuristically in more general settings (Mezard et al. 1997). In particular, the exponential is the only function compatible with basic assumptions relevant for social as well as physical systems such that the probability of events relative to two independent subsystems must multiply, while other quantities (e.g., entropy, see below) must add (Fermi 1936).

The probability distribution (2.8) is used to calculate the so-called *free energy*, from which one can derive system-level quantities such as the mean trait values m_{res} and m_{imm}.The free energy is defined as the difference between *internal energy* U, i.e., the average of H with respect to equation (2.8), and *entropy* $S = -\sum_s \Pr s \ln \Pr s$:

$$F = U - S \tag{2.9}$$

For the model in the main text one may show that (Contucci et al.)

$$\begin{aligned} U = &-\tfrac{1}{2}(J_{res}(1-\alpha)^2 m_{\text{res}}^2 + J_{\text{imm}}\alpha^2 m_{\text{imm}}^2 + 2J_{\text{int}}\alpha(1-\alpha)m_{\text{imm}}m_{res}) + \\ &-(1-\alpha)h_{\text{res}}^* m_{\text{res}} - \alpha h_{\text{imm}}^* m_{imm}. \end{aligned} \tag{2.10}$$

and

$$\begin{aligned} s = &(1-\alpha)\left(-\frac{1+m_{\text{res}}}{2}\ln\left(\frac{1+m_{\text{res}}}{2}\right) - \frac{1-m_{\text{res}}}{2}\ln\left(\frac{1-m_{\text{res}}}{2}\right)\right) \\ &+\alpha\left(-\frac{1+m_{\text{imm}}}{2}\ln\left(\frac{1+m_{\text{imm}}}{2}\right) - \frac{1-m_{\text{imm}}}{2}\ln\left(\frac{1-m_{\text{imm}}}{2}\right)\right). \end{aligned} \tag{2.11}$$

The values of m_{res} and m_{imm} are obtained from these expressions by minimizing equation (2.9), which yields equation (2.7).

Bibliography

Amit, D. (1989). *Modeling brain function*. Cambridge: Cambridge University Press.

Arbib, M. A. (2003). *The handbook of brain theory and neural networks*. MIT Press, 2nd edition.

Brown, R. (2000). *Group processes: dynamics within and between groups*. Oxford: Blackwell Academic Publishing, 2nd edition.

Byrne, D. (1971). *The attraction paradigm*. Academic Press, New York.

Byrne, D. (1997). *J. Pers. Soc. Psychol.* 14, 417–431.

Contucci, P. and Ghirlanda, S. (2007). *Qual. & Quan.* 41, 569–578.

Contucci, P., Gallo, I., and Menconi, G., http://arxiv.org/physics/0702076.

Cornelius, W. A., Martin, P. L., and Hollifield, J. F., (Eds.) (1994). *Controlling immigration: A global perspective*. Stanford, CA: Stanford University Press.

Durlauf, S. N. (1999). *Proc. Natl. Acad. Sci. U.S.A.* 96, 10582–10584.

Givens, T. and Luedtke, A. (2005). *Comp. Europ. Polit.* 3, 1–22.

Granovetter, M. S. (1978). Threshold models of collective behavior. *Am. J. Sociol.* 83, 1420–1443.

Grant, P. R. (1993). *Can. J. Behav. Sci.* 25, 28–44.

Lull, J. (2000). *Media, communication, culture*. Cambridge: Polity Press.

Macy, M. W., Kitts, J. A., Flache, A., and Benard, S. (2003). In *Dynamic social network modeling and analysis* (pp. 162–173). Washington: National Academic Press.

Mezard, M., Parisi, G., and Virasoro, M. A. (1987). *Spin glass theory and beyond*. Singapore: World Scientific.

Michinov, E. and Monteil, J.-M. (2002). *Europe. J. Soc. Psychol.* 32, 485–500.

Schelling, T. C. (1973). Hockey helmets, concealed weapons, and daylight saving: A study of binary choices with externalities. *J. Conflict Resolut.*, 32, 381–428.

Watts, Duncan J. W. (2002). *A simple model of information cascades on random networks. Proceedings of the National Academy of Science, U.S.A*, 99, 5766–5771.

Thompson, C. (1979). *Mathematical statistical mechanics*. Princeton, NJ: Princeton University Press.

Chapter 3
Society from the Statistical Mechanics Perspective

Oscar Bolina

Abstract This chapter presents an introduction to social modeling with statistical mechanics. An elementary description of spin systems is given first, then we explain how this description has been applied to binary models of the social sciences that have implications for public policies. Next we suggest other applications to research in the social sciences.

3.1 Introduction

Statistical mechanics is the physics of a large number of atoms. In any material, atoms move about under the action of forces exerted on them by the other atoms of the material.

The goal of statistical mechanics is to understand how the interactions of a collection of individual atoms give rise to the macroscopic behavior of matter.

The base for this lies in the fact that a large system of interacting atoms can be described by a small number of variables that determine the observable average behavior of the system.

The basic aspect of this theory of Physics is of a statistical nature. It is impossible (and not particularly useful) to write down and solve exactly the equations for a system containing 10^{27} atoms, which is the estimated number of atoms in the human body (see http://en.wikipedia.org/wiki/Orders_of_magnitude_(numbers)).

The methods of statistical mechanics have been widely applied in physics of many body systems.

These same methods find application in social sciences, economics, biological sciences, and other areas (Durlauf 2001, Toulouse et al. 1986). The main reason for this wide range of applicability is that statistical mechanics does not depend on the details of the system being analyzed.

O. Bolina (✉)
Kaplan Shinyway Overseas Pathway College, HangZhou 310053, P.R. China
e-mail: oscarb@kaplanshinyway.com

Part of this work was carried out during the stay of the author at the University of Idaho, Moscow.

V. Capecchi (eds.), *Applications of Mathematics in Models, Artificial Neural Networks and Arts*, DOI 10.1007/978-90-481-8581-8_3,

Socials sciences works with a variety of different models. Sociology has described models of diffusion (spread of rumors), modeled by differential equations, of social mobility, modeled by Markov chains, and of interaction networks, modeled by graph theory (Sorensen 1978). Economics has used game theory and models of general equilibrium and maximization problems. Other diverse social models have been used to study the educational effects of school policies on learning, welfare problems and policies, linear models of population and stability, group decision making, models of language competition, and cultural assimilation (Durlauf 2001, Sorensen 1978, Intriligator 1973).

In this chapter we will be interested in social interactions of populations of individuals. We describe how statistical mechanics can be used to provide a general framework for the study of individual choice and social interaction models. We do not introduce a new model. We do not try to construct a model either. We merely describe how the available machinery of statistical mechanics is capable of providing answers to problems of interest to a social scientist. Statistical mechanics provides a well-established set of rules to deal with these problems. Our emphasis is on the application of these rules to the analysis of models in the social sciences.

In this context, it is possible to quantify social interactions between individuals or between populations with parameters that are well known in statistical mechanics, write the interaction in mathematical form, and obtain definite answers by statistical mechanical methods through these well-established rules. The mathematics required is not difficult, and it can be presented in an accessible way, totally within the range of a wide and diverse audience.

Statistical mechanics works in the so-called thermodynamic limit. The thermodynamic limit means that statistical mechanics works when the system under study has an infinite number of particles. Because of this, relevant calculations are carried out for a fixed number of particles N and then N is allowed to go to infinity. In mathematical terms, we take limit $N \to \infty$ at the end.

Despite this fact, statistical mechanics can be applied to macroscopic systems containing a large – but finite – number of particles because such systems contain so many particles that they are a good approximation to the $N \to \infty$ limit for practical purposes. More can be said, however. It is possible to show that certain systems are large enough if they contain, say, 1,000 particles, where large enough means that these systems give reliable practical results as if they were in the thermodynamic limit. The same is true in the application of statistical mechanics to the social sciences. We start by presenting a (hopefully) friendly introduction to the ideas and mathematics of statistical mechanics as they are used in the physics of spin systems. Then we discuss the application of these ideas to social sciences models.

3.2 The Physics of Spin Systems

Atoms of certain elements (iron, cobalt, nickel, chromium are examples) have what is called a spin. Imagine the atom as a tiny baseball rotating along a vertical axis. If you curl the fingers of your right hand around the direction of rotation of the ball, then your thumb will represent the direction of the spin of the baseball. The atoms of iron tend to align their spins in the same direction so that all spins are parallel to one another: ↑↑↑↑. Atoms of other elements (such as chromium) tend to align their spins in opposite direction: ↑↓↑↓ (Pool 1989). In physical systems of spins a variable s is introduced to describe the spin of an atom. This variable can take on only two values +1 and −1, depending on whether an atom has spin up or down, respectively (although assigning spin +1 to spin down and −1 to spin up is equally valid). We cannot know a priori the orientation of each spin. The important point is that only these two orientations are possible. Spins of different atoms in a material interact with each other. The statistical mechanics analysis of a spin system starts by writing down the total energy of the system. We do this in the next section.

3.2.1 An Example

A simple example will help understand the structure of the problem. We consider the system of three spins only. We introduce the spin variable s_i, taking the possible values +1 or −1, where the subscript i, with $i = 1, 2, 3$, identifies the spin of the system. The interaction energy between any two spins i and j is given by

$$-J_{ij}s_i \cdot s_j$$

where J_{ij} are parameters (constants) of the model that measure the strength of the interaction. Note that the negative sign above implies that the energy of spins having the same orientation is smaller than the energy of spins having opposite orientation.

It follows that the possible interaction energies between any pairs of spins are

$$-J_{12}s_1 \cdot s_2, -J_{21}s_2 \cdot s_1, -J_{23}s_2 \cdot s_3, -J_{32}s_3 \cdot s_2, -J_{31}s_3 \cdot s_1, -J_{13}s_1 \cdot s_3$$

Because we do not know the orientation of each spin, we consider all possible orientations of the system of three spins. Any particular set of values (s_1, s_2, s_3) is called a configuration of the system. We list them below starting from (1, 1, 1) and then changing the sign of one of the spins in turn, then changing two signs, and finally arriving at (−1, −1, −1):

$$(1,1,1), (-1,1,1), (1,-1,1), (1,1,-1), (-1,-1,1),$$
$$(-1,1,-1), (1,-1,-1), (-1,-1,-1)$$

Note that there are eight possible spin configurations. Since there are two possible orientations for each spin (up or down), in general there are 2^N configurations of N spins if each spin can take on only two possible values.

The total energy of the system of three spins for each configuration $s = (s_1, s_2, s_3)$ is

$$H(s) = -J_{12}s_1s_2 - J_{13}s_1s_3 - J_{21}s_1s_2 - J_{23}s_2s_3 - J_{31}s_3s_1 - J_{32}s_2s_3 \tag{3.1}$$

In statistical mechanics – and in physics in general – the total energy (3.1) of the system is called the Hamiltonian of the system.

Note that our model is not necessarily interaction symmetric. That is why we have taken six interaction terms in equation (3.1). For each term of the form $J_{12}s_1s_2$, there is also a term of the form $J_{21}s_2s_1$. Still we observe that all equations of this formalism depend only on $J_{12} + J_{21}$, that is, on the sum of the two non-identical terms. In practice, this implies that we may well assume symmetry of the interaction and use $J_{ij} = J_{ji}$ throughout. This leads to the following simplified form of the Hamiltonian:

$$H(s) = -2J_{12}s_1s_2 - 2J_{23}s_2s_3 - J_{31}s_3s_1 \tag{3.2}$$

We now calculate the energy (3.2) explicitly for all possible configurations of the system of three spins. They are

$$\begin{aligned}
H(1,1,1) &= -2J_{12}(1)(1) - 2J_{23}(1)(1) - 2J_{31}(1)(1) = -2J_{12} - 2J_{23} - 2J_{31}\\
H(-1,1,1) &= -2J_{12}(-1)(1) - 2J_{23}(1)(1) - 2J_{31}(1)(-1) = 2J_{12} - 2J_{23} + 2J_{31}\\
H(1,-1,1) &= -2J_{12}(1)(-1) - 2J_{23}(-1)(1) - 2J_{31}(1)(1) = 2J_{12} + 2J_{23} - 2J_{31}\\
H(1,1,-1) &= -2J_{12}(1)(1) - 2J_{23}(1)(-1) - 2J_{31}(-1)(1) = -2J_{12} + 2J_{23} + 2J_{31}\\
H(-1,-1,1) &= -2J_{12}(-1)(-1) - 2J_{23}(-1)(1) - 2J_{31}(1)(-1) = -2J_{12} + 2J_{23} + 2J_{31}\\
H(-1,1,-1) &= -2J_{12}(-1)(1) - 2J_{23}(1)(-1) - 2J_{31}(-1)(-1) = 2J_{12} + 2J_{23} - 2J_{31}\\
H(1,-1,-1) &= J_{12}(1)(-1) - 2J_{23}(-1)(-1) - 2J_{31}(-1)(1) = 2J_{12} - 2J_{23} + 2J_{31}\\
H(-1,-1,-1) &= -2J_{12}(-1)(-1) - 2J_{23}(-1)(-1) - 2J_{31}(-1)(-1) =\\
&-2J_{12} - 2J_{23} - 2J_{31}
\end{aligned}$$

Note that there are only four possible different energy values for a system of three spins since $H(1,1,1) = H(-1,-1,-1)$, $H(-1,1,1) = H(1,-1,-1)$, $H(1,-1,1) = H(-1,1,-1)$, and $H(1,1,-1) = H(-1,-1,1)$. This fact will be used to simplify the calculations below.

Once the Hamiltonian of the system is obtained, we calculate the partition function of the model. This is given by

$$Z = \sum_s \mathrm{e}^{-\beta H(s)} \tag{3.3}$$

with the understanding that the sum is carried out over all possible configurations $s = (s_1, s_2, s_3))$ which, in this case, comprise all possible values ± 1 for each spin variable s_i for $i = 1,2,3$.

In equation (3.3), the parameter β is a constant related to the temperature of the system. The product βH makes the exponent in equation (3.3) a dimensionless number (Cipra 1987). Below we set $\beta = 1$.

The partition function provides a recipe to calculate other quantities of interest in statistical mechanics. The partition function of our three-spin system is

$$Z = e^{-H(1,1,1)} + e^{-H(-1,1,1)} + e^{-H(1,-1,1)} + e^{-H(1,1,-1)}$$
$$+ e^{-H(-1,-1,1)} + e^{-H(-1,1,-1)} + e^{-H(1,-1,-1)} + e^{-H(-1,-1,-1)}$$

Explicitly, this is

$$Z = e^{-(-2J_{12}-2J_{23}-2J_{31})} + e^{-(2J_{12}-2J_{23}+2J_{31})} + e^{-(2J_{12}+2J_{23}-2J_{31})}$$
$$+ e^{-(-2J_{12}+2J_{23}+2J_{31})}$$
$$+ e^{-(-2J_{12}+2J_{23}+2J_{31})} + e^{-(2J_{12}+2J_{23}-2J_{31})} + e^{-(2J_{12}-2J_{23}+2J_{31})}$$
$$+ e^{-(-2J_{12}-2J_{23}-2J_{31})}$$

We then have

$$Z = 2e^{-(-2J_{12}-2J_{23}-2J_{31})} + 2e^{-(2J_{12}-2J_{23}+2J_{31})} + 2e^{-(2J_{12}+2J_{23}-2J_{31})}$$
$$+ 2e^{-(-2J_{12}+2J_{23}+2J_{31})}$$

If we further assume that $J_{ij} = J$ for all i, j, then we are led to the following simplification of the partition function:

$$Z = 2e^{6J} + 6e^{-2J}$$

We have already seen that we cannot know a priori whether the spin variable for any particular spin will be +1 or -1. We can only measure the probability of any given configuration of spins. Statistical mechanics prescribes that the probability of a configuration $s = (s_1, s_3, s_3)$ is given by

$$\text{Prob}(s) = \frac{e^{-H(s)}}{Z} \tag{3.4}$$

Note the negative sign in the exponent. This means that lower energy configurations (which result from the alignment of spins) are configurations having higher probability. The probability of each configuration is then as follows:

$$\text{Prob}(1,1,1) = \text{Prob}(-1,-1,-1) = \frac{e^{6J}}{2e^{6J}+6e^{-2J}}$$
$$\text{Prob}(1,1,-1) = \text{Prob}(-1,-1,1) = \text{Prob}(1,-1,1) = \text{Prob}(-1,1,-1)$$
$$= \text{Prob}(-1,1,1) = \text{Prob}(1,-1,-1) = \frac{e^{-2J}}{2e^{6J}+6e^{-2J}}$$

3.3 The Spin Model in a Magnetic Field

In this section we again consider the spin model introduced above. We will streamline the notation and be more general by allowing an arbitrary number of spins N and placing our system in a region where there is an external magnetic field (Day 2002). The magnetic field tends to align the spins in the direction of field. The amount of energy of interaction between the spin and the field is of the form $-h_i s_i$, where h_i is the magnitude of the magnetic field at the position of the spin i. Here again, the negative sign favors lower energy configurations since with this choice, when h_i and

s_i are both positive, the spins tend to align in the direction of the field because the interaction energy is minimized in this case. The presence of the magnetic field just adds another term to the Hamiltonian of the system. Therefore the Hamiltonian of a system of N spin in a magnetic field of magnitude h is given by

$$H(s) = -\sum_{i,j=1}^{N} J_{ij} s_i \cdot s_j - \sum_{i=1}^{N} h_i s_i \tag{3.5}$$

where we denote a configuration of N spins by $s = (s_1, s_2 \ldots, s_N)$. The partition function of the model is, as before

$$Z = \sum_{s} \mathrm{e}^{-H(s)} \tag{3.6}$$

where the sum is carried out over all possible configurations. In statistical mechanics, the standard probability assigned to a particular configuration by $s = (s_1, s_2 \ldots, s_N)$ is

$$\mathrm{Prob}(s) = \frac{\mathrm{e}^{-H(s)}}{Z} = \frac{\mathrm{e}^{-H(s)}}{\sum_s \mathrm{e}^{-H(s)}} \tag{3.7}$$

This probability measures how likely a particular configuration is. Now suppose that we are interested in a certain quantity m of our system that depends on the spin variables. Once the configuration probabilities are known, the average value of the quantity m can be computed by

$$\langle m \rangle = \sum_{s} m \, \mathrm{Prob}(s) \tag{3.8}$$

An example of a quantity of interest in physics is the magnetization. A material is magnetized when it has a net magnetization, meaning that there are more spins pointing up (or down) than spins pointing down (or up). This is what happens – for instance – when a paper clip is rubbed with a magnet.

3.4 Social Models of Binary Choices

In this section, we describe two models of binary choice in some detail. We set the ideas using a simple referendum model and then show how the statistical mechanics formalism presented above has been applied to a model of cultural contact between two populations. All applications cited below have implications for public policies.

3.4.1 A Yes or No Answer to a Referendum Question

This is a prototypical problem for the explanation of the application of statistical mechanics in the social sciences. It can be seen as a model of binary choice, in all respects similar to the spin system described above. In this case, the values $s = +1$ or $s = -1$ of the spin variable are associated with a yes or no answer, respectively. (As before, the choice is immaterial.) The model parameter J_{ij} measures the agreement or the disagreement between individuals i and j, being positive when i and j agree and negative when i and j disagree, and the magnetic field h_i quantify a number of influences exerted on i that drive and help shape opinions coming from different groups in society. We take $h_i > 0$ when $s_i = 1$ and $h_i < 0$ when $s_i = -1$ (Contucci and Ghirland 2007).

Individuals have a preexisting opinion on the matter of referendum. Therefore, there will be an average opinion favoring an yes answer and an average opinion favoring a no answer. We denote these by m_1^* and m_2^*. These averages are not the theoretical averages given in Day (2002). They are obtained by polling. As discussion on this topic continues, individuals will change their opinion. A poll taking at a later time will record new average values m_1 and m_2. The goal is to predict the values of m_1 and m_2 and determine how these average values change with the parameters of the model.

3.4.2 Cross-cultural Interactions

We have in mind here the interaction between a resident population and a population of immigrants. In particular, we consider whether and how a cultural trait of the resident population (language, religious faith, a particular piece of clothing) will change when the two populations interact (Contucci et al.). The trait in question can be described by a $s_i = \pm 1$ spin variable in the framework of statistical mechanics. The spin variable is interpreted as the preference of an individual for that particular trait. We take $J_{ij} > 0$ and having the same value (J_{res}) for any two individuals of the resident population, we also take $J_{ij} > 0$ and having the same value (J_{imm}) for two individuals of the immigrant population, and we take $J_{ij} > 0$ and having the same value (J_{int}) for individuals of different populations (Michinov and Monteil 2002). The justification for this comes from the similarity-attraction hypothesis. (See next section for more information on this.)

We consider this model in the following context. Initially the population of one country has no or little contact with the population of the other country. Both populations have a certain trait average value – m_{res}^* and m_{imm}^*. These average values are obtained by polling in their respective countries prior to interaction between the two populations. Assume now that immigration from one country to the other has occurred. After certain time, the two populations will relax toward equilibrium. After this equilibrium has been achieved, both the resident population and the immigrant population will have new average values m_{res} and m_{imm} for that trait. These are also obtained by polling after the two populations interact.

The aim in this case is to predict the values of $m_{\rm res}$ and $m_{\rm imm}$. A second question of interest is to determine whether there are particular values of the parameters J and h of the model for which there is a transition from a cultural trait of the resident population to the immigrant population and – in particular – to determine whether there is a critical relative size of the immigration population for which the resident population average value of that trait will change (Contucci et al. 2008).

The results of Contucci and Ghirland (2007) and Contucci et al. (2007) show that when the two populations initially (before interaction) have the will to agree and have similar cultures or when the two populations initially do not have the will to agree and have dissimilar cultures, then the immigrant population causes little influence on a particular trait of the resident population in the course of their interaction. However, when the two populations initially have the will agree and have dissimilar cultures, or when they do not have the will to agree and have similar cultures, then there is a critical value of the size of the immigrant population – as measured by a parameter $\alpha = N_{\rm imm}/N$, where $N_{\rm imm}$ is the immigrant population and $N = N_{\rm imm} + N_{\rm res}$ is the total population, above which a resident population trait average value changes – and can even change to the trait average value of the immigrant population. For values of α less than this critical value, there is no significant change in the trait average value of the resident population after interaction.

We note in connection with the above two examples that statistical mechanics cannot determine the values of the parameters J_{ij} and h for a given population at a certain time. But it will predict, for a fixed set of the parameters, what the outcome will be in the sense of being able to predict the critical size of the immigrant population that will cause a change in the average value of a trait of the resident population.

The ideas outlined above can be applied to a number of social issues such as welfare policies, death penalty, gay rights, and many other that can be formulated along the lines of item 1 or 2. We also mention that spin systems have been applied to other models of the social sciences (Durlauf 2001, Brock and Durlauf 2001, Cont and Lowe 2003, Sznajd-Weron and Sznajd 2000) and in many different fields to model traffic congestion (Kulkarni et al. 1996), neural networks (Toulouse et al. 1986), and economics models (Bornholdt 2001). Also, in economics applications, the Hamiltonian is often viewed as the cost associated with cooperation or association of individuals in groups. The purpose of these individuals is then to minimize the cost of the cooperation or the association (Cont and Lowe 2003).

3.5 Hypotheses and Assumptions in Social Psychology

In the previous section we illustrated how the parameters J_{ij} can be made to reflect the similarity-attraction assumption that has been proposed in social psychology in the course of research on one type or another of the contrast between group behavior and individual behavior (Michinov and Monteil 2002). We note here that the model can also be used to actually test assumptions and hypothesis that have been made in connection with models of binary choice in the social sciences. We cite here only those hypotheses that can be discussed in mathematical form somewhat along the lines presented above.

The similarity-attraction hypothesis. According to this assumption, individuals agree (or like, or are attracted to, or reach out to) other individuals who are perceived to be similar to themselves or to share common characteristics (Michinov and Monteil 2002, Contucci et al. Forthcoming B). Following this hypothesis, we have set $J_{ij} > 0$ for ingroup interactions and $J_{ij} < 0$ for outgroup interactions in our previous analysis.

The contact hypothesis. This is a hypothesis of prejudice reduction that suggests that contact between different groups (say, interracial groups) leads to decrease in prejudice. One possible explanation for this is that contact foster positive overall attitudes between groups (Powers and Ellison 1995). An alternative explanation holds that reduction in prejudice is the result of perceived interpersonal similarities and these similarities would then decrease intergroup prejudice (Brown and Lopez 2001). Tests have been performed in which attitudes of groups of individuals are assessed by means of questionnaires and a probability analysis of the results is carried out (Sigelman and Welch 1993). One can view this as a model of binary choice where the spin variables +1 and –1 represent the categories of positive and negative attitudes of individual group members toward another group. The statistical mechanics framework outlined in this chapter offers an alternative approach to the probabilistic analysis of similar tests. Here attitudes of one group toward another would be assessed at a certain time obtaining average values m_1^* and m_2^* and then at a later time obtaining average values m_1 and m_2. These results would track the change in attitude between the two groups in terms of the parameters of the model as explained before.

A game theoretical simulation model for the contact hypothesis has been studied in Grim et al. (2005). We should mention that these ideas also apply to models of social validation that are used to study how social pressure of a group or of an authority figure influences how individuals make decisions. One area where these models can employed is in the study of how individuals go along with wrong decisions or misjudgments even if they correctly perceive them to be wrong (Sznajd-Weron and Sznajd 2000).

Self-interest hypothesis. This is a hypothesis in economics (Fehr and Schmidt 1999) that states that individuals are driven by self-interest only. Many formal models of social preference do not validate this hypothesis (Charness and Rabin 2002). Individual behavior is also motivated by reciprocal fairness (Fehr and Schmidt 1999), leading individuals to withdraw payoffs for fairness. The binary choice framework outlined above with the spin variables $\sigma = 1$ for cooperation and $\sigma = -1$ for competition can be applied here to study average opinion on tax policies, minimum wage increase, and many others and track the mood of the population regarding the prospects of these policies before they are implemented.

Bibliography

Bornholdt, S., (2001). Expectation bubbles in a spin model of markets: Intermittency from frustration across scales. *Int. J. Mod. Phys.* 12(5), 667–674.

Brock, W. and Durlauf, S. (2001). Discrete choice with social interactions. *Rev. Econ. Stud.* 68(2), 235–260.

Brown, L. M. and Lopez, G. E. (2001). Political contacts: Analyzing the role of similarity in theories of prejudice. *Polit. Psychol.* 22(2), 403–428.

Charness, G. and Rabin, M. (2002). Understanding social preferences with simple tests. *Quart. J. Econ.* 117(3), 817–869.

Cipra, B. A. (1987). An introduction to the Ising model. *Am. Math. Mon.* 94(10), 937–959.

Cont, R. and Lowe, M. (2003). Social distance, heterogeneity and social interactions. CMAP, Ecole Poly- technique, Rapport Interne. Working Paper No. 505.

Contucci, P. and Ghirland, S. (2007). Modeling Society with statistical mechanics: An application to cultural contact and immigration. *Qual. Quan.* 41(4), 569–578.

Contucci, P., Gallo, I., and Ghirlanda, S. (2007). Equilibria of culture contact derived from ingroup and outgroup attitudes. Preprint, December 2007. To appear in "Mathematics and Society" Ed. Springer. http://arxiv.org/physics/0712.1119v1

Contucci, P., Gallo, I., and Menconi, G. (2008). Phase transitions in social sciences: Two-populations mean field theory. *Int. J. Mod. Phys. B* 22(14), 1–14. http://arxiv.org/physics/0702076

Day, P. (2002). Molecular magnets: The prehistory. *Notes Rec. R. Soc. Lond.* 56(1), 95–103.

Durlauf, S. N. (2001). A framework for the study of individual behavior and social interactions. *Sociol. Methodol.* 31(1), 47–87.

Fehr, E. and Schmidt, K. M. (1999). A theory of fairness, competition, and cooperation. *Q. J. Econ.* 114(3), 817–868.

Grim, P., Selinger, E., Braynen, W., Rosenberg, R., Au, R., Louie, N., and Connelly, J. (2005). Modeling prejudice reduction: Spatialized game theory and the contact hypothesis. *Public Aff. Q.* 19(2), 95–125.

Intriligator, M. D. (1973). A probabilistic model of social choice. *Rev. Econ. Stud.* 40(4), 553–560.

Kulkarni, R. G., Stough, R. R., and Haynes, K. E. (1996). Spin glass model of congestion and emission: An exploratory step. Trans. Res. Part C: Emerg. Tech. 4(6), 407–424.

Michinov, E. and Monteil, J. M. (2002). The similarity-attraction relationship revisited: Divergence between the effective and behavioral facets of attraction. *Eur. J. So. Psychol.* 32, 485–500.

Pool, R. (1989). Strange bedfellows. *Science* 245(2), (180–204).

Powers, D. A. and Ellison, C. G. (1995). Interracial contact and black racial attitudes: The contact hypothesis and selective bias. *Soc. Forces* 74(1), 205–226.

Sigelman, L. and Welch, S. (1993). The contact hypothesis revisited: Black–white interaction and positive racial attitude. *Soc. Forces* 71(3), 781–795.

Sorensen, A. B. (1978). Mathematical models in sociology. *Ann. Rev. Sociol.* 4, 345–371.

Sznajd-Weron, K. and Sznajd, J. (2000). Opinion evolution in closed communities. *Int. J. Mod. Phys.* 11(6), 1157–1165.

Toulouse, G., Dehaene, S., and Changeux, J. P. (1986). Spin glass model of learning by selection. *Proc. Natl. Acad. Sci.* 83, 1695–1698.

Chapter 4
Objects, Words and Actions: Some Reasons Why Embodied Models are Badly Needed in Cognitive Psychology

Anna M. Borghi, Daniele Caligiore, and Claudia Scorolli

Abstract In the present chapter we report experiments on the relationships between visual objects and action and between words and actions. Results show that seeing an object activates motor information and that language is also grounded in perceptual and motor systems. They are discussed within the framework of embodied cognitive science. We argue that models able to reproduce the experiments should be embodied organisms, whose brain is simulated with neural networks and whose body is as similar as possible to humans' body. We also claim that embodied models are badly needed in cognitive psychology, as they could help to solve some open issues. Finally, we discuss potential implications of the use of embodied models for embodied theories of cognition.

4.1 Introduction

This chapter begins and ends with the conviction that cognitive neuroscience needs to broaden their objectives, making a more extensive use of models that adequately reproduce the brain its objectives and bodily characteristics of human beings. In the introduction we will briefly outline the theoretical framework of our work describing the main assumptions and claims of embodied theories of cognition. Then we will focus on some experimental studies, in which the dependent variables consist of either response times or kinematic measures. First, we will describe a study on object categorization, then three studies on language grounding; all the studies provide evidence of the strict relationship between concepts, words, and the motor system.

While describing these studies we will show that the experimental results obtained cannot be modelled without using embodied models, i.e. models that reproduce, at least in part, both the neural structure of the human brain and some of

A.M. Borghi (✉)
Department of Psychology, University of Bologna, Bologna, Italy; Institute of Cognitive Sciences and Technologies, CNR, Rome, Italy
e-mail: annamaria.borghi@unibo.it

V. Capecchi (eds.), *Applications of Mathematics in Models, Artificial Neural Networks and Arts*, DOI 10.1007/978-90-481-8581-8_4,

the crucial sensorimotor characteristics of human arms/hands. In addition, we will illustrate some studies performed within embodied cognition that led to ambiguous results. In particular, we will focus on the issue of whether reading sentences related to a given effector (e.g. hand, mouth, foot) leads to a facilitation or to an interference of responses performed with the same effector. Referring to this example, we will show that embodied models might be crucial in order to disentangle some crucial issue for the field and to formulate more precise predictions.

In Section 4.6 we will discuss potential implications of the use of embodied models for embodied theories of cognition. On one side, embodied models can represent a strong test for embodied theories of cognition. On the other side, however, assuming a very strong embodied view could render it impossible to propose a real comparison between the performance of human subjects and the performance obtained by simulated organisms.

4.2 Theoretical Framework: Embodied Theories of Cognition

Within the field of cognitive science, traditional views intend concepts and words as abstract, amodal and arbitrarily related to their referents. In the recent years, embodied views have provided a lot of evidence showing that concepts and words are not abstract, amodal and arbitrary (Fodor 1975). Rather, they are grounded in sensorimotor processes, therefore in our bodily states. Among others, Barsalou (1999) has proposed that concepts should be conceived of as simulators. In other words, concepts are seen as re-enhancement of the pattern of neural activation recorded during perception and interaction with objects and entities. Thus, for example, the concept of "dog" would consist of the re-enhancement of the neural pattern that is active while observing a dog, caressing it, listening to its barking.

Claiming that concepts imply the re-enactment of sensorimotor experiences that pertains to different modalities (vision, touch, audition, etc.) implies that concepts are modal rather than amodal. The term "amodality", which is generally used within traditional theories of cognition, entails assuming the existence of a translation process from the experience (which is modal) to the mind (which would be amodal). Bodily experience would be translated into an abstract representation mode and sensory modalities would be transducted into propositional (simil-linguistic) symbols that are stored in our mind in an arbitrary way.

According to embodied theories of cognition, modality-specific systems play a central role in representing knowledge (Barsalou 1999, Damasio 1989, Gallese and Lakoff 2005, Martin et al. 1996, Martin 2001, Martin and Chao 2001, Beauchamp et al. 2004). This does not entail that information is not distributed across different brain areas. In fact, each concept property (e.g. visual, tactile, motor property) produces significant activation in the specific neural system (for example, the visual system becomes active while processing visual properties); furthermore it also produces multi-modal activation. It means that, rather than being restricted to the modality of the specific property, neural activity is multi-modal.

For example, on verifying that "keys can be jingling" (auditory property), not just neural auditory areas are active but also the visual and the motor areas are active (Simmons et al. 2003). Therefore the dominant brain activation for each concept property does not reside only in its respective modality. Thus, the nature of conceptual knowledge seems to be modal. But, even if we assume a non-amodal view, it is essential to distinguish between supramodality and multi-modality (Gallese and Lakoff 2005). Namely, the claim that concepts are modal is compatible with two different perspectives: the view according to which concepts are supramodal and that according to which they are multi-modal.

The argument in favour of supramodality is based on the fact that the different modality-specific parts of our brain can be brought together via "association areas" (convergence zones according to Damasio 1989). These association areas integrate information that pertains to distinct modalities. In terms of neural networks, supramodality could be represented by a feed-forward network endowed with distinct modality-specific layers (e.g. audition, vision, etc.) as well as by a layer that precedes the output layer in which information from the different modality-specific areas would be integrated. Claiming that information is multi-modal (Gallese and Lakoff 2005, Fogassi and Gallese 2004) implies that information is not represented in areas that differ from the sensorimotor ones. Therefore, no integration would occur in associative areas. Accordingly, multi-modality could be represented by a feed-forward neural network in which no integration layer exists and in which the layers that concern the different sensorimotor modalities are linked by bidirectional connections.

Therefore, concepts would be directly grounded in the sensorimotor system, and different modality-specific areas would be activated during conceptual processing. The same is true for words, as words evoke their referents and re-enhance experiences with them. For example, the word "ball" would refer to a ball and evoke its bouncing sound, its visual and tactile properties and the experience of throwing it.

4.3 Embodied Models Are Necessary to Reproduce Experimental Results on Object Vision and Action

Imagine sitting in front of a computer screen in a quiet laboratory room. On the computer screen, after a briefly presented fixation cross, the photograph of a hand appears. The hand can display two different postures: a power grip, i.e. a grip adequate for grasping larger objects, such as bottles and apples, and a precision grip, adequate for grasping small objects, like pens and cherries.

The image of the hand is followed and substituted by a photo representing an object graspable with a power grip (e.g. a hammer, an orange) or a precision grip (e.g. a pencil, a strawberry). The presented objects can be either artefacts (e.g. hammer, pencil) or natural objects (e.g. apple, strawberry). Participants were instructed to press a different key on the keyboard to decide whether the object is an artefact or a natural object. Thus, the object size and its "compatibility" with the hand posture are not relevant to the task at hand. Interestingly, however, the "compatibility" between the hand and the object impacts response times. Namely, participants are significantly faster to respond when the hand and the object are compatible than when they are not, provided that, before the experiments, they are trained to reproduce with their own hands the hand posture they see.

The results found in this experiment (Borghi et al. 2007) are in keeping with an embodied theory of concepts. Namely, they suggest that vision is strictly interwoven with action, as it evokes motor information. More specifically, the results suggest that, upon viewing the image of a hand performing an action, a sort of motor resonance process is activated. Similarly, upon observing the image of an object, action-related information is activated. The results suggest that when we see somebody acting with an object, we "simulate" an action, and we take into account the possibility of a motor action even if we are not required to consider the congruency between the two visual stimuli we see, the hand and the object (for the notion of "simulation", see Gallese and Goldman 1998, Jeannerod 2007).

How could we model such a result? Would it be possible to reproduce such a situation using a model that is not embodied, i.e. with a simulated organism that is not endowed with a visual and a motor system? We believe it is not possible. Namely, modelling such an experiment with organisms that are not endowed with a neural system and a sensorimotor system roughly similar to the human ones will impede to capture important features of the human cognitive and sensorimotor systems. Therefore when we talk about embodied models, we do not refer to generic mathematical models in which the output is obtained on the basis of equations between input and output variables. Rather, we refer to *neural network models*, as these models could offer more possibilities than do the traditional mathematical models to reproduce the functional and physiological aspects of the brain. Some well-known characteristics of the real nervous system such as robustness, flexibility, generalization, recovery based on the content, learning, parallel processing can be reproduced by neural network models and sometimes also by some mathematical models. However, using neural network models, it is possible to obtain an emergent behaviour that leads the artificial brain to auto-organize its different parts, exactly as it happens in the real brain. Finally, the elaboration of information in the real nervous system is distributed, as there are many neurons involved in the same operation and a single neuron can be involved in different operations at the same time or at different times. Neural network models well reproduce this distributed elaboration of information.

4.3.1 An Example of an Experiment with a Possible Model

Consider a situation which is easier to model. Participants observe objects (artefacts or natural objects) that can be graspable either with a power or a precision grip. The task consists in deciding whether the objects are artefacts or natural objects by mimicking a precision or a power grip with a sort of joystick. The authors find a compatibility effect between the object size and the kind of grip used to respond (Tucker and Ellis 2001, Ellis and Tucker 2000). In other words, participants' response times are faster with a precision than with a power grip when subjects see cherries, strawberries, pens, etc., and RTs are faster with a power than with a precision grip when participants see apples, hammers, bottles, etc. The results indicate that seeing an object activates information about how to grasp it, even if this information is not relevant to the task, which is simply a categorization one. They confirm that vision and action are not separated but that vision incorporates a sort of simulated action.

How can we model experimental results like the described ones? Could we use simple feed-forward neural networks? Feed-forward models probably do not provide an adequate formalization for embodied theories. Namely, a great lesson of embodied theories concerns the reciprocal and circular relationship between perception, action, and cognition. The problem with feed-forward model is that they risk reproducing the traditional "sandwich" of disembodied cognitive sciences. The metaphor of the sandwich expresses clearly how perception and action were considered in traditional theories; they were intended merely as peripheral parts, having a scarce influence on the most tasty part, the inside, that is cognition. Similar to a sandwich, feed-forward neural networks are typically endowed with one or more input layers, one or more hidden unit layers and one or more output layers. However, they are not characterized by a kind of circularity among the layers which do not have recursive character.

What kind of models should be used, then? First of all, we should not use disembodied models, i.e. models that do not take into account the fact that cognition emerges from bodily experience. In the recent years, within robotics there is a trend towards humanoid robots, i.e. robots that share sensorimotor characteristics with human beings. At the same time, it is clear that for the foreseeable future there will still be substantial differences in physical embodiment between robots and humans.

Therefore, it is important that models are endowed with at least some characteristics of human reaching and grasping system and that their sensorimotor system is at least roughly similar to the human one.

In addition, it is important that models possess at least some characteristics of human neural systems. For example, studies on concepts and language grounding might have a neurophysiological basis in the recent discovery, first in monkey and then in humans, of two kinds of visuomotor neurons: canonical and mirror ones (see Gallese et al. 1996). Canonical neurons discharge for motor actions performed using three main types of prehension: precision grip, all finger prehension, and whole hand grip. Interestingly they fire also to the visual presentation of objects requiring these kinds of prehension, even when grasping movement is not required. Mirror neurons instead fire when the monkey makes or observes another monkey or an experimenter performing a goal-directed action. In addition, recent studies propose that prefrontal cortex (PFC) is as an important source of top-down biasing where different neural pathways, carrying different sources of information, compete for expression in behaviour (Miller and Cohen 2001).

Experimental results like those obtained by Tucker and Ellis (2001) should be modelled by taking into account the role played by canonical neurons as well as by the PF cortex. In synthesis, an appropriate model of experiments such as the reported ones should be an embodied model, endowed with at least some crucial characteristics of human neural structure (neural network), and it should be able to replicate the behavioural results found.

As an example, we will describe a neural network model that suggests an interpretation of the results by Tucker and Ellis (2001) in light of the general theory on the functions of the prefrontal cortex (PFC) proposed by Miller and Cohen (2001) (Caligiore et al. 2009). An artificial organism endowed with a human-like 3-segments/ 4-degree-of-freedom arm and a 21-S/19-DOF hand, and with a visual system composed of an "eye" (an RGB camera) mounted above the arm and looking down to the arm working plane has been simulated. The organism's brain is a neural network (see Fig. 4.1) formed by maps of dynamical leaky neurons (Erlhagen and Schöner 2002) that represent input and output signals on the basis of an "eye" (an RGB camera) mounted above the arm and looking down to the arm working plane. The organism's brain is a neural network (see Fig. 4.1) formed by maps of dynamical leaky neurons (Erlhagen and Schöner 2002) that represent input and output signals on the basis of population codes (Pouget and Latham 2003). The neural

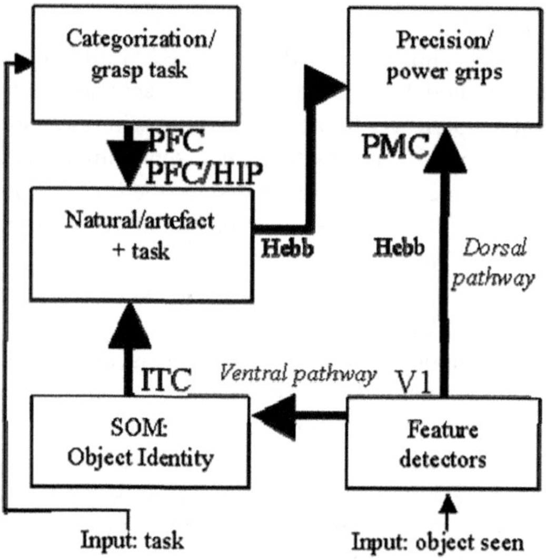

Fig. 4.1 The architecture of the neural controller. The *dorsal pathway* is formed by two neural maps, the primary visual cortex (V1) map that encodes the shape of the foveated objects through edge detection filters mimicking simple cells functions and the pre-motor cortex (PMC) map that encodes the finger postures corresponding to precision/power grip macro-actions. The *ventral pathway* includes three neural maps: the inferior temporal cortex (ITC) map that encodes objects' identity, the prefrontal cortex (PFC) map that encodes the current task (grasp/categorize) and the prefrontal cortex/hippocampus (PFC/HIP) map that encodes the representations of the task-dependent reactions to be associated with the various objects

controller of the hand acts only on the thumb and on a "virtual finger" corresponding to the four other fingers.

During the learning phase the V1–PMC connection weights are developed using an Hebb learning rule, while the organism performs randomly selected grasping actions ("motor babbling"), which mimics the acquisition of common experience, in particular the associations between big/small objects (V1) and power/precision grips (PMC), respectively. Within the ventral pathway, the V1–ITC connection weights develop the capacity to categorize objects on the basis of a learning rule that produces a self-organized map (SOM). Through an Hebb rule the PFC/HIP map learns object/task categories on the basis of input patterns from ITC and PFC. The PFC/HIP–PMC connection weights are formed using a Hebb rule which mimics the acquisition of knowledge on the task to be accomplished (e.g. during psychological experiments).

After the learning phase when the organism sees an object (e.g. a hammer), this activates the primary visual cortex (V1). V1 transmits information to two primary pathways: the dorsal stream and the ventral stream. Firmed up that the processing of visual information is task dependent, dorsal neural representation is mainly endowed with "action/perception" functions and ventral neural representation with "semantic" functions (Milner and Goodale 1995). Therefore, the dorsal neural pathway tends to trigger an action on the basis of the affordances elicited by the object (e.g. a power grip) in PMC. If the task is categorizing objects, the ventral pathway might instead evoke a different action (e.g. a precision grip in the "incompatible" condition of the target experiments) through a bias coming from the PFC, thus causing a competition between the two different tendencies within PMC. As the model assumes that the ventral pathway/PFC signal is stronger, this will cause this signal to finally prevail (thus triggering a precision grip), but the reaction times will be slower with respect to the compatible condition.

The model successfully reproduces the experimental results of Tucker and Ellis (2001) and also allows interpreting their results on the basis of the role of PFC as an important source of top-down biasing. In particular, the model shows how the PFC bias can cause organisms to perform actions different from those suggested by objects' affordances. However, affordances still exert their influence on behaviour as reflected by longer reaction times.

4.4 Embodied Models Are Necessary to Reproduce Experimental Results on Language Grounding

The evidence we reported so far concern vision and categorization of objects. In this chapter, we will consider what happens when objects are referred to by words. According to embodied views, not only concepts but also words are grounded. Thus, for example, the word "dog" would index its referent, a dog, and re-enhance the sensorimotor experience with dogs. According to this view, during language processing the same systems used for perceiving and acting would be activated. For example, while comprehending an action sentence we would "simulate" the situation it describes, activating the same neural substrate used in action.

Now imagine to complicate a bit the previously described experiment and to introduce language. Imagine participants sitting in front of a computer screen and reading sentences that appear on the screen. Sentences describe an object in a given position, as, for example, "There's a kangaroo in front of you". Once they have read the sentence, participants press a key and a noun appears; their task consists in deciding by pressing a key whether the noun refers to an object part (e.g. head, legs) or not (e.g. wood, jump). The selected parts are located either in the upper part of the object (e.g. head) or in its lower part (e.g. legs). In order to respond, in the first part of the experiment, participants are required to move upwards to press a key to respond "yes, it's a part" and to perform a movement downwards to respond "no". In the second part of the experiment, the mapping is the opposite (yes = downward movement, no = upward movement). The results show that there is a compatibility effect between the part location (upper parts, lower parts) and the direction of the movement to perform (upwards, downwards). In other words, it is faster to move upwards in order to respond to upper than to lower parts, and it is faster to move downwards to respond to lower than to upper parts (Borghi et al. 2004).

This suggests not only that object parts incorporate some sort of motor representation but also that processing a part noun implies activating the motor system. Not only objects but also words are grounded. A number of studies in the last years have shown that visual and acoustic inputs activate motor information. In the very last years, an increasing body of evidence indicates that this is not the whole story; it has been shown that language comprehension makes use of the same neural systems used for perception, action and emotion.

Since the seminal paper by Rizzolatti and Arbib (1998) on the relationship between language and motor system, a number of studies on canonical and mirror neurons have shown that these neurons might provide the neural basis underlying the language comprehension mechanism. Even if both behavioural and neural demonstrations have been provided, some issues remain to be clarified. In particular, the role played by canonical and mirror neurons during language processing is still unclear. A recently advanced proposal is that mirror neurons might be mostly involved during verb processing, while canonical neurons would be primarily activated during noun processing (Buccino, *personal communication*).

In the previous study the effect of language on motor system was investigated using reaction times and movement times. In the next study we *directly* address if the mere act of comprehending language affects the production of action, focusing on body kinematic parameters (Scorolli et al. 2009). In particular, we study a bimanual lifting action. In such an action, the motor pattern is modulated by perceptual visual cues, such as object's orientation, size and shape. Orientation is an extrinsic property of the object, as it depends on the observer and/or on the observation conditions. Instead size and shape are intrinsic properties, i.e. invariant object features. Mass is another intrinsic object property that, unlike the other ones, cannot be visually detected, because it is intrinsically linked to the action; it originates from the interaction with the object. Thus mass is a suitable property to address the characteristics of the simulation activated by language with kinematic measures. In the study, participants are standing in a quiet laboratory room, with their feet on a fixed point of the floor. They listen to sentences describing the lifting of different objects (e.g. "Move the pillow from the ground to the table"). Objects to which the words refer could be "heavy" or "light" (e.g. "tool chest" vs. "pillow"), but they do not vary in size and shape. After listening to the sentence, participants are required to lift a box placed in front of them and to rest it on a pedestal. The box can be "heavy" (mass of 12 kg) or "light" (mass of 3 kg). The kinematics of the body movements is recorded using a motion capture system. The apparatus is made up of three cameras (acquisition frequency 50–60 Hz) catching sensors movements. Sensors are placed on the outside of the participants' body, mainly on the position of the joints. After the box lifting, participants are asked a comprehension question (e.g. "Is the object on the table soft?") in order to verify whether they have listened and comprehended the sentence. The production of action is addressed focusing on the first positive maximum of elbow angular velocity, detected immediately after having grasped the box. The results show that participants are slower in case of correspondence between the weight object suggested by the sentence and the *relative* weight of the actually lifted box. As previously described, an appropriate motor lifting pattern is shaped by object's visual features such as size, shape and orientation, which in the present study are constant across the experiment. After grasping an object (box), the movement is adjusted depending also on the object mass. If language did not have any effect on motor system, changes in biomechanical parameters should have been determined only by the actual object weight. Instead we found that listening to sentences about lifting light objects leads to higher velocity values (in extending) on the actual lifting of heavy boxes compared to the lifting of the same boxes preceded by heavy sentences. Symmetrical results are obtained for the heavy boxes. Thus, the lifting simulation activated by language modulates the applied force, indirectly detected by velocity parameters. Therefore the results show that the simulation activated by language is sensitive to an intrinsic object property such as mass.

4.4.1 Examples of Possible Models

How could we model and reproduce the results of the experiment we have illustrated? Most common models of language comprehension, developed within the cognitivist tradition, are based on association frequency. One of the most influential models, latent semantic analysis (Landauer and Dumais 1997), explains word meaning in terms of the associations between one word and other words in large corpora. The higher the index of co-occurrence of words in similar texts, the higher their similarity in meaning. Even if it represents a very useful tool, this model fails when it claims to represent conceptual meaning formation. Namely, it does not take into account that words are grounded in our sensorimotor system, as it considers only the network of verbal associations in which words are embedded. For these reasons a model like this cannot capture and cannot predict the fact that an upper part is processed faster when moving upwards than when moving downwards.

Namely, these results cannot be simulated with a model that does not possess at least some features of human sensorimotor system – some form of proprioception, some kind of sensitivity to sensory inputs. In addition, the simulated organism should possess at least some features of the human motor system (e.g. reaching and grasping "devices" like an arm, a hand with fingers). For the experiment in which kinematic measures were used, the simulated body should be quite complex, in order to reproduce a lifting movement. In addition, this model should be endowed with the capacity to comprehend language by referring words to its sensorimotor experience.

Only an embodied model can reproduce the experimental results we described. Namely, reproducing the results of an experiment does not simply mean to model just a behaviour performed by a decontextualized brain simulated through a neural network but to reproduce the behaviour of an organism endowed not only with a brain but also with a body. In an ideal condition, this model should be able to reproduce learning though a mechanism of weight selection that avoids a priori hardwiring of any inhibitory or excitatory connections between or within modules. Using an embodied model has two further advantages. First, it allows one to observe rather than to infer the results. Finally, it allows reproducing the real structure of the experiment we aimed to simulate – for example, the actual button reaching behaviours could be reproduced.

A possible example of such a model is given by a self-organizing architecture developed within the MirrorBot project and based on data on language grounding (Pulvermüller 1999, 2003). In this project the model "takes as inputs language, vision and actions ... [and] ... is able to associate these so that it can produce or recognize the appropriate action. The architecture either takes a language instruction and produces the behaviour or receives the visual input and action at the particular time step and produces the language representation" (Wermter et al. 2004, 2005). The model executes predefined actions; while performing them, it learns associations between vision, action and language. Self-organizing artificial neural networks are used to associate sensor and actor data.

4.5 Embodied Models Can Help to Formulate Clearer Predictions

In the previous part of the chapter we have shown that, in order to model experimental results on concepts and language grounding, embodied models are necessary. First, models based on the assumption that the mind is a device for symbol manipulation are in contrast with embodied theories from a theoretical point of view. In addition, from a methodological point of view they are not able to capture the richness derived from the experimental setting and the experimental results.

In this part of the chapter we intend to show that embodied models might be very useful in formulating more detailed predictions that might help to disentangle unsolved issues within cognitive science. In the last years a hotly debated issue concerns the kind of relationship existing between language and the motor system. We will label it the "interference or facilitation" (IF) issue. As before, we will make an example in order to clarify what it is all about.

Consider the following study (Scorolli and Borghi 2007). Participants are sitting in a quiet laboratory in front of a computer screen. After a fixation cross, a verb appears on the screen (e.g. to kick) and then it is substituted by a noun. Verbs refer to actions typically performed with the foot and with the hand (e.g. to kick vs. to throw *the ball*), or with the mouth and with the hand (e.g. to suck vs. to unwrap *the sweet*). The task consists in deciding whether the combination between the verb and the noun makes sense or not. For example, the combination "to lick the ice cream" makes sense, while the combination "to kill the pot" does not. In order to respond that the combination makes sense, in one condition, participants are required to press a pedal with a foot, in another condition they are instructed to respond "yes" on the microphone. If the combination does not make sense, they have to refrain from responding. The results show that responses are faster in the case of correspondence between the effector used to respond and the verb–noun combination to process. Thus, responding with the foot to "foot sentences" is faster than responding by pressing a pedal to "mouth sentences"; the opposite is true with responses with the microphone.

The results suggest that when we comprehend an action sentence (or a verb–noun combination), we "simulate" the described situation, and our motor system is activated. This simulation is sensitive to the kind of effector implied by the action sentence, namely responses are faster when the effector implied by the sentence and the effector used to respond are the same than when they are not. This is in keeping with embodied theories, as it argues for a strong link between language processing and the motor system. However, why should we predict that, say, reading a foot sentence leads to facilitation in foot responses rather than to interference? If during language processing and action executing the same neural structures are activated, then this might slow down responses. The literature studies performed with tasks that slightly differ from the one we described report an interference effect (Buccino et al. 2005).

The IF issue consists in the fact that it is difficult predicting whether an interference or a facilitation effect will occur. The problem is further complicated by the fact that both interference and facilitation are compatible with an embodied account. Namely, they both indicate that language is grounded and that reading sentences leads to an activation of the motor system. However, so far it is difficult to make accurate predictions about the direction of the interaction between language and motor system. Models can help to further detail the predictions, for example, they can contribute to solve the IF issue.

4.6 Tentative Conclusions and Open Issues

In this chapter we have tried to show that embodied theories of cognitive science badly need models and that these models need to be embodied. In the first part we illustrated some behavioural experiments and showed that they can be reproduced only with embodied models. First, we reported experimental results that show that seeing an object activates its affordances, as it evokes potential actions to perform with it. Then, we described experimental evidence indicating that reading words and sentences activates the motor system – for example, reading the word "head" activates an upwards movement. In both cases we showed that the behaviour examined and the results found cannot be modelled with computational models that assume that the mind is a mechanism for symbol manipulation. Rather, adequate models can be given only by embodied artificial organisms that are endowed with neural and sensorimotor structures that at least roughly reproduce human ones.

In the second part we illustrated behavioural experiments leading to ambiguous results. As an example, we illustrated the controversial results that concern the relationship between language and the motor system – in some cases processing action-related words facilitates movements that are compatible with them, in other cases it renders them more difficult (interference vs. facilitation issue). We showed that embodied models can be a powerful means that helps to disentangle ambiguous issues and to formulate clearer predictions. The embodied cognition field has greatly expanded in the last years. In the last 10 years, much experimental evidence has been collected, but now it is crucial to formulate more detailed and precise predictions. Embodied cognition field badly needs for well-specified theories, and models can help to formulate these theories.

One last issue is worth of notice. At a very general level, embodied models might provide a powerful way to test embodied theories of cognition. Namely, comparing models whose physical (neural, sensorial, motor) structure is more or less similar to the human one will allow understanding to what extent possessing the same kind of "body" is necessary in order to understand the world and to comprehend and to use language.

From a theoretical point of view, the assumption of a very strong embodied view would lead to the avoidance of any kind of direct comparison between experiments and computer simulations. Namely, a strong embodied view could predict that only models that share the same bodily characteristics with the entities they have to reproduce (human beings) can be adequate to explain them. From this claim might derive the choice to consider the artificial world as a parallel word, with its own laws, that should (and could) not be compared with the world of human beings. Our position is that this claim can be made less strong, and a more mild embodied view can be adopted. Namely, it is possible that a certain degree of similarity between humans and their embodied models can allow capturing important aspects of human cognition and behaviour. One of the fascinating questions the research of the next years has to face is the following: To what extent do we need to be similar in body in order to share a common view of the world and to communicate with others? And again, to what extent (and for what aspects) do models need to resemble humans in order to be considered good models?

Bibliography

Barsalou, L. W. (1999). Perceptual Symbol Systems. *Behav. Brain Sci.* 22, 577–609.

Beauchamp, M. S., Lee, K. E., Argall, B. D., and Martin, A. (2004). Integration of auditory and visual information about objects in superior temporal sulcus. *Neuron* 41, 809–23.

Borghi, A. M., Bonfiglioli, C., Lugli, L., Ricciardelli, P., Rubichi, S., and Nicoletti, R. (2007). Are visual stimuli sufficient to evoke motor information? Studies with hand primes. *Neurosci. Lett.* 411, 17–21.

Buccino, G., Riggio, L., Melli, G., Binkofski, F., Gallese, V., and Rizzolatti, G. (2005). Listening to action related sentences modulates the activity of the motor system: A combined TMS and behavioral study. *Cogn. Brain Res.* 24, 355–63.

Caligiore, D., Borghi, A. M., Parisi, D., and Baldassarre, G. (2009). Affordances and compatibility effects: A neural-network computational model. In J. Mayor, N. Ruh, and K. Plunkett (Eds.), *Connectionist models of behaviour and cognition II: Proceedings of the 11th Neural Computation and Psychology Workshop* (pp. 15–26). Singapore: WorldScientific.

Damasio, A. R. (1989). Time-locked multiregional retroactivation: A systems-level proposal for the neural substrates of recall and recognition. *Cognition* 33, 25–62.

Ellis, R. and Tucker, M. (2000). Micro-affordance: The potentiation of components of action by seen objects. *Br. J. Psychol.* 91, 451–471.

Erlhagen, W. and Schöner, G. (2002). Dynamic field theory of motor preparation. *Psychol. Rev.* 109, 545–572.

Fodor J. (1975). *The language of thought*. Cambridge, MA: Harvard University Press.

Fogassi, L. and Gallese, V. (2004). Action as a binding key to multisensory integration. In G. Calvert, C. Spence, and B. E. Stein (Eds.), *Handbook of multisensory processes*. Cambridge: MIT Press.

Gallese, V., Fadiga, L., Fogassi, L., and Rizzolatti, G. (1996). Action recognition in the premotor cortex. *Brain* 119, 593–609.

Gallese, V., and Goldman, A. (1998). Mirror neurons and the simulation theory of mind reading. *Trends Cogn. Sci.* 2, 493–501.

Gallese, V. and Lakoff, G. (2005). The brain's concepts: The role of the sensorimotor system in conceptual knowledge. *Cogn. Neuropsychol.* 21, 455–479.

Jeannerod, M. (2007). *Motor cognition. What actions tell to the self.* Oxford: Oxford University Press.

Landauer, T. K. and Dumais, S.T. (1997). A solution to Plato's problem: The latent semantic analysis theory of acquisition, induction, and representation of knowledge. *Psychol. Rev.* 104, 211–240.

Martin, A., Wiggs, C. L, Ungerleider, L. G. and Haxby, G. V. (1996). Neural correlates of category specific knowledge. *Nature* 379, 649–652.

Martin, A. (2001). Functional neuroimaging of semantic memory. In R. Cabeza and A. Kingstone (Eds.), *Handbook of functional neuroimaging of cognition* (pp. 153–186). Cambridge: MIT Press.

Martin, A. and Chao, L. L. (2001). Semantic memory and the brain: Structure and processes. *Curr. Opin. Neurobiol.* 11, 194–201.

Miller, E. K. and Cohen, J. D. (2001). An integrative theory of prefrontal cortex function. *Ann. Rev. Neurosci.* 24, 167–202.

Milner, A. D., and Goodale, M. A. (1995). *The visual brain in action*. Oxford: Oxford University Press.

Pouget, A. and Latham, P. E. (2003). Population codes. In M. A. Arbib (Ed.), *The handbook of brain theory and neural networks* (2nd ed.). Cambridge, MA: The MIT Press.

Pulvermüller, F. (1999). Words in the brain's language. *Behav. Brain Sci.* 22, 253–336.

Pulvermüller, F. (2003). *The neuroscience of language: On brain circuits of words and serial order*. Cambridge: Cambridge University Press.

Rizzolatti, G. and Arbib, M. A. (1998). Language within our grasp. *Trends Neurosci.* 21, 188–194.

Scorolli, C. and Borghi, A. (2007). Sentence comprehension and action: Effector specific modulation of the motor system. *Brain res.* 1130, 119–124.

Scorolli, C., Borghi, A. M., and Glenberg, A. M. (2009). Language-induced motor activity in bimanual object lifting. *Exp. Brain Res.* 193, 43–53.

Simmons, W. K., Pecher, D., Hamann, S. B., Zeelenberg, R., and Barsalou, L. W. (2003). fMR evidence for modality-specific processing of conceptual knowledge on six modalities. *Meeting of the Society for Cognitive Neuroscience*, New York.

Tucker, M. and Ellis, R. (2001). The potentiation of grasp types during visual object categorization. *Vis. Cogn. 8*, 769–800.

Wermter, S., Weber, C., Elshaw, M., Panchev, C., Erwin, H., and Pulvermüller, F. (2004). Towards Multimodal Neural Robot Learning. *Robot. Autonom. Syst. J.* 47, 171–175.

Wermter, S., Weber, C., Elshaw, M., Gallese, V., and Pulvermüller, F. (2005). Grounding neural robot language in action. In S. Wermter, G. Palm, and M. Elshaw (Eds.), *Biomim. Neur. Learn. for Intelligent Robots* (pp. 162–181).

Chapter 5
Shared Culture Needs Large Social Networks

Luca De Sanctis and Stefano Ghirlanda

Abstract We report on a model for the emergence of shared cultural traits in a large group of individuals that imitate each other and interact in random social networks. The average size of the social network is shown to be a crucial variable ruling the emergence of a prevalent cultural trait shared by a majority of individuals. We distinguish between the case of a social network that changes while individuals develop their culture through the influence of others and the case of social networks which change slowly so that individuals reach a stable trait value before their social network changes appreciably. In both cases, no shared cultural trait emerges unless social network size is larger than a critical value. We also discuss how the formation of a shared cultural trait depends on the strength of mutual imitation, random factors that affect individuals' decisions, and external influences such as social institutions.

5.1 Introduction

One of the defining features of culture is it being shared among individuals (Kroeber 1952, Harris 1969). Many social and psychological factors influence the extent to which individuals in a group share "cultural traits," e.g., customs, beliefs, and artifacts. For instance, a group can maintain cultural traits more easily if social transmission is faithful rather than error prone (Enquist et al. 2008). How a group of individuals come to share the same cultural trait has been investigated in a number of theoretical models, e.g., about the formation of collective opinions (e.g., Schelling 1973, Thompson 1979, Durlauf 1999). These models often focus on a binary trait, such as whether to adopt a clothing item or not, or whether to favor or oppose a custom or a law. Crucially, and in agreement with social psychology (Byrne 1971, Grant 1993, Byrne 1997, Michinov and Monteil 2002), the models assume that individuals

L. De Sanctis (✉)
Department of Psychology and Mathematics, University of Bologna, Bologna, Italy
e-mail: luca.desanctis2@unibo.it

V. Capecchi (eds.), *Applications of Mathematics in Models, Artificial Neural Networks and Arts*, DOI 10.1007/978-90-481-8581-8_5,

have a tendency to imitate each other. If this tendency is strong enough, compared to other factors affecting decisions, the models predict that most individuals would make the same choice.

These results notwithstanding, many factors that potentially determine whether a group can share cultural traits remain unexplored. Here we investigate how sharing a cultural trait depends on the size of individuals' social networks, i.e., on the average number of individuals one interacts with. Thus our work follows a relatively recent interest in how features of social networks affect the collective properties of social groups, for instance, the spread of information within a group (Watts 2002). The main result we report in this chapter is that shared culture cannot exist unless social networks are larger than a critical size, which depends on how strongly individuals imitate each other.

5.2 Models

We refer to Contucci and Ghirlanda (2007) and Contucci et al. (this volume) for details of our modeling approach. We consider a group of N individuals, labeled by an integer $i = 1,..., N$. We focus on a single cultural trait that can have two forms, labeled +1 and –1. The trait value of individual i is indicated by s_i, while $s = \{S, \ldots, S_N\}$ indicates the trait configuration of the whole group. As an indicator of the extent to which individuals share the same form of the trait, we use the average trait value

$$m(s) = \frac{1}{N}\sum_{i=1}^{N} s_i \tag{5.1}$$

This quantity is 0 when the two forms of the trait are equally common. Deviation from zero, in either the positive or the negative direction, indicates that one form of the trait is more common than the other; when $m = \pm 1$, all individuals share the same form of the trait.

We assume that individuals tend to imitate each other, as it is well established in social psychology (Byrne 1971, Grant 1993, Byrne 1997, Michinov and Monteil 2002) and often assumed in models of social groups (e.g., Durlauf 1999, Contucci and Ghirlanda 2007, but see note 1). Because of this tendency, each individual can be seen as trying to minimize the extent to which she disagrees with others (note that it is not necessary to assume that this is a conscious process). Formally, we assume that each individual i intends to minimize the following measure of disagreement:

$$H_i(s) = -\sum_{j=1}^{N} J_{ij} s_i s_j \tag{5.2}$$

where Jij is the strength of the interaction between individuals i and j. Note that equation (5.2) is defined so that agreement ($s_i s_j = 1$) leads to a smaller value than does disagreement ($s_i s_j = -1$), given that $J_{ij} > 0$.[1] Therefore, a group of individuals will, as a whole, tend to minimize the function

$$H(s) = \sum_{i=1}^{N} H_i(s) = -\sum_{i,j}^{1,N} J_{ij} s_i s_j \tag{5.3}$$

Agreement with others, however, is not the only determinant of individual traits. Therefore we assume that individuals' tendency to agreement is contrasted by random "noise," which models influences on individual traits that are not explicitly considered, e.g., observation errors or spontaneous trait change. Formally, a configuration s has a probability of being attained that is proportional to $\exp(-H(s))$. Thus, a configuration s yielding a lower value of $H(s)$ has a higher probability of occurring. We denote the expected value of $m(s)$ with m according to such a probability distribution:

$$m = \frac{\sum_s m(s)\exp(-H(s))}{\sum_s \exp(-H(s))} \tag{5.4}$$

where the denominator is introduced to normalize the probability distribution.

Under the above assumptions, it is possible to calculate expected values of group-level quantities, such as equation (5.4), using the tools of statistical mechanics, a branch of theoretical physics (Thompson 1979). The result of these calculations depends crucially on the values of the J_{ij}s, i.e., the parameters that describe how individuals interact.

For instance, assuming

$$J_{ij} = J/N, \quad \forall i, j \tag{5.5}$$

means that individual tends to imitate any other individual. In this case one obtains the basic result recalled in the introduction; provided that $J > 1$, a majority of individuals will adopt the same form of the trait; the stronger the imitative interaction (larger J), the larger the majority. For $0 < J < 1$, on the other hand, the tendency to imitate others is too weak to create a majority of individuals with the same trait (Thompson 1979).

Here we want to investigate how sharing a cultural trait depends on the size of individuals' social networks. Thus we assume that each individual interacts only with some of her group fellows. To study this problem we assume

$$J_{ij} = J\nu_{ij} \tag{5.6}$$

where $J > 0$ is a common scale factor (cf. above) and the ν_{ij}s are independent Poisson variables with mean α/N, with α being a non-negative real number. This means

[1] In this chapter we consider only the case $J_{ij} \geq 0$. Negative values, however, can be used to describe a tendency to disagree with others, see Contucci et al. (this volume).

that, on average, an individual interacts with α individuals, chosen at random. It can be proved that many features of this model are independent of how the ν_{ij}s are distributed, provided some constraints on the mean and variance of the distribution are fulfilled (Starr and Vermesi 2007). In the following we focus on how the average trait value m depends on the average social network size α and on the strength of imitation J.

5.3 Results

We discuss the model under two assumptions about whether social networks can change or not. If social networks change fast, compared to the time it takes for individuals to settle on a given trait value, an individual will find herself into many different social networks before finally adopting a trait value. For example, in modern industrial societies, individuals may change acquaintances many times in their life through changes in school, job, location, and so on. On the other hand, it is also possible to study the case in which an individual's social networks do not change during the time required for the individual to stably adopt a trait value. As we will see below, these two cases share important similarities but also show some differences.

5.3.1 Fast-Changing Social Networks or Slowly Changing Traits

The main result in this case is that social network size must overcome a threshold before one form of the trait becomes more common than the other. Such a critical network size depends on the strength of imitation as follows:

$$\alpha_c = \frac{1}{2\tanh J} \tag{5.7}$$

which is illustrated in Fig. 5.1. Figure 5.2 (gray line) shows how the average trait value changes as a function of social network size. When $\alpha < \alpha_c$, the two trait values are equally common ($m = 0$). Thus if social networks are too small, no shared culture forms in this model. If $\alpha > \alpha_c$, the equilibrium in which the two trait values are equally common is replaced by two equilibria in which one form of the trait is more common than the other. As individuals' social networks get larger, more and more individuals share the same form of the trait.

5.3.2 Fixed Social Networks or Fast-Changing Traits

In the case of fixed (or slowly changing) social networks, it can be shown that social network size must exceed the same threshold as in the previous case, before one of

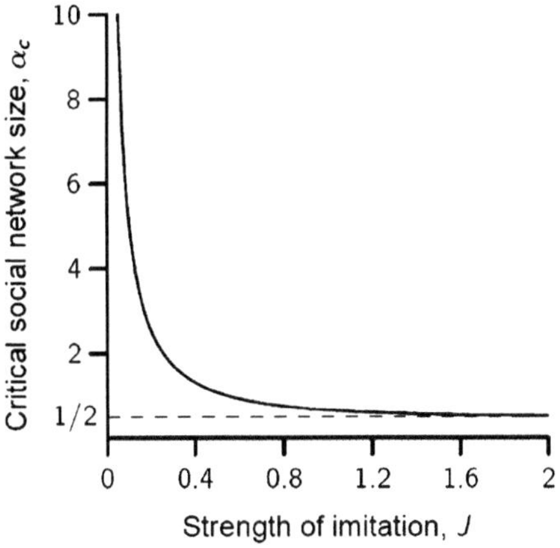

Fig. 5.1 Critical social network size vs. strength of imitation. The critical social network size is the value beyond which shared traits start to form, see Fig. 5.2

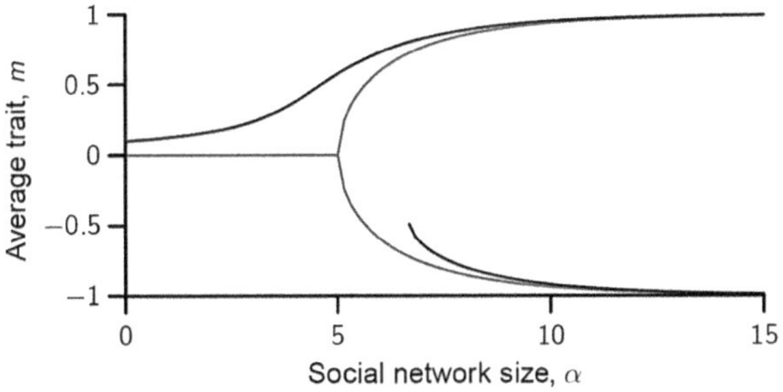

Fig. 5.2 *Gray line*: Average trait vs. social network size for a strength of imitation $J = 0.1$, resulting in a critical social network size of $\alpha_c \simeq 5$ [see equation (5.7)]. This result is obtained in the case of fast-changing social networks, but it is qualitatively similar for fixed social networks. In both cases, $m(\alpha) \sim (\alpha - \alpha_c)^{1/2}$ when α is slightly larger than α_c. *Black line*: The effect of an additional influence h on the average trait value. The figure is drawn for $J = 0.1$ and $h = 0.1$ [equation (5.9)]

the two trait values becomes more common than the other [equation (5.7)]. Also the average trait value depends on social network size in a similar way to the case of fast-changing social networks (Fig. 5.2, gray line).

A new feature, however, emerges; the group is organized in a core with a stable trait value and a periphery of small groups, loosely connected with the core and with unstable trait values. Whether or not an individual is part of the core depends on the size of her social network. Individuals whose social network is larger than $2\alpha_c$ will share the core trait value, while individuals with smaller social networks will show a fluctuating trait value (see Kolchin 1999 for an explanation of the geometry underlying this result).

5.3.3 Biased Traits and External Agencies

It is possible to study how other forces influence the average trait value by adding terms to equation (5.3). The following modification allows an additional influence h on each individual's trait:

$$H(s) = -\sum_{i,j}^{1,N} J_{ij}s_is_j - \sum_{i=1}^{N} h_is_i \tag{5.8}$$

If $h_i > 0$, then the value $s_i = 1$ is favored, if $h_i < 0$, then $s_i = -1$ is favored. The values h_i can be chosen, for instance, to describe individual preferences for one form of the trait. Here we treat the special case in which all h_is have the same value, and we assume for definiteness that the +1 form of the trait is favored. Thus we have $h_i = h > 0$:

$$H(s) = -\sum_{i,j}^{1,N} J_{ij}s_is_j - h\sum_{i=1}^{N} s_i \tag{5.9}$$

Such a situation can describe a uniform preference within the group, but also a case in which an external agency, such as an institution, promotes a particular trait (e.g., through advertisement or incentives). Two interesting effects of favoring one form of the trait over the other are shown in Fig. 5.2. First, most individuals in the group can adopt the favored trait value even when social network size is lower than would be required in the absence of the external influence. This means, for instance, that an institution can promote agreement within a group even when social networks within the group would not by themselves be sufficient to form the agreement. Second, a group of individuals with large social networks can maintain agreement on a trait that is opposed by the external influence. This is shown by the lower branch of the curve corresponding to $h = 0.1$ in Fig. 5.2 (see De Sanctis and Galla 2007 and references therein). These results have been derived analytically in the case of fast-changing social networks but are proven to be qualitatively similar for fixed social networks (De Sanctis and Guerra 2008).

5.4 Discussion

The models discussed above show that the size of social networks is an important determinant of whether a group of individuals can maintain a shared cultural trait. This result is potentially important to understand several aspects of cultural processes. For instance, it may contribute to explain why non-human primates seem unable to maintain large amounts of shared culture. Indeed, non-human primates usually learn from only a small set of individuals, often just the mother (Boesch et al. 1998). Another example concerns the formation of subcultures in contemporary societies. The basic problem here is that imitative interactions tend to erode cultural diversity. We may speculate, however, that individuals within a subgroup may maintain larger social networks within the subgroup itself than with the rest of the population. If the size of social networks external to the subgroup is small enough, it may be possible for a subgroup to maintain a different culture without completely severing ties with the rest of the population. The models above suggest that this may indeed be possible. If the subgroup is small, compared to the rest of the population, we may approximate the latter as a fixed external agency. In this case, we have seen that a subgroup with large social networks can maintain a trait value opposite to the one favored by the external agency (lower black curve in Fig. 5.2).

Acknowledgments Work supported by European Commission Contract FP6-2004-NEST-PATH-043434 (CULTAPTATION).

Appendix

Model Analysis

We are mainly interested in the expected value of the average trait defined in equation (5.1). This can be computed using the methods of statistical mechanics, a branch of theoretical physics (e.g., Thompson 1979). We summarize below a calculation given in full in De Sanctis and Guerra (2008). The statistical mechanical approach relies on calculating the so-called pressure of the model, from which group-level quantities can be easily computed. The average trait value m, for instance, can be computed as the derivative of the pressure with respect to the external influence h in equation (5.8).

The pressure is defined based on the function in equation (5.3). In the case of fixed social networks, the pressure is

$$A_N(\alpha, J, h) = \frac{1}{N}\mathbb{E}\ln\sum_s \exp(-H(s) - hNm(s)) \tag{5.10}$$

where $\mathbb{E}$ denotes expectation with respect to the random choice of individuals that interact and with respect to the values of the interactions; $\sum_s$ is the sum over all possible trait configurations. In the case of fast-changing social networks, the pressure is instead

$$\bar{A}_N(\alpha, J, h) = \frac{1}{N}\mathbb{E}_{\mathrm{v}} \ln \mathbb{E}_{\mathrm{I}}\sum_s \exp(-H(s) - hNm(s)) \tag{5.11}$$

where $\mathbb{E}_{\mathrm{I}}$ is the expectation with respect to the random choice of which individuals interact, and $\mathbb{E}_{\mathrm{v}}$ is the expectation with respect to the values of the interactions. The results discussed below for this model hold also if $\mathbb{E}_{\mathrm{v}}$ is moved inside the logarithm.

The case of fixed social networks is technically more challenging, and exact results are known only for sub-critical social network size or in the limit of large imitation strength. The model, however, is well understood by approximation techniques and numerical simulations. The case of fast-changing social networks is technically simpler, and we start from it to sketch the strategy for computing A and m. It is shown in De Sanctis and Guerra (2008) that equation (5.10) can be rewritten as

$$\bar{A}_N(\alpha,\beta) = \alpha \ln\cosh J + \frac{1}{N}\mathbb{E}_\nu \ln \sum_s \exp(K \ln(1 + m^2 \tanh J)) + Nhm)$$

where K is the Poisson random variable of mean αN. It is then convenient to define the function

$$f(m) = \ln(1 + m^2 \tanh\beta) \tag{5.12}$$

which is easily verified to be convex, that is

$$f(m) \geq f(M) + f'(M)(m - M)$$

for any given M. This allows to derive a lower bound for A by means of a trial function (easy to compute) depending on a trial value M, which is a fixed number and not a function of s. Notice also the following trivial identity:

$$\sum_M \delta_{mM} = 1$$

which instead allows to derive an upper bound for A, thanks to the obvious $\delta_{mM} \leq 1$, by means of the same trial function plus a correction which vanishes for increasingly large groups. Jointly, these bounds allow to compute A exactly for very large groups (formally, infinite). The result of this calculation is

$$\lim_{N\to\infty} \bar{A}_N(\alpha, J, h) = \sup_M \Bigg\{ \ln 2 + \alpha \ln\cosh J + \alpha \ln(1 + M^2 \tanh J) -$$

$$(2\alpha \tanh J)\frac{M^2}{1 + M^2 \tanh J} + \ln\cosh\left[(2\alpha \tanh J\frac{M}{1 + M^2 \tanh J} + h\right]\Bigg\}$$

for all values of α, J, h. The supremum condition implies

$$\frac{\mathrm{d}}{\mathrm{d}M}\left[\alpha f(M) - \alpha f'(M)M + \ln\cosh\alpha f'(M) + h\right] =$$
$$\alpha f''(M)[\tanh(\alpha f'(M) + h) - M] = 0$$

and yields the mean trait value $m = M$, which has to satisfy

$$m = \tanh\left[(2\alpha \tanh J)\frac{m}{1 + m^2 \tanh J} + h\right]$$

Let us consider for simplicity the case $h = 0$. It is easy to see that the only solution is $m = 0$ in the region

$$2\alpha \tanh J \leq 1$$

while two opposite non-zero solutions exist in the complementary region (Fig. 5.2). The model is hence solved, in the sense that we have an expression for A and (at least implicitly) for the mean opinion. The case $h > 0$ is illustrated graphically in Fig. 5.2.

Regarding the case of fixed social networks, it can be proved that A and $\bar{A}$ coincide and are equal to $\ln 2 + \ln \cosh J$ in the region where $2\alpha \tanh J \leq 1$, where the average trait value is 0. This is interpreted noticing that for sufficiently low α, individuals interact too little to influence each other enough so as to develop a common opinion, irrespective of whether social networks can or cannot change. In particular, notice that this is the case if $\alpha < 1/2$, for any strength of the mutual influence J. When $2\alpha \tanh J > 1$, then the two expressions (5.10) and (5.11) differ from $\ln 2 + \ln \cosh J$ and from one another. In both cases, if m (the positive solution, for instance) is 0 in the interval $[0, 1/2 \tanh J]$, then it deviates from 0 and reaches a certain asymptotic value as $J \rightarrow \infty$, i.e., when only the imitative process counts and two connected individuals align their opinion with probability 1. Even in this case, however, not all individuals have the same trait value, i.e., $m < 1$ unless social networks are very large (formally $\alpha \rightarrow \infty$).

The expression for the average trait is different in the case of fixed social networks, but the behavior is qualitatively the same in both models. An implicit expression for the mean opinion in the rigid model is known in the limit $J \rightarrow \infty$, where m is such that

$$m(\alpha) = 1 - \exp(- 2\alpha m(\alpha))$$

which coherently exhibits a critical value $a = 1/2$, below which m is equal to 0, and above which it is different from 0.

Lastly, we note that if we let $\alpha \rightarrow \infty$, $J \rightarrow 0$ with $2\alpha \tanh J = J'$ kept constant, both models reduce to a very simple one, in which all individuals agree on the same trait value as $J' \rightarrow \infty$, and if $J' \leq 1$, they do not agree at all ($m = 0$). This limiting model is in fact equivalent to the basic model of collective agreement mentioned in the main text [cf. Section 5.1 and text around equation (5.5)].

Bibliography

Boesch, C. M., Tomasello, B. R. W., Galef, B. G. J., Ingold, T. , McGrew, W. C., Paterson, J. D. and W. A. (1998). Chimpanzee and human cultures (with comments and reply). *Curr. Anthropol.* 39, 591–614.

Byrne, D. (1971). *The attraction paradigm.* New York: Academic Press.

Byrne, D. (1997). An overview (and underview) of research and theory within the attraction paradigm. *J. Personal. Social Psychol.* 14, 417–431.

Contucci, P., Gallo, I., and Ghirlanda, S. (2008). Equilibria of cultural contact from in- and out-group attitudes.

Contucci, P. and Ghirlanda, S. (2007). Modeling society with statistical mechanics: an application to cultural contact and immigration. *Qual. Quan.*, 41, 569–578.

De Sanctis, L. and Galla, T. (2007). Effects of noise and confidence thresholds in nominal and metric Axelrod dynamics of social influence. ArXiv:0707.3428v1.

De Sanctis, L. and Guerra, F. (2008). Mean field dilute ferromagnet I. High temperature and zero temperature behavior. ArXiv:0801.4940v2.

Durlauf, S. N. (1999). How can statistical mechanics contribute to social science?'. *Proc. Natl. Acad. Sci. USA*. 96, 10582–10584.

Enquist, M., Ghirlanda, S., Jarrick, A., and Wachtmesiter, C.-A. (2008). Cultural capacities and the logic of cumulative cultural evolution. Submitted to *Theoretical Population Biology*.

Grant, P. R. (1993). Reactions to intergroup similarity: examination of the similarity-differentiation and the similarity-attraction hypotheses. *Can. J. Behav. Sci.* 25, 28–44.

Harris, M. (1969). *The Rise of Anthropological Theory*. London: Routledge & Kegan Paul.

Kolchin, V. K. (1999). *Random graphs*. Cambridge: Cambridge University Press.

Kroeber, A. L. (1952). The concept of culture in science. *J. Gen. Edu.* I II, 182–196.

Michinov, E. and Monteil, J.-M. (2002). The similarity-attraction relationship revisited: divergence between affective and behavioral facets of attraction. *Europ. J. Soc. Psychol.* 32, 485–500.

Schelling, T. C. (1973). Hockey helmets, concealed weapons, and daylight saving: A study of binary choices with externalities. *J. Conflict Resol.* 17, 381–428.

Starr, S. L. and Vermesi, B. (2007). Some observations for mean-field spin glass models. ArXiv:0707.0031.

Thompson, C. (1979). *Mathematical statistical mechanics*. Princeton, NJ: Princeton University Press.

Watts, D. J. (2002). A simple model of information cascades on random networks. *Proc. Natl. Acad. Sci. USA*. 99, 5766–5771.

Chapter 6
Mathematical Models of Financial Markets

Claudio Gallo

6.1 Introduction

As in many fields of science, mathematics plays a major role also in finance. Spanning from macroeconomic analysis to portfolio management, from market trend evaluation/prediction to risk management, mathematics is the most powerful tool for making quantitative evaluations in finance. A huge amount of work has been done in this field, as testified by the amount of books, papers and PhD theses that can be found in the literature.

In this context, this chapter provides an overview on some fruitful applications of mathematical modelling to financial topics. These applications have had and still have a wide impact on society (investment funds, insurances, market movements, etc.). Here, some issues regarding financial modelling are briefly discussed. At first, the focus is on the use of mathematics for building predictive models for financial market trend. Quantitative predictions have a direct consequence both on asset allocation and on the risk to which a portfolio is exposed. Then, the basic concepts regarding risk modelling are described by introducing the classical VaR models. Since risk has not only to be estimated but also to be limited, proper investment strategies aimed at decouple portfolio return from the market trend are mentioned. This is obtained through "hedging" which is the key factor for both large and small portfolios. In particular, the main ideas regarding cointegration and its collaborative application with pair-trading strategies are viewed as an important alternative for building home-made hedging strategies for small capitals.

C. Gallo (✉)
Imaging & Numerical Geophysics, Energy & Environment Department, Center for Advanced Studies, Research and Development in Sardinia (CRS4), Pula CA, Italy
e-mail: fender@crs4.it

V. Capecchi (eds.), *Applications of Mathematics in Models, Artificial Neural Networks and Arts*, DOI 10.1007/978-90-481-8581-8_6,

6.2 Models for Financial Market Predictions

The possibility of predicting financial market trends represents the chimaera for every trader/investor since the beginning of times. The capability of predicting market evolution would imply the possibility of achieving maximum investment profits. As nobody owns the crystal ball, different approaches have been developed and applied by traders, investors, fund managers and economists: (1) technical analysis; (2) statistical correlations; (3) quantitative analysis; (4) econophysics; (5) fundamental analysis; (6) fractal analysis; (7) physical similitude; (8) nonlinear analysis; (9) astrological analysis; and (10) others. This list includes only most known techniques and many books are available in the literature on these methods. Although some readers may be sceptical regarding some of them, it should be kept in mind that the objective of the modeller is the match between predictions and actual market data.

Let us take a step further. Suppose we have developed our "market prediction machine" and implemented a suitable asset allocation strategy according to the machine prediction. Our portfolio is now exposed to market oscillations. This implies a risk of big losses, as we have no guarantees that our prediction is correct. How big is the risk we are exposing to? Is it measurable? Apart from market prediction accuracy, risk is not generally an easily measurable quantity for a number of reasons: market phenomena are nonlinear, generally not Gaussian, and not fully stochastic. It is important to bear in mind that when evaluating risk, we may choose different definitions which would lead to different results:

- Risk can be defined as the probability of occurrence of a negative event (this is called the "optimistic" formulation and this is what financial promoters use when trying to convince investors to subscribe a particular financial instrument they sell)
- Risk can be defined as the probability of occurrence of a negative event multiplied by the extent of the damage caused (this is the pessimistic formulation, i.e. the risk considered in an a posteriori fashion)

Risk evaluation has become a hot topic in recent years due to globalization of financial markets, increase of market volatility and explosive growth of financial derivatives. Risk managers work to estimate the minimum amount of capital required to cover portfolio potential losses. VAR (value at risk, Jorion 2001) models are a widely known statistical tool for risk evaluation and accepted by the new Basilea 2 rules (Bank of International Settlements 2004). These models are based on an analysis of the price time series of the financial instruments composing the asset of the portfolio. The VaR is defined as the maximum loss not exceeded with a given probability defined as the confidence level, over a given period of time. According to "quantitative risk management" (McNeil et al. 2005: 38), given some confidence level $\alpha \in (0,1)$, the VaR of the portfolio at the confidence level α is given by the smallest number l such that the probability that the loss L exceeds l is not larger than $(1 - \alpha)$:

$$VaR_\alpha = \inf\{l \in \Re : P(L > l) \leq 1 - \alpha\} = \inf\{l \in \Re : F_L(l) \geq \alpha\} \tag{6.1}$$

In probabilistic terms VaR is a quantile of the loss distribution. VaR is widely applied in finance for quantitative risk management for many types of risk. VaR, however, does not give any information about the severity of loss by which it is exceeded. Furthermore, this formula is used assuming that market movement is a Gaussian process. However, real markets teach (see, for example, the book of Taleb 2003 or the book of Dunbar 2000) that the probability of occurrence of "extreme" events is much higher than that predicted by Gaussian models. Thus, a modified version of the VAR model, the so-called modVaR, has been introduced in order to account for the third and fourth moments of the yield distribution. Modified VARs provide sensitive differences from the classical VaR only for abrupt market movements of the market, while no significant difference appears under standard conditions. VARs and VAR-like models, however, do not chase the problem of reducing the risk of asset allocation. This can be achieved by exploiting some specific allocation strategies, as described below.

The SHORT Investment: One way to circumvent the risk of market crash is the use of short selling with which investors can speculate on market descents. On the one hand, this seems to be a parachute on market crashes. On the other hand, we are exposing ourselves to the risk of virtually unlimited loss (imagine you have sold MICROSOFT at the end of 1998, etc.). Thus, short selling can ride market descents, but the problem of following wrong predictions is still unsolved.

6.3 Exiting from the Trend

The risk of undergoing big losses due to inaccuracy of market predictions under both ascending and descending trends is a real problem. The so-called black swans, namely, unexpected and violent market movements, may cause portfolio default. Furthermore, as discussed by Taleb (2003), the probability of extreme events is generally much higher than that predicted by the classical Gaussian model. More suitable statistical distributions should be used such as lognormal, Pareto–Levy, that is, fat-tail distributions. But let us go back to the main objective. Is it possible to operate in order to reduce the risk of large losses or portfolio default? We may reformulate the question as follows: Is it possible to allocate an asset whose behaviour is independent from the ongoing trend? This would imply that we are freed from the problem of making reliable predictions. The solution to our problem can be condensed in the following word: "hedging". A hedge is an investment that is taken out specifically to reduce or cancel out the risk in another investment. Hedging is a strategy designed to minimize exposure to an unwanted business risk, while still allowing the business to profit from an investment activity. It is not in the purpose of this work to describe in detail the characteristics of hedging strategies. It is worthy of giving some information of the following financial instruments widely used in hedging:

- Options, that are special contracts defined as right but not the obligation, to buy (for a call option) or sell (for a put option) a specific amount of a given stock, commodity, currency, index or debt, at a specified price (the strike price) during a specified period of time.
- Combined LONG and SHORT strategies implemented on the basis of significant statistical relationships.

Basic Ideas on Options: According to the given definition, an option can be viewed as a sort of insurance that will cover the losses of counter-trend investments. Although the concept is easy to understand, the correct evaluation of the price of an option is a complicated task. This depends on the time to expiration, market volatility (the range of oscillation of the price within a given time period – the wider the price variation, the higher the volatility) and risk-free interest rate. The initial formula for the correct pricing of options was given by Fisher Black and Myron Scholes (1973) for which they were appointed the Nobel Prize. Then, further studies contributed to develop this formula to adapt it to different financial products such as futures, stocks, commodities. The price of the underlying stock S_t is assumed to follow a geometric Brownian motion with constant drift μ and volatility σ (Black and Scholes 1973):

$$dS_t = \mu S_t\, dt + \sigma S_t\, dW_t \tag{6.2}$$

Other assumptions are needed: (1) It is possible to short sell the underlying stock; (2) there are no arbitrage opportunities; (3) trading in the stock is continuous; (4) there are no transaction costs or taxes; (5) all securities are perfectly divisible (e.g. it is possible to buy 1/100th of a share); (6) it is possible to borrow and lend cash at a constant risk-free interest rate; (7) the stock does not pay a dividend. The above lead to the following formula for the price of a European call option with exercise price K on a stock currently trading at price S, i.e. the right to buy a share of the stock at price K after T years. The constant interest rate is r and the constant stock volatility is σ

$$C(S, T) = S\Phi(d_1) - Ke^{-rT}\Phi(d_2) \tag{6.3}$$

where

$$d_1 = \frac{\ln(S/K) + (r + \sigma^2/2)T}{\sigma\sqrt{T}}$$

$$d_2 = \frac{\ln(S/K) + (r + \sigma^2/2)T}{\sigma\sqrt{T}} = d_1 - \sigma\sqrt{T}$$

Here Φ is the standard normal cumulative distribution function. Similarly, the price of a put option reads as follows:

$$P(S, T) = Ke^{-rT}\Phi(-d_2) - S\Phi(-d_1) \tag{6.4}$$

The above formula is not easy to handle and it holds only under ideal conditions. More complicated and closer-to-real-market formulas have been derived by testing the initial model on real data. When managing a complete portfolio with hundreds of positions with different financial instruments such as stocks, futures, currencies and options, the complexity of hedging operations becomes huge.

LONG and SHORT Combined Trades: This discipline has achieved increasing importance in last two decades as soon as computers have become more and more powerful. It applies mathematics, statistics, and other stochastic calculus to finance in order to find correlations and other relationships that could be exploited in asset allocation. Generally, quantitative analysts exploit market divergences, that is transient perturbations of an underlying equilibrium or situations that starting from contingent situation evolve naturally towards a "minimum" energy status, such as the bond yield curves; the expiration of an option (short selling of option); shares of companies that work in the same sector but give a feedback of the underlying (see, for example, the case of the stock EXXON and TOTAL giving a response to crude-oil price variations). Also in this case, the planning of portfolio strategies based on financial engineering requires a big computational effort and almost real-time corrections of the asset allocation. This type of analyses requires a strong mathematical and computational background. Famous hedge funds are managed by skilled risk managers and asset-allocation gurus, but this may not be enough for guaranteeing profit and capital preservation. Actually, hedge fund results are various and span between great successes to complete defaults. Two famous examples of hedge-fund defaults are the long-term capital management fund (LTCM) whose default occurred in 1997 has been well documented in the book of Dunbar (2000) and the default of the Amaranth fund that went on default due to an excessive exposition to natural gas open positions. Thus, we conclude that even when we put our money in theoretically safe investments we cannot make risk disappear completely.

In the next paragraph, the basic ideas of a recent investment approach are presented. This is aimed at introducing an interesting alternative for small investors to implement their own home-made hedging-oriented strategy. This approach is based on the binomial cointegration and pair trading.

6.4 Cointegration and Pair Trading

Where does the term "cointegration" come from? This was formulated in the early 1970s for the first time by Prof. Clive Granger who was awarded the Nobel Prize for economy in 2003 for his research on cointegration (Engle and Granger 1987, Engle and Lee 1999). But what is cointegration? To introduce this concept, we may start with the simple example of a man taking his dog out for a walk (Fig. 6.1).

Consider how the man and his pet are moving: their centre of mass follows a straight path, while the two trajectories are sort of random walk. This type of

Fig. 6.1 Sketch of the path of the man–dog system

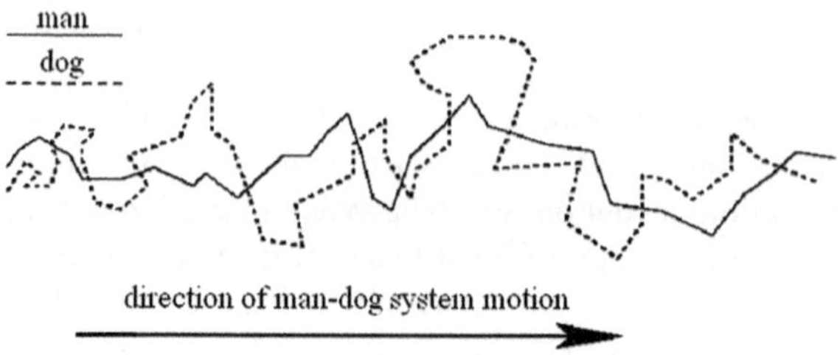

reciprocal movement can be found in a number of couples of stocks, futures and commodities. The components of the couple seem to act independently when considered separately, but they show a cointegrated behaviour when considered in couples.

An interesting example is shown in Fig. 6.2 where the daily "close" historical series of two insurance Italian bluechips, Alleanza and Generali, are shown (prices of Alleanza are normalized to make it comparable with Generali). Based on what we see from Fig. 6.2, we may informally define cointegration as *a statistical characteristic relating two (or more) historical series whose properly weighted sum follows a straight trajectory*. The verification of existence of cointegration (Boswijk 1995) between two time series is quite complicated (the interested reader is addressed to the bibliography of this work for further reading). It is worth mentioning that cointegration requires a precondition to be verified. Time series that are liable to be linked by cointegration must be unit root (Dickey and Fuller 1979, Phillips and Perron 1988). A time series is said to be integrated of order 1 (namely, unit root and indicated as $I(1)$), if, although not having constant average and variance, the time series obtained calculating its first-order difference is $I(0)$ (namely, the series is integrated

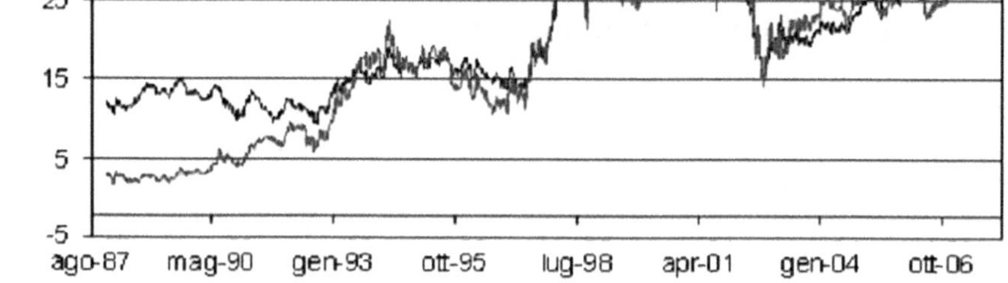

Fig. 6.2 Plot of the prices of Generali and Alleanza (normalized)

of zero order), that is, both its average and variance are constant. This concept may be translated directly in terms of stock market: historical prices can be considered as $I(1)$ if the derived yield series is $I(0)$.

If cointegration (Harris 1995, Harris and Sollis 2003) holds, we can rely on a statistical support for the existence of a strong correlation between two stocks. Thus, we can apply a pair-trading strategy (Ross 1995, Ganapathy 2004, Gallo and Acheri 2007). What is peculiar of this type of strategy is that two opposite positions are opened simultaneously, that is, if we go LONG for one stock we go SHORT for its cointegrated companion. It has to be remarked that verifying the existence of cointegration is crucial for the success of the pair-trading strategy because it gives a statistical guarantee that our expectation that the "liason" between the two stocks verified on the base of past history will probably hold also in the future.

6.5 Final Remarks

Mathematical modelling of financial markets is not a trivial business, although it is achieving increasing attention. Several topics have been considered in this work. Mathematical models for predicting market evolution have become highly sophisticated, but they imply a trend-following asset allocation. If the prediction results to be wrong we happen to be positioned against the ongoing trend and we may incur in big losses or even at default. This caused risk analysis and modelling to become one of the milestones of financial management. In this context, VaR and VaR-derived models have become fundamental in every financial context. Banks and fund managers apply these models for calculating the amount of liquidity needed for bounding potential portfolio losses to a certain percentage with a given confidence level. Although risk evaluation is important, the importance of hedging has been stressed. Several approaches and techniques have been mentioned to diminish the risk. These are aimed at making our portfolio market trend independent. Options and pair-trading techniques have been seen as examples of market neutral techniques. In particular, pair trading seems to be a suitable technique for home-made hedge fund-like strategies for managing also small portfolios. To this aim, the basics of cointegration have been overviewed in the framework of pair trading. Due to its characteristics, cointegration is seen to be crucial for setting up a LONG–SHORT strategy by giving a statistical support to the expectations that two "coupled" stocks will continue to show a correlated trend in the future. This is exactly what we do expect when we implement a trading strategy based on its passed history.

Bibliography

Bank of International Settlements (June 2004). *International convergence of capital measurement and capital standard – A revised framework.* Press & Communications CH-4002 Basel, Switzerland.

Black, F. and Scholes, M (1973). The pricing of options and corporate liabilities. *J. Polit. Econ.* 813, 637–654.

Boswijk, P. H. (1995). *Identifiability of cointegrated systems*. Technical Report, Tinbergen Institute.
Dickey, D. A. and Fuller, W. A. (1979). Distribution of the estimators for autoregressive time series with a unit root. *J. Am. Stat. Assoc*. 74, 427–431.
Dunbar, N. (2000). *Inventing money: The story of long-term capital management and the legends behind it.* Wiley & Sons.
Engle, R. F. and Granger, C. W. J. (1987). Co-integration and error correction: Representation, estimation, and testing. *Econometrica* 55, 251–276.
Engle, R. and Lee, G. J. (1999). A permanent and transitory component model of stock return volatility. In R. Engle and H. White, (Eds.), *Cointegration, causality, and forecasting: A festschrift in honor of Clive W. J. Granger*, Oxford University Press, 475–497.
Gallo, C. and Acheri, A. (2007). *Cointegration for pair trading – Principi e Analisi di Cointegrazione per la Speculazione Finanziaria con il Metodo del Pair-Trading*. Casa editrice: Lulu (www.lulu.com).
Ganapathy, V. (2004). *Pairs trading: Quantitative methods and analysis*. Wiley & Sons.
Harris, R. I. D. (1995). *Using cointegration analysis in econometric modelling*. Prentice Hall.
Harris, R. and Sollis, R. (Eds.) (2003). *Applied time series modelling and forecasting*. Wiley & Sons.
Jorion, P, (2001). *Value at Risk: The new benchmark for managing financial risk*, 2nd ed., McGraw-Hill Trade.
McNeil, A. J., Frey, R. and Embrechts, P. (2005). *Quantitative risk management: Concepts, techniques, and tools.* Princeton University Press.
Phillips, P. C. B. and Perron, P. (1988). Testing for a unit root in time series regression. *Biometrika* 75, 335–346.
Ross, J. (1995). *Trading spread & seasonals*. Ross Trading.
Taleb, N. (2003). *Giocati dal caso*. Casa editrice: il Saggiatore.

Chapter 7
Tackling Climate Change Through Energy Efficiency: Mathematical Models to Offer Evidence-Based Recommendations for Public Policy

Federico Gallo, Pierluigi Contucci, Adam Coutts, and Ignacio Gallo

Abstract Promoting and increasing rates of energy efficiency is a promising method of reducing CO_2 emissions and avoiding the potentially devastating effects of climate change. The question is: How do we induce a cultural or a behavioural change whereby people nationally and globally adopt more energy-efficient lifestyles?

We propose a new family of mathematical models, based on a statistical mechanics extension of discrete choice theory, that offer a set of formal tools to systematically analyse and quantify this problem. An application example is to predict the percentage of people choosing to buy new energy-efficient light bulbs instead of the old incandescent versions; in particular, through statistical evaluation of survey responses, the models can identify the key driving factors in the decision-making process, for example, the extent to which people imitate each other. These tools and models that allow us to account for social interactions could help us identify tipping points that may be used to trigger structural changes in our society. The results may provide tangible and deliverable evidence-based policy options to decision makers.

We believe that these models offer an opportunity for the research community, in both the social and the physical sciences, and decision makers, both in the private and the public sectors, to work together towards preventing the potentially devastating social, economic and environmental effects of climate change.

7.1 Introduction

Climate change is one of the greatest environmental, social and political challenges facing humankind. In order to avoid and prevent climate change, we need to significantly reduce global CO_2 and greenhouse gas emissions over the next couple of

---

P. Contucci (✉)
Department of Mathematics, University of Bologna, Bologna, Italy; Centre for the Study of Cultural Evolution, Stockholm University, Stockholm, Sweden
e-mail: contucci@dm.unibo.it

V. Capecchi (eds.), *Applications of Mathematics in Models, Artificial Neural Networks and Arts*, DOI 10.1007/978-90-481-8581-8_7,

decades. Energy efficiency offers a method by which this can be achieved and that offers a number of social and economic advantages. For example, it does not require us to reduce our standard of living and could result in significant financial savings.

Therefore, we are faced with an enormous problem: Can we achieve a national and global cultural, behavioural change – structural change – whereby people decide, out of their own volition, to adopt more energy-efficient behaviours and lifestyles? The purpose of this chapter is to present a tool that will help decision makers achieve this goal, in particular, to induce our society to make a transition towards a sustainable way of life.

For the sake of analysis, one may view this issue as a binary choice problem; nationally or globally a population may choose to either continue an energy-inefficient lifestyle or replace it with an energy-efficient one. One key difficulty with this problem statement is that it is too vague and general. However, we can overcome this difficulty by breaking the problem into smaller, more tractable, components that can be clearly specified, quantified and attacked.

Figure 7.1 shows a schematic illustration of the approach. As an example, we could focus on energy efficiency measures and view them individually as binary choices, for instance, buying new energy-efficient light bulbs instead of the energy-guzzling incandescent bulbs. In this way, the apparently intractable problem of shifting our society's behaviour from an energy-inefficient lifestyle to sustainable one is reduced to simpler problems such as inducing people in *specific geographical areas* and from *specific socio-economic backgrounds* to change *specific choices*, such as buying energy-efficient bulbs.

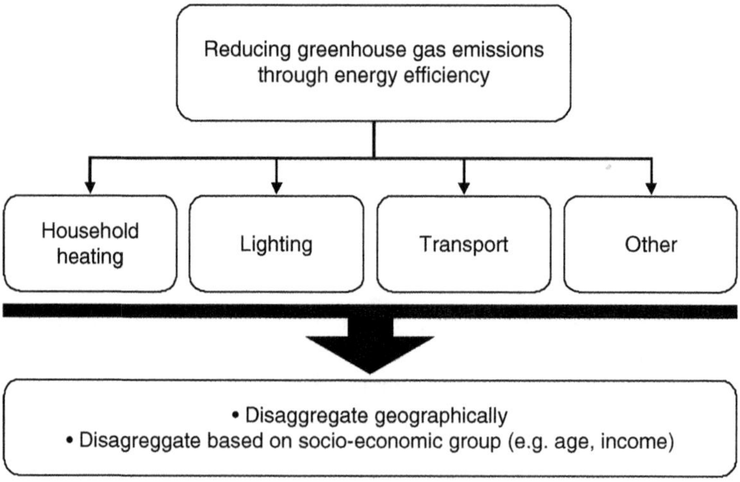

Fig. 7.1 Schematic illustration of how the goal of achieving a global culture change may be broken into smaller components that are easier to analyse. The models presented in this chapter offer a rigorous, quantitative methodology to obtain the evidence to inform policy makers

The purpose of this chapter is to introduce a new multidisciplinary "family" of models that may help policy makers tackle the above problem. In particular, these models may help decision makers adopt policy options that will induce widespread behaviour change, and perhaps even structural or cultural change. To this end, this family of models offers two specific tools to decision makers:

1. First, *a framework to systematically deconstruct this apparently intractable problem into smaller more manageable pieces*, as shown in Fig. 7.1. This would allow researchers to focus on and analyse one specific problem at the time: find the most relevant policy option and then move to the next problem. It is important to note that this is also possible because these choices are generally independent of each other, for example, the choice of buying energy-efficient light bulbs may be assumed to be independent of the mode of transport used to go to work.
2. Second, these models offer a *rigorous and quantitative bottom-up tool* to identify and understand the key incentives that drive people's decisions. As will be shown in the following sections, the end product of this analysis is a formula – known as a utility function that describes people's preferences in a given context. This formula can be designed so that it includes variables, or policy levers, that decisions makers can manipulate to induce behaviour change. An example could be the level of taxation on a given consumer product, say energy-efficient light bulbs. As will be explained later in more detail, this utility function is obtained empirically from data.

The remainder of this chapter is structured as follows. Section 7.2 introduces the behavioural models. Section 7.3 provides details of energy efficiency in the context of climate change and gives further evidence of the benefits of using the above behavioural models in this context. Finally, Section 7.4 concludes and proposes some ideas for further research.

7.2 Behavioural Models: Beyond "Rational Man" and *Homo Economicus*

This section presents a family of behavioural models that can be directly applied to the above-stated problem of increasing energy efficiency through behaviour change. These models have been developed to overcome the main limitations of the *Homo Economicus* or "Rational Man" model (Persky 1995), including the following:

3. Access to limited information and emotions and
4. Imitation and social interactions.

Section 7.2.1 gives an overview of discrete choice theory, which is an econometric tool that has been used for over three decades to understand people's preferences in issues ranging from transport to health care. This model not only describes the

Predicted Share	**55.8%**	**22.9%**	**14.9%**	**6.3%**
(Std. Error)	*(11.4%)*	*(10.7%)*	*(3.7%)*	*(2.5%)*
Actual Share	**59.9%**	**21.7%**	**12.2%**	**6.2%**

Fig. 7.2 Discrete predictions against actual use of travel modes in San Francisco, 1975 (Source: McFadden 2001)

Table 7.1 Prediction success table, journey to work (pre-BART model and post-BART choices)

Cell counts		Predicted choices			
Actual choices	Auto alone	Carpool	Bus	BART	Total
Auto alone	255.1	79.1	28.5	15.2	378
Carpool	74.7	37.7	15.7	8.9	137
Bus	12.8	16.5	42.9	4.7	77
BART	9.8	11.1	6.9	11.2	39
Total	352.4	144.5	94.0	40.0	631

rational aspects of human choice but also accounts for factors such as emotions or imperfect information.

The following section presents a more recent extension of this model that allows us to rigorously account for imitation in human behaviour, including social norms and peer pressure. Based on well-established theories in mathematical physics, these models predict the existence of tipping points and structural changes (see Fig. 7.2). This could potentially be used to devise highly cost-effective social policies to induce cultural change as well as behaviour change at the individual level. For example, we may find that a small subsidy on the costs of cavity wall insulation may induce enough people to change their behaviour and hit a critical mass whereby, through imitation, suddenly a large fraction of the population decide to insulate their homes just because their societal peers seem to be doing it.

7.2.1 Bounded Rationality and Emotion: Discrete Choice Analysis

Discrete choice analysis is a well-established research tool that has been applied to real social phenomena for more than 30 years. Due to the development of this theory, Daniel McFadden was awarded the Nobel Prize in Economics in 2000, for bringing economics closer to quantitative scientific measurement. Figure 7.2 shows an example where the model prediction was 98% accurate.

The purpose of discrete choice is to describe people's behaviour. It is an econometric technique to infer people's preferences based on empirical data.

In discrete choice the decision maker is assumed to make choices that maximise their own benefit. Their "benefit" is described by a mathematical formula, a utility function, which is derived from data collected in surveys. This utility function includes rational preferences but accounts for elements that deviate from rational behaviour.

Discrete choice models, however, do not account for "peer pressure" or "herding effects"; individual decisions are assumed to be driven by influences such as prices of goods and overall quality of services. In other words, discrete choice assumes that people's decisions are unaffected by the choices made by other people. We shall see in Section 7.2.2, however, that there are good reasons, both empirical and theoretical, to believe that mutual influence between people themselves might have a crucial and quantifiable role in the overall behaviour of society.

It is nonetheless a fact that the standard performance of discrete choice models is close to optimal for the analysis of many phenomena where peer influence is perhaps not a major factor in an individual's decision; Fig. 7.3 shows an example of this. Figure 7.2 compares predictions and actual data concerning the use of travel modes before and after the introduction of new rail transport system called BART in San Francisco, 1975. We see a remarkable agreement between the predicted share of people using BART (6.3%) and the actual measured figure after the introduction of the service (6.2%).

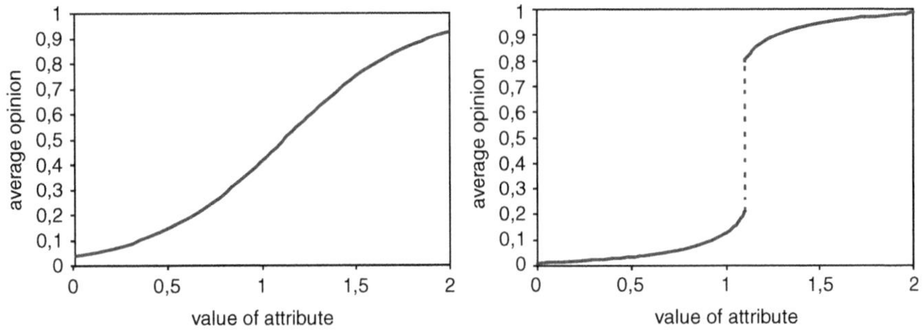

Fig. 7.3 The diagram on the right illustrates how structural changes are unavoidably linked to the interactions between decision makers. This is a fundamental improvement in traditional discrete choice analysis

7.2.1.1 Theory

In discrete choice, each decision process is described mathematically by a utility function, which each individual seeks to maximize. As an example, a binary choice could be to either cycle to work or catch a bus. The utility function for choosing the bus may be written as follows:

$$U = \sum_a \beta_a x_a + \sum_a \lambda_a y_a + \varepsilon \tag{7.1}$$

The variables x_a are attributes that describe the alternatives, for example, the bus fare or the journey time. On the other hand, y_a are socio-economic variables that define the decision maker, for example, their age, gender or income. It is this latter set of parameters that allows us to zoom in on specific geographical areas or socio-economic groups.

The β_a and λ_a are parameters that need to be estimated empirically, through survey data. The key property of these parameters is that they quantify the relative importance of any given attribute in a person's decision; the larger its value is, the more this will affect a person's choice. For example, we may find that certain people are more affected by the journey time than the bus fare; therefore changing the fare may not influence their behaviour significantly. Section 7.2.1.2 will explain how the value of these parameters is estimated from empirical data.

It is an observed fact (Luce and Suppes 1965, Ariely 2008) that choices are not always perfectly rational. For example, someone who usually goes to work by bus may one day decide to cycle instead. This may be because it was a nice sunny day, or for no particular reason. This unpredictable component of people's choices is accounted for by the random term ϵ.

The functional distribution of ϵ may be assumed to be of different forms, giving rise to different possible models; if, for instance, ϵ is assumed to be normal, the resulting model is called a *probit* model, and it does not admit a closed-form solution.

Discrete choice analysis assumes ϵ to be extreme-value distributed, and the resulting model is called a *logit* model (Ben-Akiva and Lerman 1985). In practice this is very convenient as it does not impose any significant restrictions on the model but simplifies it considerably from a practical point of view. In particular, it allows us to obtain a closed-form solution for the probability of choosing a particular alternative, say catching a bus rather than cycling to work:

$$P = \frac{e^V}{1 - e^V} \tag{7.2}$$

where V is the deterministic part of the utility U in equation (7.1), i.e.

$$V = \sum_a \beta_a x_a + \sum_a \lambda_a y_a$$

In words, this describes the rational preferences of the decision maker.

As will be explained later on, equation (7.2) is analogous to the equation describing the equilibrium state of a perfect gas of heterogeneous particles; just like gas particles react to external forces differently depending, for instance, on their mass and charge, discrete choice describes individuals as experiencing heterogeneous influences in their decision making, according to their own socio-economic attributes, such as gender and wealth. This offers a mathematical and intuitive link between econometrics and physics, more specifically statistical mechanics. The importance of this "lucky coincidence" cannot be overstated, and some of the implications will be discussed later on in more detail.

7.2.1.2 Empirical Estimation

Discrete choice may be seen as a purely empirical model. The utility function given by equation (7.1) is very general; it may be seen as describing the decision process of an archetypal human being. In order to specify the actual functional form associated with a specific group of people facing a specific choice, empirical data are needed. The actual utility function is then specified by estimating the numerical values of the parameters β_a and λ_a. As mentioned earlier, these parameters quantify the relative importance of the attribute variables x_a and y_a. For example, costs are always associated with negative parameters; this means that the higher the price of an alternative, the less likely the people to choose it. This makes intuitive sense. What discrete choice offers is a quantification of this effect.

There are two types of data that may be used to estimate the values of the parameters β_a and λ_a:

1. Revealed preference data and
2. Stated preference data.

Revealed preference refers to choices that people have made in the past. For example, "roadside interviews" collect information about people's actual travel choices, including the chosen route, time of day and the mode of transport.

On the other hand, stated preference data are based on hypothetical questions. For example, businesses may be interested to learn about people's preferences in view of the imminent launch of a new product.

Once the data have been collected, the model parameters may be estimated by standard statistical techniques. In practice, maximum likelihood estimation methods are used most often (see, e.g. Ben-Akiva and Lerman 1985, Chapter 4).

7.2.1.3 Applications

Discrete choice has been used to study people's preferences since the 1970s (McFadden 2001). Initial applications focused on transport (Train 2003, Ortuzar and Wilumsen 2001). These models have been used to develop national and regional transport models around the world, including the United Kingdom, the Netherlands (Fox et al. 2003), as well as Copenhagen (Paag, Daly, Rohr 2001).

Since then discrete choice has also been applied to a range of social problems, for example, health care (Gerard et al. 2003, Ryan and Gerard 2003), telecommunications (Takanori and Koruda 2006) and social care (Ryan et al. 2006).

In particular, discrete choice is especially well suited to inform policy making. This is due to a number of reasons. First, the fact that it is rooted in empirical data and its rigorous and transparent methodology make it a trustworthy tool to inform evidence-based policy making. Second, the utility functions that are produced allow researchers to test concrete policy scenarios by varying variables such as the level of taxation.

7.2.2 Imitation and Social Interactions: Statistical Mechanics

A key limitation of discrete choice theory is that it does not formally account for social interactions and imitation. In discrete choice, each individual's decisions are based on purely personal preferences and are not affected by other people's choices. However, there is a great deal of theoretical and empirical evidence to suggest that an individual's behaviour, attitude, identity and social decisions are influenced by that of others through vicarious experience or social influence, persuasions and sanctioning (Akerlof 1997, Bandura 1986). These theories specifically relate to the interpersonal social environment including social networks, social support, role models and mentoring. The key insight of these theories is that individual behaviours and decisions are affected by their relationships with those around them – with parents, peers and so on.

Mathematical models taking into account social influence have been considered by social psychology since the 1970s (see Scheinkman 2008 for a short review). In particular, influential works by Schelling (1978) and Granovetter (1978) have shown how models where individuals take into account the mean behaviour of others are capable of reproducing, at least qualitatively, the dramatic opinion shifts observed in real life (for example, in financial bubbles or during street riots). In other words, they observed that the *interaction* built into their models was unavoidably linked to the appearance of *structural changes* on a phenomenological level in the models themselves.

Figure 7.3 compares the typical dependence of average choice with respect to an attribute parameter, such as cost, in discrete choice analysis (left), where the dependence is always a continuous one, with the typical behaviour of an interaction model of Schelling or Granovetter kind (right), where small changes in the attributes can lead to a drastic jump in the average choice, reflecting structural changes such as the disappearing of equilibria in the social context.

The research course initiated by Schelling was eventually linked to the parallel development of the discrete choice analysis framework at the end of the 1990s when Brock and Durlauf (2001, 2007) suggested a direct econometric implementation of the models considered by social psychology. In order to accomplish this, Brock and Durlauf had to delve into the implications of a model where an individual takes into account the behaviour of others when making a discrete choice; this could be done only by considering a new utility function which depended on the choices of all other people.

Such a new utility function was built by starting from the assumptions of discrete choice analysis. The utility function reflects what an individual considers desirable; if we hold (see, e.g. Bond and Smith 1996) that people consider desirable to conform to people they interact with, we have that, as a consequence, an individual's utility increases when he agrees with other people.

Symbolically, we can say that when an individual i makes a choice, his utility for that choice increases by an amount J_{ij} when another individual j agrees with him, thus defining a set of interaction parameters J_{ij} for all couples of individuals. The new utility function for individual i hence takes the following form:

$$U_i = \sum_j J_{ij}\sigma_j + \sum_a \beta_a x_a{}^{(i)} + \sum_a \lambda_a y_a{}^{(i)} + \varepsilon \tag{7.3}$$

where the sum $\sum_j$ ranges over all individuals, and the symbol σ_j is equal to 1 if j agrees with i and 0 otherwise. Analysing the general case of such a model is a daunting task, since the choice of another individual j is itself a random variable, which in turn correlates the choices of all individuals.

This problem, however, has been considered by statistical mechanics since the end of the nineteenth century, throughout the twentieth century, until the present day. Indeed, the first success of statistical mechanics was to give a microscopic explanation of the laws governing perfect gases, and this was achieved, thanks to a formalism which is strictly equivalent to the one obtained by discrete choice analysis in equation (7.2).

The interest of statistical mechanics eventually shifted to problems concerning interaction between particles, and as daunting as the problem described by equation (7.3) may be, statistical physics has been able to identify some restrictions on models of this kind to make them tractable, while retaining great descriptive power as shown, e.g. in the work of Pierre Weiss (Weiss 1907) regarding the behaviour of magnets.

The simplest way devised by physics to deal with such a problem is called a *mean field* assumption, where interactions are assumed to be of a uniform and global kind, leading to manageable closed-form solution. Such an assumption leads to a model coherent with the models of Schelling and Granovetter and is shown by Brock and Durlauf to be closely linked to the assumption of *rational expectations* from economic theory, which assumes that the observed behaviour of an individual must be consistent with his belief about the opinion of others.

By assuming *mean field* or *rational expectations*, we can rewrite equation (7.3) in the tamer form:

$$U_i = Jm + \sum_a \beta_a x_a{}^{(i)} + \sum_a \lambda_a y_a{}^{(i)} + \varepsilon \tag{7.4}$$

where m is the average opinion of a given individual, and this average value is coupled to the model parameters by a closed-form formula.

If we now define V_i to be the deterministic part of the utility, similarly as before,

$$V_i = Jm + \sum_a \beta_a x_a{}^{(i)} + \sum_a \lambda_a y_a{}^{(i)}$$

we have that the functional form of the choice probability, given by equation (7.3)

$$P_i = \frac{e^{V_i}}{1 - e^{V_i}}$$

remains unchanged, allowing the empirical framework of discrete choice analysis to be used to test the theory against real data. This sets the problem as one of heterogeneous interacting particles, and the physics of such mean field systems has been shown to be analytically tractable (see, e.g. Contucci et al. 2007).

Though the mean field assumption might be seen as a crude approximation, since it considers a uniform and fixed kind of interaction, one should bear in mind that statistical physics has built throughout the twentieth century the expertise needed to consider a wide range of forms for the interaction parameters J_{ij}, of both deterministic and random nature, so that a partial success in the application of mean field theory might be enhanced by browsing through a rich variety of well-developed, though analytically more demanding, theories.

Nevertheless, an empirical attempt to assess the actual descriptive and predictive power of such models has not been carried out to date; the natural course for such a study would be to start by empirically testing the mean field picture, as it was done for discrete choice in the 1970s (see Fig. 7.2), and to proceed by enhancing it with the help available from the econometrics, social science and statistical physics communities.

It is worthwhile to remark that the kind of cross-bred models considered in this chapter would allow to give a quantitative estimate of the role of social interactions in a decision-making process. This is a relevant fact, since statistical mechanics tells us that a model involving social interactions is capable of exhibiting deep structural changes that may result, for instance, in a sudden fall in demand of a commodity due to a slight increase in its price.

These structural changes, known as *phase transitions* in physics, cannot be predicted by standard discrete choice analysis, due to the regularity of the equations arising from it. On the other hand, it is a fact that sudden dramatic changes can be observed in the behaviour of large groups of people.

Therefore, by successfully implementing the kind of models considered here, researchers may gain the ability to study quantitatively a whole new range of human phenomena. As a consequence, policy makers working in areas where the interaction between individuals could play a key role, such as increasing energy efficiency of households, may acquire a valuable new tool.

7.3 Application – Energy Efficiency and Climate Change

This type of models can be applied to any problem involving individuals making choices out of a finite set of alternatives. Applications over the past three decades include transport, health care and communications. Here we focus on climate change, specifically on energy efficiency, for two reasons. First, this is one of the greatest challenges facing mankind; second, the binary nature of the choices involved, i.e. energy-efficient versus energy-inefficient behaviour, makes climate change a perfectly suited field of application.

After decades of intense scientific debate, it has now been demonstrated beyond reasonable doubt that climate change and global warming are indeed taking place. It is almost unanimously accepted that human greenhouse gas emissions play a key role (Stern 2007). Given the current and projected levels of greenhouse gas emissions, climate models predict temperatures to rise significantly over the course of the next century. If nothing is done to reduce the emissions, serious consequences are predicted for our planet, including mass extinctions, sea level rises, increase in the occurrences of extreme weather events such as hurricanes, flooding and severe drought, just to name a few (see, for example, the IPCC's Fourth Assessment Report 2007).

In recent years, thanks also to a growing popular awareness, the debate has moved to the top of political agenda. No country denies the existence of the problem, and many are already taking action to reduce emissions.

The famous Kyoto agreement in 1997 resulted in a set of emission targets for a number of developed countries. Since this agreement is set to expire in 2012, governments have been actively working to reach a new agreement for the post-Kyoto framework. The UN Conference on Climate Change that took place in December 2007 in Bali resulted in a "Roadmap", whereby the international community agreed to begin negotiations towards a new global deal on climate change. Many countries are already taking unilateral action. For example, the United Kingdom is about to introduce a new Climate Change Bill, which will commit the nation to a legally binding target of emission reductions.

Once the international post-Kyoto emission reduction targets are agreed, the question will be how to achieve the emission reductions. Figure 7.4 shows the various available options for reducing greenhouse gas emissions. Reducing the global population is not an option, although working on reducing population growth may be. Alternatively, we can reduce emissions per capita. We could do this by reducing our level of consumption. Although this is clearly one of the causes of the problem, it is unlikely that this option would produce significant emission reductions in the

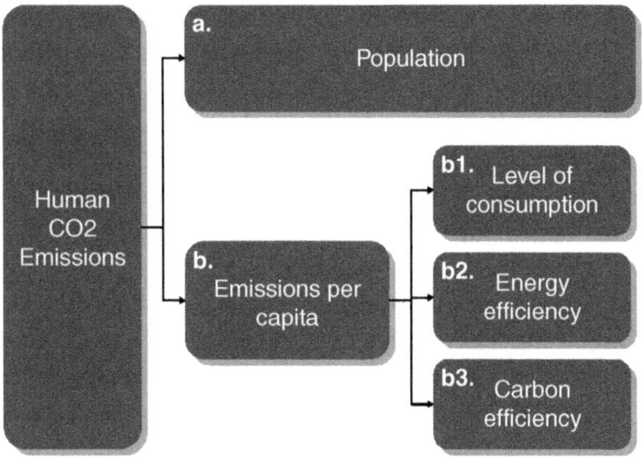

Fig. 7.4 All the ways to reduce greenhouse gas emissions

short term. This is in part because it would require the world to significantly change the current way of life as well as the existing global economic system. Another alternative is to improve the carbon intensity of our energy sources. For example, by replacing coal power plants with wind farms. A lot of work is being done in this direction.

The last option is to increase energy efficiency. This option has a number of significant advantages. For example, it can potentially lead to significant financial savings. Some models estimate that globally up to US $500 billion could be saved yearly by 2030, US $90 billion of which in the United States alone (Creyts et al. 2007). This would result from, for example, lower energy bills after thermally insulating homes or switching to energy-efficient lighting. Moreover, higher energy efficiency would reduce the stress on the other options discussed above, for example, if no extra energy is required, then there is no need to build a wind farm instead of a coal power plant.

The models presented in this chapter, together with the framework for deconstructing this apparently unmanageable problem into smaller manageable chunks, offer a systematic, robust and transparent approach to tackling the problem of climate change. Moreover, from a research perspective, climate change offers a testing ground to further develop and improve this family of models that can be applied to problems in most policy areas.

7.3.1 Case Study – United Kingdom

Up to now, governments have mostly adopted top-down policies to increase energy efficiency which are focused on particular actions and technologies. For example, condensing boilers became mandatory in the United Kingdom in 2005 and the energy regulators in the United Kingdom require that any energy suppliers undertake a pre-agreed level of activity to improve energy efficiency and save emissions in the domestic sector; the scheme is known as Carbon Emissions Reduction Target (DEFRA 2008). Neither governments nor energy companies have yet engaged in incentivising individuals to change their behaviour. In fact, energy bill structures still reward customers who use more energy by offering them a lower per unit tariff. Regulating companies to undertake energy efficiency activities has the effect of subsidising these activities and potentially undermining any attempts to develop a profit-driven market in these activities. Customers who know the energy companies are obliged to offer insulation, energy efficiency appliances and energy-efficient light bulbs may be less inclined to pay for these things themselves.

The current set of regulations in the domestic sector is set to expire in 2011, and some energy companies (including Scottish and Southern Energy, the second largest supplier of electricity and natural gas in the United Kingdom) are demanding a less proscriptive regulatory approach. This means that they are asking for a legally binding target from the government to reduce their customers' demand but with the freedom to meet that target in the most efficient way. A similar policy is expected to be introduced in the large commercial sector in 2010 – the Carbon Reduction Commitment – which caps participants' emissions from their downstream use of energy.

To put this in the context of the models presented in this chapter, it is likely that new policies could be introduced in the United Kingdom to create a *new market in energy efficiency*. In this case large energy providers, and potentially new start-up companies, will be looking for ways to induce large segments of the population to adopt more energy-efficient behaviours in order to reduce their demand.

Practically, decision makers want to know, for instance, what should government do in order to induce the population to buy energy-saving light bulbs. The government could invest towards lowering the cost of each light bulb or educating towards energy-saving lifestyles; on the other hand, money will be saved by reducing CO_2 emissions, for example, by generating carbon credits to be sold on the international carbon market or avoiding penalties for non-compliance to international agreements such as the Kyoto Protocol. How to balance the choice crucially depends on predicting the percentage of people that will turn to energy-saving light bulbs. That is what a statistical mechanics model can achieve after a suitable estimation of the parameters involved, which include, in particular, the measure of what is the imitation strength between peers concerning buying habits.

More concretely, the private sector will play a major role in tackling climate change, and companies are already looking for ways to contribute to the solution as well as to make significant profits. For example, Philips is developing and delivering energy-efficient light bulbs to the market. An achievable energy saving of up to 40% on all the lighting currently installed globally would save 106 billion Euros. This equates to 555 million tonnes of CO_2 per year, which corresponds to 1.5 billion barrels of oil per year or the annual output of 530 medium-sized power stations producing 2 TWh per year (Verhaar 2007).

There is therefore an opportunity for government and business to work together towards inducing behaviour change towards sustainable behaviour by the consumer. The family of models presented in this chapter offers a tool to provide evidence and inform decision makers and help them make the right choices.

7.4 Beyond Climate Change: Why Focus on Behavioural and Cultural Change to Achieve Policy Goals?

The majority of public and social policies are based on theoretical assumptions about human behaviour. However, these are rarely made explicit or tested against the available data. There are a number of factors that have encouraged the growing academic and especially policy interest in how to induce behavioural change amongst a population in order to generate sustainable and cost-effective social improvements.

Delivering and achieving sustainable and major policy outcomes such as climate change require greater engagement and participation from a national population–

"you can't leave it all up to the government" – rather than traditional ways of delivering public services or policies. Higher levels of spending and better-run public services can achieve improved outcomes. However, in order to achieve sustainable lasting outcomes and social improvements, much depends on changes in individual personal behaviour, for example, in achieving population improvements in health and well-being this means individuals adopting a better diet and taking up more exercise, and in education on children's willingness to learn and parents' willingness to help them learn (Knott et al. 2007).

There are also strong moral and political arguments for encouraging personal responsibility and behavioural change amongst a population. Most of the dominant traditions of social and political thought emphasise individuals' and communities' ability to take control and act in their own best interests as goods in themselves. They see it as better for governments to empower citizens and provide a social and economic context in which citizens on their own are able to make informed decisions regarding their behaviour.

And lastly policy interventions based on behavioural change can be significantly more cost-effective and preventive than traditional service delivery. There is good evidence from across a range of policy areas – for example, in health, education, crime – of the cost-effectiveness of behaviour-based social interventions (for example, altering an individual's diet that reduces and prevents the risk of cardiovascular disease is a more efficient and cheaper way than is dealing with the consequences of poor diet with heart surgery).

7.5 Discussion

Climate change is now hovering near the national and global political agenda. Motivated by increasing public awareness, pressure from environmental organizations and a growing body of scientific evidence, decision makers are now working hard to reach an international deal to reduce greenhouse gas emissions and therefore avoid the devastating social, economic and environmental impacts of climate change. Emission targets are expected to become increasingly stricter over the next years and decades. Consequently this means that governments and companies will look for the most cost-effective ways of meeting these by providing the social and economic context in which people are able and willing to make informed choices regarding their lifestyles.

This chapter argued that increasing energy efficiency has a number of advantages, including potential savings worth hundreds of billions of dollars annually by 2030, and will therefore play a key role. It is expected that new regulations will allow the creation of new markets in energy efficiency, whereby profits would be made by incentivising consumers to adopt energy-efficient behaviours. There is already demand from energy companies, such as Scottish and Southern Energy in the United Kingdom, for such policies. Moreover, companies such as Philips would profit from selling new energy-efficient bulbs.

This means that there is a growing demand for behavioural models that can help contribute to better understand, in concrete and measurable ways, the drivers behind consumer choices. In particular, there is interest in models that may help policy makers trigger structural changes in the way people behave. Given the nature of the problem of climate change, this demand is set to grow dramatically in the next few years.

This chapter presented a family of models that can address this issue. These models combine the practicality and reputation of well-established econometric tools with the flexibility and rigor of advanced mathematical tools produced by decades of research in the physical sciences. Perhaps more importantly, these models will bring together the insights from experts in both the physical and social sciences.

Moreover, the models presented in this chapter are consistent with the concept of personal responsibility and may be used to empower individuals to make choices that are consistent with their personal interests as well as with the common good. Perhaps these models may help government create a society that spontaneously protects the private as well as the public good in a way that reduces government interference but avoids market failures and "tragedy of the commons" scenarios (Schelling 1978).

Acknowledegments F.G. and A.C. would like to thank Bryony Worthington and James Fox for their contributions and the useful discussions. I.G. acknowledges partial support from the CULTAPTATION project of the European Commission (FP6-2004-NEST-PATH-043434).

Bibliography

Akerlof, G. (1997). Social distance and economic decisions. *Econometrica* 65, 1005–1027.

Ariely, D. (2008). *Predictably irrational – the hidden forces that shape our decisions*. London: Harper Collins.

Bandura A. (1986). *Social foundations of thought and action: A social cognitive theory*. Englewood Cliffs, NJ: Prentice Hall.

Ben-Akiva M. and Lerman, S. R. (1985). *Discrete choice analysis*. Cambridge MA: The MIT Press.

Bond, R. and Smith, P. B. (1996). Culture and conformity: A meta-analysis of studies using Asch's (1952b,1956) line judgment task. *Psychol. Bull.* 119, 111–137.

Brock, W. and Durlauf, S. (2001). Discrete choice with social interactions. *Rev. Econ. Stud.* 68, 235–260.

Brock, W. and Durlauf, S. (2007). Identification of binary choice models with social interactions. *J. Economet.* 140, 52–75.

Contucci, P., Gallo, I., and Ghirlanda, S. (2007). Equilibria of culture contact derived from ingroup and outgroup attitudes, *arXiv: 0712.1119*.

Contucci, P. and Ghirlanda, S. (2007). Modeling society with statistical mechanics: An application to cultural contact and immigration. *Qual. Quan.* 41, 569–578.

Contucci, P. and Giardina, C. (2008). Mathematics and social sciences: A statistical mechanics approach to immigration. *ERCIM News* 73, 34–35.

Creyts, J., Derkach, A., Nyquist, S., Ostrowski, K., and Stephenson, J. (2007). Reducing U.S. greenhouse emissions: how much and at what cost? *McKinsey & Company Report*, http://www.mckinsey.com/clientservice/ccsi/greenhousegas.asp

DEFRA (2008). Household energy supplier obligations – The carbon emissions reduction target. Published on the DEFRA website: http://www.defra.gov.uk/environment/climatechange/uk/household/supplier/index.htm

Fox, J., Daly, A. J, and Gunn, H. (2003). *Review of RAND Europe's transport demand model systems*. Published on RAND's website: http://rand.org/pubs/monograph_reports/MR1694

Gerard, K., Shanahan, M., and Louviere, J. (2003). Using stated preference discrete choice modelling to inform health care decision-making: A pilot study of breast screening participation. *Appl. Econ.* 359, 1073–1085.

Granovetter, M. (1978). Threshold models of collective behavior. *Am. J. Sociol.* 83, 1420–1443.

IPCC (2007). Fourth assessment report: climate change 2007. Published on the IPCC's website: http://www.ipcc.ch/ipccreports/assessments-reports.htm

Knott, D., Muers, S., and Aldridge, S., (2007). *Achieving cultural change: A policy framework.* The strategy unit, Cabinet Office, UK Government.

Luce, R. and Suppes, P. (1965). Preferences, utility and subjective probability. In R. Luce,, R. Bush, Galenter E. (Eds.) *Handbook of mathematical psychology* (Vol. 3) New York: Wiley.

McFadden, D. (2001). Economic choices. *Am. Econ. Rev.* 91, 351–378.

Ortuzar, J. and Wilumsen, L. (2001). *Modell. Trans.* Chichester, UK: Wiley.

Paag, H., Daly, A.J., and Rohr, C. (2001). Predicting use of the Copenhagen harbour tunnel. In H. David (Ed.), *Travel behaviour research: the leading edge*. Pergamon.

Persky, J. (1995). Retrospectives: The ethology of Homo Economicus. *J. Econ. Perspect.* 92, 221–23.

Ryan, M. and Gerard, K. (2003). Using discrete choice experiments to value health care programmes: Current practice and future research reflections. *Appl. Health Econom. Health Pol.*, 21, 55–64.

Ryan, M., Netten, A., Skatun D., and Smith, P. (2006). Using discrete choice experiments to estimate a preference-based measure of outcome – An application to social care for older people. *J. Health Economics*, 255, 927–944.

Scheinkman, J. A. (2008). Social interactions. *The New Palgrave Dictionary of Economics* (2nd edn.) Palgrave Macmillan.

Schelling, T. (1978). Micromotives and macrobehavior. New York: *W. W. Norton & Company*.

Stern, N. (2007). *The economics of climate change – The stern review*. Cambridge: Cambridge University Press.

Takanori, I. and Koruda, T. (2006). Discrete choice analysis of demand for broadband in Japan. *J. Regul. Econ.* 291, 5–22.

Train, K. (2003). *Discrete choice methods with simulation.* Cambridge: Cambridge University Press.

Verhaar, H. (2007). Reducing CO_2 emissions by 555 Mton through Energy Efficiency Lighting. Presented at the UNFCCC Conference in Bali, December 8.

Weiss, P. (1907). L'hypothèse du champ moléculaire et la propriété ferromagnétique. *J. de Phys.* 4 série VI, 661–690.

Chapter 8
An Application of the Multilevel Regression Technique to Validate a Social Stratification Scale

Simone Sarti and Marco Terraneo

Abstract This chapter applies the multilevel regression technique in order to validate the ranking of occupational categories in a reputational scale of social desirability. Such attention to the differences inherent in work roles resumes the topic of the unequal distribution of material and symbolic rewards within societies. A tool widely used by sociologists to grasp the distributive inequalities associated with jobs is the occupational stratification scale or the hierarchical ordering of occupations.

The aim of the model presented in this chapter is to validate an occupational stratification scale constructed in 2007 on the basis of the scale developed by de Lillo-Schizzerotto in 1985. The scale consists of 110 occupational categories constructed as the aggregate of 676 occupations (described in detail) which 2000 interviewees were asked to evaluate in terms of their social desirability. The ordering of the scale is validated through decomposition of the heterogeneity of the evaluations. The multilevel model shows that the 110 categories explain large part of this heterogeneity, also with the socio-demographic characteristics of the interviewees remaining equal.

8.1 Introduction to the Stratification Scale

Many of the contemporary sociological theories that concern themselves with social stratification in the advanced societies consider occupation to be the most relevant dimension on which to define the social positions of individuals (Treiman 1977, Erikson and Goldthorpe 1992, Wright 1997, Schizzerotto 2002, de Lillo 2007). The substantial reasons for this view relate to the conviction that occupational and social inequalities broadly overlap, with the consequence that studying work activities and jobs yields information which sheds important light on the structure of

S. Sarti (✉)
Department of Sociology and Social Research, University of Milan "Bicocca", Milan, Italy
e-mail: simone.sarti@unimib.it

V. Capecchi (eds.), *Applications of Mathematics in Models, Artificial Neural Networks and Arts*, DOI 10.1007/978-90-481-8581-8_8,

social inequalities. It is evident that this approach to the study of social stratification is sound if it is able to show that social and occupational inequalities are closely connected. In our view, although developments in sociological theory (see e.g., Beck 2000, Castells 2000, Savage 2000) have raised doubts on the matter, the occupation maintains its explanatory capacity as a key dimension interpretation of the differences among the life chances of individuals, given that it is still the principal source of material and symbolic resources for the majority of persons (Cobalti and Schizzerotto 1994, Crompton 1993, Pisati 2000).

Work is therefore a key factor in understanding the features of social stratification. Indeed, the occupation is one of the most important social and economic characteristics that society assigns to individuals when they assume adult roles. It furnishes information about the technical and social skills possessed by a participant in the labor market, as well as about the current difficulties and future economic prospects of the members of a given society (Hauser and Warren 1996).

From this it follows that focusing on differences among work roles throws light on the unequal distribution of rewards in society. The structure of inequalities can be studied from various perspectives, for instance, from the relational perspective which addresses power relations between individuals and groups. However, it should be stressed that this study is concerned solely with the distributive aspect of the phenomenon. Numerous material and non-material advantages constitute distributive inequalities (Grusky 2001). The most significant of them can be grouped into three categories: economic privileges (amount of wealth and income, level of vocational qualification, career opportunities, etc.); cultural and symbolic privileges (level of formal and informal education, predominant consumption patterns, etc.); and political privileges (level and number of positions occupied in political parties, trade unions, employers' organizations, etc.). A tool widely used by sociologists to grasp the distributive inequalities associated with jobs is the occupational stratification scale, or the hierarchical ordering of occupations.

In 2005 a group of universities,[1] engaged in a project co-funded by the Italian Ministry of Universities and Research (PRIN2003) entitled "The Social Evaluation of Occupations," conducted a survey on the social desirability[2] of occupations which led to construction of an occupational stratification scale for Italy. The

---

[1]Specifically, the Universities of Milano-Bicocca, Piemonte Orientale "Amedeo Avogrado", "Federico II" of Naples, and Trento.

[2]We use the term "social desirability" to denote the concept underlying our scale because we believe that reputational scales measure the objective social advantages and disadvantages associated with occupations (de Lillo and Schizzerotto 1985), and not prestige, as frequently argued (for instance by Treiman 1977). We believe, in fact, that the critique to the functionalist approach about the study of social inequalities is correct when it maintains that interviewees do not judge occupations as socially better in light of norms or values. Consequently, it is entirely misleading to establish an association between the social hierarchy of work roles and some sort of classification of individual abilities and merit (Cobalti and Schizzerotto 1994). Our view is borne out by a study on the criteria used by interviewees to evaluate the social positions of occupations in 2005, which found that prestige was not the only dimension underlying the ratings given to those positions (Arosio and De Luca 2007).

research adhered closely to the criteria already adopted in 1985 by de Lillo and Schizzerotto (1985) when conducting the first systematic study in Italy on the perception and evaluation of occupations.[3]

Given the aim of this study, the first priority is to describe, albeit briefly, the research design which led to the construction of the 2005 scale of the social desirability of occupations (SIDES2005).[4] The universe of occupations from which selection was made for evaluation by the interviewees amounted to around 19,000 in 2005. Chosen for evaluation by the sample were 676 occupations representative of 118 occupational categories referring to the entire Italian labor market. These categories could not be directly submitted to rating by the interviewees for two reasons: first, one of the hypotheses to be tested was the homogeneity of the categories; second, the subjects were able to evaluate individual jobs, but not abstract constructs like occupational categories. Given the impossibility for each interviewee to grade 676 occupational titles, the sample – composed of 2000 subjects representative by gender, age, and geographical zone of residence of the active Italian population aged between 24 and 65 – was asked to grade 20 occupations chosen at random from among the representative ones. Each occupation received 60 evaluations.

After the occupations had been ordered by the interviewees, a score called the "index of desirability" – was calculated for each of them. This measure fulfilled the twofold requirement of being a cardinal variable and covering the entire set of evaluations made by the interviewees on all the occupations proposed to them. The index was based on the assumption that the subjects did not compare all the occupations simultaneously but rather performed a sequence of pairwise comparisons in which each occupation was compared with each of the others. As for the scale constructed in 1985, the formula used to calculate the index was the following:

$$Ip = \frac{2N_i + N_e}{2\,(N-1)} \times 100 \tag{8.1}$$

where N is the number of objects that the subject had to grade; N_i is the number of objects one rank below that of the object for which the score was being calculated; N_e is the number of objects with a rank equal to that of the object examined; $(N-1)$ is the number of pairwise comparisons possible for each object, so that $2\,(N-1)$ represents the maximum value of elementary scores; and where, moreover, the factor 100 is used only to have Ip vary from 0 to 100 (de Lillo and Schizzerotto 1985).

The SIDES 2005 stratification scale will be thoroughly described in both theoretical and methodological terms in a book currently being prepared by the teams

[3]For a comparison of the 1985 and 2005 scales which sought to determine whether and how the image of the occupational stratification has changed in Italy over the past twenty years see Sarti and Terraneo (2007).

[4]The SIDES2005 stratification scale will be thoroughly described in both theoretical and methodological terms in a book currently being prepared by the teams at the Universities which took part in the PRIN2003 project. Some aspects of the scale have already been discussed in a special issue of *Quaderni di Sociologia*, 45, 2007.

at the Universities which took part in the PRIN 2003 project. Some aspects of the scale have already been discussed in a special issue of *Quaderni di Sociologia*, 45, 2007.

The final step in defining the scale was the attribution of scores to the occupational categories. This was done by calculating for each category the mean of the averages of the scores given to each occupation in that category. The internal homogeneity of each category was controlled by variance analysis and Snedecor's F-test. Following considerations of a substantive and statistical nature, the occupational categories were reduced to 110.[5]

Because presentation of the SIDES 2005 scale would be beyond the scope of this chapter, for solely exemplificatory purposes, Table 8.1 reports one of the scale's 110 categories and the occupation scores calculated using the above formula. The mean of the average scores is the score associated with the category.

Table 8.1 Example of one category with the relative occupations and scores

Manual workers in services	Score	Std. dev.
Family helper	10.6	14.52
Concierge	13.7	13.02
Bill poster	8.8	16.85
Cleaner	10.1	17.46
Docker	8.2	13.81
Mean category score	10.3	

Table 8.2 instead sets out the 17 macro groups derived from the further aggregation of the 110 categories. As will be seen, the macro categories well reproduce the fundamental features of Italy's occupational stratification: positioned at the top of the hierarchy are jobs that combine high income, serious decision-making responsibilities, and strong impact on social life, also outside the work context, while partial possession or the lack of these characteristics pushes occupations toward the bottom of the scale.

8.2 Validation of the Ordering of the Categories

It should be clear from the previous section's description of how the SIDES 2005 scale was constructed that the score for each of the 110 categories resulted from a two-step aggregation procedure: first calculated was the "advantageousness" score of each occupation as the average of the scores attributed by 60 valuators; then calculated was the mean of the average scores for the occupations in each category. Overall, therefore, the 2000 interviewees expressed 40,000 evaluations (recall that each interviewee was asked to order 20 different jobs) which were then condensed

[5] See again note 4.

Table 8.2 Hierarchy of the 17 occupational macro categories of 2005

Macro categories	Score
Top managers	85.8
Employers with 50+ employees	79.6
Politicians	75.3
Professional employees	71.3
Employers with 15–49 employees	70.1
Middle managers	69.1
Independent professionals*	67.4
Employers with 4–14 employees	58.3
Members of the armed forces	57.8
Clergymen	57.7
Intermediate white-collars	56.6
Teachers	54.1
Self-employed workers with 1–3 employees	46.9
Supervisors of manual workers	43.4
Routine non-manual employees	39.3
Self-employed workers without employees	37.4
Manual and non-manual workers	24.6

*The category "independent professionals" comprises both the traditional independent professions (lawyer, doctor, architect, surveyor, etc.) and the self-employed occupations similar to them (musician, sports coach, theater actor, etc.)

into only 110 categories which, when ordered, defined the position of each category in the occupational hierarchy. It is evident that the category scores were not insensitive to the variability inherent in the evaluations of the occupations, so that it was necessary to validate the 110-category scale. Put otherwise: the 110-category scale could be regarded as accurately representing occupational stratification in Italy if it was certain that the variability observed among the categories explained the variability connected to the opinions on occupations.

The heterogeneity in the ratings of occupations was due to three main factors. The first was the different evaluations received by each occupation. The 60 judgments obtained by each job obviously differed from interviewee to interviewee, so that the variability for every occupation could be very pronounced. For example, the railway ticket inspector obtained an average score of 34.6 and a standard deviation of 15.2 (with an observed score range from 10 to 60). The second source of heterogeneity was the diversity of the occupations constituting each category. In this case the variability was due, as said, to the fact that the category score was the mean of the scores for the occupations belonging to the category. Occupations in the same category naturally had different scores: for example, the category of self-employed workers in food retailing with 1–3 employees obtained a score of 34.5, which resulted from the mean of the scores obtained by the rotisserie owner (37.9), ice-cream maker (36.8), baker (34.9), grocer (34.0), and greengrocer (29.0).

The third source was the socio-demographic characteristics of the valuators. The subjects requested to order the occupations had characteristics, both ascribed and acquired, which may have influenced their opinions. In our data set, again by way of example, the bank cashier obtained four points more from male interviewees than from female ones; twelve points more from lower-educated subjects than from those possessing higher qualifications (elementary certificate holders against graduates); nine points more from younger subjects (aged between 25 and 34) than from more elderly ones (aged between 55 and 64); ten points more from residents of the South than from those in the North.

Validation of the categories in the scale of social desirability therefore required maintaining control over the heterogeneity associated with various factors (those listed above); this heterogeneity derives from the way in which the survey was structured (see Fig. 8.1). In fact, the survey started with collection of the scores given by the interviewees to the occupations. The judgments expressed by the 2000 valuators could be conditioned by their socio-demographic characteristics. For every occupation, the scores of the 60 evaluations constituted its mean score, for a total of 466 occupations rated during the survey.[6] Finally, the occupations were aggregated into homogeneous categories, both in terms of the similarity of work content and the desirability score obtained. This produced a set of occupational categories (110) arranged on the scale of social desirability.

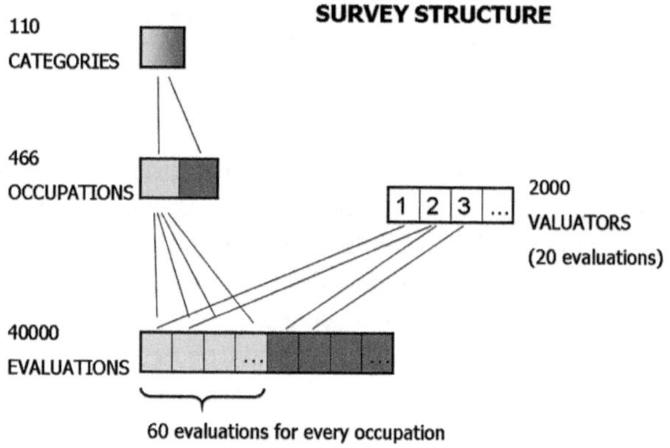

Fig. 8.1 The structure of the survey carried out to construct the SIDES 2005 scale

Given these premises, we asked ourselves the following question: how could we determine whether the differences among the scores for the categories on the scale indeed represented different positions in the occupational hierarchy, rather than

[6]The overall number of occupations reported in the figure is 466, and not the 676 as previously indicated. The reason for the discrepancy is as follows. The research design envisaged that some occupations would be evaluated depending on the kind of contract; instead other occupations would be judged according to whether the incumbent was a man or a woman. During the analysis phase, the occupations subject to multiple evaluation were treated as follows: as regards the employment contract only considered were judgments related to occupations pursued on a permanent basis; as regards the gender of the occupation's incumbent, the score was obtained as the average of the scores given by male and female respondents. This choice entailed a reduction in the overall number of jobs.

being the result of the variability associated with the evaluation of the occupations, which in its turn reflected the structure of the survey and the socio-demographic characteristics of the valuators?

Given the hierarchical form and the plurality of contexts assumed by the survey's structure, we believed that applying the multilevel regression technique to our data, by virtue of the assumption on which it is based, would furnish an answer to this question, and therefore validate the SIDES 2005 scale of social desirability.

8.3 The Multilevel Technique Applied to the Stratification Scale

As said, the technique adopted to decompose the heterogeneity in the data was multilevel regression, which is a development of linear regression (Goldstein 1995, Snijders and Bosker 1999). This technique, in fact, makes it possible to formalize a multivariate model in which account can be taken of the levels of aggregation in which the data are organized. "With clustering, regression methods that assumes independent observations provide inefficient and possibly biased coefficient estimates, and associated confidence intervals that are too narrow" (Mason 2001: 14989).

Often, in fact, social phenomena and the variables that operationalize them are structured hierarchically, so that the more elementary units of analysis are embedded in different contexts. The latter may assume different forms: they may concern spatial areas (like countries), temporal sequences (surveys repeated over time), and also social aggregations (for instance, educational institutions).[7] The hierarchical structure of the levels can be shaped according to the intentions of the researcher and the intrinsic characteristics of the contexts. It is thus possible to explain, for instance, the achievement in terms of grades awarded to pupils by considering different times of the year (e.g., examinations) at the second level and school-class membership at the third level.

The aim of multilevel analysis is therefore to estimate the effects exerted by the context through hierarchically structured regressions. In practice, this technique estimates the parameters of the equations and their residuals in function of the level, that is, taking account of how the regression coefficients vary within the different levels.

As regards the application presented here, we have three levels organized as follows: at the first level, the 40,000 evaluations expressed by the interviewees; at

[7] A classical example demonstrating the need to consider the contexts within which individuals' act is provided by education. In a study of the 1970s, conducted using standard regression analysis, Bennett (1976) found a statistically significant relation between the "formal" model of education and better student performance. Subsequently Aitkin et al. (1981) repeated the analyses on the same data controlling for the classes to which the students belonged. The result of inserting a higher level of aggregation was the disappearance of the effect of "formal" teaching on pupil progress. In practice, shown to be more important for student performance were the skills of the teacher (common to all the students in the same class), not the teaching method (Goldstein 1995).

the second, the 466 occupations evaluated; and at the third, the 110 categories into which the scale was finally structured.

We will therefore have a general equation in which the score of the evaluation is equal to its average value plus a certain residual, which will vary – or better will be distributed differently – according to the level.

On the whole, the evaluation score is expressed as if there is a single level (called *micro*), the i, from the regression equation:

$$P_i = \beta_0 + e_i \tag{8.2}$$

where P_i is the score for evaluation i, β_0 is the overall expected value (which holds for all the levels), and e_i is the residual for every ith evaluation.

The technique therefore enables estimation of the beta parameter by decomposing the residuals relative to the different levels (i, j, and k) by the means of the equations (called *macro*, i.e., relative to the levels above the first one), where

u_{0jk} are the residuals estimated for every jth context of the second level (the 466 occupations);

v_{0k} are the residuals estimated for every kth context of the third level (the 110 categories).

The estimate of the beta parameter that takes account of the *micro* and *macro* dimensions of the model will therefore be equal to the estimate of the parameter plus the residuals distinguishes at the different levels:

$$\beta_{0ijk} = \beta_0 + e_{0ijk} + u_{0jk} + v_{0k} \tag{8.3}$$

where beta is equal to the estimate of the expected overall value plus the residual at level of the evaluation, plus the residual at the level of the occupations, plus the residual at the level of the categories.

Schematically, the decomposition of the residuals comes about as shown in Fig. 8.2.

Besides estimation of the parameters, it is of extreme importance to evaluate the distribution of the residuals and the heterogeneity explained by them at the various levels (Leyland and McLeod 2000).

The first-level variance relative to the residuals e_{0ijk} is denoted with Ω_e, while the variances at the other levels are denoted, respectively, by Ω_u for the second level and by Ω_v for the third level.

A low residual variance indicates very small residuals, so that the deviations added to the overall average value are of little magnitude.

By contrast, the greater the residual variance at a particular level, the higher is the "noise" (stochastic or related to variables not considered) relative to that level. The residuals of that level to be added to β_0 will strongly influence the estimate β_{0ijk}.

From the substantive point of view with regard to our analysis, organization of the data into this three-level structure enabled us to construct an ordering of the average scores of the 110 categories purged of heterogeneity at the level of the evaluations and at the level of the occupations.

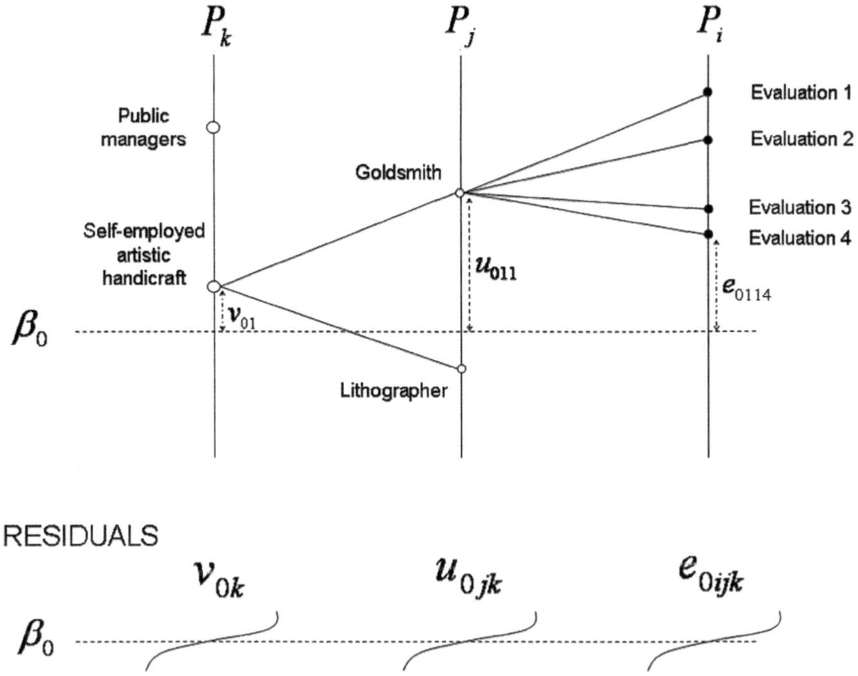

Fig. 8.2 Decomposition of the residuals according to the level

In substance, the residuals at the third level (k) added to the expected overall value of the estimate of the parameter made it possible to construct the ordering of the 110 occupational categories taking account of the heterogeneity captured in the first two levels (at the level of the evaluations and the occupations). We were thus able to appraise the extent to which the occupational categories at the third level were able to explain the residual variance at the second level. More prosaically, this meant measuring the extent to which the 110 categories were "good substitutes" for the 466 occupations, which was the main aim of the analysis.

Accordingly, the next section comments on the results obtained with the various models employed.

8.4 Results of the Analysis

The analyses were performed with the support of the MLWIN software and consisted of four models. The first of them, which had two levels, was a simple test to establish the basis for the comparison with the other models. The second model, with three levels, was the expression with the closest bearing on the analytical approach described above (see Table 8.3). The third and the fourth models, also

Table 8.3 Hierarchical organization of the model

Level	Unit	Number
First – I	Evaluations	40,000
Second – J	Occupations	466
Third – K	Categories	110

with three levels, incorporated the further hypothesis that the socio-demographic characteristics of the interviewees influenced their evaluation of the occupations.

We now describe the various models. The first of them, which we shall call "model A," considered only the first two levels, i.e., the evaluations and the occupations, bearing in mind that, given the structure of the survey, each occupation was subject to 60 evaluations by 60 different interviewees.

As said, "model A" was the basis for evaluation of the subsequent models. Inspection of the output reported in Fig. 8.3 shows that the estimate of the parameter β_0, the average score attributed to the occupations, was 52.747 with a standard deviation equivalent to 0.944. Hence the interval of confidence at 0.05 was more or less two points from the point estimate.

$$\textbf{punt\_val}_{ijk} \sim \mathrm{N}(XB, \Omega)$$
$$\textbf{punt\_val}_{ijk} = \beta_{0ij}\textbf{const}$$
$$\beta_{0ij} = 52.747(0.944) + u_{0jk} + e_{0ijk}$$

$$\left[u_{0jk}\right] \sim \mathrm{N}(0, \Omega_u) : \Omega_u = \left[408.719(27.139)\right]$$

$$\left[e_{0ijk}\right] \sim \mathrm{N}(0, \Omega_e) : \Omega_e = \left[397.194(3.382)\right]$$

*-2*loglikelihood(IGLS Deviance)* = **249797.000(28096 of 28096 cases in use)**

Fig. 8.3 Model A – estimates of the model and the structure of the (two-level) model

The residual variance at the first level was around 397, while that at the second level was around 409. This latter value indicates the heterogeneity Ω_u at the level of occupations. That is to say, it is a measure of the extent to which the occupations were evaluated differently.[8]

The residual variance at the first level, Ω_e, was instead the noise present in the data relatively to the single purged evaluations of the second level; that is, bearing in mind the fact that the evaluations, in groups of 60, concerned the same occupation.

[8] Ω_u describes the heterogeneity of the distribution of the deviations from the general average of each of the 466 occupations – for example, the extent of the differences among a carpenter, bill poster, newspaper editor – bearing in mind that the score for each occupation derived from 60 evaluations.

$$\text{punt\_val}_{ijk} \sim \mathrm{N}(XB, \Omega)$$
$$\text{punt\_val}_{ijk} = \beta_{0ijk}\text{const}$$
$$\beta_{0ijk} = 52.914(1.885) + v_{0k} + u_{0jk} + e_{0ijk}$$

$$\left[v_{0k}\right] \sim \mathrm{N}(0,\ \Omega_v) : \Omega_v = \left[386.280(52.663)\right]$$

$$\left[u_{0jk}\right] \sim \mathrm{N}(0,\ \Omega_u) : \Omega_u = \left[9.388(1.204)\right]$$

$$\left[e_{0ijk}\right] \sim \mathrm{N}(0,\ \Omega_e) : \Omega_e = \left[397.205(3.379)\right]$$

*-2*loglikelihood(IGLS Deviance)* = **248781.800(28096 of 28096 cases in use)**

Fig. 8.4 Model B – estimates of the parameters and the structure of the (three-level) model

The next step was to estimate another model, "model B", in Fig. 8.4, which also took account of the existence of a third level: the 110 categories in which the occupations were embedded. The parameters were therefore estimated with reference to a structure with three levels: the evaluations within the occupations and the occupations within the categories.

The estimate of the parameter β_0 is similar to the previous one. The most important aspect to be stressed concerns the variances of the residuals; in fact, the insertion of a third level diminished the variance at the second level, that of the occupations. The variance Ω_u decreased from around 409 to only 9 points. The residual variance of the new level $\Omega_v$was 386. This means that bearing in mind that the occupations were embedded within the categories gave rise to large residuals at the third level, considerably decreasing those at the second. While in the two-level model the second level had, in terms of percentages, a 50.7% residual variance on the total of residual variance, now the variability was reduced to 1.2%, while for the third level it was 48.7%.[9] Hence, the correlation between two evaluations within the same category was 0.487.

On considering only variability above the first level, "model B" showed that the third level explained 97.6% of the heterogeneity, obtained as 48.7 / (1.2 + 48.7). This means that the correlation between two occupations within the same category was 0.976.

From the substantial point of view, therefore, the categories well explain – or more precisely, they explain in the same way as the occupations – the heterogeneity of the evaluation scores.

These results corroborate the hypothesis that the SIDES 2005 110-category scale functions well as a synthesis of the hundreds of occupations surveyed.

[9] The percentages measure the intra-unit correlation indicating the ability of the contexts in the different levels to explain variability (Goldstein 1995, Leyland and McLeod 2000). For instance, on two levels the variability explained by the second level is calculated as $\rho = \frac{\Omega_u}{\Omega_e + \Omega_u}$.

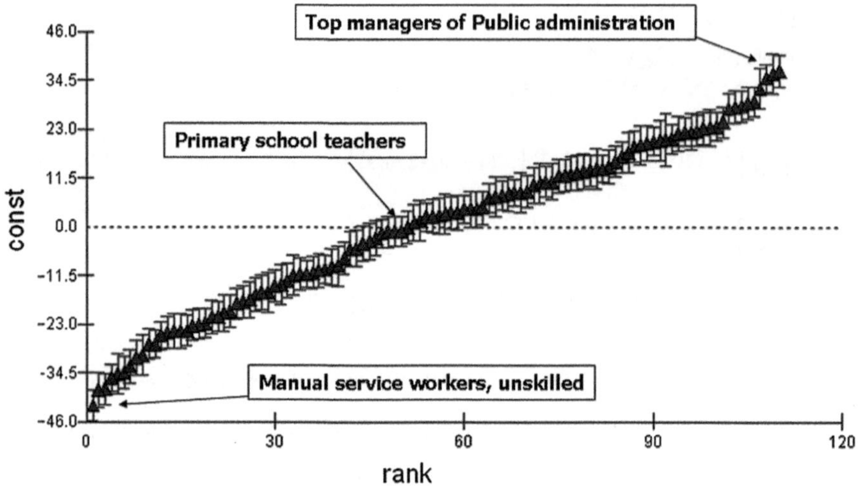

Fig. 8.5 Model B – ordering of the occupational categories, third-level residuals, and respective intervals of confidence

Figure 8.5 reports the third-level residuals each of the 110 contexts of the level k, i.e., the occupational categories, and it shows the ordering of the scale purged of heterogeneity at the first and second levels. In this case the residuals are the deviations from the general average score of the individual occupational categories. For instance, considering only the residuals v_k, the category of "manual service workers, unskilled" has a score equal to 52.9 + (– 43), i.e., around ten points, and occupies the lowest position in the scale. We may therefore expect the ordering of the categories to be largely the same as the one constructed from the simple average category scores. As exemplified by the labels of some categories in Fig. 8.5, the scale fully retains the ordering.

Even more interesting is the graph of the residuals at second level. It will be recalled that these are the residuals of each single occupation, considering that some occupations belong to the same category at the third level. The occupations with negative residuals received below-average evaluations in comparison to the other occupations in the same category. The occupations with positive deviations were instead evaluated on average better than the other occupations in the same category.

This raises some interesting considerations. For example, jobs which involve the handling or the working of gold tend to receive better scores regardless of occupational position (whether the worker is self-employed or a dependent employee, whether she/he has no, few, or many employees). By contrast, occupations in particularly fatiguing work, or with negative connotations, like blast furnace work or cleaning, tend to receive worse evaluations.

It should be specified, however, that inspection of the range of values on the axis of ordinates and the exiguousness of the residual variance at the second level (Ω_u equal to around 9) show that the residuals are extremely small (Fig. 8.6). In fact,

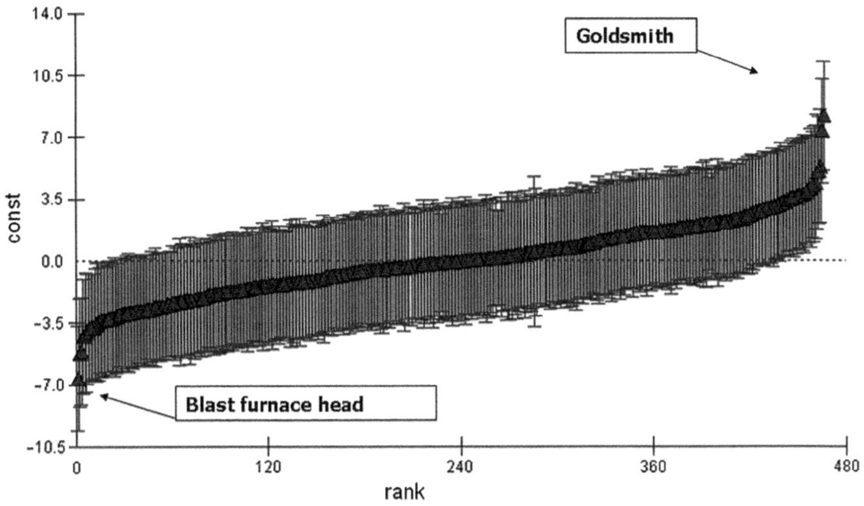

Fig. 8.6 Model B – second-level residuals and respective intervals of confidence

the great majority of the latter are between more and less four points and have such wide intervals of confidence that the differences are negligible.

The third and the fourth models considered the socio-demographic characteristics of the interviewees. The hypothesis tested was whether these characteristics systematically influenced the interviewees' evaluations of the occupations. Consequently, added to the equation of the previous model were a number of regressors describing socio-demographic characteristics (Table 8.4).

The variables gender, age-class (25–34, 35–44, 45–54, and 55–65 years old), educational qualification (elementary certificate, lower secondary certificate, upper secondary diploma, and degree), and geographical area of residence (north, center, and south) were inserted into the hierarchical structure at the second level, i.e., as control variables which might influence the evaluations.

Table 8.4 Hierarchical organization of the model

Level	Unit	Number	Regressors
First – I	Evaluations	40,000	
Second – J	Occupation	466	Socio-demographic characteristics
Third – K	Categories	110	

In the third model, "model C," the estimates of the parameters of the regressors were performed while keeping the contexts constant. By contrast, in the fourth model, "model D," the regressors were freed at the level of the second-level contexts (random-slope model).

Table 8.5 Estimates and standard deviations of the various models

		Model A	Model B	Model C	Model D
	β_0	52.75 (0.944)	52.66 (0.171)	51.15 (1.947)	51.29 (1.965)
Level I	Ω_e	397.2 (3.4)	397.2 (3.8)	396.6 (3.4)	390.1 (3.6)
Level J	Ω_u	408.7 (27.1)	9.4 (1.2)	9.4 (1.2)	2.5 (1.9)–25.6 (9.0)*
Level K	Ω_v	–	386.3 (52.7)	386.4 (52.7)	387.9 (52.8)
–2*log (likelihood)		249.797	248.781	248.736	248.601
Δ_A –2*log (likelihood)		*0*	*– 1016*	*– 45*	*– 135*

*Range of the variable estimates according to the parameters

Space precludes exhaustive treatment of these models.[10] However, the results of all the models analyzed are summarized in Table 8.5.

As far as the aims of this study are concerned we merely point out that the amount of the residual variances, at all the levels, and the connected distribution of the residuals are substantially unchanged with respect to "model B."

We may therefore conclude from the estimates in the outputs (and from the relative standard deviations) that no significant effects were exerted by the socio-demographic variables on evaluation of the occupations.[11]

8.5 Conclusions

The aim of this study has been to test the parsimony of the SIDES 2005 stratification scale, which consists of 110 occupational categories whose scores were obtained from the numerous occupations evaluated by the sample of interviewees. The purpose of these categories is to synthesize the perceptions of Italians concerning the social desirability of the occupations that make up the labor market.

Given the structure of the scale, we considered multilevel regression to be the method best suited to decomposing the heterogeneity inherent in the data according to the various levels into which the information collected was organized. We expected that the level of the occupational categories would be a valid "substitute" for the occupations, or in other words, that the variability of the categories would effectively explain the variability of the occupations.

As shown by the results of the analyses performed, and particularly as described in regard to "model B," the variability of the third level, that of the categories of the scale, explained almost all the variance that in "model A," with only two levels, was attributable to the occupations.

[10]Detailed information about the models can be obtained from the authors upon request. For technical details see Snijders and Bosker (1999).

[11]Similar conclusions have been reached by Meraviglia and Accornero (2007).

Tests on more complex models, which we have been unable to treat thoroughly here for reasons of space, suggested that the introduction as control variables of certain socio-demographic characteristics of the valuators did not generate any substantial variation.

Acknowledgments We are grateful to Mario Lucchini for his suggestions in regard to multilevel analysis. However, responsibility for any errors or omissions is ours alone.

Bibliography

Arosio, L. and De Luca, S. (2007). I criteri di valutazione della desiderabilità sociale delle occupazioni. *Quaderni di Sociologia*, LI, 45.

Aitkin, M. et al. (1981). Teaching styles and pupil progress: A re-analysis. *Br. J. Edu. Psychol.* 512, 170–186.

Beck, U. (2000). *What is globalization?* Cambridge: Polity Press.

Bennett, S. N. (1976). *Teaching styles and pupil progress*. London: Open Books.

Castells, M. (2000). *The rise of the network society*. Oxford: Blackwells.

Cobalti, A. and Schizzerotto A. (1994). *La mobilità sociale in Italia*. Bologna: il Mulino.

Crompton, R. (1993). *Class and stratification*. Cambridge, MA: Polity Press.

De Lillo, A. (2007). *A che servono le scale di stratificazione?* In D. Gambardella (Ed.)

De Lillo, A. and Schizzerotto, A. (1985). *La valutazione sociale delle occupazioni. Una scala di stratificazione occupazionale per l'Italia contemporanea*. Bologna: il Mulino.

Erikson, R. and Goldthorpe, J. H. (1992). *The constant flux: A study of class mobility in industrial societies*. Oxford: Clarendon Press.

Gambardella, D. (Ed.) (2007). *Genere e valutazione delle occupazioni*. Roma: Carocci.

Goldstein, H. (1995). *Multilevel Statistical Models* (2nd edn.). London: Edward Arnold.

Grusky, D. B. (2001). Social stratification. In *International encyclopedia of the social & behavioral sciences* (pp. 14443–14452). Oxford: Pergamon.

Leyland, A. H. and McLeod, A. (2000). *Mortality in England and Wales, 1979–1992*. Glasgow: MRC Social and Public Health Sciences Unit.

Hauser, R. M. and Warren, J. R. (1996). Socioeconomic indexes for occupations: A review, update, and critique. In *centre for demography and ecology working paper* (n. 96–01). University of Wisconsin-Madison.

Meraviglia, C. and Accornero, L. (2007). La valutazione sociale delle occupazioni nell'Italia contemporanea: una nuova scala per vecchie ipotesi. In *Quaderni di Sociologia*, LI, 45.

Mason, W. M. (2001). Statistical analysis: Multilevel method. In Smelser N. J. and Baltes P. B. (Eds.), *International encyclopedia of the social and behavioral sciences* (pp. 14988–14994). Amsterdam: Elsevier Science.

Pisati, M. (2000), *La mobilità sociale*. Bologna: il Mulino.

Savage, M. (2000). *Class analysis and social transformation*. Buckingham: Open University Press.

Sarti, S. and Terraneo, M. (2007). Stabilità e mutamento della scala di stratificazione occupazionale in Italia. *Quaderni di Sociologia*, LI, 45.

Schizzerotto, A. (2002). *Vite ineguali*. Bologna: il Mulino.

Snijders, T. A. B. and Bosker, R. (1999). *Multilevel analysis*. London: Sage Publications.

Treiman, D. J. (1977). *Occupational prestige in comparative perspectives*. New York, Academic Press.

Wright, E. O. (1997). *Class counts: Comparative studies in class analysis*. Cambridge: Cambridge University Press.

Chapter 9
The Academic Mind Revisited: Contextual Analysis via Multilevel Modeling

Robert B. Smith

> *To organize our material [on the causes of teachers' apprehension] we followed the well-established idea that all human experiences are determined by two broad groups of elements: the characteristics of the people themselves and those of the environment in which they live and work.*
>
> *Paul F. Lazarsfeld and Wagner Thielens, Jr. (1958, 159–160)*

Abstract Contemporary studies of the politics of American professors compare their political preferences to those of the American public. That some professors exhibit more liberal attitudes than the public leads critics to ask whether this difference biases teaching and enforces political correctness that stifles the study of controversial topics. To provide an alternative substantive and methodological paradigm for future studies of academia – one that focuses on social contexts, mechanisms, and outcomes – this chapter briefly reviews Lazarsfeld and Thielens's *The Academic Mind: Social Scientists in a Time of Crisis*. They studied the effects of McCarthyism on academia, documenting how contextual and personal variables influenced the professors' apprehension, i.e., worry and caution. This chapter then applies multilevel statistical modeling to their pivotal three-variable contextual tables, showing how contemporary statistical methods can advance their analysis by close inspection of tabular data. Multilevel models can incorporate simultaneously the effects of numerous contextual and individual variables, providing measures of effects and appropriate tests of significance for the clustered data.

The political sociology of higher education is enjoying a renaissance in the United States. In their comprehensive review of the field, Gross and Simons' (2007) findings may be paraphrased roughly as follows: Recent studies focus on political differences among professors and on how the attitudes of academics differ from

R.B. Smith (✉)
Social Structural Research Inc., Cambridge, MA 02140, USA
e-mail: rsmithphd@comcast.net

V. Capecchi (eds.), *Applications of Mathematics in Models, Artificial Neural Networks and Arts*, DOI 10.1007/978-90-481-8581-8_9,

those of the public at large. Some on the Right believe that the Left has captured academia and that instruction is consequently biased. Others question these assertions believing that academics exhibit a variety of political beliefs and that many professors do not express their personal politics in the classroom. Given the research aim of either documenting or debunking such assertions, the typical study follows the logic of a public opinion survey: It samples individual professors and compares their responses to those of the public; it does not emphasize the effects of institutional and departmental contexts. Some studies exhibit methodological flaws of sampling design, questionnaire construction, measurement, data analysis, and interpretation, and they do not examine closely the influence processes and social mechanisms that shape faculty opinion.

Contrarily, as the above epigraph suggests, some social scientists assume that a person's behavior depends on three factors: (1) the person's dispositions, which are perceptions, attitudes, desires, beliefs, and capabilities; (2) how the social environment impinges on that person; and (3) the interactions between these predisposing and environmental factors. A *contextual study* includes variables concerning both the person and the environment; *contextual effects* are the cross-level interactions between the personal and environmental variables, and the study of these interactions defines *contextual analysis*.

9.1 Lazarsfeld's Contextual Analysis

Herbert Blumer (1956) critiqued survey research studies for ignoring the effects of context and networks and for merely describing relationships among aggregated psychological variables, linking one attribute of a respondent to other attributes. Taking up this challenge, Lazarsfeld and Thielens developed a paradigm for contextual analysis that culminated in their 1958 book, *The Academic Mind: Social Scientists in a Time of Crisis*. Probing the pressing social problem of the effects of McCarthyism on academia, the investigators asked: How did the climate of fear—generated globally by the cold war against communism and manifested locally on college campuses by attacks on the character of individual teachers because of their alleged political beliefs—affect colleges and universities and their social science teachers?

By reviewing the study design, measures, and results of this classic contextual analysis, and by applying recently developed statistical methods to its data, this chapter aims to underscore the importance of contextual analysis for contemporary studies of the politics of professors and to tighten the linkage between contextual analysis and multilevel statistical modeling.

The investigators hypothesized that variables at the level of the individual teacher (level-1) and at the level of the academic institution (level-2), along with their cross-level interactions, affected the key outcome variable, namely, a teacher's apprehension about being singled-out and punished for expressing his or her political beliefs. Because they thought that apprehension was jointly determined by variables at the level of the academic institution and by variables at the level of the teacher, they therefore randomly sampled 165 educational institutions and 2,451 teachers of the social sciences within these institutions (Lazarsfeld and Thielens 1958, 371–377). These data, which are available in data archives for secondary analysis, characterize the population of social scientists and academic institutions during April and May 1955, a period when the effects of McCarthyism were still evident. The investigators used the empirical findings to draw inferences about the population of American academic social scientists during that time period. Because apprehension was the key outcome, they referred to this survey informally as the "teachers' apprehension study."

9.1.1 Apprehension and Its Correlates

To develop measures of apprehension, the investigators first conducted detailed exploratory interviews. They asked the interviewees to describe any experiences as a teacher that made them feel uneasy about their academic freedom, induced worry about how their political views could affect their professional advancement, or made them cautious about expressing potentially controversial thoughts. On the basis of these detailed interviews, the investigators then created questionnaire items that assessed worry and caution, the two dimensions they had defined for apprehension. Below, I mark with "a" (for apprehension) the statements that formed the final six-item apprehension index.

To assess worry, the questions Lazarsfeld and Thielens asked are as follows (1958, 76): Have you ever worried or wondered that (a) students could pass on warped views of what you have said leading to false ideas about your political beliefs? (a) potential employers might ask others about your political biases in teaching? (a) there may be gossip in the community about you because of your politics? (a) expression of your political opinions could jeopardize your promotion or job security? your political beliefs could make you unpopular with the alumni? and the college administration may keep a political file or dossier on you and on other faculty members?

Whereas the questions about worry directly tapped the teacher's state of mind, the following questions about caution ascertained whether or not the teacher had acted in ways that would prevent potential controversies about his or her political beliefs. To assess caution, the questions Lazarsfeld and Thielens asked are essentially as follows (1958, 78): Have you at least occasionally: made statements or told anecdotes that made it very clear that you are neither an extreme leftist or rightist? refrained from participating in some political activity so as not to embarrass the trustees or the administration? refrained from discussing political topics with colleagues in order not to embarrass them? (a) not recommended readings that could lead to criticism that these were too controversial? (a) toned down your writing because you worried that they might cause controversy?

The worry and caution indexes are strongly correlated—the ordinal measure of association gamma (γ) = 0.70. Nonetheless, the investigators chose the six items that most directly indicate the underlying sentiment of occupational apprehension, the dimension along which the respondents could best be classified.[1] By simply summing the dichotomized replies to the six items, the investigators created an index that ranges from zero (no apprehension) to six (considerable apprehension). They grouped the scores as low (0, 1) = 54%, medium (2, 3) = 33%, and high (4–6) = 13%, and, most often, because only counter–sorters and not computers were then generally available, they dichotomized this variable, analyzing the determinants and consequences of high plus medium = 1 versus low = 0 apprehension.

Having built the index of apprehension, the investigators then turned to validating it by clarifying its relationships with other variables. They found that "vulnerable" teachers, those who had been involved in a personal incident or who were members of a controversial organization, were more likely to exhibit a high degree of apprehension, with personal incidents having the stronger average effect.[2] Other correlations with apprehension were as follows: the higher the teachers' levels of apprehension (at least through scores 0–4), the more likely the teachers were to protest bans on controversial speakers and on debates about admission of communist China to the United Nations; to read left-of-center journals like *The Nation, The New Republic*, and the now defunct *The Reporter*; and to be alert to issues of academic freedom and civil liberties (Lazarsfeld and Thielens 1958, 92–112). At each level of vulnerability, teachers who were more concerned about civil liberties were also more likely to exhibit high apprehension (Lazarsfeld and Thielens 1958, Fig. 4-8, 109).

In order to relate a teacher's apprehension to the college context, the investigators formed a typology of academic institutions based on size (the number of students) and type of organization (private, public, teachers colleges, Protestant, and Catholic). The nine types are private (large and small), public (very large, large, small), teachers colleges, Protestant, Catholic (large and small). The investigators found that teachers at small Catholic institutions and small public institutions

[1]To calculate gamma (γ) first define A as the number of concordant pairs of observations (++ or −−) and B as the number of discordant pairs of observations (+- or -+). Then, gamma = (A − B)/(A + B). For Table 3-3 (1958, 81): A = 1,184 × 423 = 500,832; B = 125 × 719 = 89,875; A − B = 410,957; A + B = 590,707; γ = 410,957/590,707 = .70.

[2]Rough estimates of the average effects of these variables can be calculated by simply taking a simple average of the two conditional relationships. For the data of their Fig. 3-7 the roughly estimated average effect of involvement in an incident on apprehension, controlling for membership in a controversial organization = ((75% − 56%) + (71% − 36%))/2 = (19% + 35%)/2 = 27%. The roughly estimated average effect on apprehension of membership in a controversial organization, controlling for involvement in an incident = ((75% − 71%) + (56% − 36%))/2 = (4% + 20%)/2 = 12%. The roughly estimated interaction effect on apprehension of not being involved in an incident but belonging to a controversial organization is the difference between these differences divided by 2. It equals (20% − 4%)/2 = (35% − 19%)/2 = 8%. These rough estimates do not take into consideration the different sample sizes and the limitations of the linear probability model.

were less apprehensive than those at the other types of institutions (see Lazarsfeld and Thielens, Fig. 3-8, 90); these other institutions exhibited little difference in apprehension. Attacks were more frequent at institutions of higher quality, but a protective administration could reduce its faculty's amount of apprehension induced by such attacks (Lazarsfeld and Thielens 1958, 167–174). At the same time, a teacher's breadth of permissiveness (rather than conservatism) increased apprehension.

9.1.2 *Assessing Permissiveness*

A salient determinant of a professor's apprehension was the scope of his or her permissiveness. Permissive professors were more likely to permit freedom of expression for leftist political views on campus, whereas the more conservative professors were less likely to do so. Indicators of a permissive outlook were that a professor would not fire a teacher who admittedly is a communist and would allow the young Communist League on campus. Indicators of a conservative outlook were that a professor would not allow Owen Lattimore to speak on campus (Lattimore was an expert on China whom Senator Joseph McCarthy accused of being a spy for the Soviet Union); would fire a store clerk who admitted to being a Communist; would not allow the Young Socialist League on campus; and considered it a luxury to have a radical teacher for the college. From these indicators the investigators created a bipolar index of permissiveness versus conservatism (see their pages 125–127 for the details). Teachers classified as highly permissive gave two permissive replies and no conservative replies. Teachers classified as highly conservative were at the other extreme, giving two or more conservative and no permissive replies. The other teachers exhibited different combinations so that scores on the permissiveness index ranged from 0 = clearly conservative (14%); 1 = somewhat conservative (14%); 2 = somewhat permissive (29%); 3 = quite permissive (21%); and 4 = highly permissive (22%). A trichotomous index results when the two categories at either extreme are combined.

The investigators clarified the meaning of permissiveness by relating its index to a number of indicators that distinguished the political left from the political right; these measures were similar to those they used to validate their apprehension index. Compared with their conservative counterparts, permissive teachers were more likely to vote Democratic, read liberal magazines, belong to professional and controversial organizations, favor classroom discussion of political topics, support academic freedom, be professionally productive, say their own academic freedom had been threatened, say they had been reported to higher authorities, and acknowledge they felt pressures to conform politically (Lazarsfeld and Thielens 1958, 132–156). Not surprisingly, they also were more likely to exhibit apprehension, which was in part a consequence of their permissiveness. Because the investigators conceptualized permissiveness versus conservatism as a basic attitudinal predisposition, they viewed permissiveness as a predetermining variable that induced apprehension—worry and caution—rather than assuming the opposite direction of effect, or reciprocal influence.[3] Thus,

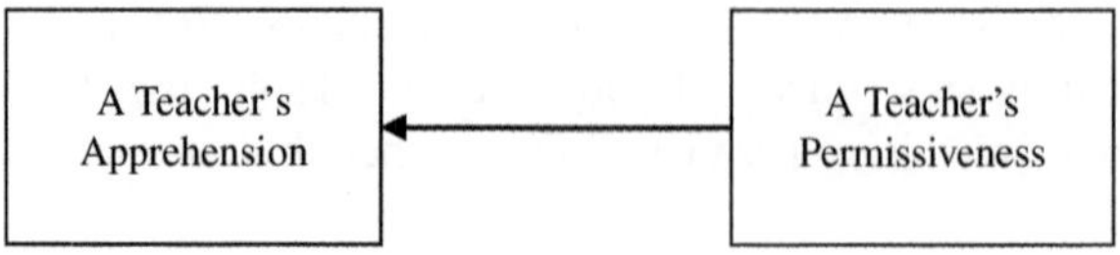

The investigators depicted these relationships in a bar chart (Lazarsfeld and Thielens 1958, Fig. 6–15) similar to that in Fig. 9.1; both charts clearly show that apprehension increases with increases in permissiveness. These variables are measured at level-1, but *The Academic Mind* also reports the effects of incidents, a level-2 contextual variable that characterized the academic institutions.

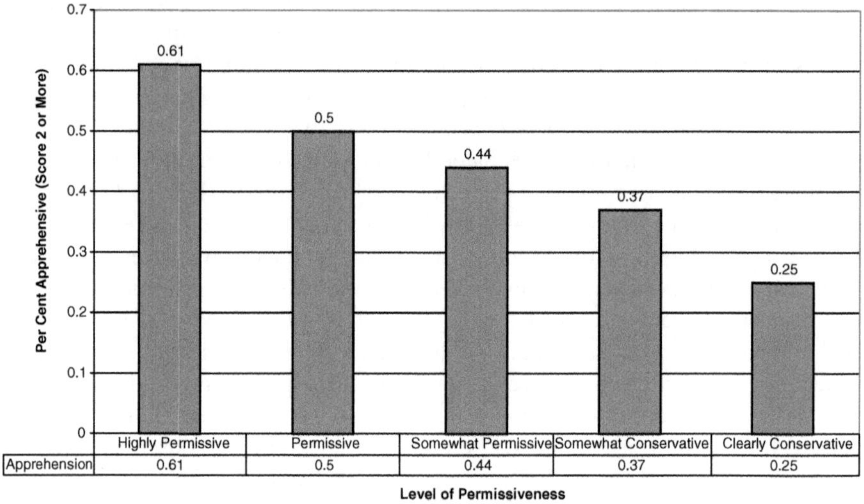

Fig. 9.1 Permissive teachers are more apprehensive than conservative teachers (Data from Lazarsfeld and Thielens, Fig. 6.15, p. 153)

[3]The direction of the effect between permissiveness and apprehension has perplexed some scholars (personal communication). Lazarsfeld and Thielens assumed that permissiveness led to apprehension (Fig. 7-13). Implicitly, they may have conceptualized permissiveness–conservatism as roughly analogous to the cluster of variables indicative of authoritarianism. The conservative pole of permissiveness is somewhat analogous to political and economic conservatism whereas the openness-to-ideas aspect of permissiveness suggests stronger commitments to anti-authoritarian democratic values. If authoritarianism is a variable of personality, then, given this analogy, it is logical to assume that apprehension is in part a manifestation of permissiveness, rather than the opposite. This leaves open the possibility of mutual effects.

9.1.3 Institutional Incidents

The investigators clarified their use of the word "incident" as follows (Lazarsfeld and Thielens 1958, 44):

> it describes an episode, long or short, in which an attack, accusation, or criticism was made against a teacher, a group of teachers, or a school as a whole.... This [overt] act might be a listing of the names of supposedly "pink" professors in the gossip column of a local newspaper, a student going to a dean with a charge against a teacher, or a teacher reporting that another man had been passed over for promotion because of his politics.

To interpret how the institutions affected their faculties' apprehension, the investigators applied an "attack and defense" model, which holds that a strong defense can mitigate the effects of an attack. At the time of the study, right-wing attacks on teachers and their institutions induced apprehension, but if the institution's administrators defended their faculty from these incidents, their defense alleviated this apprehension. The investigators measured such incidents by relying on reports from their interviewees. They distinguished corroborated from uncorroborated reports and deleted from their contextual analysis those teachers who had personally experienced an attack or another incident. They then characterized the institutions by their count of corroborated incidents (Lazarsfeld and Thielens 1958, 259).

The count of academic freedom incidents that characterized a teacher's institution was crucial in engendering apprehension, as this diagram depicts:

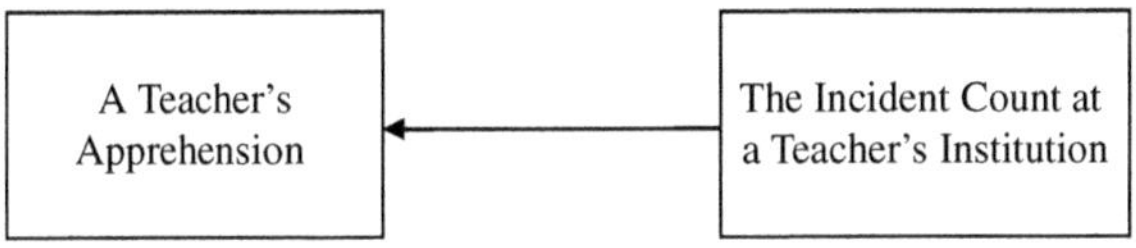

Using data from Fig. 10-9 of the *Academic Mind*, Fig. 9.2 compares the effects of incidents on the apprehension of 1,878 teachers for three types of institutions—those with 0, 1, or 2 or more (hereafter, 2+) corroborated incidents. This figure exemplifies a *comparative analysis* because it shows how the categories of a level-2 variable shape the amounts of a level-1 variable. The teachers included in this analysis had not experienced a personal attack or other political difficulties themselves. Even so, as the number of corroborated incidents at a teacher's institution increased, the amount of the apprehension among the teachers at that institution also increased. When there are zero corroborated incidents, the baseline (intercept) level of apprehension is 37%. When there is one incident, then the mean level of apprehension increases by 7 percentage points to 44%. When there are 2+ incidents, then the mean level of apprehension increases from the baseline value by 16 percentage points to 53%. Moreover, when the incidents increase from 1 to 2+, the increase in apprehension is 9 percentage points. All of these differences are statistically significant.

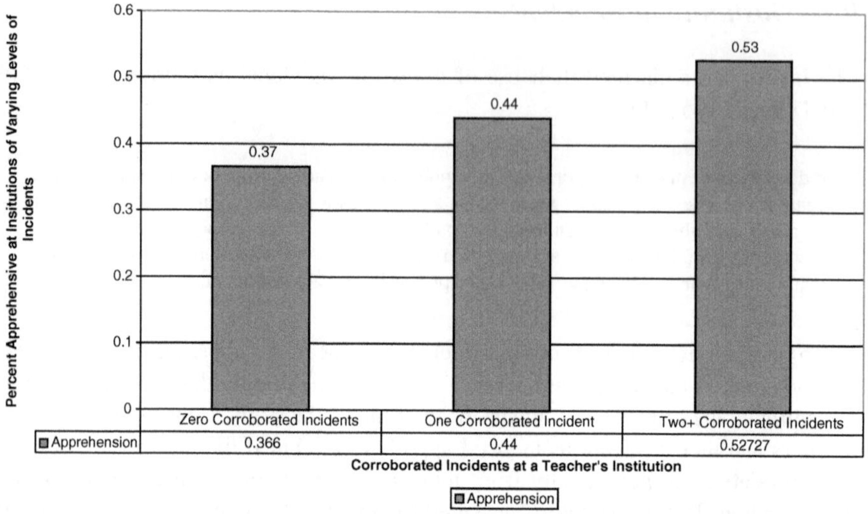

Fig. 9.2 The greater the number of corroborated academic freedom incidents at a teacher's insititution, the higher the teachers' apprehension at that institution (Data from Lazarsfeld and Thielens, Fig. 10-9, p. 259)

Lazarsfeld and Thielens put together the micro-level relationship depicted in Fig. 9.1 and the macro-comparative, cross-level relationship of Fig. 9.2 by first sorting the data on the teachers into three groups: clearly permissive (highly and quite permissive), somewhat permissive, and conservative (somewhat and clearly conservative). Then, for each of these groups, they cross-tabulated a teacher's level of apprehension with the number of corroborated incidents at that teacher's institution and they looked for interaction effects.

Figure 9.3 below depicts these relationships quantitatively (it uses the data of the investigators Fig. 10-9 and my estimates from the multilevel models). Holding constant an institution's count of incidents, one set of relationships links the two micro-level variables: the higher the professor's permissiveness the higher the apprehension. Holding constant permissiveness, the cross-level set of relationships compares the amount of apprehension at institutions with varying incident counts: for each amount of permissiveness, the greater the number of corroborated incidents at a teacher's institution, the greater the amount of apprehension at that institution, even though the teachers included in this figure did not experience attacks or political problems themselves. The institutional context induced apprehension controlling for the effects of permissiveness.

The effects of context are as follows: the different institutions had different impacts on apprehension, which depended upon the extent of the teachers' permissiveness or conservatism. The apprehension of conservative teachers increased linearly with the increased number of incidents; the increases for the other teachers were less steep. When there were 2+ incidents, then there was very little difference (1 percentage point) between somewhat permissive and conservative teachers.

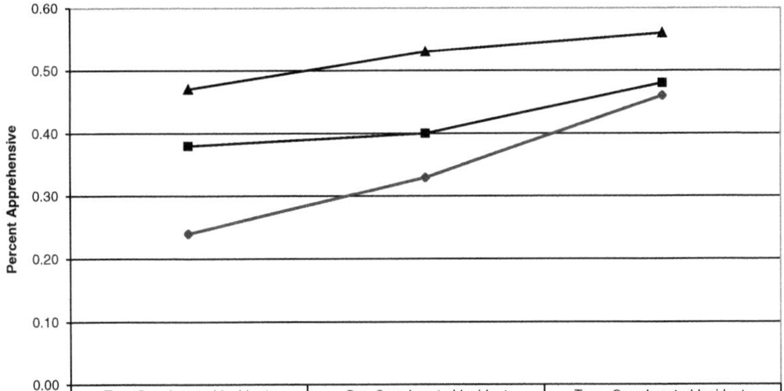

	Zero Corroborated Incidents	One Corroborated Incident	Two+ Corroborated Incidents
Conservative	0.24	0.33	0.46
Somewhat Permissive	0.38	0.40	0.48
Clearly Permissive	0.47	0.53	0.56

Incidents at a Teacher's Institution

Conservative — Somewhat Permissive — Clearly Permissive

Fig. 9.3 At each level of permissiveness, the greater the number of corroborated academic freedom incidents at a teacher's institution, the higher the percentage of apprehensive teachers at that institution (From Lazarsfeld and Thielens, Fig. 10-9)

When there were no incidents, then the difference was much larger (14 percentage points). When the teachers were not predisposed toward apprehension by their basic conservative political orientation, then the institutional context of incidents induced the greater change in apprehension: for conservative teachers the change was 22 percentage points compared with 10 percentage points for somewhat permissive teachers and 9 percentage points for clearly permissive teachers — context matters! Diagrammatical representation is shown below.

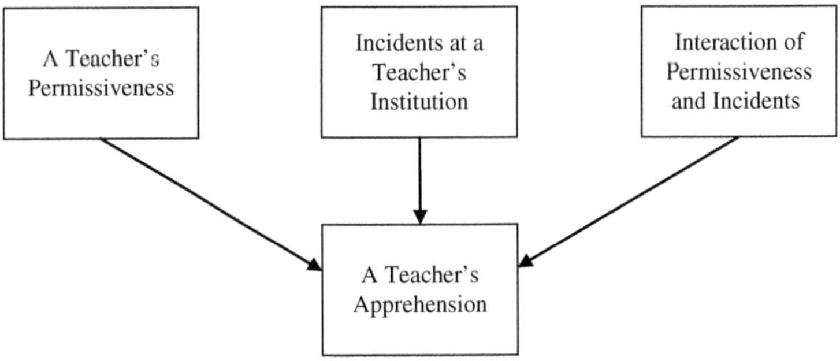

Lazarsfeld and Thielens synthesized the level-1 relationship between permissiveness and apprehension and the cross-level relationships by cross-tabulating the three variables. Their technology—counter-sorters and close inspection of data—limited the number of variables that they could consider simultaneously and prevented them from quantifying the sizes of the effects and from testing these effects for statistical significance; today's technology transcends these limitations. Our next task is to understand how multilevel statistical methods can be applied to advance their methods and especially those of contemporary investigators of the politics of professors.

9.2 Developing Multilevel Statistical Models

To develop models for the data of Fig. 9.3, I closely follow the logic, conceptualizations, mathematical symbols, and equations of Raudenbush and Bryk (2002, 16–37); the expositions of Singer and Willett (2003, 76–85); the insights of Gelman and Hill (2007); and the SAS procedures for estimation using Proc Mixed and Proc Glimmix (Littell et al. 2006, 526–566). A strategy for building a two-level multilevel statistical model suggests that one should first explore how the response variable varies across the level-2 units; if the distribution is flat, then a multilevel model most probably is not required. In either case, one should then specify an equation that links level-1 variables. If the data suggest that a multilevel model is appropriate, then the intercepts and slopes of the level-1 variables become the response variables in equations that include level-2 variables. The two sets of equations may be estimated separately; or one may substitute the level-2 relationships into the level-1 equation and then estimate the coefficients of the combined equation. I prefer the latter approach because, after the combined equation is simplified, it resembles the familiar single-equation regression model but includes additional stochastic elements.

For data sets in which missingness is minimal I follow these nine steps: (1) explore the data, when feasible dividing the sample data into portions for exploratory and confirmatory analyses; (2) formulate and estimate a baseline unconditional means model that does not include covariates—this model clarifies how the intercepts vary across categories of the level-2 grouping variable and provides statistics for comparing subsequent models; (3) formulate and estimate a model that includes the level-1 response variable (here, apprehension) and at least one level-1 explanatory variable (here, permissiveness); (4) formulate level-2 equations that are linked to the level-1 coefficients and that include at least one level-2 explanatory variable (here the latter is the category of institutional incidents into which the teachers are grouped—synonyms of *grouped* are *clustered* or *contained*); (5) create a combined model by substituting the level-2 equations into the level-1 equation and simplify; (6) estimate the coefficients of the variables in the combined model and assess the model's goodness of fit; (7) test the preferred model against other alternative models; (8) replicate the analysis using alternative statistical procedures; and, if feasible (9), replicate the analysis with other data.

The data of Fig. 9.3, which we will now model by applying multilevel analysis, present the effects of the covariates—permissiveness, incidents, and their interactions—on the measure of apprehension. As mentioned earlier, at the time of this survey computers were rare and data analysts relied on counter-sorters to provide the needed cross-tabulations. Consequently, survey researchers formed dichotomies and trichotomies from their continuous variables; in general there is no pressing need to do so now. By assuming that apprehension is truly a normally distributed continuous variable, and by applying a linear multilevel regression model (here, a linear probability model), the subsequent statistical modeling develops a paradigm that can be applied whenever it is reasonable to assume that the response variable is continuous with normally distributed residuals. Such models can be estimated directly using SAS's Proc Mixed or Proc Glimmix (2005). For the latter, by specifying that the response distribution is normal and the linkage between the set of covariates and the response distribution is made by the identity function (i.e., equality); this is the canonical specification for a linear regression model. In step (8), acknowledging the gaps between the assumptions of the estimated multilevel models and the form of the data, I use logistic regression to reestimate the models more appropriately by treating apprehension as a binary response proportion.[4] Such models can be estimated in Proc Glimmix by specifying that the response distribution is binomial and the linkage between this response distribution and the set of covariates is made by the logit function; this is the canonical specification for a logistic regression model.

9.2.1 Step 1: Exploring the Data

This multilevel modeling strategy might not seem intuitive because it requires that the intercepts and slopes of a level-1 equation become response variables in a set of equations that contain level-2 variables—the *hyperparameters* of the macro-level variables are assumed to influence the coefficients of the micro-level variables. Close inspection of the relationships in Fig. 9.3 may make this approach more intuitive; please note the following: When there are no incidents, the three trace lines have different intercepts, which are 0.24, 0.38, and 0.47, respectively, for the conservative, somewhat permissive, and the clearly permissive teachers—this indicates that the macro variable affects the level-1 intercepts. The change from 0 to 1 institutional incident induces changes in apprehension (the slopes of the first line segments) of 0.09, 0.02, and 0.06. Moreover, the change from 1 to 2+ incidents

[4]Although binary response variables are best analyzed using a logistic regression model, the linear probability regression model is easy to implement and can be applied to explore the data when the dichotomized response variable has near equal proportions in categories 0 or 1 as is the case here. Moreover, some sociologists state that proportions are easier to interpret than the logits and odds ratios of logistic regression (Cole 2001, Davis 2001, Hellevick 2009); sociologists have developed a core body of methods based on the linear probability model (Lazarsfeld 1961, 1971, Coleman 1964, Davis 1975, 1980); statisticians have provided some corrections that ameliorate its shortcomings (Fleiss 1981, Goldberger 1991); and the linear probability model can be readily transformed into a logistic regression model (Coleman 1981), as will be done later in this chapter. Thus, in modeling these data I will first apply a linear probability model that assumes that the proportion apprehensive varies continuously from 0 to 1 and that the error terms are asymptotically normally distributed, then I will apply the logit model that has much better statistical properties for analyzing dichotomous responses.

Table 9.1 Intercepts and Slopes for the Effects of Permissiveness on Apprehension in Different Institutional Contexts Assessed by Counts of Academic Freedom Incidents

	Estimates	Confidence interval bounds		t	p
		Lower	Upper		
Overall incidents					
Intercept	0.30	0.26	0.34	14.4	< 0.0001
Slope	0.11	0.09	0.14	7.9	< 0.0001
Incidents = zero					
Intercept	0.25	0.19	0.30	8.9	<0.0001
Slope	0.12	0.07	0.16	5.3	< 0.0001
Incidents = one					
Intercept	0.31	0.24	0.39	8.7	< 0.0001
Slope	0.10	0.06	0.15	4.2	<0.0001
Incidents = two +					
Intercept	0.44	0.34	0.55	8.3	< 0.0001
Slope	0.06	−0.001	0.12	1.7	0.08

induces changes in apprehension (the slopes of the second line segment) of 0.13, 0.08, and 0.03, respectively. Adding together each pair (i.e., 0.09 + 0.13, etc.) and dividing by 2, the average overall slope estimates are about 0.11, 0.05, and 0.045—this indicates that the macro variable influences the level-1 slopes.

Furthermore, the regression coefficients of Table 9.1 suggest that, within institutions characterized by different incident counts (level-2), the relationships between permissiveness and apprehension (the level-1 variables) differ. If the institutions have no incidents, then the intercept value of apprehension is 0.25 and the effect of permissiveness on apprehension is 0.12 ($p < 0.0001$). If there is one incident, then the intercept is 0.31 and the effect of permissiveness on apprehension is 0.10 ($p < 0.0001$). But if there are 2+ incidents, then the intercept is the highest (0.44) but the effect of permissiveness on apprehension is the lowest, 0.06, and not statistically significant ($p = 0.08$). Thus, the level-2 variable has effects on the intercepts and slopes of the level-1 relationships, and these impacts provide an intuitive rationale for the baseline and subsequent models.

9.2.2 Step 2: The Baseline Unconditional Means Model

Assuming for now that the teachers' apprehension is a normally distributed variable, at least asymptotically, and that the teachers are contained within the category of their institution's incidents, the unconditional means model specifies the following parameters that when estimated provide baseline information for the assessment of subsequent models: the variance $\sigma_{\mathrm{I}}^2 = \tau_{00}$ between categories of institutional incidents; the residual variance σ_{T}^2 of teachers within categories of institutional incidents; the intraclass correlation ρ, the reliability of the sample mean in any incident category j, and the grand mean apprehension score. Here, I follow the convention that the lowest-level unit is denoted by *i*, the next highest unit by *j*, and the next highest unit by *k*, etc., and that the level-2 covariance parameters are symbolized by $\tau_{00}, \tau_{01} = \tau_{10}$, and τ_{11}; I will define these concepts later.

The empirical data we are modeling have only three categories of institutions, those with $j = 0,1$, or 2+ incidents; symbolically, $j = 0,1,\ldots,J$ types of institutions based on their incident count. Because Lazarsfeld and Thielens wanted to study the effects of incidents on professors who did not experience a personal attack, they removed from this dataset those teachers who had suffered a personal attack or who had experienced other repressive actions because of their politics. The investigators grouped the 1,878 remaining teachers as follows: 754 teachers in institutions with 0 incidents, 629 in institutions with 1 incident, and 495 in institutions with 2+ incidents. The multilevel model assumes that these teachers are contained within the categories of institutional incidents, that is, the number of teachers contained in each institutional incident category *j* is $i = n_0, n_1, \ldots, n_j$.

The simplest equation for the apprehension score Y_{ij} for teacher *i* contained in incident category *j* is

$$Y_{ij} = \beta_{0j} + r_{ij} \tag{9.1}$$

The right-hand side of equation (9.1) comprises the intercept β_{0j}, which represents for each incident category *j* the true population mean amount of apprehension $(\beta_{0j} = \mu_{Yj})$, and the level-1 residual r_{ij}, which represents the effects of other variables on the apprehension of individual *i* in institutional group *j; r_{ij}* is assumed to be distributed normally ($\sim N$) with a mean of zero and a constant level-1 variance σ_T^2. More formally, $r_{ij} \sim N(0,\sigma_T^2)$)—the subscript T refers to the teachers and the symbol $\sim$ means distributed as.

At level-2, the intercept β_{0j} for each category of institutional incidents (the category's true mean of apprehension) is portrayed as the sum of the population grand mean amount of apprehension γ_{00} plus random deviation from that mean quantified by μ_{0j} for each category of incidents:

$$\beta_{0j} = \gamma_{00} + \mu_{0j} \tag{9.2}$$

where $\mu_{0j} \sim N(0,\tau_{00} = \sigma_I^2)$—the subscript I of the variance refers to the institutional incidents but τ_{00} is a more convenient symbol than σ_I^2. Substitution of equation (9.2) into equation (9.1) produces this multilevel model:

$$Y_{ij} = \gamma_{00} + \mu_{0j} + r_{ij} \tag{9.3}$$

where $\mu_{0j} \sim N(0,\tau_{00} = \sigma_I^2)$ and $r_{ij} \sim N(0,\sigma_T^2)$. This equation states that the apprehension score *Y* of a teacher *i* in institutional incident category *j* equals the grand mean level of apprehension γ_{00} plus random deviations from that mean μ_{0j} due to differences between the categories *j* of institutional incidents plus the residuals of the *i*th teacher grouped in the *j*th institutional incident category.

The results in Table 9.2 (and later in Table 9.3) are based on full maximum likelihood estimation of the parameters of the equations; this method enables us to compare the fit of successive models of the data. For the baseline model 1 the estimate of the grand mean amount of apprehension is 0.44 on the zero to one scale, with lower and upper confidence limits of 0.28 and 0.61, respectively. The variance components indicate that the estimate of the variance between institutional incident categories is $\hat{\tau}_{00} = \hat{\sigma}_{\mathrm{I}}^2 = 0.004$ ($z = 1.1$, not significant). This parameter is very small, especially when compared with the estimate of the residual variance of teachers grouped within their institution's incidents category, which is $\hat{\sigma}_{\mathrm{T}}^2 = 0.242$, ($z = 30.6$, very significant). The ^ sign over each variance symbol indicates that its value is a sample estimate of the population parameter. To assess the proportion of variance in Y that is between the categories of a variable like incidents, Raudenbush and Bryk (2002, 24) recommend the use of the intraclass correlation $\hat{\rho} = \hat{\sigma}_{\mathrm{I}}^2/(\hat{\sigma}_{\mathrm{I}}^2 + \hat{\sigma}_{\mathrm{T}}^2) = \hat{\tau}_{00}/\left(\hat{\tau}_{00} + \hat{\sigma}_{\mathrm{T}}^2\right)$. Here it equals 0.016—about 1.6% of the variance in apprehension is between the categories of institutional incidents—a noticeable percentage, even though the z score for $\hat{\tau}_{00} = \hat{\sigma}_{\mathrm{I}}^2$ indicates a lack of statistical significance. Most multilevel models exhibit a much higher initial percentage of variance between the level-2 units, which other level-2 variables may reduce to insignificance. Lazarsfeld and Thielens grouped the apprehension scores so that about 0.46 of the teachers had higher apprehension and 0.54 had lower apprehension, rather than allowing this variable to range across all of the values of apprehension. Their dichotomization of this response variable reduces the variance that is between categories of institutional incidents.

Raudenbush and Bryk (2002, 72) also suggest calculating the reliability of the sample mean in any level-2 unit j by substituting the estimated variance components into this equation:

$$\hat{\lambda}_j = \text{Reliability } (\bar{Y}.j) = \hat{\sigma}_i^2/[\hat{\sigma}_i^2 + (\hat{\sigma}_{\mathrm{T}}/n_j)] \tag{9.4}$$

$$= \hat{\tau}_{00}/[\hat{\tau}_{00} + (\hat{\sigma}_T^2/n_j)]$$

For the three categories of institutional incidents, the simple average of the reliability scores is $\bar{\lambda} = 0.91((1.92 + 0.91 + 0.89)/3)$, which indicates that the sample means are very reliable indicators of the true means of the institutional incidents.

Table 9.2, and Table 9.3 later on, reports these measures of goodness of fit of the various models: the –2 log-likelihood (–2LL), which is the deviance of the model; Akaike's (1974) information criterion (AIC); and Schwarz's (1978) Bayesian information criterion (BIC). Most simply, the deviance of the model is defined as the difference between the –2LL of the current model and the –2LL of the saturated model, which is zero. Thus, the –2LL of the current model is a measure of how poorly this model fits the data relative to the saturated model that fits the data perfectly. The AIC and the BIC are designed to prevent an investigator from artificially reducing the deviance by adding to the model many variables that have small effects. Both of these statistics thus penalize the investigator for building models that lack parsimony, with the BIC being more punitive than the AIC. The AIC adjusts the

Table 9.2 Linear Probability Models for the Effects on Apprehension of Permissiveness and Institutional Academic Freedom Incidents, Maximum Likelihood Estimates from Proc Glimmix

	Model 1: Baseline, random intercepts	Model 2: Permissiveness, random intercepts	Model 3: Permissiveness and incidents, random intercepts	Model 1a: Baseline, no random intercepts	Model 2a: Permissiveness, no random intercepts	Model 3a: Permissiveness and incidents, no random intercepts	Model 4a: Permissiveness| incidents, no random intercepts
Random effects							
$\tau_{00} = \hat{\sigma}_I^2$	0.0039	0.0017	–	Zero	Zero	Zero	Zero
SE	0.0035	0.0017	–	–	–	–	–
Z	1.114	1.000	–	–	–	–	–
Pr Z	–	–	–	–	–	–	–
$\hat{\sigma}_T^2$	0.242	0.236	0.236	0.246	0.238	0.236	0.236
SE	0.008	0.008	0.008	0.008	0.008	0.008	0.008
Z	30.62	30.60	30.60	30.75	30.62	30.60	30.56
Pr Z	–	–	–				
Model fit criteria (PQ Option)							
- 2 Residual log likelihood	2671.1	2624.2	2616.1	2693.0	2631.4	2616.1	2612.4
Akaike's information (AIC)	2677.1	2634.2	2628.1	2697.0	2639.4	2628.1	2632.4
Schwarz's Bayesian (BIC)	2674.4	2629.7	2622.7	2708.1	2661.6	2661.3	2687.7
Fixed effects							
Intercept	0.44	0.52	0.58	0.434	0.52	0.58	0.56
t	11.7	17.9	24.4	37.95	30.8	24.4	20.1
Pr > | t |	0.007	0.003	–	<.0001	<.0001	<0.0001	<0.0001
(Lower, Upper)	(0.281, 0.607)	(0.395, 0.645)	–	(0.412, 0.456)	(0.490, 0.557)	(0.530, 0.623)	(0.505, 0.614)
Permissiveness (Very is base)							
Conservative	–	–0.204	–0.198	–	–0.2256	–0.198	–0.095
t	–	–6.86	–6.64	–	–7.75	–6.64	–1.34
Pr > | t |	–	<0.0001	<.0001	–	<0.0001	<0.0001	0.180
(Lower, Upper)	–	(–0.262, –0.145)	(–0.257, –0.140)	–	(–0.283, –0.169)	(–0.257, –0.140)	(–0.234, 0.043)
Moderate	–	–0.105	–0.097	–	–0.115	–0.097	–0.078
t	–	–3.87	–3.73	–	–4.45	–3.72	–1.55
Pr > | t |	–	<0.0001	0.0002	–	<0.0001	0.0002	0.122
(Lower, Upper)	–	(–0.152, –0.050)	(–0.149, –0.046)	–	(–0.166, –0.064)	(–0.149, –0.046)	(–0.176, 0.021)

Table 9.2 (continued)

	Model 1: Baseline, random intercepts	Model 2: Permissiveness, random intercepts	Model 3: Permissiveness and incidents, random intercepts	Model 1a: Baseline, no random intercepts	Model 2a: Permissiveness, no random intercepts	Model 3a: Permissiveness and incidents, no random intercepts	Model 4a: Permissiveness| incidents, no random intercepts
Incidents (2 or more is base)							
Institutions with Zero	–	–	–0.11	–	–	–0.11	0.00
t	–	–	–3.9	–	–	–3.9	–2.1
Pr > | *t* |	–	–	–	–	–	0.0001	0.035
(Lower, Upper)	–	–	–	–	–	(–0.17,–0.056)	(–0.17, –0.006)
	–						
Institutions with One	–	–	–0.058	–	–	–0.057	–0.0289
t	–	–	–1.96	–	–	–1.95	–0.71
Pr > | *t* |	–	–	–	–	–	0.051	0.476
(Lower, Upper)	–	–	–	–	–	(–0.116, 0.0001)	(–0.108, 0.050)
Cross Level Interactions							
Institutions with Zero Incidents							
Conservative	–	–	–	–	–	–	–0.137
t	–	–	–	–	–	–	–1.63
Pr > | *t* |	–	–	–	–	–	–	0.103
(Lower, Upper)	–	–	–	–	–	–	(–0.301, 0.027)
Moderate	–	–	–	–	–	–	–0.013
t	–	–	–	–	–	–	–0.19
Pr > | *t* |	–	–	–	–	–	–	0.846
(Lower, Upper)	–	–	–	–	–	–	(–0.142, 0.116)
Institutions with One Incident							
Conservative	–	–	–	–	–	–	–0.107
t	–	–	–	–	–	–	–1.23
Pr > | *t* |	–	–	–	–	–	–	0.218
(Lower, Upper)	–	–	–	–	–	–	(–0.277, 0.063)
Moderate	–	–	–	–	–	–	–0.053
t	–	–	–	–	–	–	–0.79
Pr > | *t* |	–	–	–	–	–	–	0.432
(Lower, Upper)	–	–	–	–	–	–	(–0.184, 0.079)

Note: Data from Lazarsfeld and Thielens, Fig. 10-9, p. 259

–2LL according to the number of parameters the model uses, and the BIC takes into account the sample size as well. SAS calculates the AIC and BIC so that smaller values indicate the better models. The formula for the AIC = –2LL + 2 × the dimension of the model. In the baseline model there are three dimensions: the two variance components and the intercept. Consequently, AIC = 2,671.1 + 6 = 2,677.1. The formula for the BIC = –2LL + the dimension of the model × ln(n). Here n = three "subjects" and the ln(n) = 1.0986. Therefore, for the baseline model the BIC = 2,671.1 + 3(1.0986) = 2,677.1 + 3.2958 = 2,674.4. If more complex models actually fit the data better than simpler models, then for successive models their AIC and BIC ought to become smaller, as the models become more complex.

9.2.3 Step 3: The Level-1 Model

Before assessing the effects on apprehension of the institutional contexts, it is best to let a teacher's permissiveness explain as much apprehension as it can. The level-1 equation (9.5) includes the teacher's amount of permissiveness (X_{ij}) as a level-1 continuous covariate:

$$Y_{ij} = \beta_{0j} + \beta_{1j}X_{ij} + r_{ij} \tag{9.5}$$

where r_{ij} is the teacher-level residual and σ_{T}^2 is the variance of $r_{ij} - r_{ij} \sim N(0, \sigma_{\mathrm{T}}^2)$.

The set of level-2 equations for the intercept and the coefficient on permissiveness, assuming that each has a random component, are

$$\beta_{0j} = \gamma_{00} + \mu_{0j} \tag{9.6a}$$

$$\beta_{1j} = \gamma_{10} + \mu_{1j} \tag{9.6b}$$

Here γ_{00} and γ_{10} are institutional-level coefficients and μ_{0j} and μ_{1j} are institutional-level random effects: μ_{0j} designates that the intercepts β_{0j} can vary across the categories of institutional incidents and μ_{1j} designates that β_{1j}, the influence of permissiveness on apprehension, can also vary across categories of incidents. The inclusion of these random effects complicates the representation of the covariance parameters as follows (Raudenbush and Bryk 2002, 35–36, Singer 1998, 333, Singer and Willett 2003, 61–63):

$$\begin{pmatrix} \mu_{0j} \\ \mu_{1j} \end{pmatrix} \sim N\left[\begin{pmatrix} 0 \\ 0 \end{pmatrix}, \begin{pmatrix} \tau_{00} & \tau_{01} \\ \tau_{10} & \tau_{11} \end{pmatrix}\right] \tag{9.7}$$

Expression (9.7) states that the two level-2 residuals are distributed bivariate normal with means of zero and variance components τ_{00} and τ_{11}, the former is the variance of the intercepts and the latter is the variance of the slopes; the covariance of τ_{00} and τ_{11} is $\tau_{01} = \tau_{10}$.

The model for the effect of permissiveness on apprehension is derived by substituting the level-2 equations (9.6a) and (9.6b) into the level-1 equation (9.5) and rearranging terms to obtain equation (9.8), which has three parts:

$$Y_{ij} = \left[\gamma_{00} + \gamma_{10}X_{ij}\right] + \left[\mu_{0j} + \mu_{1j}X_{ij} + r_{ij}\right] \tag{9.8}$$

The response variable Y_{ij} refers to the amount of apprehension of teacher i when contained in institutional incident category j. The first set of brackets encloses the model's structural variables (the intercept and slope for permissiveness); the second set of brackets encloses the stochastic elements. Table 9.2 reports the sample estimates for the non-zero parameters of model 2—two covariance parameters—τ_{11} and τ_{01} $(= \tau_{10})$ are zero and are not reported. That $\tau_{11} = 0$ implies that the slope coefficients for the effect of permissiveness on apprehension do not vary much across categories of incidents and therefore the covariance between τ_{00} and $\tau_{01} = (= \tau_{10})$ also is zero. Compared with model 1, the baseline model, the variance between institutional incident categories $\tau_{00} = \hat{\sigma}_{\mathrm{T}}^2 = 0.0017$, ($z = 1.000$, not significant) is now smaller, whereas the estimate of the residual variance of teachers within their institution's incidents category—$\hat{\sigma}_{\mathrm{T}}^2 = 0.236$—is about unchanged and is very statistically significant ($z = 30.6$). The addition of the effect of the permissiveness covariate, which model 2 estimates as a binary (0, 1) indicator variable, reduces the –2LL, AIC, and BIC by, respectively, 1.76, 1.60, and 1.67 percentage change points.

The indicator variable coding quantifies the effects of permissiveness on apprehension using the very permissive teachers as the base category. Compared with the very permissive teachers, moderates have lower apprehension by -0.105 ($p < 0.0001$) and conservatives have lower apprehension by -0.204 ($p < 0.0001$). The least-square means of apprehension express these different effects: the mean apprehension for conservatives = 0.30, for moderates = 0.41, and for the very permissive = 0.52. These values are about the same as the subsequent effects, when incidents are introduced into the model as a level-2 covariate.

9.2.4 Step 4: Adding a Level-2 Covariate

Given that we found in step 1 that differences in the level-2 categories of institutional incidents had some influence on the level-1 intercept and slopes, it is reasonable to specify equations (9.9a) and (9.9b) that relate the intercept and slope coefficients, β_{0j} and β_{1j} to the categories of institutional incidents symbolized by W_j:

$$\beta_{0j} + \gamma_{00} + \gamma_{01}W_j + \mu_{0j} \tag{9.9a}$$

$$\beta_{1j} = \gamma_{10} + \gamma_{11}W_j + \mu_{1j} \tag{9.9b}$$

Equation (9.9a) states that the intercept β_{0j} in the level-1 equation equals a new value of the conditional intercept γ_{00} that reflects the effect of W_j, plus the effect on B_{0j} of W_j that operates through the regression coefficient γ_{01}, plus the random effect μ_{0j} that implies that the intercepts vary across the categories of incidents. Equation (9.9b) states that the slope coefficient β_{1j} for the effect of permissiveness on apprehension equals a new value of the conditional intercept γ_{10}, plus the effect on β_{1j} of W_j that operates through the regression coefficient γ_{11}, plus the random effect μ_{1j} that implies that the effect of permissiveness on apprehension varies across the categories of incidents.

9.2.5 Step 5: The Combined Multilevel Model

Our modeling strategy suggests that we should combine the equations by substituting equations (9.9a) and (9.9b) into the level-1 equation (9.5), collect the terms forming the combined model, and then explicate the assumptions concerning the random effects:

$$
\begin{aligned}
Y_{ij} &= \beta_{0j} + \beta_{1j}X_{ij} + r_{ij} \\
Y_{ij} &= (\gamma_{00} + \gamma_{01}W_j + \mu_{0j}) + (\gamma_{10} + \gamma_{11}W_j + \mu_{1j})X_{ij} + r_{ij} \qquad (9.10) \\
Y_{ij} &= \left[\gamma_{00} + \gamma_{10}X_{ij} + \gamma_{01}W_j + \gamma_{11}W_jX_{ij}\right] + \left[\mu_{0j} + \mu_{1j}X_{ij} + r_{ij}\right]
\end{aligned}
$$

where $r_{ij} \sim N(0,\sigma^2_{\mathrm{T}})$ and $\begin{pmatrix}\mu_{0j}\\ \mu_{1j}\end{pmatrix} \sim N\left[\begin{pmatrix}0\\0\end{pmatrix}, \begin{pmatrix}\tau_{00} & \tau_{01}\\ \tau_{10} & \tau_{11}\end{pmatrix}\right]$. When the parameters of equation (9.10) are estimated, given the earlier results about the covariance parameters, it is reasonable to expect that the variance for slopes τ_{11} and the covariance between intercepts and slopes $\tau_{01}(=\tau_{10})$ will equal zero (and they do) and that the already small variance τ_{00} between categories of institutional incidents will be further reduced, becoming zero.

9.2.6 Step 6: Estimate the Parameters of the Combined Model

Ignoring for the moment the cross-level interaction in equation (9.10), the results in Table 9.2 for model 3 for the effects of indicator variables for permissiveness and incidents on apprehension indicate that the estimates of the random effects τ_{11} and $\tau_{01}(=\tau_{10})$ are in fact zero and the introduction of incidents as a covariate reduces the variance between categories of institutional incidents to $\tau_{00} = 0.0000000$. Thus, τ_{00} can be removed from the model, which I have done in models 1a through 4a. Model 3 is a multilevel model that specifies a random intercept and a level-1 residual error r_{ij}. Model 3a is an analogous linear probability model that only specifies a level-1 residual error r_{ij}, which is conceptualized as the dispersion of the model. The elimination of this $\tau_{00} = 0$ allows the tests of significance to be calculated for the intercept and for the institutional incidents and improves the fit statistics. In model 3a, institutions with zero incidents engender less apprehension by $-.11 (p = 0.0001)$ compared with institutions with 2+ incidents, and institutions with 1 incident engender less apprehension by $-.058$ ($p = 0.0505$) also compared with institutions with 2+ incidents; the least-squares means for the categories of incidents are 0.36, 0.42, and 0.48.

The algorithm for the type III test quantifies the significance of each covariate by first calculating the overall fit of the model with all of the covariates included. Then it assesses the difference made by deleting each covariate from the full model one at a time. The type III tests indicate that the effects of permissiveness ($p < 0.0001$) and incidents ($p = 0.0005$) are very statistically significant and remain significant when the cross-level interactions are estimated, as in model 4a.

Model 4a elaborates model 3a by examining the joint effects on apprehension of permissiveness and institutional incidents, and their interactions, when the variables are coded as indicator variables. It reports the estimates of the effects of all of the fixed variables of equation (9.10) including the cross-level interaction, but all of the τ coefficients are zero—the only random effect is the level-1 residual σ_T^2. Consequently, the statistical model is a linear probability regression model. Holding constant the level of institutional incidents, the conservative teachers tend to have less apprehension than the moderately permissive and the very permissive, but these differences are not statistically significant. Moreover, the type III test indicates that the effect of the permissiveness $\times$ incidents interaction is not statistically significant ($p = 0.45$); the inclusion of this non-significant effect increases the BIC by 26.4 from model 3a. But the overall lack of significance of the permissiveness $\times$ incidents interaction masks some important contextual effects that will become apparent when we examine the differences among the least-square means later in this chapter.

9.2.7 Step 7: Testing the Preferred Model Against Alternative Models

Figure 9.4 plots the values of the –2LL, the AIC, and the BIC from Table 9.2 for the baseline model 1a to the more complex model 4a that includes the cross-level effects of permissiveness and incidents. The introduction of the teachers' permissiveness in model 2a significantly reduces all three measures of fit from the baseline model. The addition of the institutional incidents in model 3a significantly decreased the –2LL and the AIC, but not the BIC. When the interaction term that is not statistically significant is added to form model 4a, then the BIC strongly penalizes this model by increasing considerably beyond the value for model 3a, and the AIC also increases, but slightly. Taking into consideration all three fit statistics, model 3a fits the data best but model 4a includes some statistically significant contextual effects. A very similar pattern of results characterizes the logistic equation models of Table 9.3.

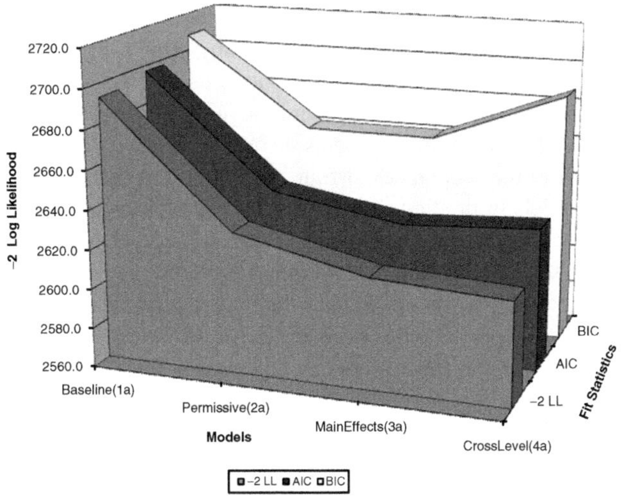

Fig. 9.4 Comparison of fit statistics for four linear probability models, maximum likelihood estimates from Proc Glimmix

9.2.8 Step 8: Replicate the Analysis Using Alternative Statistical Procedures

Gelman and Hill (2007, 70) state, and I agree, "logistic regression is the standard way to model binary outcomes (that is, data y_i that take on the values 0 or 1)." Logistic regression and multilevel logistic regression models are based on the logit transformation. The logit transform for the binary proportion apprehensive (A) is defined as logit (A) = ln (A/(1 − A)) = the natural log (ln) of the odds of being classified as apprehensive. This quantity is set equal to the right-hand side of an equation that contains the covariates and stochastic elements. Paralleling equation (9.1) for a continuous response variable, equation (9.11) states that the logit of the proportion of teachers classified as exhibiting apprehension when teacher i is grouped in incident category j is

$$\text{logit}(\text{A}_{ij}) = \ln(\text{A}_{ij}/(1 - \text{A}_{ij})) = \beta_{0j} + r_{ij} \tag{9.11}$$

By first setting $u = \beta_{0j} + r_{ij}$ and then exponentiating the simplified equation (9.11), we can derive an expression (9.12) that directly produces estimates of the binary proportion A_{ij} :

$$\begin{aligned} (\text{A}_{ij}/(1 - A_{ij})) &= \text{e}^{\text{u}} \\ \text{A}_{\text{ij}} &= \text{e}^{\text{u}} - \text{A}_{\text{ij}} \times \text{e}^{\text{u}} \\ \text{A}_{ij} + \text{A}_{ij} \times \text{e}^{\text{u}} &= \text{A}_{ij}(1 + \text{e}^{\text{u}}) = \text{e}^{\text{u}} \\ \text{A}_{ij} &= \text{e}^{\text{u}}/(1 + \text{e}^{\text{u}}) = 1/(1 + 1/\text{e}^{\text{u}}) \end{aligned} \tag{9.12}$$

Paralleling the linear probability models analyzed earlier, Table 9.3 presents a series of logistic regression models on the untransformed logit scale. The effects in these models can be expressed as proportions using SAS's ilink option on the least-square means statement, thereby implementing the logic of equation (9.12). The models in the first set of three models include a variance that is between level-2 units; the models in the second set of four models do not include this insignificant variance. The models in the first set are two-level models estimated by GLIMMIX using pseudo log-likelihood. The models in the second set are single-level models estimated by GENMOD using maximum likelihood. For both sets of models I specified the response distribution as binomial and the link as logit.

For the first set, model 1 is the baseline multilevel model in which the intercept is specified as random and the variance components are specified as unstructured. Two parameters are estimated on the natural logarithm scale: the variance between the institutions with different incident counts, $\tau_{00} = \hat{\sigma}_I^2 = 0.101$ (standard error = se = 0.108, not significant), and the variance of teachers within the institutions with different incident counts $\sigma_T^2 = 1.0$ (se = 0.033, very significant). This latter parameter is conceptualized as the dispersion of the model—the estimate of 1 indicates that the model is not being fit to over-dispersed data. The pseudo log-likelihood is 8002.9 and the intercept is $-.2268 = u$ on the log scale ($p = 0.355$) and exp ($u = -.2268$) = 0.779 on the odds scale. That the value of the odds is less than 1 suggests that a smaller proportion of teachers are in category 1 of apprehension than in category 0 of apprehension. The odds can be expressed as the proportion apprehensive by this expression:Odds/(1 + Odds) = $\mathrm{e^u}/(1 + \mathrm{e^u}) = 0.797/(1 + 0.797) = 0.444$, which is an estimate of the proportion of teachers with a score of 1 on apprehension.

Because the teachers are conceptualized as being grouped according to their own institution's count of academic freedom incidents—0, 1, 2+—to obtain estimates of the levels of apprehension for these incident levels, it is necessary to adjust the intercept by the estimates of the random effects. These adjustments are zero incidents = −0.3052 ($p = 0.116$), one incident = −0.00596 ($p = 0.98$), and two+ incidents = 0.3112 ($p = 0.112$); note that these random effect estimates sum to zero and that their sample variance (0.1875/2 = 0.095) approximates the value of the variance that is between levels of incidents (0.101). Intuitively, the negative signs should result in lowering the predicted proportion of teachers exhibiting apprehension whereas the positive sign should raise the predicted proportion exhibiting apprehension, and they do: For institutions with zero incidents u_0 = intercept+random effect = −0.2268+ −0.3052 = −0.6320 and the proportion apprehensive = $\hat{A}_0 = \mathrm{e^{u0}}/(1 + \mathrm{e^{u0}}) = 0.53152/1.53152 = 0.347$. For institutions with one incident u_1 = intercept + random effect = −0.2268 + −0.00596 = −0.23276 and the proportion apprehensive = $\hat{A}_1 = \mathrm{e^{u1}}/(1+\mathrm{e^{u1}}) = 0.79234/1.79234 = 0.442$. For institutions with two or more incidents u_2 = intercept+random effect = −0.2268+0.3112 = +0.0844 and the proportion apprehensive = $\hat{A}_{2+} = \mathrm{e^{u1}}/(1 + \mathrm{e^{u1}}) = 1.08806/2.08806 = 0.521$. These estimates are very close to the actual proportions: 0.366, 0.442, and 0.527.

Table 9.3 Logistic Regression Models for the Effects on Apprehension of Permissiveness and Institutional Academic Freedom Incidents. Residual PL and Maximum Likelihood Estimates from Proc Glimmix

Logistic regression models Random effects	Model 1: Baseline, random intercepts residual PL*	Model 2: Permissiveness, random intercepts residual PL*	Model 3: Permissiveness and incidents, random intercepts residual PL*	Model 1a: Baseline, no random intercepts ML Estimates	Model 2a: Permissiveness, no random intercepts ML Estimates	Model 3a: Permissiveness and incidents, No random intercepts ML Estimates	Model 4a: Permissiveness| incidents, no random intercepts ML Estimates
$\tau_{00} = \hat{\sigma}_I^2$	0.101	0.048	5.00E-08	Zero	Zero	Zero	Zero
SE	0.108	0.055	371394	–	–	–	–
Z	0.936	0.866	0.000	–	–	–	–
Pr Z	–	–	–	–	–	–	–
$\hat{\sigma}_T^2$	1.000	1.000	1.002	1.000	1.000	1.000	1.000
SE	0.033	0.033	0.033	–	–	–	–
Z	30.62	30.60	30.60	–	–	–	–
Pr Z	–	–	–	–	–	–	–
Model fit criteria (PQ Option)							
– 2 Residual log –likelihood	8002.9	8054.3	8061.3	2570.6	2509.0	2493.9	2489.4
Akaike's information (AIC)	8008.9	8064.3	8075.3	2572.6	2515.0	2503.9	2507.4
Schwarz's Bayesian (BIC)	8025.5	8092.0	8114.0	2578.2	2531.6	2531.6	2557.2
Effects							
Intercept	–0.227	0.08	0.31	–0.266	0.09	0.31	0.24
t	–1.2	0.144	3.2	–5.7	1.4	3.2	2.1
Pr > | t |	0.355	0.637	–	0.0001	0.175	0.002	0.040
(Lower, Upper)	(–1.043, 0.590)	(–0.541, 0.700)	–	(–0.357,–0.174)	(–0.042, 0.232)	(.119, 0.504)	(.011, 0.465)
Permissiveness (Very is base)							
Conservative	–	–0.867	–0.843	–	–0.951	–0.843	–0.381
t	–	–6.61	–6.48	–	–7.49	–6.48	–1.31
Pr > | t |	–	<.0001	<.0001	–	<.0001	<.0001	0.192
(Lower, Upper)	–	(–1.111, –0.603)	(–1.098, –0.588)	–	(–1.20,–0.70)	(–1.098, –0.588)	(–0.953, –0.191)
Moderate	–	–0.403	–0.394	–	–0.465	–0.394	–0.312
t	–	–3.71	–3.62	–	–4.34	–3.62	–1.5
Pr > | t |	–	0.0002	0.0003	–	<.0001	0.0003	0.133
(Lower, Upper)	–	(–0.616,–0.190)	(–0.608,–0.181)	–	(–0.675,–0.255)	(–0.608,–0.181)	(–0.719, 0.095)

Table 9.3 (continued)

Logistic regression models / Random effects	Model 1: Baseline, random intercepts residual PL*	Model 2: Permissiveness, random intercepts residual PL*	Model 3: Permissiveness and incidents, random intercepts residual PL*	Model 1a: Baseline, no random intercepts ML Estimates	Model 2a: Permissiveness, no random intercepts ML Estimates	Model 3a: Permissiveness and incidents, No random intercepts ML Estimates	Model 4a: Permissiveness| incidents, no random intercepts ML Estimates
Incidents (2 or more is base)							
Institutions with Zero	–	–	–0.471	–	–	–0.471	–0.355
t	–	–	–3.86	–	–	–3.86	–2.051
Pr > | *t* |	–	–	–	–	–	0.0001	0.041
(Lower, Upper)	–	–	–	–	–	(–0.71,–0.232)	(–0.695,–0.015)
Institutions with One	–	–	–0.234	–	–	–0.234	–0.116
t	–	–	–1.9	–	–	–1.9	–0.7
Pr > | *t* |	–	–	–	–	–	0.058	0.486
(Lower, Upper)	–	–	–	–	–	(–0.475, 0.008)	(–0.443, 0.211)
Cross Level Interactions							
Institutions with Zero Incidents							
Conservative	–	–	–	–		–	–0.66
t	–	–	–	–		–	–1.86
Pr > | *t* |	–	–	–	–		–	0.063
(Lower, Upper)	–	–	–	–		–	(–1.36, 0.036)
Moderate	–	–	–	–		–	–0.059
t	–	–	–	–		–	–0.22
Pr > | *t* |	–	–	–	–		–	0.828
(Lower, Upper)	–	–	–	–		–	(–0.595, 0.477)
Institutions with One Incident							
Conservative	–	–	–	–		–	–0.456
t	–	–	–	–		–	–1.25
Pr > | *t* |	–	–	–	–		–	0.21
(Lower, Upper)	–	–	–	–		–	(–1.168, 0.257)
Moderate	–	–	–	–		–	–0.215
t	–	–	–	–		–	–0.78
Pr > | *t* |	–	–	–	–		–	0.438
(Lower, Upper)	–	–	–	–		–	(–0.761, 0.33)

Notes:
Residual PL is the default estimation procedure for GLMMs. It is appreviated as RSPL in SAS. R=Residual, S= Subject Specific, PL = Pseudo–Likelihood. Fit statistics based on PLs are not useful for comparing models that differ in their pseudo–data.
Data from Lazarsfeld and Thielens, Fig. 10-9, pp. 259

Although the random effects in model 1 are small and not significant, it is instructive to elaborate the analysis by continuing to designate the institutional incident counts as random and then introducing a teacher's permissiveness as a level-1 covariate that is coded as an indicator variable. For binary proportions A_{ij} the relevant multilevel model has this form, which parallels equation (9.8):

$$\text{logit}(A_{ij}) = \ln(A_{ij}/(1 - A_{ij})) = [\gamma_{00} + \gamma_{10}X_{ij}] + [\mu_{0j} + \mu_{1j}X_{ij} + r_{ij}] \quad (9.13)$$

A_{ij} is the probability teacher *i* in institutional incident category *j* has an apprehension score of 1 (rather than 0). The transformed response variable logit (A_{ij}) refers to the log odds that teacher *i* in institutional incident category *j* has apprehension equal to 1. If the right-hand side of equation (9.13) is set equal to *u*, then the estimated probability that teacher *i* in institutional incident category *j* has an apprehension score of 1 is $\hat{A}_{ij} = e^u/(1 + e^u)$.

The first set of brackets in equation (9.13) enclose the model's structural variables (the intercept and slopes for the indicator-coded permissiveness variable); the second set of brackets enclose the stochastic elements. Model 2 of Table 9.3 reports the sample estimates for the parameters of this model; two covariance parameters τ_{11} and $\tau_{01}(=\tau_{10})$ are zero. That $\tau_{11} = 0$ implies that the slope coefficients for the effects of permissiveness on apprehension do not vary across categories of incidents and that the covariance between τ_{00} and $\tau_{01}(=\tau_{10})$ also is zero. Compared with the baseline model, the variance on the logit scale between institutional incident categories $\tau_{00} = \hat{\sigma}_I^2 = 0.0477$ (se $= 0.0551$, not significant) is even smaller than in model 1, whereas the estimate of the residual variance of teachers within their institution's incidents category is about unchanged, $\hat{\sigma}_T^2 = 1$ ($z = 30.6$), indicating that the modeled data are not over-dispersed. The addition of the effect of the fixed permissiveness covariate does not reduce the pseudo –2LL; it is larger: 8054.3 compared with 8002.9. This increased pseudo –2LL, when a very statistically significant predictor is added to the model, is consistent with the view that it is not appropriate to compare fit statistics across models based on pseudo log-likelihoods.

Model 3 introduces into the model the effects of institutions with different incident counts, estimating this equation:

$$\text{Logit}(A_{ij}) = \ln(A_{ij}/(1-A_{ij})) = [\gamma_{00}+\gamma_{10}X_{ij}+\gamma_{01}W_j]+[\mu_{0j}+\mu_{1j}X_{ij}+r_{ij}] \quad (9.14)$$

The fixed portion states that the logit of the probability that the apprehension of teacher *i* grouped by his or her institution's incident count *j* is 1 equals the sum of the intercept, the effect of the teacher's own level of permissiveness, and the effect of the incidents. The variance between institutional incident counts is now miniscule: $\hat{\sigma}_I^2 = 5.00 \times 10^{-8}$ and the model does not estimate well: the pseudo log-likelihood is 8061.3, which is much higher than that for the baseline model. Moreover, SAS does not report the significance probabilities of the effects of the indicator-coded institutional incident categories. It is best to re-specify the model so that it does not include the variance between the institutional incidents. This change reduces the model to what is called a population average model that SAS estimates using Proc

Genmod, the generalized linear models procedure. Models 1a through 4a of Table 9.3 report the maximum likelihood estimates.

Inspection of the data for these four models indicates that the variance that is between institutions is now set to zero and that the variance among professors within their institution' incident count is 1—the models are not over-dispersed. The effects on the logit scale generally indicate that permissiveness and the institutional incidents exhibit the same patterns as found earlier with the linear probability model. The main effects of the categories of permissiveness and the categories of institutional incidents are statistically significant, but the interactions of these variables in model 4a fail to achieve significance. The estimates of all three fit statistics—the deviance (–2LL), AIC, and BIC—are all smaller in model 2a compared with model 1a; the estimates of the deviance and AIC of model 3a are smaller than those of model 2a. Moreover, the deviance of model 4a is smaller than that of model 3a, but the AIC and especially the BIC exhibit significant increases.

Figure 9.5 depicts these relationships among these fit statistics emphasizing that the BIC decisively prefers model 3a to model 4a, as it did earlier for the linear probability model. But our close examination of the differences between the least-square means of model 4a for both the linear probability and the logistic regression models will uncover some important contextual effects that are absent in model 3a. This indicates that a too heavy reliance on the fit statistics can lead to false-negative results. Although the patterns for Figs. 9.4 and 9.5 are very similar, the comparable –2LL for the logistic regression models are always less than that for the

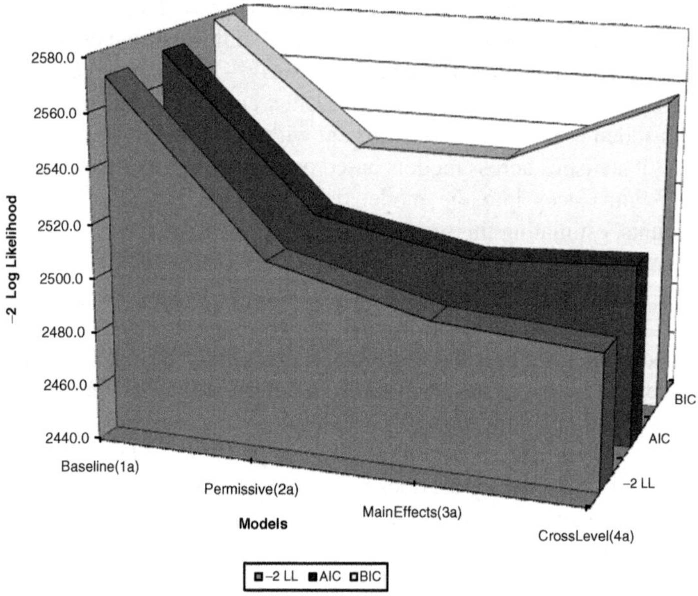

Fig. 9.5 Comparison of fit statistics for four logistic regression models, maximum likelihood estimates from Proc Genmod via Proc Glimmix

Table 9.4 Effects on Teachers' Apprehension of Institutions With Different Counts of Academic Freedom Incidents, For Teachers with Different Levels of Permissiveness, Maximum Likelihood Estimates from Proc Glimmix

a. Linear probability estimates

	Institutional academic freedom incidents		
	0 compared to 1	1 compared to 2+	0 compared to 2+
Conservative (Not Permissive)	–0.09	–0.14	–0.23
	$p = 0.09$	$p = 0.08$	$p = 0.002$
Moderately Permissive	–0.02	–0.08	–0.10
	$p = 0.67$	$p = 0.13$	$p = 0.047$
Very Permissive	–0.06	–0.03	–0.09
	$p = 0.16$	$p = 0.48$	$p = 0.035$

b. Logistic regression estimates

	0 compared to 1	1 compared to 2+	0 compared to 2+
Conservative (not permissive)	–0.44	–0.57	–1.01
	$p = 0.06$	$p = 0.08$	$p = 0.001$
Moderately permissive	–0.08	–0.33	0.41
	$p = 0.66$	$p = 0.14$	$p = 0.051$
Very permissive	–0.24	–0.12	–0.35
	$p = 0.18$	$p = 0.49$	$p = 0\ .04$

linear probability model. This suggests that the logistic models more closely fit the data than the linear probability models.

Proc Glimmix and other multilevel modeling programs can estimate the statistical significance of the differences between the least-square means; such differences may be easier to interpret than the coefficients on the covariates. Using this option, the two panels of Table 9.4 quantify the contextual effects of the institutional academic freedom incidents on the teachers' apprehension for teachers with different amounts of permissiveness for, respectively, the linear probability (panel 4a) and the logistic regression models (panel 4b). For each amount of permissiveness, apprehension is significantly lower when there are zero academic freedom incidents compared with two or more such incidents.

Earlier, when we interpreted the data of Fig. 9.3 by close inspection, we found that the apprehension of conservative teachers increased rather uniformly as the number of institutional incidents increased. The multilevel models produce similar results; note the first row in each panel of Table 9.4. In panel 4a, for conservative teachers when there are 0 academic freedom incidents at their institution their apprehension is lower by -0.09 ($p = 0.09$) than when there is only 1 incident and lower by $-.14$ ($p = 0.08$) when the incidents change from 1 to 2+, for an overall 0 to 2+ difference of -0.23 ($p = 0.002$) units on the apprehension scale. The incremental and overall changes for moderately permissive and very permissive teachers are much less. In panel 4b, the logistic regression estimates on the logit scale corroborate this pattern.

Table 9.5 Effects on Teachers' Apprehension of Differences in Teachers' Permissiveness, For Institutions With Different Counts of Academic Freedom Incidents, Maximum Likelihood Estimates from Proc Glimmix

Institutional academic freedom incidents	Conservative compared to moderately permissive	Moderately permissive compared to very permissive	Conservative compared to very permissive
a. Linear probability estimates			
0	–0.14 $p = 0.001$	–0.09 $p = 0.03$	–0.23 $p < 0.0001$
1	–0.07 $p = 0.18$	–0.13 $p = 0.003$	–0.20 $p < 0.0001$
2+	–0.02 $p = 0.82$	–0.08 $p = 0.12$	–0.095 $p = 0.18$
b. Logistic regression estimates			
0	–0.67 $p = 0.001$	–0.37 $p = 0.04$	–1.04 $p < 0.0001$
1	–0.31 $p = 0.18$	–0.53 $p = 0.005$	–0.84 $p < 0.0001$
2+	–0.07 $p = 0.83$	–0.31 $p = 0.13$	–0.38 $p = 0.19$

Moreover, as institutional incidents increase, the differences in apprehension between conservative and very permissive teachers decline—the institutional context makes the initially divergent teachers more similar; see Table 9.5. In panel 5a, when there are 0 incidents, then the professor's permissiveness tends to determine the amount of apprehension. When there is one incident, then the main difference is between the very permissive and the other categories. When there are two or more incidents, then there is very little difference in apprehension for the different amounts of permissiveness. Comparing the very permissive to the conservative professors, when there are zero incidents there is a difference of $-0.23(p < 0.0001)$ in apprehension; when there is 1 incident the difference is -0.20 ($p < 0.0001$), but when there are 2+ incidents the difference is smaller (–0.10) and not statistically significant ($p = 0.10$) . The context of 2+ incidents makes the teachers more similar with respect to their apprehension. The logistic regression estimates of panel 5b corroborate this pattern.

9.2.9 Step 9: Replicate the Analysis with Other Data

Lazarsfeld and Thielens ended their data analysis by interpreting their Fig. 10-10 (1958: 261). They grouped professors by the protectiveness of their institution's administration, and for each of the four levels of administrative protectiveness,

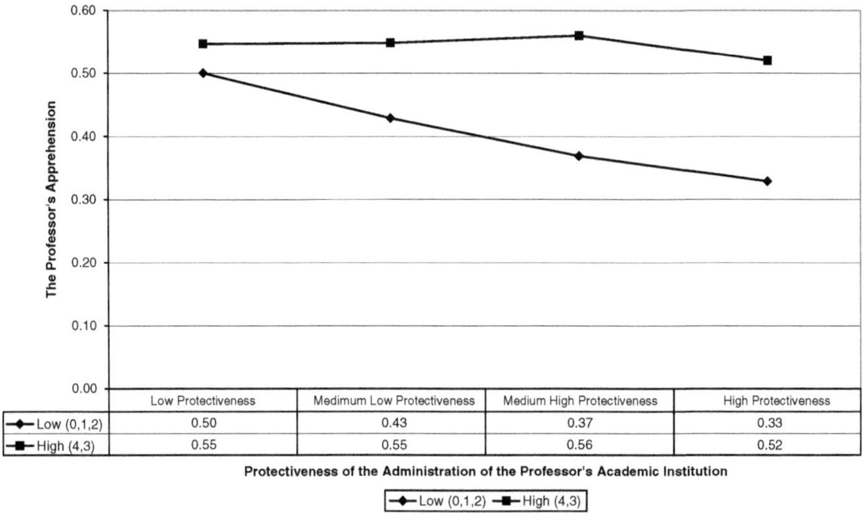

Fig. 9.6 Protective administrations alleviate the apprehension of the less permissive professors (i.e., Low) but not of the more permissive professors (i.e., High), least-squares means from Proc Glimmix (Data from Lazarsfeld and Thielens, Fig. 10-10, p. 261)

they depicted the relationships between binary measures of the professors' permissiveness and apprehension. Contextual and personal characteristics interacted: the administration's protectiveness only alleviated the apprehension of the less permissive professors. Modeling their data, I found that the variance between categories of protectiveness is miniscule. I then applied logistic regression to obtain the least-square means and tests of statistical significance; Fig. 9.6 plots the means. As administrative protectiveness increases, the difference in apprehension between the more and less permissive professors also increases. At low protectiveness the difference is 0.05 ($p = 0.46$); at medium low, 0.12 ($p = 0.003$); at medium high, 0.19 ($p < 0.0001$); and at high, 0.19 ($p = 0.0007$). Thus, as the investigators stated (1958: 260) "apprehension increases with the number of incidents on campus and is relieved by an administration's protective performance." Even so, the academic freedom incidents narrowed the scope of American higher education.

9.3 Conclusion

Contemporary studies of the politics of American professors compare the politics of professors to those of the American public. That some professors exhibit more liberal attitudes than the public leads critics to ask whether this difference biases teaching and enforces political correctness that stifles the study of controversial topics. The typical study de-contextualizes the professors by not focusing on the social structures, processes, and mechanism that engender the political outlooks and activities of academics.

To provide an alternative substantive and methodological paradigm for future studies, this chapter has briefly reviewed Lazarsfeld and Thielens's classic contextual study, *The Academic Mind*, and showed how contemporary statistical methods for multilevel modeling can in principle advance their method of close inspection of tabular data. These new methods can provide estimates of the effects of numerous level-1 and level-2 variables, tests of significance, and model fit for different response distributions. The investigators studied how the cold war against communism and radical right-wing McCarthyism engendered fear at academic institutions. They identified the mechanism for the interplay of stimulus, predisposition, and response: the count of corroborated incidents at an institution (the stimulus) combined with the teachers' political attitudes, their leaning toward permissiveness or conservatism (the predisposition), to produce the amounts of apprehension—assessed by worry and caution—about infringements to one's academic and political freedoms (the response).

Lazarsfeld and Thielens's pivotal contextual analysis combined (1) a level-1 relationship between permissiveness and apprehension, (2) a comparative relationship between an institution's incident count and its teachers' apprehension, and (3) a contextual interaction effect between permissiveness and incidents as these variables jointly determined apprehension. The effects of institutional contexts were indicated by the varying effects on apprehension among teachers with different amounts of permissiveness at institutions with different counts of incidents: for conservative teachers apprehension increased linearly from low values to fairly high values as the number of incidents increased; for the more permissive teachers the amounts of apprehension were high from the start, even when there were no incidents and, as incidents increased, their apprehension increased, but only moderately.

Because of the limitations of cross tabular analysis, Lazarsfeld and Thielens could not simultaneously analyze all of the variables in their summarizing qualitative theory (1958, Fig. 7-13, 188). Their scheme views apprehension as jointly determined by the quality of the school, the permissiveness of the faculty, the pressures impinging on the institution, and the administration's shortcomings. The quantification of this qualitative theory is a challenging problem for contemporary multilevel modelers.

Bibliography

Akaike, H. (1974). A new look at statistical model identification. *IEE Transact. Auto. Cont. AIC* 19, 716–723.

Blumer, H. (1956). Sociological analysis and the variable. *Am. Sociol. Rev.* 21 (December), 683–690.

Cole, S. (Ed.) (2001). *What's wrong with sociology*? New Brunswick: Transaction Publishers.

Coleman, J. S. (1964). *Introduction to mathematical sociology*. New York: Free Press.

Coleman, J. S. (1981). *Longitudinal data analysis*. New York: Basic Books.

Davis, J. A. (1975). Analyzing contingency tables with linear flow graphs: *d* systems. In D. R. Heise (Ed.), *Sociological methodology 1976* (pp. 111–145). San Francisco: Jossey-Bass.

Davis, J. A. (1980). Contingency table analysis: Proportions and flow graphs. *Qual. Quan.* 14, 117–153.
Davis, J. A. (2001). What's wrong with sociology?. In S. Cole (Ed.), *What's wrong with sociology?* (pp. 99–119). New Brunswick: Transaction Publishers.
Fleiss, J. L. (1981). *Statistical methods for rates and proportions.* New York: Wiley.
Gelman, A., and Hill, J. (2007). *Data analysis using regression and multilevel/hierarchical models.* New York: Cambridge University Press.
Goldberger, A. (1991). *A course in econometrics.* Cambridge: Harvard University Press.
Gross, N. and Simmons, S. (2007). The social and political views of American professors. Harvard Sociology Department, Working Paper, September 24.
Hellevick, O. (2009). Linear versus logistic regression when the dependent variable is a dichotomy. *Qual. Quan.* 43, 59–74.
Lazarsfeld, P. F., and Wagner Thielens, Jr. (1958). *The academic mind.* New York: Free Press.
Lazarsfeld, P. F. (1961). The algebra of dichotomous systems. In Solomon H. (Ed.), *Studies in item analysis and prediction.* Stanford: Stanford University Press. Reprinted in *Continuities in the language of social research*, edited by Paul F. Lazarsfeld, Ann K. Pasanella, and Morris Rosenberg, 193–207. New York: Free Press, 1972.
Lazarsfeld, P. F. (1971). Regression analysis with dichotomous attributes. In P. F. Lazarsfeld, A. K. Pasanella, and M. Rosenberg (Ed.), *Continuities in the language of social research* (pp. 208–214). New York: Free Press.
Littell, R. C., Milliken, G. A., Stroup, W. W., Wolfinger, R.D., and Schabenberger, O. (2006). *SAS for mixed models*, (2nd Ed.). Cary NC: SAS Institute.
Raudenbush, S W., and Bryk, A. S. (2002). Hierarchical linear models: Applications and data analysis methods, (2nd Ed.). Newbury Park, CA: Sage.
SAS Institute. (2005). *The Glimmix procedure, November.* Cary NC: SAS Institute.
Schwarz, G. (1978). Estimating the dimension of a model. *Anna. Stat.* 6, 461–464.
Singer, J. D., (1998). Using SAS PROC MIXED to fit multilevel models, hierarchical models, and individual growth models. *J. Educ. Behav. Stat.* 244, 323–355.
Singer, J. D., and Willett, J. B. (2003). *Applied longitudinal data analysis.* New York: Oxford University Press.

Part II
Mathematics and Neural Networks

Chapter 10
The General Philosophy of the Artificial Adaptive Systems

Massimo Buscema

Abstract This chapter has the objective of describing the structure and placing in a taxonomy the artificial adaptive systems (AAS). These systems form part of the vast world of artificial intelligence (AI), nowadays called more properly artificial sciences (AS). Artificial sciences mean those sciences for which an understanding of natural and/or cultural processes is achieved by the recreation of those processes through automatic models. In particular, natural computation tries to construct automatic models of complex processes, using the local interaction of elementary microprocesses, simulating the original process functioning. Such models organise themselves in space and time and connect in a nonlinear way to the global process they are part of, trying to reproduce the complexity through the dynamic creation of specific and independent local rules that transform themselves in relation to the dynamics of the process. Natural computation constitutes the alternative to classical computation (CC). This one, in fact, has great difficulty in facing natural/cultural processes, especially when it tries to impose external rules to understand and reproduce them, trying to formalise these processes in an artificial model. In natural computation ambit, artificial adaptive systems are theories which generative algebras are able to create artificial models simulating natural phenomenon. The learning and growing process of the models is isomorphic to the natural process evolution, that is, it is itself an artificial model comparable with the origin of the natural process. We are dealing with theories adopting the "time of development" of the model as a formal model of "time of process" itself. Artificial adaptive systems comprise evolutive systems and learning systems. Artificial neural networks are the more diffused and best-known learning system models in natural computation. For this reason we present in this chapter an application of new artificial adaptive systems to a very hard and pragmatic topic: drug trafficking. That because we think that "real world" is often the best theory.

M. Buscema (✉)
Semeion Research Center, Via Sersale, Rome, Italy
e-mail: m.buscema@semeion.it

V. Capecchi (eds.), *Applications of Mathematics in Models, Artificial Neural Networks and Arts*, DOI 10.1007/978-90-481-8581-8_10,

10.1 Artificial Adaptive Systems

Artificial adaptive systems (AAS) form part of the vast world of natural computation (NC). Natural computation (NC) is a subset of the artificial sciences (AS). Artificial sciences mean those sciences for which an understanding of natural and/or cultural processes is achieved by the recreation of those processes through automatic models.

In the AS, the computer is what writing represents for *natural language*: The AS consist of *formal algebra* for the generation of *artificial models* (structures and processes), in the same way in which natural languages are made up of semantics, syntax and pragmatics for the generation of *texts*.

In natural languages, writing is achieving *independence of the word from time*, through *space*; in the AS, the computer is the achievement of *independence of the model from the subject*, through automation.

Exactly as through writing a natural language can create *cultural objects* that were unthinkable before writing (stories, legal texts, manuals, etc.), in the same way the AS can create through the computer *automatic models* of unthinkable complexity.

Natural languages and artificial sciences, without writing and the computer, are therefore limited. But a writing not based on a natural language or an automatic model not generated by formal algebra is a set of scribbles (Fig. 10.1).

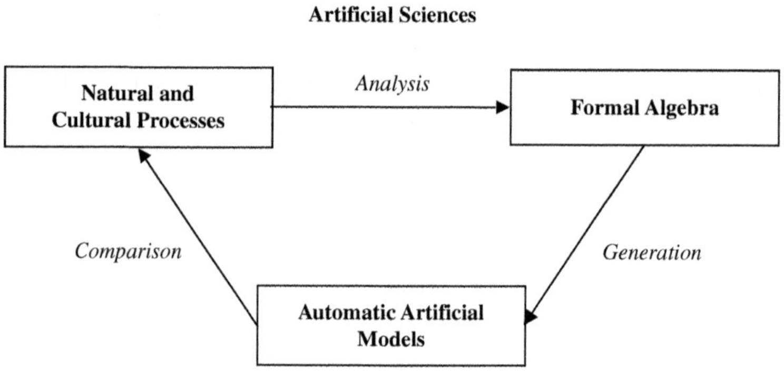

Fig. 10.1 The diagram shows how the analysis of natural and/or cultural processes, that need to be understood, starts from a theory which, adequately formalised (formal algebra), is able to generate automatic artificial models of those natural and/or cultural processes. Lastly, the generated automatic artificial models must be compared with the natural and/or cultural processes of which they profess to be the model and the explanation

In the AS, the understanding of any natural and/or cultural process occurs in a way that is proportional to the capacity of the automatic artificial model to recreate that process. The more positive the outcome of a comparison between original process and model generated is, the more likely it is the artificial model has explained the functioning rules of the original process (see Fig. 10.2).

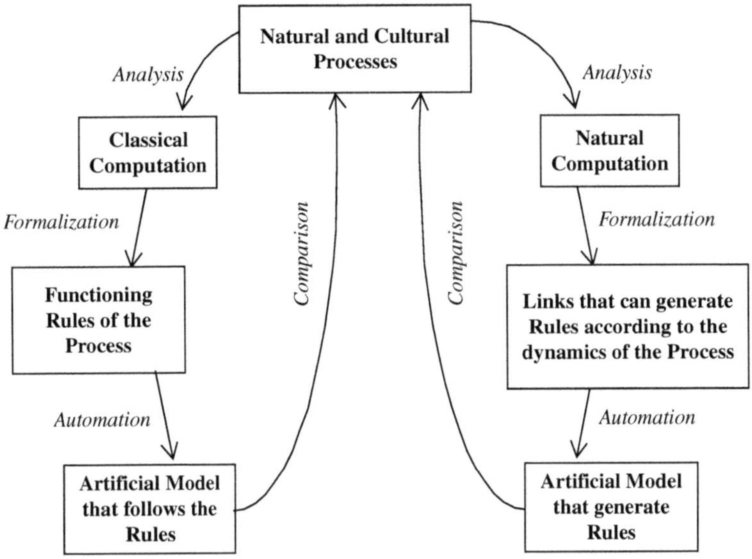

Fig. 10.2 The diagram shows in more detail the formalisation, automation and comparison between natural and/or cultural processes and automatic artificial models seen from two points of view (classical computation and natural computation). Each point of view can be seen as a cycle that can repeat itself several times. This allows to deduce that the human scientific process characterising both the cycles resembles more the natural computation than the classical computation one

However, this comparison cannot be made simple mindedly. Sophisticated analysis tools are needed to make a reliable comparison between original process and artificial model.

Most of the analysis tools useful for this comparison consist of comparing the dynamics of the original process and the dynamics of the artificial model when the respective conditions in the surroundings are varied. In sum, it could be argued that

1. on varying the conditions in the surroundings, *the more* varieties of response dynamics are obtained both in the original process and in the artificial model *and*
2. *the more* this dynamics between original process and artificial model is homologous,
3. *the more* probable it is that the artificial model is a good explanation of the original process.

In Fig. 10.3, we propose a taxonomic tree for characterisation of the disciplines that, through natural computation and classic computation, make up the artificial sciences system.

Natural Computation (NC) means that part of the artificial sciences (AS) that tries to construct automatic models of natural and/or cultural processes through the

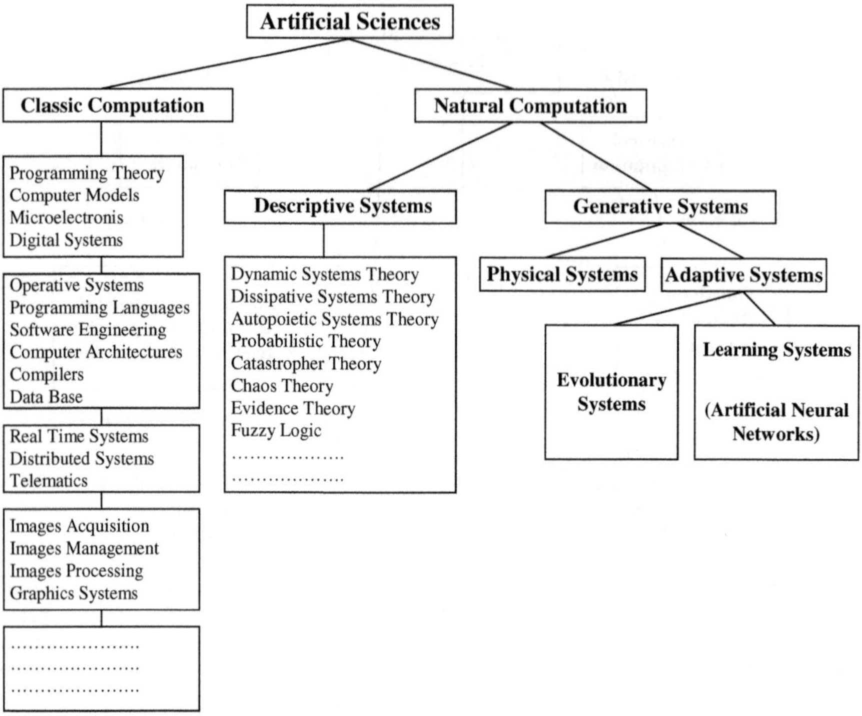

Fig. 10.3 Taxonomic tree of the disciplines that make up the artificial sciences system

local interaction of non-isomorphic microprocesses in the original process. In NC, it is therefore assumed that

1. any process is the more or less contingent result of more basic processes tending to self-organise in time and space;
2. none of the microprocesses is in itself informative concerning the function that it will assume with respect to the others, nor the global process of which it will be part.

This computational philosophy, very economic for the creation of simple models, can be used effectively to create any type of process or model that is inspired by complex processes or by processes regarding which the classic philosophies came up against considerable problems.

NC in fact deals with the construction of artificial models not simulating the complexity of natural and/or cultural processes through rules, but through commitments that, depending on the space and time through which the process takes form, autonomously create a set of contingent and approximate rules.

NC does not try to recreate natural and/or cultural processes by analysing the rules, through which it is wanted to make them function, and formalising them into an artificial model. On the contrary, NC tries to recreate natural and/or cultural processes by constructing artificial models able to create local rules dynamically, capable of change in accordance with the process itself.

The links that enable NC models to generate rules dynamically are similar to the Kantian transcendental rules: These are rules that establish the conditions of possibility of other rules.

In NC, a dynamic such as *learning to learn* is implicit in the artificial models themselves, while in classical computation it needs further rules. The following are part of natural computation:

- *Descriptive Systems* (DS): These are those disciplines that have developed, whether or not intentionally, *formal algebra* that has proved particularly effective in drawing up appropriate functioning links of artificial models generated within NC (for example, the theory of the dynamic systems, the theory of autopoietic systems, fuzzy logic).
- *Generative Systems* (GS): These are those theories of NC that have explicitly provided formal algebra aimed at generating artificial models of natural and/or cultural processes through links that create dynamic rules in space and in time.

In turn, generative systems can be broken down into the following:

- *Physical Systems* (PS): This means grouping those theories of natural computation whose *generative algebra* creates artificial models comparable to physical and/or cultural processes, only when the artificial model reaches given evolutive stages (limit cycles type). While not necessarily the route through which the links generate, the model is itself a model of the original process. In brief, in these systems the generation time of the model is not necessarily an artificial model of evolution of the process time (for example, fractal geometry).
- *Artificial Adaptive Systems* (AAS): This means those theories of natural computation whose generative algebra creates artificial models of natural and/or cultural processes, whose birth process is itself an artificial model comparable to the birth of the original process. They are therefore theories assuming the emergence time of the model as a formal model of the process time itself.

In short: for these theories, each phase of artificial generation is a model comparable to a natural and/or cultural process.

Artificial adaptive systems in turn comprise the following (see Fig. 10.4):

- *Learning Systems (Artificial Neural Networks* – ANNs): These are algorithms for processing information that allow to reconstruct, in a particularly effective way, the approximate rules relating a set of "explanatory" data concerning the considered problem (the input), with a set of data (the output) for which it is requested to make a correct forecast or reproduction in conditions of incomplete information.

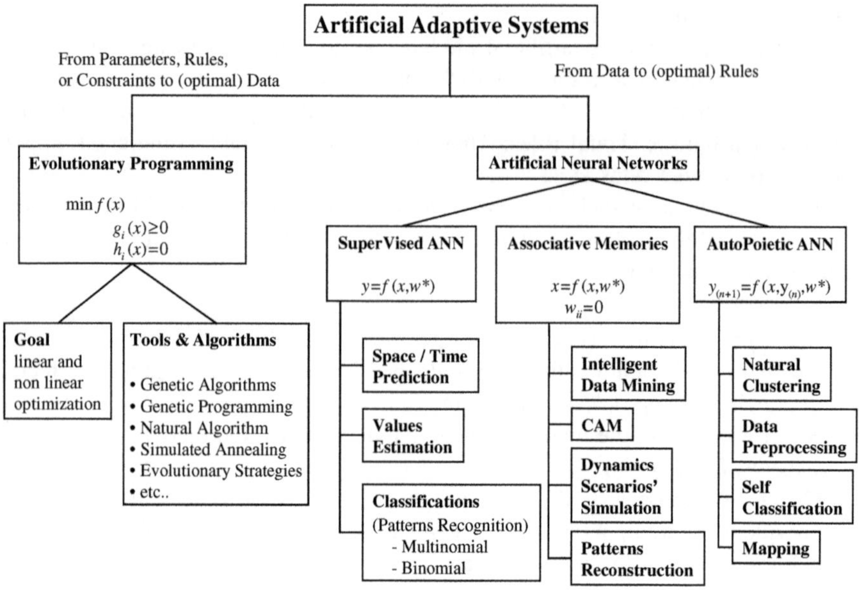

Fig. 10.4 Artificial adaptive systems – general diagram

- *Evolutionary Systems* (ES): This means the generation of adaptive systems changing their architecture and their functions over time in order to adapt to the environment into which they are integrated or comply with the links and rules that define their environment and, therefore, the problem to be simulated. Basically, these are systems that are developed to find data and/or optimum rules within the statically and dynamically determined links and/or rules.

The development of a genotype from a time t_i to a time $t_{(i+n)}$ is a good example of the development over time of the architecture and functions of an adaptive system.

10.2 A Brief Introduction to Artificial Neural Networks

10.2.1 Architecture

ANNs are a family of methods stimulated by the workings of the human brain. Currently ANNs comprise a range of very different models, but they all share the following characteristics:

- The fundamental elements of each ANN are the *nodes*, also known as processing elements (PE), and their *connections*.
- Each node in an ANN has its own *input*, through which it receives communications from the other nodes or from the environment, and its own *output*, through

which it communicates with other nodes or with the environment. Finally it has a function, $f(\cdot)$, by which it transforms its global input into output.
- Each connection is characterised by the force with which the pair of nodes excite or inhibit each other: Positive values indicate excitatory connections and negative ones indicate inhibitory connections.
- Connections between nodes may change over time. This dynamics triggers a *learning process* throughout the entire ANN. The way (the law by which) the connections change in time is called the "learning equation".
- The overall dynamics of an ANN is linked to *time*. In order to change the connections of the ANN properly, the environment must act on the ANN several times.
- The ANNs environment is constituted by the data. Thus, in order to process them, data must be subjected to the ANN several times.
- The overall dynamics of an ANN depends exclusively on the local interaction of its nodes. The final state of the ANN must, therefore, evolve "spontaneously" from the interaction of all of its components (nodes).
- Communications between nodes in every ANN tend to occur in *parallel*. This parallelism may be *synchronous* or *asynchronous* and each ANN may emphasise it in a different way. However, any ANN *must* present some form of parallelism in the activity of its nodes.
- From a theoretical viewpoint this parallelism does not depend on the hardware on which the ANNs are implemented.

Every ANN must present the following architectural components:

- Type, number of nodes and their properties
- Type, number of connections and their location
- Type of signal flow strategy
- Type of learning strategy

10.2.1.1 The Nodes

There can be *three types* of ANN nodes, depending on the position they occupy within the ANN.

- Input nodes: These are the nodes that (also) receive signals from the environment outside the ANN.
- Output nodes: These are the nodes whose signal (also) acts on the environment outside the ANN.
- Hidden nodes: These are the nodes that receive signals only from other nodes in the ANN and send their signal only to other nodes in the ANN.

The number of input nodes depends on the way the ANN is intended to *read* the environment. The input nodes are the ANN's *sensors*. When the ANN's environment consists of data the ANN should process, the input node corresponds to a sort of data *variable*.

The number of output nodes depends on the way one wants the ANN to *act* on the environment. The output nodes are the *effectors* of the ANN. When the ANN's environment consists of data to process, the output nodes represent the variables sought or the results of processing.

The number of hidden nodes depends on the complexity of the function one intends to map between the input nodes and the output nodes.

The nodes of each ANN may be grouped into classes of nodes sharing the same properties.

Normally these classes are called layers.

Various types can be distinguished:

- Monolayer ANNs: all nodes of the ANN have the same properties.
- Multilayer ANNs: The ANN nodes are grouped in functional classes; e.g. nodes (a) sharing the same signal transfer functions and (b) receiving the signal only from nodes of other layers and send them only to new layers;
- Node-sensitive ANNs: Each node is specific to the position it occupies within the ANN; e.g. the nodes closest together communicate more intensely than they do with those further away.

10.2.1.2 The Connections

There may be various types of connections: monodirectional, bidirectional, symmetrical, antisymmetrical and reflexive (Fig. 10.5):

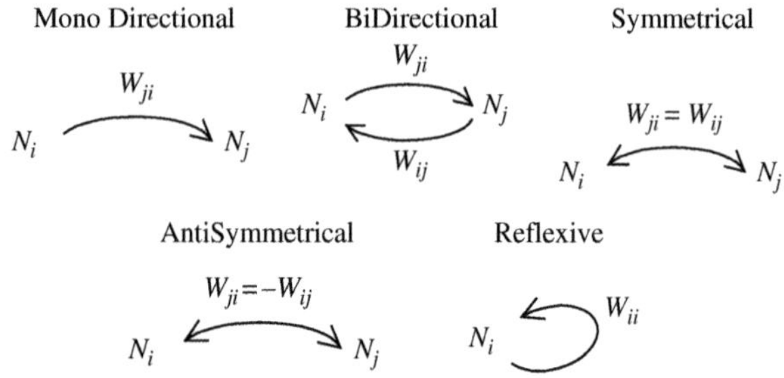

Fig. 10.5 Types of possible connections

- The number of connections is proportional to the memory capabilities of the ANN. Positioning the connections may be useful as methodological preprocessing for the problem to be solved, but it is not necessary. An ANN where the connections between nodes or between layers are not all enabled is called an ANN with *dedicated connections*; otherwise it is known as a *maximum gradient* ANN.

In each ANN the connections may be

- Adaptive: They change depending on the learning equation
- Fixed: They remain at fixed values throughout the learning process
- Variable: They change deterministically as other connections change

10.2.1.3 The Signal Flow

In every ANN the signal may proceed in a direct fashion (from input to output) or in a complex fashion.

Thus we have two types of flow strategy:

- *Feed forward ANN*: The signal proceeds from the input to the output of the ANN passing all nodes only once.
- *ANN with feedback*: The signal proceeds with specific feedbacks, determined beforehand or depending on the presence of particular conditions.

The ANNs with feedback are also known as *recurrent ANNs* and are the most plausible from a biological point of view. They are often used to process timing signals and they are the most complex to deal with mathematically.

In an industrial context, therefore, they are often used with feedback conditions determined a priori (in order to ensure stability).

10.2.2 The Learning

Every ANN can learn over time the properties of the environment in which it is immersed or the characteristics of the data which it presents, in one of two ways (or mixture of both):

- By reconstructing approximately the probability density function of the data received from the environment, compared with preset constraints
- By reconstructing approximately the parameters which solve the equation relating the input data to the output data, compared with preset constraints

The first method is known in the context of ANNs as *vector quantisation*; the second method is *gradient descent*. The vector quantisation method articulates the input and output variables in *hyperspheres* of a defined range. The gradient descent method articulates the input and output variables in *hyperplanes*.

The difference between these two methods becomes evident in the case of a feed forward ANN with at least one hidden unit layer. With vector quantisation the hidden units encode *locally* the more relevant traits of the input vector.

At the end of the learning process, each hidden unit will be a *prototype* representing one or more relevant traits of the input vector in definitive and exclusive form.

With gradient descent, the hidden units encode *in a distributed manner* the most relevant characteristics of the input vector.

At the end of the learning process, each hidden unit will tend to represent the relevant traits of the input in a fuzzy and non-exclusive fashion.

Summing up, the vector quantisation develops a *local* learning and the gradient descent develops a *distributed* or *vectorial* learning.

Considerable differences exist between the two approaches:

- Distributed learning is computationally more efficient than local learning. It may also be more plausible biologically (not always or in every case).
- When the function that connects input to output is nonlinear, distributed learning may "jam" on local minimums due to the use of the gradient descent technique.
- Local learning is often quicker than distributed learning.
- The regionalisation of input on output is more sharply defined using vector quantisation than when using gradient descent.
- When interrogating an ANN trained with vector quantisation, the ANN responses cannot be different from those given during learning; in the case of an ANN trained with gradient descent the responses may be different from those obtained during the learning phase.
- This feature is so important that families of ANNs treating the signal in two steps have been designed: First with the quantisation method and then with the gradient method.
- Local learning helps the researcher to understand how the ANN has interpreted and solved the problem and distributed learning makes this task more complicated (though not impossible).
- Local learning is a competitive type and distributed learning presents aspects of both competitive and cooperative behaviours between the nodes.

10.2.3 Artificial Neural Networks Typology

ANNs may in general be used to resolve three types of complex problems and consequently they can be classified into three subfamilies.

10.2.3.1 Supervised ANNs

The first type of problem that an ANN can deal with can be expressed as follows: Given N variables, about which it is easy to gather data, and M variables, which differ from the first and about which it is difficult and costly to gather data, assess whether it is *possible to predict* the values of the M variables on the basis of the N variables.

These family of ANNs are named *supervised* ANNs (SV) and their prototypical equation is

$$y = f(x, w^*) \tag{10.1}$$

where y is the vector of M variables to predict and/or to recognise (target), x is the vector of N variables working as networks inputs, w is the set of parameters to approximate and $f()$ is a nonlinear and composed function to model.

When the M variables occur subsequently in time to the N variables, the problem is described as a *prediction* problem; when the M variables depend on some sort of typology, the problem is described as one of *recognition* and/or *classification.*

Conceptually it is the same kind of problem: Using values for some *known variables* to predict the values of other *unknown variables.*

To correctly apply an ANN to this type of problem we need to run a *validation protocol.*

We must start with a good sample of cases, in each of which the N variables (known) and the M variables (to be discovered) are both *known* and *reliable.*

The sample of complete data is needed in order to

- *train* the ANN and
- *assess* its predictive performance.

The validation protocol uses *part* of the sample to *train* the ANN (training set), while the *remaining cases* are used to assess the *predictive capability* of the ANN (testing set or validation set).

In this way we are able to test the reliability of the ANN in tackling the problem *before* putting it into operation. An example of this kind of network is reproduced in the Fig. 10.6.

10.2.3.2 Dynamic Associative Memories

The second type of problem that an ANN can be expressed is as follows: Given N variables defining a data set, find out its optimal connections matrix able to define each variable in terms of the others and consequently to approximate the hypersurface on which each data point is located.

This second sub-family of ANNs is named *dynamic associative memories (DAM).*

The specificity of these ANNs is incomplete patterns reconstruction, dynamic scenarios simulation and possible situations prototyping.

Their representative equation is

$$x^{[n+1]} = f(x^{[n]}, w^*) \tag{10.2}$$

where $x^{[n]}$ is the N variables evolution in internal time of ANN, w^* is connection matrixes approximating the parameters of the hypersurface representing the data set

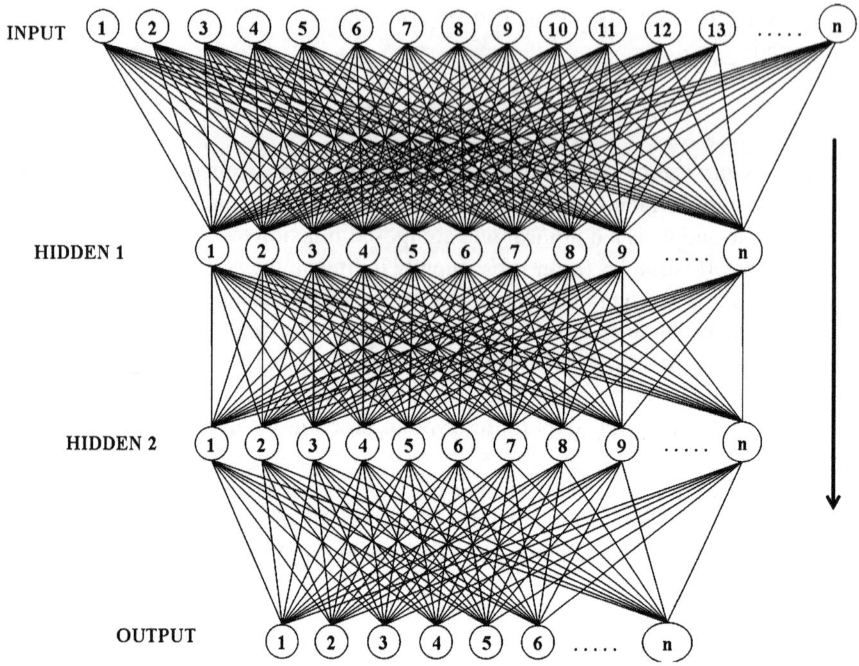

Fig. 10.6 Example of supervised ANN

and *f*() is some suitable nonlinear and eventually composed function governing the process.

DAM ANNs need to be submitted to a validation protocol named "data reconstruction blind test" after the training phase. In this test the capability of a DAM ANN to rebuild complete data from uncompleted ones is evaluated from a quantitative point of view. An example of this kind of network is reproduced in Fig. 10.7.

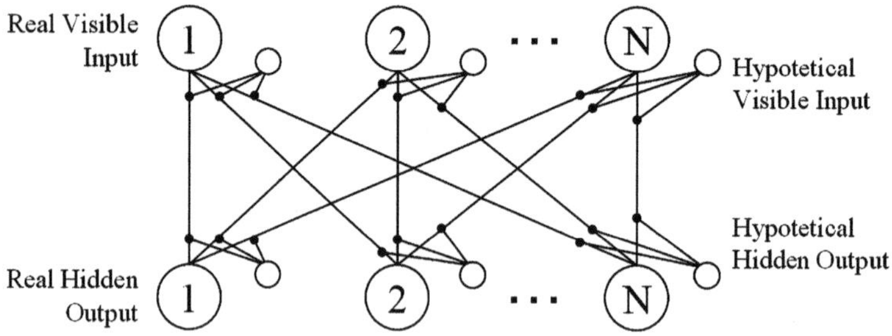

Fig. 10.7 Example of dynamic associative memory – new recirculation ANN

10.2.3.3 Autopoietic ANNs

The third type of ANNs can be described as follows: Given *N* variables, define *M* records in a data set, how these variables are distributed and how these records are naturally clustered in a small projection space *K* ($K<<N$) according to their most important relationships.

These ANNs are named as unsupervised (US) or autopoietic ANNs. Their specificity is the nonlinear extraction of the similarities among records in a database, using all the variables at the same time. One important feature of these ANNs is also the possibility that some of them have to visualise in a two- or three-dimensional map the geographical similarities among records and among variables.

The prototypical equation of the US ANNs is

$$y^{[n+1]} = f(y^{[n]}, x, w^{*}) \tag{10.3}$$

where y is the projection result along the time, x is the input vector (independent variables) and w is the set of parameters (codebooks) to be approximated.

In US ANNs, the codebooks (w) after the training phase represent an interesting case of cognitive abstraction: In each codebook the ANN tends to develop its abstract cognitive representation of some of the data which it learnt. An example of this kind of network (self-organising maps) is reproduced in the Fig. 10.8. The following Table 10.1 synthesizes the different typologies of ANNs.

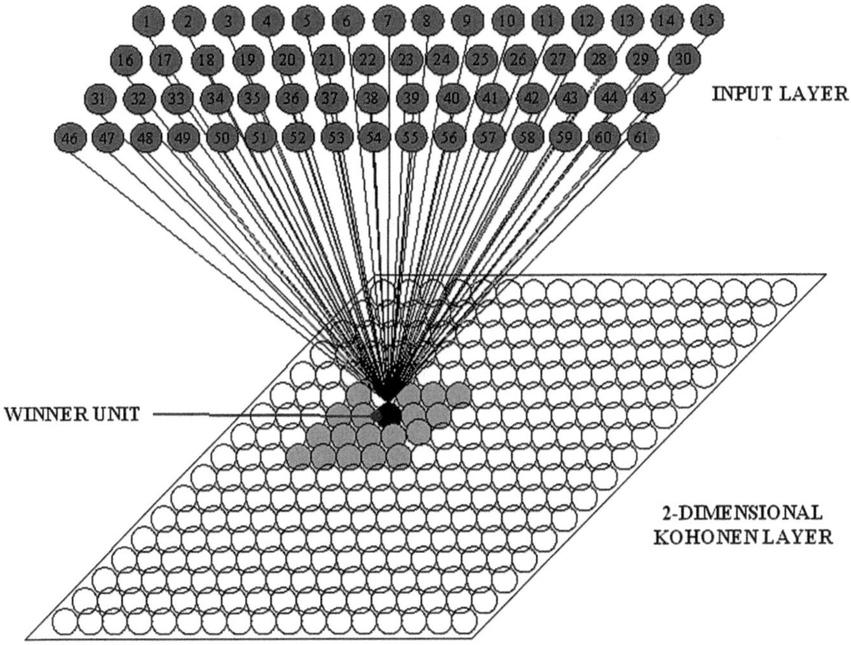

Fig. 10.8 Example of unsupervised ANN – self-organising map

Table 10.1 Differences between traditional GA and GenD

Traditional GAs	GenD
• Assesses individual health • Creates a wheel of probabilities	• Assesses individual health • Calculates the average • Calculates the variance • Creates a band around the average
• Creates a new population based on the wheel of probabilities criterion	• Creates a vulnerability list based on the average criterion
• Undertakes a fixed % of marriages according to the wheel of probabilities – (the best marry)	• Undertakes a variable % of marriages according to the vulnerability list (number) and the average (quality) – ("normal" individuals marry)
• Each marriage has N crossover and hybridises parents' genes (produces possible improvements)	• Each marriage has N crossover and consists of a search for possible states between parents and the population (produces possible improvements and increases biodiversity)
• The percentage of mutations is fixed and serves to produce biodiversity	• The percentage of mutations is variable, depending on marriages not undertaken, and serves to offer a final opportunity only to some of the most vulnerable individuals
• Biodiversity is provided on the basis of errors (mutations) and decreases as the average rises	• Biodiversity is generated by marriages and rises as the average goes up
• The system tends towards stability	• The system becomes more unstable as it approaches stability
• There is no evolution of evolution	• There is evolution of evolution
• Worst and average individuals tend not to reproduce	• Worst and best individuals tend not to reproduce

10.3 A Brief Introduction to Evolutionary Algorithms

The genetic algorithms (GAs) constitute a subset of the evolutionary algorithms, a generic term that indicates a range of systems of problem resolution based on the use of computer, similar to the evolutionary processes.[1] Apart from the genetic algorithms, they include evolutionary programming, evolutionary strategies, classifying systems, genetic programming and genetic doping algorithms.

In general, the algorithms used in the disciplines of artificial intelligence work on the research of a global minimum or maximum in a finite space on the basis of bounds on the space of the solutions. From a formal point of view we can state that, given an element X belonging to a Cartesian space D (where n is the cardinality of D, then X is a vector) and given a function $f{:}D \rightarrow R$ called objective function, then the research of the global optimum is the research of an X^* maximising this

[1] Written with Massimiliano Capriotti.

function, that is $X^* \in D$ and $\forall X \in D{:}f(X) \leq f(X^*)$. Factors as the presence of more points of local maximum, bounds on the domain D, that is the nonlinearity, can make the research very difficult and the problem could not be solvable in an acceptable time. Then we use algorithms of a heuristic type that, even solving the problem with degrees of uncertainties and not assuring the convergence of the search of the solution in some cases, require much less time of convergence.

It results from here the distinction between "strong" and "weak" methods. The former methods are oriented to the solution of a specific problem, on the basis of the knowledge of the particular domain and of the inner representation of the system under examination. The good solutions obtained are hardly adaptable to other tasks and with unsatisfying results. The weak methods use less knowledge of the domain; they are not oriented to a specific target and solve a wide range of problems. The evolutionary algorithms are algorithms based on a heuristic research and considered as weak methods. However, the new typology of the weak evolutionary methods has recently introduced methods having initially little knowledge of the domain but that during their evolution acquire a greater awareness of the problem, implementing some characteristics of the strong methods ("emerging intelligence")

10.3.1 Genetic Algorithm

Between the end of the 1950s and the beginning of the 1960s the researchers in the field of evolutionary computation began taking interest in the natural systems convinced that they could build a model for the new algorithms of optimisation. In this optics, the mechanisms of the evolution can be adapted in order to face some of the most interesting computational problem, related to the search for the solution among a large number of alternatives. For instance, to solve the problem of proteins design with the help of the computer, it is necessary to build an algorithm that locates a protein with certain characteristics among a very high number of possible sequences of amino acids. Similarly, we can search a group of rules or equations that allow to foresee the behaviour of the financial markets. Algorithms of this type have to be adaptive, because they "interact" with a changing environment.

From this point of view the organisms can be considered as very good problem solvers. As they are able to survive in their environment, they develop behaviours and skills that are the result of the natural evolution. The biologic evolution is similar to a method of research inside a very large number of solutions, constituted by the set of all genetic sequences, whose results, that is the desired solutions, are highly adapted organisms, with a strong capacity of survival and reproduction in a changeable environment that will transmit their genetic material to the future generations. Essentially, the evolution of a species is ruled thus by two fundamental processes: the natural selection and the sexual reproduction. The latter determines the recombination of the genetic material of the parents generating an evolution much more rapid than the one that might be obtained if all the descendants contained simply a copy of genes of one parent, modified randomly by a mutation. It is a process with a high degree of parallelism: It does not work on a species at the time, but it tries and changes millions of species in parallel.

In short, a genetic algorithm (GA) is an iterative algorithm that operates on a population of individuals encoding the possible solutions of a given problem. The individuals are evaluated through a function that measures the capacity to solve the problem and identifies the most suitable individuals for reproduction. The new population evolves on the basis of random operators, inspired to the sexual reproduction and to the mutation. The complete cycle is repeated until reaching a given criteria of stop. The use of these algorithms is essentially linked to the programming of the artificial intelligence in robotics, to the bio-computation, to the study of the evolution of the parallel cell systems, to particular problems of management and systems of optimisation in engineering.

Thus GAs have the following strong points:

- Possibility to solve complex problems without knowing the precise method of solution
- Capacity of auto-modification on the basis of the mutation of the problem
- Capacity of simulating some phenomena given a structure and operative modalities similar to those of the biological evolution

The first attempts of designing instruments of optimisation, the evolutionary strategies of Rechemberg and the evolutionary planning of Fogel Owens and Walsh, did not produce interesting results as the tests of biology of the first 1960's highlighted the operator of the mutation rather than the reproductive process for the generation of new genes. In the mid-1960s John Holland's proposal marked a meaningful progress, whose genetic algorithms underlined for the first time the importance of the sexual reproduction.

In some applications, the GAs find good solutions in reasonable times. In others, they might take days, months or even years to find an acceptable solution. But since they work with populations of independent solutions, it is possible to distribute the computational load on more computers, producing simultaneously different hypothesis with the consequent reduction of the calculation time.

10.3.2 Natural Evolution and Artificial Evolution

10.3.2.1 Natural Evolution

The modalities of action of the Darwinian principle of the natural selection can be summarised as follows:

The natural evolution acts on the genetic material (genotype) of an individual and not on his physical characteristics, the phenotype. Each variation that promotes the adaptation of an individual emerges from the genetic property, not from what the parents have learnt in their life.

The natural selection favours the reproduction of the individuals that improves the adaptability to the changing environment and eliminates the individuals with less reproductive potentials. From the genetic point of view, the natural selection promotes those particular genetic combinations that give birth to a more efficient organism, selecting the genotype, not the phenotype.

The reproduction is the central core of the evolutionary process: The generational variability of a species is determined by the genetic recombination and by the little random mutations of the genetic code. The differences between individual and parents are established. The variability is an essential condition of the evolution.

Natural evolution operates over entire populations through cyclic and generational processes and is determined exclusively by the environment and by the interactions among various organisms.

The terminology used draws inspiration directly from the studies on the natural biological evolution.

The combination of the Darwinian hypothesis with genetics gave birth to principles that constitute the basis of populations genetics, that is the explanation of the evolution of the populations at a genetic level.

A population is defined as a group of individuals of the same species operating and crossing in the same place.

In biology the chromosomes are the filaments of DNA acting as project for the organism. Each chromosome is composed of genes, each of them encoding a particular protein that determines in turn the specific characteristics of the organism, as it happens for the colour of the eyes. The positions of the genes inside the chromosome are called locus and the different configurations of the proteins are called *alleles*. Most of the organisms have more than a chromosome, whose set is called *genome*. With *genotype* is meant the set of the genes of the genome. The final result of the evolution, that is the individual, is called *phenotype*.

The sexual reproduction consists in the recombination (crossover) of the genetic material of the parents that produces a new complete genetic material for the progeny. Mutations on single parts of DNA may occur. The *fitness* is the suitability of the individual, the probability that he/she lives enough to reproduce. The natural selection promotes the individuals having the most suitable phenotypes as parents – encoded from particular genotypes – for the next generation. It can be directional, if it helps the increase of frequency of an extreme form of the character; stabilising, if it helps the individuals carrying an intermediate form of a certain character; and diverging, if the extreme forms of a character are favoured at the expense of the intermediate ones.

The evolution is based on the following mechanisms:

- Mutation of allele: Primary source of genetic variability
- Genetic flux: Variation of the frequencies of the alleles, due to the migratory movements of some individuals, with a consequent introduction or removal of certain genotypes.

- Genetic drift: Unpredictable variations in the frequency of the alleles if a population have a small number of components. Actually, from a probabilistic point of view it is easier that less probable events happen in a small population with bigger effects.

10.3.2.2 Artificial Evolution

In the terminology of genetic algorithms the chromosome encodes a candidate solution of a given research problem. In Holland's model with a binary encoding, the chromosome identifies a string of bits; the genes are the bits of the string; and the alleles, as property of the genes, can be 1 or 0. The *crossover* is the recombination of the genetic material of two parents composed by a single chromosome and the mutation in the random variation of the value of the alleles in each *locus* of the chromosome. The phenotype is the meaning of the chromosome that is the decoding of the candidate solution of the problem. In common applications the individuals at a single chromosome used, thus, in terms of genotype, chromosome and individual are equivalent. When the coding of the chromosome represents directly a candidate solution, as in some applications where the chromosome is a string of real numbers rather than the bits, the terms genotype and phenotype can coincide, too.

10.3.2.3 The Holland Model

Stating that the genetic algorithms are adaptive complex procedures finalised to the resolution of research and optimisation problems is equivalent to saying that they are procedures searching for the maximum point of a certain function, when it is too complex to be rapidly maximised with analytical techniques and when a procedure exploring randomly the space of the solutions is inconceivable. The GAs select the best solutions and recombine them with different modalities so that they evolve towards a maximum point. The function to be maximised is called *fitness*. The term has many aspects: it may mean "adaptation", "adaptability", "biologic success", "competition".

The original model by Holland is based on a population of n strings of bits with a fixed length l (n, $l\hat{I}$ N), generated randomly. The set of the binary strings with a length l has 2^l elements and represents the space of the solutions of the problems. Each string (genotype) is the binary coding of a candidate solution (phenotype). In general, the function of *fitness* is given in the following form:

$$F = f(x_1, x_2, ..., x_n)$$

Through this function, at each genotype g_i of the initial population $P(t = 0)$ is associated with a value $F_i = F(g_i)$ which represents the capacity of the individual to solve the given problem. In order to determine the value of adaptability, the function of *fitness* receives a genotype in input; it decodes it into the corresponding phenotype and tests it on the given problem. Once the phase of evaluation of the individuals belonging to the initial population is concluded, a new population $P(t+1)$ of new n candidate solutions, obtained applying the operators of selection, crossover, mutation and inversion, is generated.

Selection

Within a population, a probability of selection linked to the fitness is associated with each individual. The selection of operator generates a random number $c\in)1,0($ which determines which individual will be chosen. The chosen individual is copied in the so-called *mating pool*. The mating pool is filled with n copies of the selected individuals, at the time $P(t=0)$. The new population $P(t+1)$ is obtained through the operator of crossover, mutation and inversion. The operator of selection, choosing the individuals that have the possibility to generate descendants with a high fitness, plays the role of the natural selection for the living organisms in the context of genetic algorithm.

Crossover

Within the mating pool two individuals called parents and a point of cut called point of crossover are randomly chosen. The portions of genotype on the right of the crossover point are exchanged generating two descendants, as in Fig. 10.9:

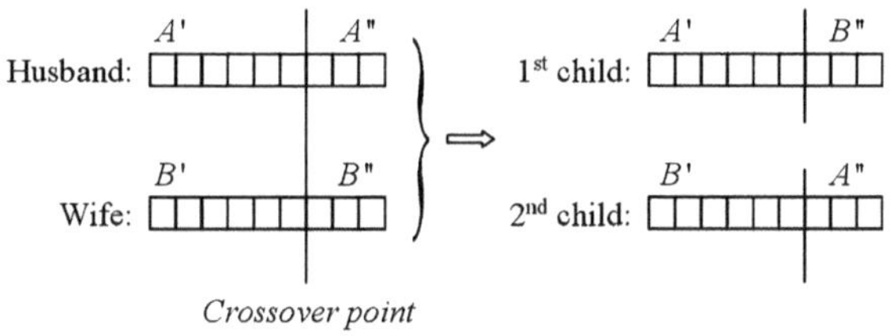

Fig. 10.9 The crossover operator

The so-called operator of *one-point crossover* is applied $n/2$ times to obtain n descendants on the basis of a given probability p. If the crossover is not applied, the descendants coincide with the parents.

Another technique used is the *two-point crossover*: The individuals are not represented by linear strings, but by circles. A portion of circle of an individual is substituted with the one of another, selecting two points of crossover.

The *uniform crossover* states that for each couple of parents a binary string of the same length called *mask* is generated. The descendant is generated by copying the bit of the father or of the mother if the corresponding position of the mask is, respectively, 0 or 1.

The crossover is a metaphor of the sexual reproduction where the genetic material of the descendants is a combination of one of the parents.

Mutation

This operator is inspired to the rare variation of elements of the living creatures' genome during the evolution. On the basis of a little probability p, the value of the bits of each individual is changed (from 0 to 1 and vice versa).

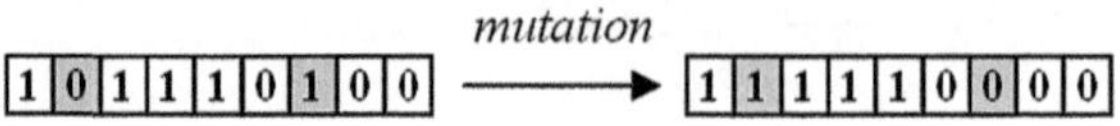

As it happens in nature, the mutation adds a "noise" or a randomness to the whole procedure, in order to assure that starting from a population generated randomly there are no points of a space of the solutions that are not explored.

Inversion

On the basis of a fixed probability p, two points in the string are chosen. The string encodes the individual and inverts the bits between two positions.

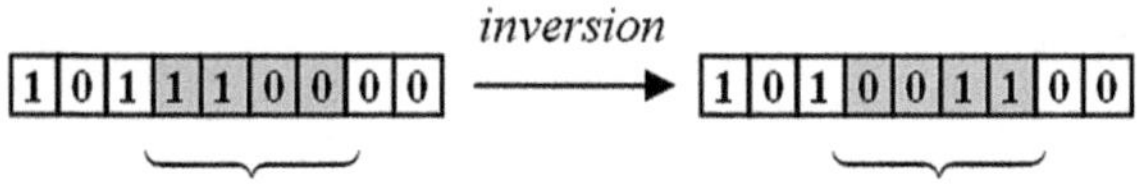

In an initial large population it is difficult to estimate which values of the probability of crossover and mutation will give the best performances. The experience shows that there is a strong dependence on the type of problem. Generally the probability of crossover is between 60 and 80%, while in the case of mutation, it fluctuates between 0.1 and 1%. If the probabilities an individual is selected for the reproduction are proportional to its fitness (if f is the value of fitness of a solution and F is the sum of the values of fitness of all the population, the probability might be f/F), it is probable that, after the crossover, the best individuals are recombined with the consequent loss of the best chromosome. In order to avoid this and to speed up the convergence times, the best individual of a generation may be cloned. Through this technique, called *elitism*, which keep a high number of populations, it is possible to clone more individuals in the next generation, proceeding for the others in the classical way.

10.3.2.4 Types of Encoding of Artificial Genome

In general, it is possible to encode the solutions of a problem with binary strings. In other cases, representations of higher level are used and operators of crossover and mutation able to operate on such representations are defined. Besides the binary encoding, an other type is used, and it is based on the real numbers.

The binary encoding is important not only from the historical point of view but also because the more relevant theoretical results have been obtained with models based on it. The structure of the data is a vector of bit with a length equal to l, which associated a space of 2^l possible solutions. We need to define a function that encodes the genotype, or parts of it, in one or more of the real values. The most used operator of crossover is, in this case, the crossover n points (n points of cut).

The encoding based on floating point numbers is the most natural for problems of optimisations of real parameters. The structure of the data is a vector of length l where each element is a real number. Each candidate solution is a point in the space of the research, and it is not necessary to foresee decoding functions of the genotype. The operator of crossover can be the classic one point of cut, but for the mutation operator, the elements of another vector are added, in order to alter the genes of the individuals.

10.3.3 Other Evolutionary Algorithms

10.3.3.1 The Evolutionary Programming

The evolutionary programming (EP) is a stochastic strategy of optimisation similar to GAs, based on the definition of population, fitness and on the selection of the best. But while these try mainly to simulate the operators of crossover and mutation as it happens in nature, the evolutionary programming concentrates on the connection existing between parents and sons. The basic method consists in three steps: to choose randomly an initial population (the bigger is the number of individuals, the faster we arrive to the convergence); each individual is copied in a new population and to each son a mutation with a specific probability is applied; the fitness of each individual is calculated and through a tournament with stochastic selection N possible solutions are chosen.

In particular, each individual of the population is an FSM (finite states machine), formed by a series of inner states belonging to a finite alphabet. The FSM receives in input a series of symbols and gives back in output a series of states, on the basis of the current states and input. The objective is the forecast of the next configuration of the system, not through the operator of crossover (as in the GAs), but entrusting exclusively to the mutation: it alters the initial state, modifies the transition or changes an inner state. The basic characteristic of this type of algorithms is that the sons have a similar behaviour to their parents.

10.3.3.2 The Evolutionary Strategies

The evolutionary strategies are techniques similar to the previous one, but developed originally for problems concerning civil and structural engineering. The principal difference consists in the selection of the individuals in the EP: They are selected for the mutation with a certain probability that is proportional to the fitness as it happens in the GAs, while in this case the worst individuals are rejected deterministically. The method of optimisation is based on the choice of a strategy that is then applied to a population. The two main strategies are known as strategy plus $(m + l)$ and strategy comma (m,l). In the first case, the parents can participate to the selection in the next generation and in the second, it is only possible to select the sons when the parents die. m represents the number of individuals in the population, while l is the number of sons conceived for each generation. An individual in the population consists of a genotype that represents a point in the research space (that is the space of possible solutions). To each point it is possible to associate

- object variables xi on which the operators of crossover and mutation will be applied until an optimal solution of the problem is reached
- strategy variables Si that determine the "mutability" of xi. They represent the standard deviation of a Gaussian distribution $(0, Si)$. With an expectation value equal to zero the parents will produce on average, sons that are similar to them. This strategy works because sooner or later the individual, with a good value of the objective function (the one to be optimised), will be favoured and that recombining among them will probably make better sons. The value of the objective function $f(x)$ represents the phenotype (fitness) we will take into consideration in the selection. In the plus strategy the better m individuals over $(m + l)$ will survive and will become parents in the next generation, while in the *comma* the selection it happens only among the sons.

10.3.3.3 The Classifying Systems

The classifying systems are operators working in an environment from which they receive input that classifies according to rules which permit them to generate output of instructions to be followed. The instructions belong to the type *if–then*. For example, the problem might be the optimisation of a productive process done by machinery managed by a computer: This receives from its sensors a series of inputs like the temperature of the machinery, the external pressure, the type of material and it acts according to starting rules. Such instructions are not fixed, but if they are encoded in a binary form, they evolve like populations of a GA and their fitness is the performance of the machinery.

10.3.3.4 The Genetic Programming

The technique of the genetic programming is similar to the genetic algorithms, but in this case the population is not constituted by bit strings, but by programs that evolve, combine, reproduce or change when they are executed, in order to create other programs that constitute better solutions of a specific problem. These programs are encoded with a tree structure where the inner nodes are functions and the leaves are the terminal symbols of the program. For example, the expression *IF (TIME>10) THEN return 1+2+3 ELSE return 1+2+4* can be rewritten as *+ (1 2 (IF>TIME 10)3 4))* (language LISP) and transferred in a tree as in the figure:

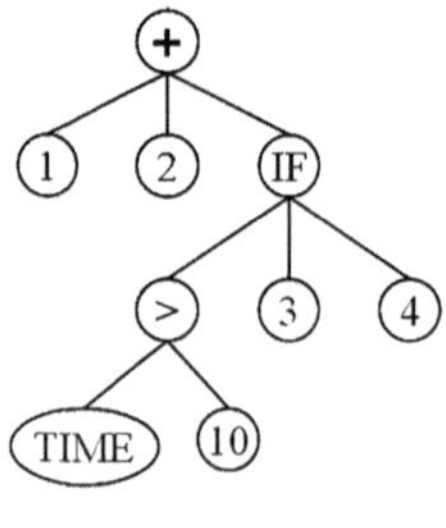

The space of research is constituted by all the programs composed by the terminals and by the functions defined for a specific problem.

The genetic programming has a degree of complexity greater than the genetic algorithms, because programming requires the selection of many more parameters, such as the generation of the initial population, the set of the basic functions and terminals, the type of selection, the dimension of the population and the maximum number of generations, and the criteria of termination.

The operator of crossover is the dragging force of the algorithm: We take at random two subtrees from selected individuals on the basis of their fitness and we recombine them giving birth to two son trees, with parameters establishing limits on the maximum dimension of the population's tree. Other operators, such as the mutation, permutation, editing, encapsulating and decimation, are used in particular cases. In general, the operators determine the syntactic accuracy of the generated trees, but not the semantic correctness. The fitness penalising the trees does not respect the semantic conditions, in order to favour the growth of semantically correct trees.

If the genetic algorithms optimise a solution defined and parameterised by the user, and thus the optimisation works on the representation of the parameters of a function whose structure is known, in the genetic programming we work at a higher level as the user defines the elements of a grammar (operators and terminal symbols) used to generate functions that have to evolve. The optimisation of the fitness consists then not only in the manipulation of the code of the parameters, but above all in that of the functions.

The extension of the research space (the space of all the functions that satisfy the grammar defined by the user) and the less efficiency of the mapping in the memory of the representation used allow the genetic programming to require a higher computational load and a high occupation of memory. It results in a lower usage of the genetic algorithms and the necessity to realise a parallel implementation of these algorithms on environments of a distributed type.

10.3.3.5 Comparison with Other Techniques

As in GAs, there are other techniques of general approach that operates starting from a fitness function that has to be maximised. Some of them are applicable only to limited domains, such as the dynamic programming, where the fitness function is the sum of the fitness functions calculated in each phase of the problem and there is no interaction among the various phases.

In the method of the gradient the information on the gradient of the function are used to lead the direction of the research. However, the function must be continuous; otherwise the derivative cannot be calculated. In general, these methods are called *hill climbing* and in case of functions with only one peak – or less for multi-modal functions – it is not sure that the first hill climbed peak is the highest. In the following figure there is an example of the problem: starting from a random point *X*, with *uphill* movements the maximum *B* is localised, but *A* and *C* are not.

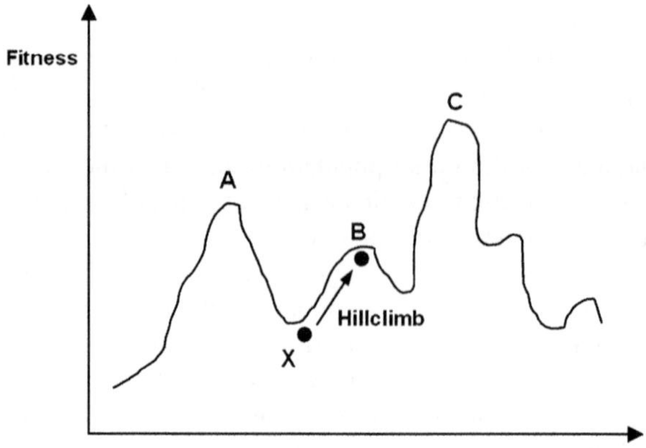

In the iterative research the method of the gradient is combined with the random research, where the points of the research space are randomly chosen. Once the peak is found, the climb starts again from another point randomly chosen. The technique has the advantage to be simple and it gives good results with functions that obviously do not have many local maxima. However, since each test is isolated, a total figure of the form of the domain is not obtained and while the random search continues, the same tests led both in regions where high values of fitness are not found and in regions with a low value of fitness continue to be allocated. A genetic algorithm, instead, operates starting from an initial random population and carries out attempts in regions with a higher fitness. It might be a disadvantage if the maximum is found in a little region surrounded by regions with a low fitness. But this type of function is hardly optimised with any method.

The technique of the simulated annealing is a modified version of the hill climbing. From a random point a random movement is operated: If this brings to a higher point, it is accepted with a probability $p(t)$, where t is the time. At the beginning, the value of $p(t)$ is close to 1 but it gradually tends to 0. If at the beginning each movement is accepted, the probability of accepting a negative movement decreases with the passage of time. Sometimes the negative movements are needed to avoid local maxima, but if they are too many, they may deviate from the maximum. In general, this technique works with only one candidate solution at a time; it does not build a total figure of the research space and the information of the previous movements, used to lead us towards the solution, are not saved.

10.3.4 The Genetic Doping Evolutionary Algorithm

In genetic algorithms (GAs) the principle of reproduction assumes an evolutionary criteria external to the system that in each generation identifies the best and the worst individuals.[2]

[2] Tóth and Lõrincz (1995).

Such criteria recall much more the technique of the exams in school, rather than an evolutionary principle intrinsic to the natural evolution. Similarly, the percentages of crossover and mutations foreseen in every generation cannot be two fixed parameters, established from outside (by the experimentalist); it is preferable to figure them out as adaptive parameters linked to the health of the whole "population" in each generation.

Besides, in the traditional GA the crossovers have fixed rules, typical of the overpopulated and advanced societies (monogamies, prohibition of incest, etc.). It would be proper that a population in a phase of "cultural starting" had more flexible sexual rules and proportioned to its rapid expansion and genetic differentiation.

Just like the traditional genetic algorithms, GenD is able to find solutions to problems of optimisation conceiving the possible solutions as individuals of restricted populations, letting the population evolve, generation after generation, on the basis of specific genetic operators and a selection based on fitness – more suitable individuals – and to the consequent disappearance of the worst ones. After a certain number of generations, the resulted population includes, like the better, a good approximation of the solution to the problem of optimisation. Unlike the traditional genetic algorithms, the evolution of GenD is due to its inner instability, which generates a continuous evolution and a natural increase of the biodiversity, thanks to specific characteristics such as the conceptualisation of the population as structured organisation of individuals (tribes), the definition of an evolutionary law is enough on the fitness of such organisation and the usage of the genetic operators.

10.3.4.1 Theory

In order to increase the speed and the quality of the solutions that have to be optimised, the algorithm GenD makes the evolutionary process of the artificial populations more natural and less centred on the culture of the individual liberalism.

In the first phase the algorithm calculates the fitness score of each individual on the basis of the function we want to optimise. The value of the average health of the whole population is not a simple index. In GenD the average health constitutes first the criteria of *vulnerability*, and lastly those of *connectivity* of all the individuals of the population. It results that the basic unit of the algorithm is not the individual, unlike the classical GAs and many other evolutionary algorithms.

The reference unit is the species, acting on the evolution of the individuals in terms of the average health for each generation.[3]

The feedback loop among the individuals and the average health of the population (species) allows the GenD to transform, in evolutionary terms, the whole population from a sparse set of individuals (like the traditional models) into a dynamic structure of subjects.

[3]Eldredge (1995).

10.3.4.2 The Criteria of Vulnerability

All the individuals whose health is less or equal to the average health of the population are registered into a list of vulnerability. They are not eliminated, they continue participating to the process, but are flagged.

The number of vulnerable individuals establishes automatically the maximum number of crossovers allowed in that generation. The number of possible crossovers in each generation, thus, is variable and it is a function of the average health of the population.

The whole population has this possibility. The maximum number of random calls to the coupling is calculated so that all the individuals flagged as vulnerable might, theoretically, be substituted by new individuals. When the type of used crossover operator generates only a new individual, this number corresponds to the number of vulnerable individuals; otherwise, it is equal to its half when the type of the crossover operator used generates two individuals.

10.3.4.3 Criteria of Connectivity

In order to let a coupling generate offspring, at least one of the proposed individual must have a fitness whose value is close to the average fitness of the whole population (average $\pm\ k$, where $2k$ defines the width of the coupling band).

In alternative, GenD may adopt other criteria of connectivity. Each couple of individuals may generate offspring if the fitness of at least one of the two is greater than the average fitness. The individual that satisfies the condition is named "candidate qualified for the crossover".

The effects of these two criteria are similar: The normal distribution of the fitness of each individual with respect of the average fitness operates a band of dynamic crossover in each generation.

The algorithm *GenD*, thus, assumes that the individuals "sui generis", that is too weak or too healthy, tend not to marry among each other. In practice, the crossovers are not suitable for the best or the worst. It is the "most normal" subjects that tend to crossover. Furthermore, there are no restrictions on crossovers: each individual may marry whoever he/she chooses.

The offspring of each crossover occupies the places of the subjects marked in the list of vulnerability. It may happen, therefore, that a weak individual has the possibility to continue existing through his own offspring.

10.3.4.4 The Criteria of the Last Chance

The number of possible crossovers is a function of the number of subjects marked as vulnerable; the latter is a function of the average health of the population. The criteria of coupling, however, urge the system to have a number of crossovers not necessarily giving birth to offspring. The difference between possible crossovers and realised crossovers defines the number of mutations. That is, the subjects present in the list of vulnerability, that were not substituted by the offspring generated by the realised crossovers, are changed. A last chance to re-enter in the evolutionary game is granted to this variable number of weak subjects through a mutation.

10.3.4.5 The New Crossover

The criteria of coupling allow crossovers only if at least one of the individuals of the couple is a qualified candidate for the crossover: that is, if he/she enjoys of a health close to the average health of the population (first type) or greater (second type). If we indicate with F_i the health of the ith individual, with $\overline{F}$ the average health of the population, with σ^2 the variance of the health of the population, then $F_i$is a candidate qualified for the marriage of the first type if

$$\left(\overline{F} - k\right) \leq F_i \leq \left(\overline{F} + k\right)$$
$$k = 1 - \sigma^2$$

while he/she is a candidate of the second type if $F_i \geq \overline{F}$.

However, in *GenD* the coupling does not consist in the simple interchange of genes between husband and wife around a crossover point, i.e.

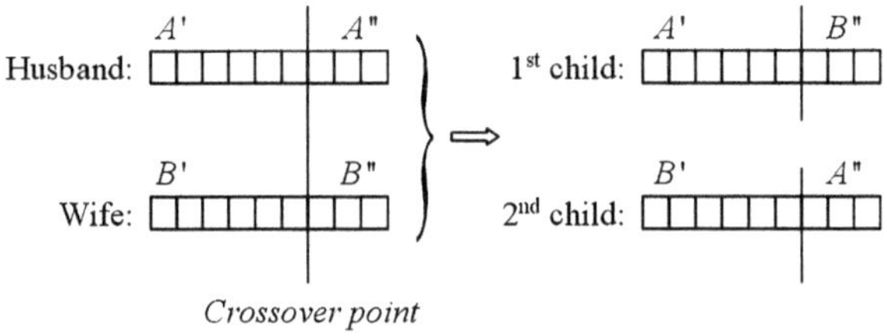

The coupling of genes between parents is carried out in a selective way, in two manners:

1. A logic crossover: when the repetitions are allowed
2. An opportunistic crossover: when the repetitions are not allowed

The Logic Crossover

The logic crossover comprises four cases:

1. Health of the father and mother greater than the average health of the whole population:

$$\left(F_{\mathrm{F}} > \overline{F}\right) \text{and} \left(F_{\mathrm{M}} > \overline{F}\right)$$

2. Health of both parents lower than the average health of the whole population:

$$\left(F_{\mathrm{F}} < \overline{F}\right) \text{and} \left(F_{\mathrm{M}} < \overline{F}\right)$$

3. and 4. Lower health of one of the parents and the one of the other greater than the average health of the whole population:

$$\left(F_{\mathrm{F}} > \overline{F}\right) \text{ and } \left(F_{\mathrm{M}} < \overline{F}\right) \text{ or } \left(F_{\mathrm{F}} < \overline{F}\right) \text{ and } \left(F_{\mathrm{M}} > \overline{F}\right)$$

In the first case, the generation of two sons (suppose for simplicity the case with two sons and only one crossover point) happens in the traditional way:

$$\left(F_{\mathrm{F}} > \overline{F}\right) \text{ and } \left(F_{\mathrm{M}} > \overline{F}\right): \underbrace{\begin{matrix} A' + A'' \\ B' + B'' \end{matrix}}_{\text{parents}} \Rightarrow \underbrace{\begin{matrix} A' + B'' \\ B' + A'' \end{matrix}}_{\text{children}}$$

In the *second case*, the generation of two sons happens through the *negation* ($\sim$) of the parents' genes:

$$\left(F_{\mathrm{F}} < \overline{F}\right) \text{ and } \left(F_{\mathrm{M}} < \overline{F}\right): \underbrace{\begin{matrix} A' + A'' \\ B' + B'' \end{matrix}}_{\text{parents}} \Rightarrow \underbrace{\begin{matrix} \sim A' + \sim B'' \\ \sim B' + \sim A'' \end{matrix}}_{\text{children}}$$

In the third and fourth cases, only the parent whose health is greater than the average health transmits his own genes, while the genes of the other are denied:

$$\left(F_{\mathrm{F}} > \overline{F}\right) \text{ and } \left(F_{\mathrm{M}} < \overline{F}\right): \underbrace{\begin{matrix} A' + A'' \\ B' + B'' \end{matrix}}_{\text{parents}} \Rightarrow \underbrace{\begin{matrix} A' + \sim B'' \\ \sim B' + A'' \end{matrix}}_{\text{children}}$$

or

$$\left(F_{\mathrm{F}} < \overline{F}\right) \text{ and } \left(F_{\mathrm{M}} > \overline{F}\right): \underbrace{\begin{matrix} A' + A'' \\ B' + B'' \end{matrix}}_{\text{parents}} \Rightarrow \underbrace{\begin{matrix} \sim A' + B'' \\ B' + \sim A'' \end{matrix}}_{\text{children}}$$

The concept of genetic negation, in *GenD*, does not correspond to the cancellation of the weaker parent's genes and therefore to their replacement carried out randomly. It deals instead with a genetic substitution carried out with the criteria of a moving window running from right or left the alternative genetic options for each single gene in each specific position.

If, for example, a certain gene shows only two alternatives $g[0, 1]$, then the *moving window* has the following form:

↓	1	0
T	0	1

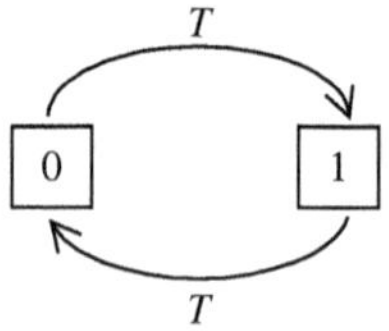

In the same way we will proceed with a gene that presents four possible states; $g[A, B, C, D]$:

↓	A	B	C	D
T	B	C	D	A

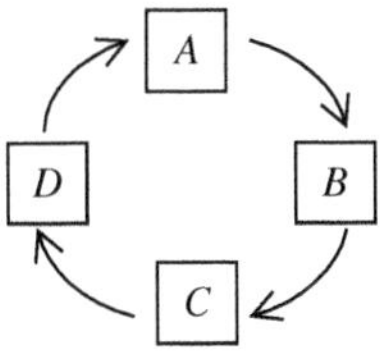

The criterion of the negation through the moving window is applicable also when the various possible states of a gene are not ordered among them. This method, in fact, is based on the systematic exploration of the phase space and on keeping the same systematic criteria.

The Opportunistic Crossover

This operator acts when the repetitions are not allowed. The parents are overlapped with respect to a random crossover point. After, the offspring is generated selecting the most effective gene of the parents. This operation is repeated until all the genes of the offspring are completed.

Table 10.2 Semantics and syntax of ANNs

(A)	Type	Dynamic	Properties
Nodes	• Input • Output • Hidden	Type of equation I → O	• No layer (each node is distinct from every other) • Multilayer (each node is the same as those of its own layer) • Monolayer (each node is the same as the others)
Connections	• Symmetrical • Antisymmetrical • Monodirectional • Bidirectional • Reflexive	• Adaptive • Fixed • Variables	• Maximum connections • Dedicated connections
(B)	**Flow strategy**		**Learning strategy**
Type of ANN	• Feed forward • With parametric or adaptive feed back • Intranode • Intralayer • Among layers • Among ANNs		• Approximation of the function • Gradient descent • Vector Quantisation • Learning conditions of the function • Supervised • Dynamic associative memories • Unsupervised or autopoietic

This rule may be considered as a variant of the algorithm Greedy.[4] In short, the number of marriages and mutations in GenD are not external fixed parameters established from outside, but adaptive variables defining themselves from inside, starting from the global trends of the population system. The above Table 10.2 summarizes the difference between classic genetic algorithm and GenD.

References

Tóth, G. J. and Lõrincz, A. (1995). Genetic algorithm with migration on topology conserving maps. *Neural Netw. World* 2, 171–181.

Eldredge, N. (1995). *The great debate at the high table of evolutionary theory*. New York: John Wiley & Sons.

Reetz, B (1993). Greedy solutions to the travelling sales persons problem. *Advanced Technology for Developers* 2, 8–14.

[4]Reetz (1993).

Chapter 11
Auto-contractive Maps, the *H* Function, and the Maximally Regular Graph (MRG): A New Methodology for Data Mining

Massimo Buscema and Pier L. Sacco

Abstract In this chapter we introduce

1. a new artificial neural network (ANN) architecture, the auto-contractive map (auto-CM);
2. a new index to measure the complexity of a-directed graphs (the *H* index); and
3. a new method to translate the results of data mining into a graph representation (the maximally regular graph).

In particular, auto-CMs squash the nonlinear correlation among variables into an embedding space where a visually transparent and cognitively natural notion such as "closeness" among variables reflects accurately their associations.

Through suitable optimization techniques that will be introduced and discussed in detail in what follows, "closeness" can be converted into a compelling graph-theoretic representation that picks all and only the relevant correlations and organizes them into a coherent picture.

- The architecture of auto-contractive map (equations, topology, and parameters) was ideated by Massimo Buscema at Semeion Research Center from 2000 to 2007. Auto-contractive map is implemented in Buscema (2002, 2007) and Massini (2007b).
- The pruning algorithm was ideated by Giulia Massini at Semeion Research Center in 2006. The pruning algorithm is implemented in Massini (2007a) and Buscema (2008).
- The *H* function was ideated by Massimo Buscema at Semeion Research Center in 2007. The *H* function is implemented in Buscema (2008).

M. Buscema (✉)
Semeion Research Center, Via Sersale, Rome, Italy
e-mail: m.buscema@semeion.it

The "*B*" matrix operator was ideated by Massimo Buscema at Semeion Research Center in 1999. The "*B*" operator is implemented in Buscema (2002).

V. Capecchi (eds.), *Applications of Mathematics in Models, Artificial Neural Networks and Arts*, DOI 10.1007/978-90-481-8581-8_11,

- The delta H function was ideated by Massimo Buscema and Pierluigi Sacco at Semeion Research Center in 2007. The delta H function is implemented in Buscema (2008).
- The maximally regular graph (MRG) was ideated by Massimo Buscema at Semeion Research Center in 2007. The MRG is implemented in Buscema (2008).

11.1 Introduction and Motivation

Investigating the pattern of correlations among large numbers of variables in large databases is certainly a quite difficult task that is seriously demanding in both computational time and capacity. The statistically oriented literature has developed a variety of methods with different power and usability, all of which, however, share a few basic problems; among them the most outstanding are the nature of the a priori assumptions that have to be made on the data-generating process, the near impossibility to compute all the joint probabilities among the vast number of possible couples and n-tuples that are in principle necessary to reconstruct the underlying process' probability law, and the difficulty of organizing the output in an easily grasped, ready-to-access format for the non-technical analyst. The consequence of the first two weaknesses is the fact that when analyzing poorly understood problems characterized by heterogeneous sets of potentially relevant variables, traditional methods can become very unreliable when not unusable. The consequence of the last one is that, also in the cases where traditional methods manage to provide a sensible output, its statement and implications can be so articulated to become practically unuseful or, even worse, easily misunderstood.

In this chapter, we introduce a new methodology based on an artificial neural network (ANN) architecture, the auto-contractive map (auto-CM), which allows for basic improvements in both robustness of use in badly specified and/or computationally demanding problems and output usability and intelligibility. In particular, auto-CMs "spatialize" the correlation among variables by constructing a suitable embedding space where a visually transparent and cognitively natural notion such as "closeness" among variables reflects accurately their associations. Through suitable optimization techniques that will be introduced and discussed in detail in what follows, "closeness" can be converted into a compelling graph-theoretic representation that picks all and only the relevant correlations and organizes them into a coherent picture. Such a representation is not actually constructed through some form of cumbersome aggregation of two-by-two associations between couples of variables, but rather by building a complex global picture of the whole pattern of variation. Moreover, it fully exploits the topological meaningfulness of graph-theoretic representations in that actual paths connecting nodes (variables) in the representation carry a definite meaning in terms of logical interdependence in explaining the data set's variability. We are aware of the fact that these techniques are novel and therefore not entirely understood so far in all of their properties and implications and that further research is called for to explore them. But at the same time we are convinced that their actual performance in the context of well-defined, well-understood problems provides an encouraging test to proceed in this direction.

11.2 The Auto-contractive Map

We begin our analysis with a relatively concise but technically detailed presentation of the ANN architecture that provides the basis for all of the subsequent analysis: the auto-contractive map (auto-CM). The auto-CM is characterized by a three-layer architecture: an input layer, where the signal is captured from the environment; a hidden layer, where the signal is modulated inside the auto-CM; and an output layer, through which the auto-CM feeds back upon the environment on the basis of the stimuli previously received and processed (Fig. 11.1).

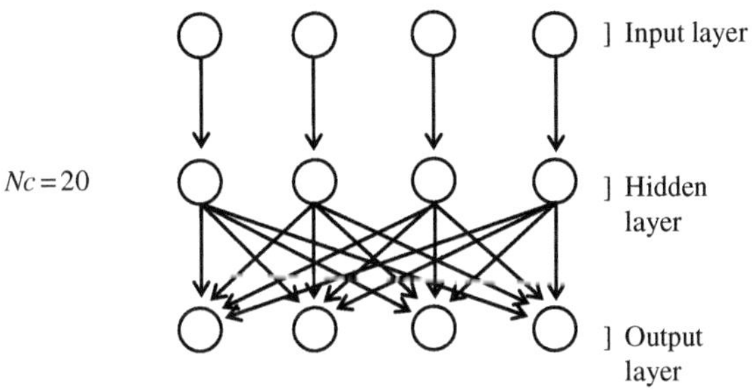

Fig. 11.1 An example of an auto-CM with $N = 4$

Each layer contains an equal number of N units, so that the whole auto-CM is made of $3N$ units. The connections between the input and the hidden layers are mono-dedicated, whereas the ones between the hidden and the output layers are fully saturated, i.e., at maximum gradient. Therefore, given N units, the total number of the connections, N_c, is given by $N_c = N(N+1)$.

All of the connections of auto-CM may be initialized either by assigning a same, constant value to each or by assigning values at random. The best practice is to initialize all the connections with a same, positive value, close to zero.

The learning algorithm of auto-CM may be summarized in a sequence of four characteristic steps:

1. Signal transfer from the input into the hidden layer
2. Adaptation of the values of the connections between the input and the hidden layers
3. Signal transfer from the hidden to the output layer
4. Adaptation of the value of the connections between the hidden and the output layers

Notice that steps 2 and 3 may take place in parallel.

We write as $m^{[s]}$ the units of the input layer (sensors), scaled between 0 and 1; as $m^{[h]}$ the units of the hidden layer; and as $m^{[t]}$ the units of the output layer (system target). We moreover define $\mathbf{v}$, the vector of mono-dedicated connections; $\mathbf{w}$, the matrix of the connections between the hidden and the output layers; and n, the discrete time that spans the evolution of the auto-CM weights or, put another way, the number of cycles of processing, counting from zero and stepping up one unit at each completed round of computation: $n \in N$.

In order to specify steps 1–4 that define the auto-CM algorithm, we have to define the corresponding signal forward transfer equations and the learning equations as follows:

a. Signal transfer from the input to the hidden layer:

$$m_{i(n)}^{[h]} = m_i^{[s]} \left(1 - \frac{v_{i(n)}}{C}\right) \tag{11.1}$$

where C is a positive real number not lower than 1, which we will refer to as the contraction parameter (see below for comments), and where the subscript (n) has been omitted from the notation of the input layer units, as these remain constant at every cycle of processing.

b. Adaptation of the connections $v_{i(n)}$ through the variation $\Delta v_{i(n)}$, which amounts to trapping the energy difference generated according to (11.1):

$$\Delta v_{i(n)} = \left(m_i^{[s]} - m_{i(n)}^{[h]}\right) \cdot \left(1 - \frac{v_{i(n)}}{C}\right) \tag{11.2}$$

$$v_{i(n+1)} = v_{i(n)} + \Delta v_{i(n)} \tag{11.3}$$

c. Signal transfer from the hidden to the output layer:

$$\mathrm{Net}_{i(n)} = \sum_{j=1}^{N} m_{j(n)}^{[h]} \cdot \left(1 - \frac{w_{i,j(n)}}{C}\right) \tag{11.4}$$

$$m_{i(n)}^{[t]} = m_{i(n)}^{[h]} \left(1 - \frac{\mathrm{Net}_{i(n)}}{C}\right) \tag{11.5}$$

d. Adaptation of the connections $w_{i,j(n)}$ through the variation $\Delta w_{i,j(n)}$, which amounts, accordingly, to trapping the energy difference as to (11.5):

$$\Delta w_{i,j(n)} = \left(m_{i(n)}^{[h]} - m_{i(n)}^{[t]}\right) \cdot \left(1 - \frac{w_{i,j(n)}}{C}\right) \cdot m_{j(n)}^{[h]} \tag{11.6}$$

$$w_{i,j(n+1)} = w_{i,j(n)} + \Delta w_{i,j(n)} \tag{11.7}$$

Even a cursory comparison of (11.1) and (11.5) and (11.2), (11.3) and (11.6), (11.7), respectively, clearly shows how both steps of the signal transfer process are guided by the same (contraction) principle, and likewise for the two weight adaptation steps (for which we could speak of an energy entrapment principle).

Notice how the term $m^{[h]}_{j_{(n)}}$ in (11.6) makes the change in the connection $w_{i,j_{(n)}}$ proportional to the quantity of energy liberated by node $m^{[h]}_{i_{(n)}}$ in favor of node $m^{[t]}_{i_{(n)}}$. The whole learning process, which essentially consists of a progressive adjustment of the connections aimed at the global minimization of energy, may be seen as a complex juxtaposition of phases of acceleration and deceleration of velocities of the learning signals (adaptations $\Delta w_{i,j_{(n)}}$ and $\Delta v_{i_{(n)}}$) inside the ANN connection matrix. To get a clearer understanding of this feature of the auto-CM learning mechanics, begin by considering its convergence condition:

$$\lim_{n\to\infty} v_{i_{(n)}} = C \tag{11.8}$$

Indeed, when $v_{i_{(n)}} = C$, then $\Delta v_{i_{(n)}} = 0$ (according to (11.2)) and $m^{[h]}_{j_{(n)}} = 0$ (according to (11.1)) and, consequently, $\Delta w_{i,j_{(n)}} = 0$ (as from (11.6)): the auto-CM then converges.

There are, moreover, four variables that play a key role in the learning mechanics of auto-CM. Specifically,

(1) $\varepsilon_{i_{(n)}}$ is the contraction factor of the first layer of auto-CM weights:

$$\varepsilon_{i_{(n)}} = 1 - \frac{v_{i_{(n)}}}{C}$$

As is apparent from (11.1), the parameter C modulates the transmission of the input signal into the hidden layer by "squeezing" it for given values of the connections; the actual extent of the squeeze is indeed controlled by the value of C, thereby explaining its interpretation as the contraction parameter. Clearly, the choice of C and the initialization of the connection weights must be such that the contraction factor is a number always falling within the]0, 1[range and decreasing at every processing cycle n, to become infinitesimal as n diverges.

(2) $\eta_{i,j_{(n)}}$ is, analogously, the contraction factor of the second layer of auto-CM weights which, once again given the initialization choice, falls strictly within the unit interval:

$$\eta_{i,j_{(n)}} = 1 - \frac{w_{i,j_{(n)}}}{C}$$

As for the previous layer, the value of the contraction factor is modulated by the contraction parameter C.

(3) $\varphi_{i_{(n)}}$ is the difference between the hidden and the input nodes:

$$\varphi_{i(n)} = m_i^{[s]} - m_{i(n)}^{[h]}$$

It is a real function of n, and it always takes positive, decreasing values in view of the contractive character of the signal transfer process.

(4) $\lambda_{i(n)}$ is, likewise, the difference between the output and the hidden nodes:

$$\lambda_{i(n)} = m_{i(n)}^{[h]} - m_{i(n)}^{[t]}$$

It is, by the same token, a real function with positive values, decreasing in n.

The second step to gain insight into the auto-CM learning mechanics is to demonstrate how, during the auto-CM learning phase, $\Delta v_{i(n)}$ describes a parabola arc, always lying in the positive orthant. To see this, re-write (11.2) as follows:

$$\begin{aligned}\Delta v_{i(n)} &= \left(m_i^{[s]} - m_i^{[s]}\left(1 - \tfrac{v_{i(n)}}{C}\right)\right)\cdot\left(1 - \tfrac{v_{i(n)}}{C}\right)\\ &= m_i^{[s]}\cdot\tfrac{v_{i(n)}}{C}\left(1 - \tfrac{v_{i(n)}}{C}\right)\end{aligned} \tag{11.2a}$$

Remembering how $\varepsilon_{i(n)}$ was defined, we can write $v_{i(n)}\big/C = 1 - \varepsilon_{i(n)}$ and then further re-write (11.2a) as a function of the contraction factor $\varepsilon_{i(n)}$:

$$\begin{aligned}\Delta v_{i(n)} &= m_i^{[s]}(1 - \varepsilon_{i_{(n)}})\cdot(1 - (1 - \varepsilon_{i(n)}))\\ &= m_i^{[s]}(1 - \varepsilon_{i(n)})\cdot\varepsilon_{i(n)}\end{aligned} \tag{11.2b}$$

Keeping in mind the definition of $\varepsilon_{i(n)}$ and letting the values of the input layer units decrease along the unit interval, one can easily check that the $\Delta v_{i(n)}$ parabola arc (11.2b) meets the following condition:

$$0 < \Delta v_{i(n)} < \varepsilon_{i(n)} \le C\cdot\varepsilon_{i(n)} \tag{11.2c}$$

Equation (11.2c) tells us that the adaptation of the connections between the input and hidden layers, $\Delta v_{i(n)}$, will always be smaller than the adaptation that $v_{i(n)}$ needs to reach up C. Actually, $v_{i(n+1)} = v_{i(n)} + \Delta v_{i(n)} = C - C\cdot\varepsilon_{i(n)} + \Delta v_{i(n)}$, but from (11.2c) we know that $\Delta v_{i(n)} - C\cdot\varepsilon_{i(n)} \le 0$, which proves our claim. As a consequence, $v_{i(n)}$ will never exceed C. However, the convergence condition requires that $\lim_{n\to\infty} v_{i(n)} = C$, which in turn implies the following:

$$\lim_{n\to\infty}\varepsilon_{i(n)} = 0,\ \lim_{n\to\infty} m_{i(n)}^{[h]} = 0,\ \lim_{n\to\infty} m_{i(n)}^{[t]} = 0,\ \lim_{n\to\infty}\varphi_{i(n)} = m_i^{[s]},\ \text{and}$$

$$\lim_{n\to\infty}\lambda_{i(n)} = 0 \tag{11.8}$$

In view of the contractive character of the signal transmission process at both of the auto-CM's layer levels, combining (11.1) and (11.5) we can also write

$$m_{i_{(n)}}^{[t]} \leq m_{i_{(n)}}^{[h]} \leq m_i^{[s]} \quad (11.1-5)$$

and in particular, we can reformulate them as follows:

$$m_{i_{(n)}}^{[h]} = m_i^{[s]} \cdot \varepsilon_{i_{(n)}} \quad (11.1a)$$

and

$$m_{i_{(n)}}^{[t]} = m_i^{[s]} \cdot \varepsilon_{i_{(n)}} \cdot \left(1 - \frac{\mathrm{Net}_{i_{(n)}}}{C}\right) \quad (11.5a)$$

We are now in the position to clarify the relationship between $\Delta v_{i_{(n)}}$ and $\Delta w_{i,j_{(n)}}$. From (11.1-5), we can stipulate

$$m_{i_{(n)}}^{[h]} = m_i^{[s]} - \varphi_{i_{(n)}} \quad (11.1b)$$

where $\varphi_{i_{(n)}}$ is a small positive real number and

$$m_{i_{(n)}}^{[t]} = m_{i_{(n)}}^{[h]} - \lambda_{i_{(n)}} \quad (11.5b)$$

where $\lambda_{i_{(n)}}$ is another small positive real number. As already remarked, such small positive numbers must become close to 0 as n diverges. We can also write

$$m_{i_{(n)}}^{[t]} = m_i^{[s]} - (\varphi_{i_{(n)}} + \lambda_{i_{(n)}}) \quad (11.5c)$$

At this point, we can easily reformulate (11.2) as follows:

$$\Delta v_{i_{(n)}} = \left(m_i^{[s]} - m_{i_{(n)}}^{[h]}\right) \cdot \left(1 - \frac{v_{i_{(n)}}}{C}\right) = \varphi_{i_{(n)}} \cdot \varepsilon_{i_{(n)}} \quad (11.2d)$$

And, likewise, (11.6) as follows:

$$\begin{aligned} \Delta w_{i,j_{(n)}} &= \left(m_{i_{(n)}}^{[h]} - m_{i_{(n)}}^{[t]}\right) \cdot \left(1 - \frac{w_{i,j_{(n)}}}{C}\right) \cdot m_{j_{(n)}}^{[h]} \\ &= \lambda_{i_{(n)}} \cdot \eta_{i,j_{(n)}} \cdot m_j^{[s]} \cdot \varepsilon_{i_{(n)}} \end{aligned} \quad (11.6b)$$

noting that

$$\lim_{\varepsilon \to 0} \Delta w_{i,j_{(n)}} = 0 \quad (11.6e)$$

Plugging (11.6b) into (11.7) and remembering the definition of the contraction factor $\eta_{i,j_{(n)}}$ yields

$$w_{i,j_{(n+1)}} = C \cdot \left(1 - \eta_{i,j_{(n)}}\right) + \lambda_{i_{(n)}} \cdot \eta_{i_{(n)}} \cdot m_j^{[s]} \cdot \varepsilon_{i_{(n)}} \quad (11.7a)$$

Finally, from (11.7a) and (11.8), we can conclude that

$$\lim_{n\to\infty} w_{i,j(n)} = C \cdot (1 - \eta_{i,j(n)}) \tag{11.7b}$$

In a nutshell, the learning mechanics of the auto-CM boils down to the following. At the beginning of the training, the input and hidden units will be very similar (see (11.1)) and, consequently, $\Delta v_{i(n)}$ will be very small (see (11.2d)), while for the same reason $\lambda_{i(n)}$ (see its definition above) at the beginning will be very big and $\Delta w_{i,j(n)}$ bigger than $\Delta v_{i(n)}$ (see (11.2d) and (11.6b)). During the training, while $v_{i(n)}$ rapidly increases as the processing cycles n pile up, $m_{i(n)}^{[h]}$ decreases, and so do accordingly $\lambda_{i(n)}$ and $\varepsilon_{i(n)}$. Consequently, $\Delta w_{i,j(n)}$ rolls along a downward slope, whereas $\Delta v_{i(n)}$ slows down the pace of its increase. When $\lambda_{i(n)}$ becomes close to zero, this means that $m_{i(n)}^{[h]}$ is now only slightly bigger than $m_{i(n)}^{[t]}$ (see (11.5b)). $\Delta v_{i(n)}$ is accordingly getting across the global maximum of the equation $\Delta v_{i(n)} = m_i^{[s]}(1-\varepsilon_{i(n)})\cdot\varepsilon_{i(n)}$, so once the critical point has been hit, $\Delta v_{i(n)}$ will in turn begin its descent toward zero.

It may be convenient to illustrate the above auto-CM mechanics at work by means of a numerical simulation on a toy data set. Specifically, consider the following 3-bit data set (Table 11.1).

Table 11.1 Three-bit data set

3 bits	Var 1	Var 2	Var 3
Rec 1	0	0	0
Rec 2	0	0	1
Rec 3	0	1	0
Rec 4	0	1	1
Rec 5	1	0	0
Rec 6	1	0	1
Rec 7	1	1	0
Rec 8	1	1	1

After 48 epochs of processing, auto-CM, with $C = 1$, reaches a thorough learning of the data set (i.e., RMSE = 0.0000).

Denoting by **v** the three weights of the first layer, at the end of the training we have that

$v(1)$	1.00
$v(2)$	1.00
$v(3)$	1.00

whereas the weights of the second layer turn out to be (with the main diagonal not trained)

$w(1,1)$	0.00
$w(1,2)$	0.89
$w(1,3)$	0.89
$w(2,2)$	0.00
$w(2,3)$	0.89
$w(3,3)$	0.00

In Table 11.2, we report the dynamics of the training of the weights of the first layer and of the only three weights of the second layer that connect different nodes ($w(1,2)$, $w(1,3)$, $w(2,3)$).

It is apparent that, as expected, all weights monotonically converge. Consider, as a further useful illustration (Fig. 11.2), the graph of the dynamics of weights $v(1,1)$ and $w(1,2)$ and compare it with the graph showing their updation (i.e., the respective adaptations) during the training phase (Fig. 11.3).

We can clearly trace these graphs back to the dynamics described in (11.8) to (11.7b) and to the simple reconstruction of the mechanics spelled out just above.

We can make similar remarks by considering the graph of the history of the values taken by the first hidden node and by the first output node (Fig. 11.4). Once again, the relaxation dynamics that has by now become typical of auto-CM is apparent.

A further important remark is that we can see the second layer connections of auto-CM as the place where the energy liberated by the nodes, moving from one layer to another, is *trapped*. Figure 11.5, showing the dynamics of the contractive factors ε,η and of the signal differences φ,λ, provides a clear illustration of this effect.

We can easily see from Fig. 11.5 how, as n piles up, energy is accumulated in the passage from the input to the hidden layer (the dynamics of φ) to be subsequently released in the passage from the hidden to the output layer (the dynamics of λ). Meanwhile, the contraction factors progressively die down, although with very idiosyncratic patterns.

11.3 Experimenting with the Auto-contractive Map

Now that we have understood how the learning mechanics of the auto-CM actually works, we are ready to explore its performance in carrying out tasks of interest. To this purpose, we now move our attention from the algorithmic structure of the auto-CM to its actual behavior in relevant circumstances. In particular, we start by addressing the following basic issues:

a. How it behaves with respect to specific typologies of inputs
b. How and whether it stabilizes its own output
c. How its connections manage to stabilize

Table 11.2 Dynamics of the training

3 bits	$v(1)$	$v(2)$	$v(3)$	$w(1,2)$	w **(1,3)**	w **(2,3)**
Epoch 1	0.000161	0.000161	0.000161	0.370855	0.370856	0.370857
Epoch 2	0.000259	0.000259	0.000259	0.533956	0.533957	0.533959
Epoch 3	0.000418	0.000418	0.000418	0.627853	0.627855	0.627857
Epoch 4	0.000672	0.000672	0.000672	0.689412	0.689414	0.689416
Epoch 5	0.001083	0.001083	0.001083	0.733061	0.733064	0.733066
Epoch 6	0.001742	0.001742	0.001742	0.765688	0.765692	0.765695
Epoch 7	0.002803	0.002803	0.002803	0.791018	0.791022	0.791026
Epoch 8	0.004508	0.004508	0.004508	0.811242	0.811248	0.811253
Epoch 9	0.007242	0.007242	0.007242	0.827736	0.827743	0.827750
Epoch 10	0.011617	0.011617	0.011617	0.841397	0.841407	0.841416
Epoch 11	0.018589	0.018589	0.018589	0.852828	0.852841	0.852854
Epoch 12	0.029631	0.029631	0.029631	0.862436	0.862454	0.862471
Epoch 13	0.046947	0.046947	0.046947	0.870492	0.870515	0.870539
Epoch 14	0.073678	0.073678	0.073678	0.877163	0.877195	0.877227
Epoch 15	0.113961	0.113961	0.113961	0.882545	0.882589	0.882633
Epoch 16	0.172487	0.172487	0.172487	0.886696	0.886753	0.886811
Epoch 17	0.253100	0.253100	0.253100	0.889672	0.889746	0.889820
Epoch 18	0.356198	0.356198	0.356198	0.891592	0.891682	0.891773
Epoch 19	0.475946	0.475946	0.475946	0.892666	0.892770	0.892875
Epoch 20	0.599992	0.599992	0.599992	0.893172	0.893285	0.893400
Epoch 21	0.713680	0.713680	0.713680	0.893370	0.893487	0.893608
Epoch 22	0.806393	0.806393	0.806393	0.893435	0.893554	0.893677
Epoch 23	0.874853	0.874853	0.874853	0.893453	0.893573	0.893697
Epoch 24	0.921696	0.921696	0.921696	0.893458	0.893578	0.893702
Epoch 25	0.952067	0.952067	0.952067	0.893459	0.893579	0.893703
Epoch 26	0.971068	0.971068	0.971068	0.893459	0.893579	0.893703
Epoch 27	0.982688	0.982688	0.982688	0.893459	0.893579	0.893703
Epoch 28	0.989697	0.989697	0.989697	0.893459	0.893579	0.893703
Epoch 29	0.993887	0.993887	0.993887	0.893459	0.893579	0.893703
Epoch 30	0.996380	0.996380	0.996380	0.893459	0.893579	0.893703
Epoch 31	0.997859	0.997859	0.997859	0.893459	0.893579	0.893703
Epoch 32	0.998735	0.998735	0.998735	0.893459	0.893579	0.893703
Epoch 33	0.999252	0.999252	0.999252	0.893459	0.893579	0.893703
Epoch 34	0.999558	0.999558	0.999558	0.893459	0.893579	0.893703
Epoch 35	0.999739	0.999739	0.999739	0.893459	0.893579	0.893703
Epoch 36	0.999846	0.999846	0.999846	0.893459	0.893579	0.893703
Epoch 37	0.999909	0.999909	0.999909	0.893459	0.893579	0.893703
Epoch 38	0.999946	0.999946	0.999946	0.893459	0.893579	0.893703
Epoch 39	0.999968	0.999968	0.999968	0.893459	0.893579	0.893703
Epoch 40	0.999981	0.999981	0.999981	0.893459	0.893579	0.893703
Epoch 41	0.999989	0.999989	0.999989	0.893459	0.893579	0.893703
Epoch 42	0.999993	0.999993	0.999993	0.893459	0.893579	0.893703
Epoch 43	0.999996	0.999996	0.999996	0.893459	0.893579	0.893703
Epoch 44	0.999998	0.999998	0.999998	0.893459	0.893579	0.893703
Epoch 45	0.999999	0.999999	0.999999	0.893459	0.893579	0.893703
Epoch 46	0.999999	0.999999	0.999999	0.893459	0.893579	0.893703
Epoch 47	0.999999	0.999999	0.999999	0.893459	0.893579	0.893703
Epoch 48	1.000000	1.000000	1.000000	0.893459	0.893579	0.893703

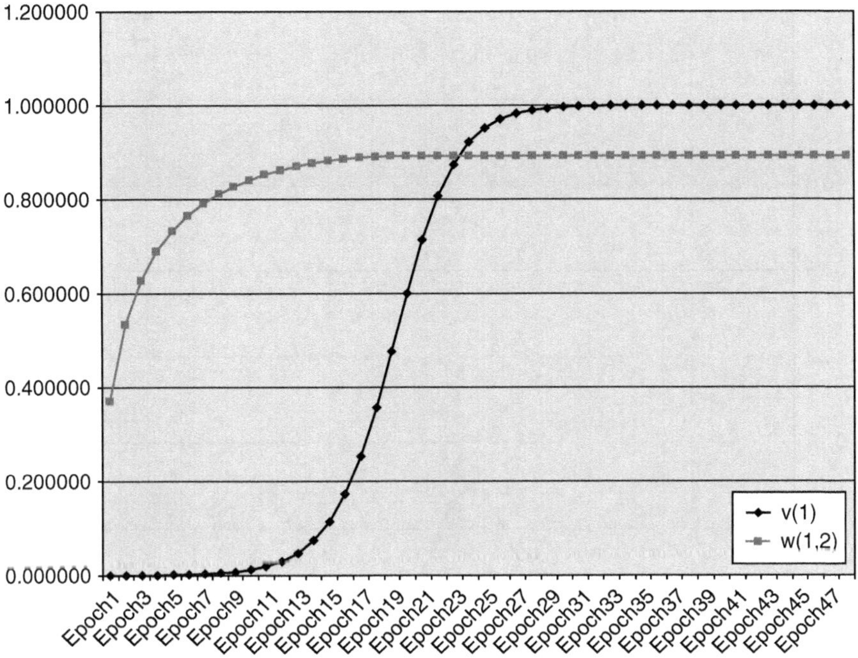

Fig. 11.2 Dynamics of weights $v(1,1)$ and $w(1,2)$

To develop these points, we have chosen another toy problem whose nature fits particularly well some of the qualifying characteristics and properties of this ANN, thereby allowing to highlight them in an easy and simple way. Our input set consists of 9 patterns, each one composed of 121 nodes, which consist of sketchy pictures of human faces, each one bearing a different expression (Fig. 11.6).

Given the structure of the input, the auto-CM has been shaped in the following way:

- 121 input nodes
- 121 hidden nodes
- 121 output nodes
- 121 connections between inputs and hidden
- 14,641 connections (i.e., 121 $\times$ 121) between the hidden and output units

All the 14,762 connections have been initialized using the same value (0.01). The signal transfer and the learning equations used here are the ones already described in (11.1), (11.2), (11.3), (11.4), (11.5), (11.6), and (11.7). The learning process has been carried out presenting the nine patterns to the auto-CM in a random way. We have meant the notion of *epoch* in its more traditional meaning, namely each epoch

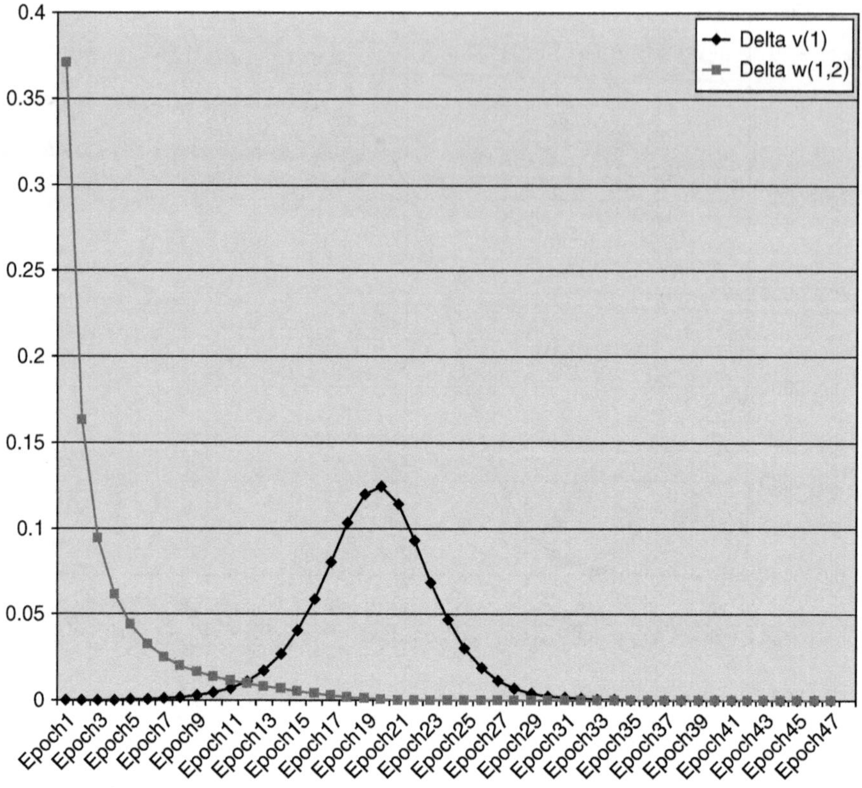

Fig. 11.3 Dynamics of updating weights $v(1,1)$ and $w(1,2)$ during the training phase

amounts to a complete presentation to the ANN of all the training patterns in the input set.

The ANN's performance during the training process may be divided into five characteristic phases.

In a *first phase* of the period of training, the output of all the nine patterns tends to assume the value 1 for all the input nodes that belong to the non-empty intersection of all the patterns and the value 0 for all the rest of the output nodes. This phase may be thought of as a phase of research of the *common traits* among the whole set of the input patterns. An example of such an output is shown in Fig. 11.7.

In a *second phase*, each input vector triggers a response that corresponds to the union of all the patterns as the characteristic output. Here, the ANN may be regarded as undertaking a phase of exploration and characterization of the *overall variability* of the input patterns (Fig. 11.8).

In a *third phase*, each input pattern is reproduced in the output vector by the auto-CM exactly as it is. This is clearly the phase of the sorting out of the specificity (i.e., of the *identification*) of each item in the input set.

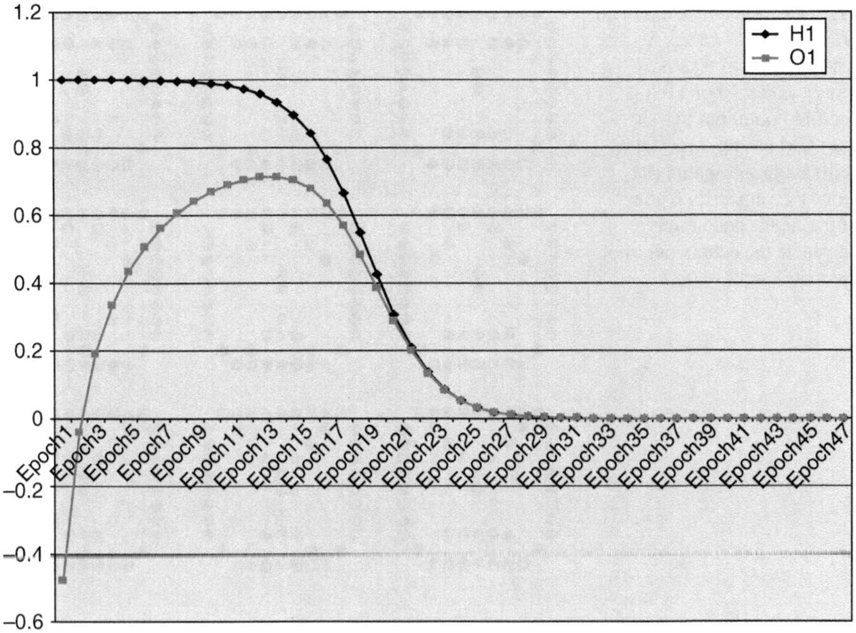

Fig. 11.4 Graph of the history of the values taken by the first hidden node and by the first output node

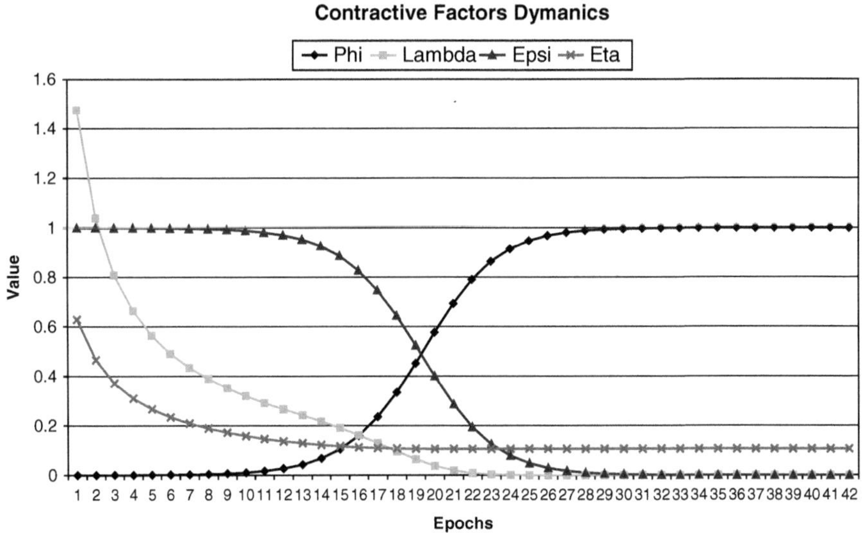

Fig. 11.5 Dynamics of the contractive factors

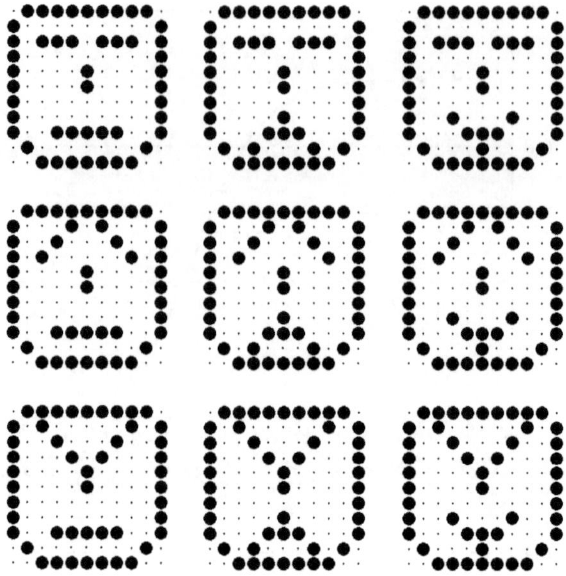

Fig. 11.6 Each face has been drawn within a matrix X whose cells can take only binary values (0 or 1). It is useful to point out that the auto-CM has no information at all about the spatial (let alone the semantic) features of the inputs and simply considers the actual values of the matrix cells

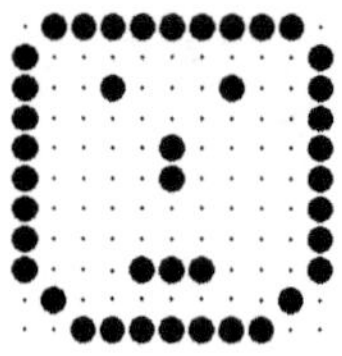

Fig. 11.7 Output for all of the nine input patterns after two epochs

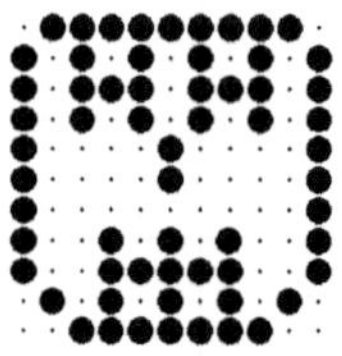

Fig. 11.8 Output response as the union of all input patterns after around 10 epochs

In a *fourth phase*, the output vector contains only all those entries of each specific input pattern that do not lie in the common intersection of all patterns. In other words, it selects the difference between the actual face and the "intersection" face generated at phase 1. This has to do with characterizing the differential traits that have to be looked after for the *discrimination* among the various patterns (Fig. 11.9).

In the *last phase*, every input produces a null (zero) output. The ANN has acquired all the necessary and useful elements for the pattern recognition task and has consequently ceased to learn, becoming unresponsive to the training stimuli as

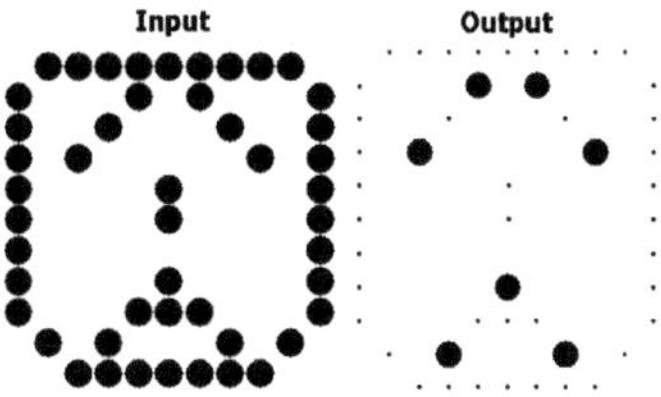

Fig. 11.9 Each pattern generates as output only its specific features, after around 100 epochs

if it had "lost interest" in them. This amounts to a *self-validation* of the auto-CM, which thereby acknowledges that the learning process has come to an end.

If this highly organized and systematic sequence of behavioral responses of the auto-CM may seem surprising, even more so is the outcome of the analysis of the structure of the 14,641 stabilized connections established between the hidden and the output layers of the ANN. In fact, such connections actually make up a single, global picture that evidently presents fractal characteristics. The picture clearly draws out the "union" face found in phase 2, i.e., the one summarizing the overall variability of traits of all the faces included in the input set. But this time the "big face" is no longer made of single pixels, but in turn of smaller faces, arranged in ways that encompass – in a highly structured, symmetrical way – all the above-discussed learning phases. And the way in which the small faces are chosen to represent details of the big faces is highly pertinent. To all of the points of the "big face" that correspond to the "intersection face" found out in phase 1 of the process, there corresponds an "intersection face." The "union face" is pictured only in the "big face" but is never found in the smaller ones, in that it corresponds to the overall variability and it is pointless to assign it at any specific point of the "big face." The rest of the points of the "union face" host faces that resemble the original input patterns, placed in locations that correspond to their typical differential traits, but no one is really identical to any of the actual input patterns. In particular, in the various "small faces" one can find all the "expressions of the face" and all the "expressions of the eyes" occurring in the nine training patterns. Specifically, if the "expression of the mouth" is equal to the expression of the mouth of any of the training patterns, then the "expression of the eyes" is the *union* of all the expressions of the eyes of the corresponding training patterns. Similarly, if the "expression of the eyes" is equal to the one of any training pattern, then the expression of the mouth is the *union* of all the expressions of the mouths of the corresponding training patterns.

This ingenious "cognitive" scheme ultimately represents a *fractal immersion* of the N-dimensional space of the input into the N^2-dimensional space associated with the weights matrix of the auto-CM (Fig. 11.10).

In spite of the specificity of this particular set of inputs and of the related tasks, the insights developed here hold more generally and characterize the auto-CM's performance. In particular, it turns out that one of the auto-CM's specialties is that of finding out, within a given set of input patterns, the global statistics of the associations among the underlying variables. Also the peculiarities of the matrix of the hidden–output connections have been reproduced in hundreds of tests with very diverse input classes of all kinds.

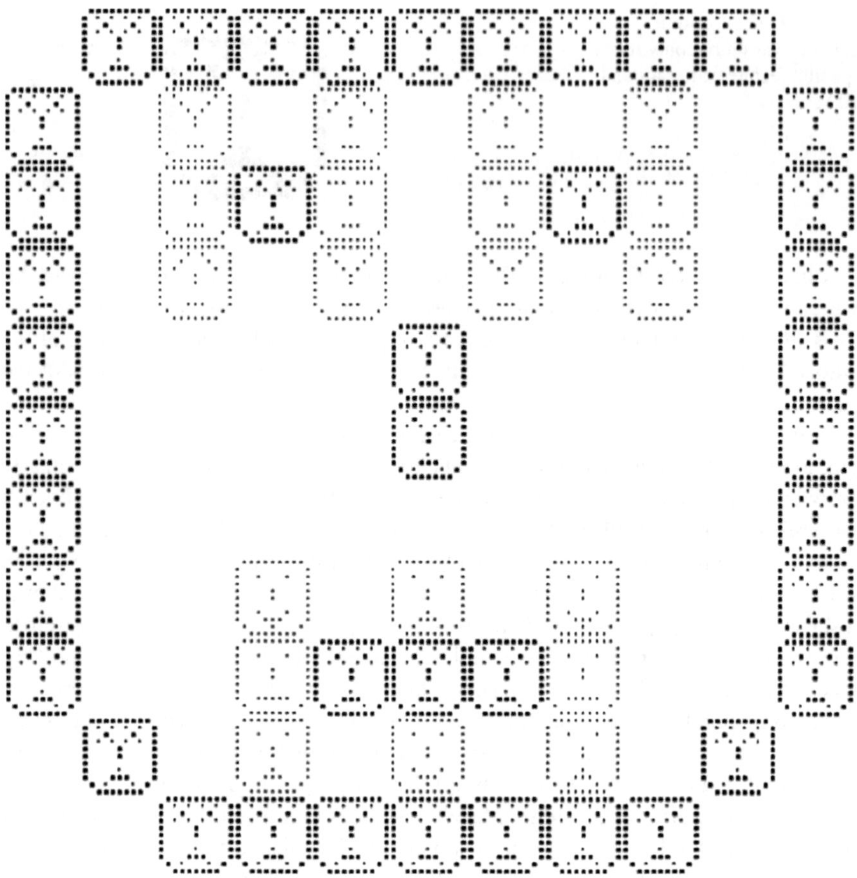

Fig. 11.10 The matrix of values of the hidden–output connections according to the *B*-operator (see text)

11.4 Auto-CMs: A Theoretical Discussion

There are a few important peculiarities of auto-CMs with respect to more familiar classes of ANNs that need special attention and call for careful reflection:

- Auto-CMs are able to learn also when starting from initializations where all connections are set at the same value, i.e., they do not suffer the problem of the symmetric connections.
- During the training process, auto-CMs always assign positive values to connections. In other words, auto-CMs do not allow for inhibitory relations among nodes, but only for different strengths of excitatory connections.
- Auto-CMs can learn also in difficult conditions, namely when the connections of the main diagonal of the second layer connection matrix are removed. In

the context of this kind of learning process, auto-CMs seem to reconstruct the relationship occurring between each couple of variables. Consequently, from an experimental point of view, it seems that the ranking of its connections matrix translates into the ranking of the joint probability of occurrence of each couple of variables.

- Once the learning process has occurred, any input vector, belonging to the training set, will generate a null output vector. So, the energy minimization of the training vectors is represented by a function through which the trained connections absorb completely the input training vectors. Thus, auto-CM seems to learn how to transform itself in a "dark body."
- At the end of the training phase ($\Delta w_{i,j} = 0$), all the components of the weights vector **v** reach the same value:

$$\lim_{n \to \infty} v_{i_{(n)}} = C \tag{11.8}$$

The matrix **w**, then, represents the auto-CM knowledge about the whole data set.

One can use the information embedded in the **w** matrix to compute in a natural way the joint probability of occurrence among variables:

$$p_{i,j} = \frac{w_{i,j}}{\sum_{j=1}^{N} w_{i,j}} \tag{11.9}$$

$$P(m_j^{[s]}) = \sum_{i}^{N} p_{i,j} = 1 \tag{11.10}$$

The new matrix **p** can be read as the probability of transition from any state variable to anything else:

$$P(m_i^{[t]} \,|\, m_j^{[s]}) = p_{i,j} \tag{11.11}$$

- Alternatively, the matrix **w** may be transformed into a non-Euclidean distance metric (semi-metric) when we train the auto-CM with the main diagonal of the **w** matrix fixed at value N.

Now, if we consider N as a limit value for all the weights of the **w** matrix, we can write

$$d_{i,j} = N - w_{i,j} \tag{11.12}$$

The new matrix **d** is again a squared symmetric matrix, where the main diagonal entries are null (i.e., they represent the zero distance of each variable from itself) and where the off-diagonal entries represent "distances" between each couple of variables. We will expand on this interpretation below.

11.4.1 The Contractive Factor

We now discuss in more detail the "spatial" interpretation of the squared weights matrix of the auto-CM. Consider each variable of the data set as a vector made by all of its values. In this perspective, one can see the dynamic value of each connection between any two variables as the local velocity of their mutual attraction caused by the degree of similarity of their vectors. The more the vectors' similarity, the more their speed of attraction in the corresponding space. When two variables are attracted to each other, they "contract" proportionally the original Euclidean space between them and reshape it accordingly. The limit case is when two variables are identical: the space contraction should be infinitive and the two variables would collapse into the same point.

We can extract from each weight of a trained auto-CM this specific contractive factor:

$$F_{i,j} = \left(1 - \frac{w_{i,j}}{C}\right)^{-1}, \quad 1 \leq F_{i,j} \leq \infty \tag{11.9a}$$

Equation (11.9a) is interesting for three reasons:

- It is the inverse of the contractive factor that rules the auto-CM training.
- In view of (11.3b), each mono-connection v_i at the end of the training will reach the value C. In this case, the contractive factor will diverge because the two variables connected by the weight are indeed the same variable.
- Considering instead (11.7b), each weight $w_{i,j}$ at the end of the training will always be smaller than C. This means that the contractive factor for each weight of the matrix will always stay bounded. To visualize this claim within our spatial reference space, notice that, in the case of weight $w_{i,i}$, the variable is of course connected with itself, but the same variable has also received the influences of the other variables (remind that the matrix **w**is a squared matrix where each variable is linked to the other), and consequently there will remain enough difference to prevent contractive collapse.

At this point, we are in a position to calculate the contractive distance between each variable and the other, by suitably adjusting the original Euclidean distance by the specific contractive factor (11.9a).

The Euclidean distance among the variables in the data set is given by the following equation:

$$d_{i,j}^{[\text{Euclidean}]} = \sqrt{\sum_{k}^{R} (x_{i,k} - x_{j,k})^2} \tag{11.10a}$$

where R is the number of the records of the assigned data set; $x_{i,k}$ and $x_{j,k}$ are the ith value and the jth value of the variables in the kth record, respectively, whereas the auto-CM distance matrix among the same variables is given by

$$d_{i,j}^{[\text{auto-CM}]} = \frac{d_{i,j}^{[\text{Euclidean}]}}{F_{i,j}} \tag{11.11a}$$

Equation (11.11a) makes it explicit how the similarity attraction effect deforms the original Euclidean embedding space and paves the way for a fruitful characterization and interpretation of the "spatializing" properties of auto-CM, to which we now turn.

11.4.2 Auto-CM and Minimum Spanning Tree

Equation (11.12) transforms the squared weights matrix of auto-CM into a squared matrix of distances among nodes. Each distance between a pair of nodes may therefore be regarded as the weighted edge between these pair of nodes in a suitable graph-theoretic representation, so that the matrix **d** itself may be analyzed through the graph theory toolbox.

A graph is a mathematical abstraction that is useful for solving many kinds of problems. Fundamentally, a graph consists of a set of vertices and a set of edges, where an edge is an object that connects two vertices in the graph. More precisely, a graph is a pair (V, E), where V is a finite set and E is a binary relation on V, to which it is possible to associate scalar values (in this case, the distances $d_{i,j}$).

V is called a vertex set whose elements are called vertices. E is a collection of edges, where an edge is a pair (u, v) with u, v belonging to V. In a directed graph, edges are ordered pairs, connecting a source vertex to a target vertex. In an undirected graph, edges are unordered pairs and connect the two vertices in both directions, hence in an undirected graph (u, v) and (v, u) are two ways of writing the same edge.

The graph-theoretic representation is not constrained by any a priori semantic restriction: it does not say what a vertex or edge actually represents. They could be cities with connecting roads or web pages with hyperlinks, and so on. These semantic details are irrelevant to determine the graph structure and properties; the only thing that matters is that a specific graph may be taken as a proper representation of the phenomenon under study, to justify attention on that particular mathematical object.

An adjacency matrix representation of a graph is a two-dimensional $V \times V$ array, where rows represent the list of vertices and columns represent edges among vertices. To each element in the array is assigned a Boolean value saying whether the edge (u, v) is in the graph.

A distance matrix among V vertices represents an undirected graph, where each vertex is linked with all the others but itself (Table 11.3).

At this point, it is useful to introduce the concept of minimum spanning tree (MST).

The minimum spanning tree problem is defined as follows: Find an acyclic subset T of E that connects all of the vertices in the graph and whose total weight (viz., the total distance) is minimized, where the total weight is given by

Table 11.3 Adjacency matrix of a distance matrix

	A	B	C	D	...	Z
A	0	1	1	1	1	1
B	1	0	1	1	1	1
C	1	1	0	1	1	1
D	1	1	1	0	1	1
:	1	1	1	1	0	1
Z	1	1	1	1	1	0

$$d(T) = \sum_{i=0}^{N-1} \sum_{j=i+1}^{N} d_{i,j} \quad \forall d_{i,j} \tag{11.13}$$

T is called a spanning tree and the MST is the T whose weighted sum of edges attains the minimum value:

$$\mathrm{MST} = \mathrm{Min}\{d(T_k)\} \tag{11.14}$$

Given an undirected graph G, representing a matrix of distances d, with V vertices, completely linked to each other, the total number of their edges (E) is

$$E = \frac{V \cdot (V-1)}{2} \tag{11.15}$$

and the number of its possible spanning trees is

$$T = V^{V-2} \tag{11.16}$$

Kruskal (1956) found out an algorithm to determine the MST of any undirected graph in a quadratic number of steps, in the worst case. Obviously, the Kruskal algorithm generates one of the possible MSTs. In fact, in a weighted graph more than one MSTs are possible.

From a conceptual point of view, the MST represents the *energy minimization* state of a structure. In fact, if we consider the atomic elements of a structure as vertices of a graph and the strength among them as the weight of each edge, linking a pair of vertices, the MST represents the minimum of energy needed so that all the elements of the structure preserve their mutual coherence. In a closed system, all the components tend to minimize the overall energy. So the MST, in specific situations, can represent the most probable state for the system to tend.

To determine the MST of an undirected graph, each edge of the graph has to be weighted. Equation (11.12) shows a way to weight each edge whose nodes are the variables of a data set and where the weights of a trained auto-CM provide the (weight) metrics.

Obviously, it is possible to use any kind of auto-associative ANN or any kind of linear auto-associator to generate a weight matrix among the variables of an assigned data set. But it is hard to train a two-layer auto-associative back-propagation ANN with the main diagonal weights fixed (to avoid auto-correlation problems). In most cases, the root mean square error (RMSE) stops to decrease after a few epochs, especially when the orthogonality of the records is relatively high, a circumstance that is frequent when it is necessary to weight the distance among the records of the assigned data set. In this case, it is necessary to train the transposed matrix of the data set. By the way, if a linear auto-associator is used for the purpose, all of the nonlinear association among variables will be lost.

Therefore, auto-CM seems to be the best choice to date to compute a complete and a nonlinear matrix of weights among variables or among records of any assigned data set.

11.4.3 Other Algorithms for MST

In principle, as we just remarked, it could be possible to use any algorithm to weight the graph edges, although the final outcome will be in general quite different. It is therefore useful to review briefly some of the most used options in the current practice.

Linear correlation: To begin with, it is necessary to calculate the linear correlation between each pair of variables of the assigned data set:

$$R_{i,j} = \frac{\sum_{k=1}^{N}(x_{i,k} - \bar{x}_i)\cdot(x_{j,k} - \bar{x}_j)}{\sqrt{\sum_{k=1}^{N}(x_{i,k} - \bar{x}_i)^2 \cdot \sum_{k=1}^{N}(x_{j,k} - \bar{x}_j)^2}}, -1 \le R_{i,j} \le 1;\ i,j \in [1,2,...,M] \tag{11.17}$$

where $R_{i,j}$ is the linear correlation between any couple of variables x_i and x_j of the assigned data set; $\bar{x}_i$ the mean value of any variable x_i; N the number of records of the assigned data set; and M the number of variables of the assigned data set.

Equation (11.17) will generate a symmetric squared matrix with null diagonal, providing the linear correlation between each variable and any other.

Through (11.18), the correlation matrix is transformed into a matrix of linear distances among the variables:

$$d_{i,j}^{[R]} = \sqrt{2\cdot(1 - R_{i,j})} \tag{11.18}$$

At this point, following the same steps as above, the assigned data set can be reformulated as an undirected weighted graph, where MST optimization is applicable.

Prior probability: One starts by calculating the prior probability of co-occurrence between any couple of variables of the assigned data set:

$$A_{i,j} = -\ln\frac{(1/N^2)\cdot\sum_{k=1}^{N}x_{i,k}\cdot(1 - x_{j,k})\cdot\sum_{k=1}^{N}(1 - x_{i,k})\cdot x_{j,k}}{(1/N^2)\cdot\sum_{k=1}^{N}x_{i,k}\cdot x_{j,k}\cdot\sum_{k=1}^{N}(1 - x_{i,k})\cdot(1 - x_{j,k})}$$
$$-\infty \le A_{i,j} \le +\infty,\ x \in [0,1],\ i,j \in [1,2,...,M] \tag{11.19}$$

where $A_{i,j}$ is the association strength between any couple of variables x_i and x_j of the assigned data set; x_i the value of any variable scaled between 0 and 1; N the number of records of the assigned data set; and M the number of variables of the assigned data set.

One goes on in a by now familiar way by transforming the matrix of association among variables into a nonlinear distance matrix:

$$d_{i,j}^{[A]} = \text{Max } A - A_{i,j} \tag{11.20}$$

where Max A is the maximum A matrix value.

Euclidean distance: the Euclidean distance among variables is easy to compute. It is necessary at first to scale all entries between 0 and 1 and then to transpose the matrix of the assigned data set:

$$d_{i,j}^{[E]} = \sqrt{\sum_{k=1}^{M} (x_{i,k} - x_{j,k})^2} \ , i,j \in [1,2,\ldots,N],\ x \in [0,1] \tag{11.21}$$

where $d_{i,j}^{[E]}$ is the Euclidean distance among any couple of variables; x_i the value of any record scaled between 0 and 1; N the number of variables of the assigned data set; and M the number of records of the assigned data set.

All of the above options have the advantage of being very fast computationally, but their common, serious limit is to define the distance among variables or records by just picking them in couples. This means that each weight explains the association between two variables or records, but it does not take into account the additional influence that other variables or records could exert on that specific couple. This situation is quite similar, say, to the case of 10 children all playing together in a swimming pool. If one would pretend to explain their global behavior by making the statistics of the interaction between all possible pairs of children, this would amount to skip all of the external constraints that the concomitant positions and movements of the other children are imposing on each given couple at each given moment. By skipping this crucial information, the actual mutual behavior of each couple will be poorly understood, and a fortiori this will also be the case for the global picture that is built through the aggregation of such partial two-by-two views.

As an alternative to traditional methods, however, one could make use of other ANN architectures, such as the following.

Auto-associative BP: A back-propagation without a hidden unit layer and without connections on the main diagonal can be used also to compute a metric among variables (Fig. 11.11).

This is an ANN featuring an extremely simple learning algorithm:

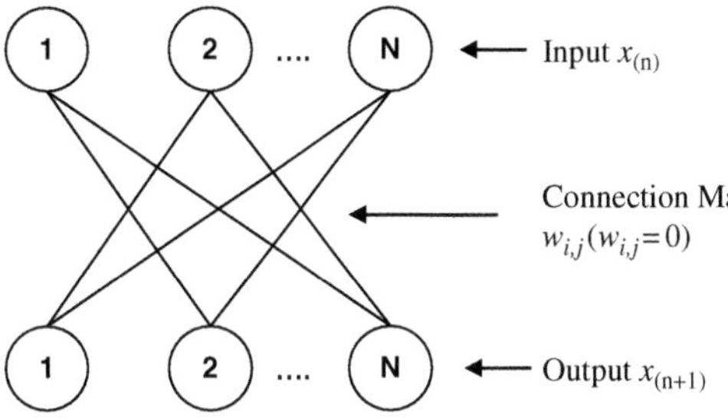

Fig. 11.11 Two-layer auto-associative back-propagation with $w_{i,i} = 0$

$$\begin{aligned} \text{Output}_i &= f\left(\sum_j^N \text{Input}_j \cdot W_{i,j} + \text{Bias}_i\right) \\ &= \frac{1}{1+\exp\left(-\left(\sum_j^N \text{Input}_j \cdot W_{i,j} + \text{Bias}_i\right)\right)}, W_{i,i} = 0 \end{aligned} \tag{11.22}$$

$$\begin{aligned} \delta_i &= (\text{Input}_i - \text{Output}_i) \cdot f'(\text{Output}_i) \\ &= (\text{Input}_i - \text{Output}_i) \cdot \text{Output}_i \cdot (1 - \text{Output}_i) \end{aligned} \tag{11.23}$$

$$\Delta W_{i,j} = \text{LCoef} \cdot \delta_i \cdot \text{Input}_j,\ \text{LCoef} \in [0,1] \tag{11.24}$$

$$\Delta \text{Bias}_i = \text{LCoef} \cdot \delta_i \tag{11.25}$$

$$W_{i,j}^{[n+1]} = W_{i,j}^{[n]} + \tfrac{1}{2} \cdot \left(\Delta W_{i,j} + \Delta W_{j,i}\right), \quad \text{Bias}_i^{[n+1]} = \text{Bias}_i^{[n]} + \Delta \text{Bias}_i \tag{11.26}$$

Auto-BP is an ANN featuring $N^2 - N$ inter-node connections and N biases inside every exit node, for a total of N^2 adaptive weights. It is an algorithm that works similar to logistic regression and can be used to establish the dependency of every variable from each other.

At the end of the training phase, to proceed as before with MST optimization, it is necessary to convert each connection in a nonlinear symmetric distance (semi-metric):

$$V_{i,j} = V_{j,i} = \tfrac{1}{2} \cdot (W_{i,j} + \text{Bias}_i + W_{j,i} + \text{Bias}_j), \quad d_{i,j}^{[Bp]} = \text{Max } V - V_{i,j} \tag{11.27}$$

where $\text{Max } V = \text{Max}\{V_{i,j}\}$ and then one follows the by now usual route.

The advantage of auto-BP is due to its learning speed, which is due to the small size of its connections and to the simplicity of both its topology and its algorithm. Moreover, at the end of the learning phase, the connections between variables, being direct, have a clear conceptual meaning. Every connection indicates a relationship of faded excitement, inhibition, or indifference between every pair of variables or records.

The disadvantage of auto-BP is, on the contrary, its limited convergence capacity, due to that same topological simplicity. That is to say, complex relationships between variables may be approximated or ignored. Auto-BP, then, only partially overcomes, at best, the limitations of the previous options.

11.4.4 Some Qualitative Features of MST Optimization

Once we have a distance matrix among nodes, $d_{i,j}^{[\ldots]}$ with $i,j \in [1,2,\ldots,N]$, the MST of the implicit graph is easy to define, by means of the Kruskal algorithm. The MST adjacency matrix, then, has to be analyzed.

The easiest criterion to study the adjacency matrix is to rank the number of links of each node; this algorithm defines the *connectivity* of each node:

$$C_i = \sum_{j}^{N} l_{i,j} \tag{11.28}$$

where

$$\begin{aligned} &\text{if } l_{i,j} \in \text{MST then } l_{i,j} = 1 \\ &\text{if } l_{i,j} \notin \text{MST then } l_{i,j} = 0 \\ &l_{i,j} = \text{ possible direct connection between node}_i \text{ and node}_j \end{aligned}$$

- Nodes with only one link are named *leaves*. Leaves define the boundaries of the MST graph.
- Nodes with two links are named *connectors*.
- Nodes with more than two connections are named *hubs*. Each hub has a specific degree of connectivity:

$$\text{HubDegree}_i = C_i - 2 \tag{11.29}$$

A second indicator qualifying an MST graph is the *clustering strength* of each of its nodes. It is proportional to the number of its links and to the number of links of the nodes directly connected to it:

$$S_i = \frac{C_i^2}{\sum_{j=1}^{C_i} C_j} \tag{11.30}$$

A third indicator is the *degree of protection* of each node in any a-directed graph. This indicator defines the rank of centrality of each node within the graph, when an iterative pruning algorithm is applied. This algorithm was found and applied for the first time as a global indicator for graph complexity by Giulia Massini at Semeion Research Center in 2006 (Massini 2007a):

```
Rank = 0;
Do
{
Rank + +;
Consider_All_Nodes_with_The_Minimum_Number_of_Links();
Delete_These_Links();
Assign_a_Rank_To_All_Nodes_Without_Link(Rank);
Update_The_New_Graph();
Check_Number_of_Links();
}whileat_least_a_link_is_present
```

(11.31, Pruning Algorithm)

The higher the rank of a node, the bigger the centrality of its position within the graph. The latest nodes to be pruned are also the kernel nodes of the graph. In this chapter, this algorithm is generalized to measure the global complexity of any kind of graph.

11.5 Graph Complexity: The *H* Function

The pruning algorithm can be used also to define the *quantity of graph complexity* of any graph. If we take μ as the mean number of nodes without any link, at each iteration, as the pruning algorithm is running, we can define the hubness index, H_0, of a graph with N nodes. In order to properly define this quantity, we need to introduce a few preliminary concepts. We define a cycle or iteration of the pruning algorithm as a given round of application of the algorithm. At each cycle, there corresponds a gradient, which can be different from cycle to cycle. Insofar as two subsequent cycles yield the same gradient, they belong to the same pruning class. As the gradient changes from one cycle to the other, the previous class ends and a new one begins. We are now in a position to define hubness as follows:

$$H_0 = \frac{\mu \cdot \varphi - 1}{A}, \quad 0 < H_0 < 2 \tag{11.32}$$

where

$$\mu = \frac{1}{M}\sum_i^M Nd_i = \frac{A}{M}, \quad \varphi = \frac{1}{P}\sum_j^P S_{TGj}$$

A is the number of links of the graph ($N - 1$ for trees); M the number of cycles of the pruning algorithm; P the number of pruning classes; Nd_i the number of nodes without link at the jth iteration; and S_{TGj} the class j pruning gradient.

Using H_0 as a global indicator, it is possible to define to what extent a graph is *hub oriented*. We show below three possible cases when $N = 6$ (N is the number of nodes):

- Case 1: $H_0 = 0.2$, – the tree is for $\frac{1}{5}$ hub oriented

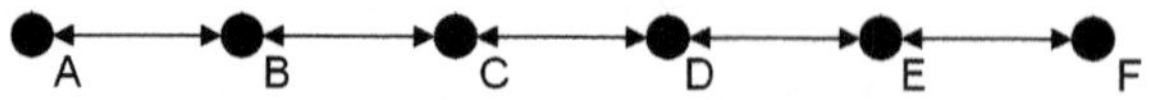

- Case 2: $H_0 = 1$ – the tree is completely hub oriented

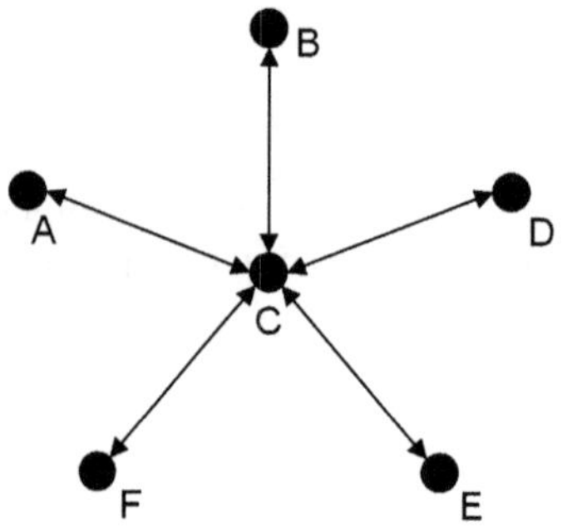

- Case 3: $H_0 = 0.4$ – the tree is for $\frac{2}{5}$ hub oriented

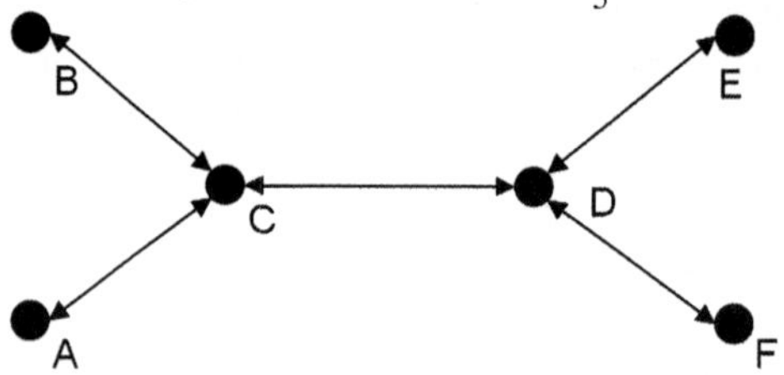

The simple equation (11.32) turns out to be correct also in the limit case of a tree with only three nodes. In this case, $H_0 = 1$ applies, as this type of tree is the limit case where a hub collapses into a chain. This limit case has relevance when the number of nodes x is odd and their topology is a chain. Indeed,
IF

- S is the progressive index for pruning cycles,
- G the gradient of the erased nodes at cycle j,
- L the number of links erased at cycle j;
- N^* the number of erased nodes at cycle j

THEN

$$\left|\begin{array}{cccc} S & G & L & N* \\ 1 & 1 & 2 & 2 \\ 2 & 1 & 2 & 2 \\ \vdots & \vdots & \vdots & \vdots \\ \frac{(x-1)}{2} & 1 & 2 & 3 \end{array}\right| \tag{11.33}$$

$$\varphi^{[C]} = 1, \mu^{[C]} = \frac{2x}{x-1}$$

$$N^{[C]} = x$$

$$H_0^{[C]} = \frac{\mu^{[C]} \cdot \varphi^{[C]} - 1}{N^{[C]} - 1} = \frac{x+1}{(x-1)^2} = \frac{1}{x-1} \cdot \frac{x+1}{x-1} \tag{11.34}$$

In other words

$$\lim_{x \to \infty} H = 0 \tag{11.35}$$

So, in the case of a "chain tree" composed of an odd number of nodes, the last pruning cycle has to delete three nodes, representing the limit case where "hub tree" and "chain tree" collapse into each other. In this condition, a "chain tree" will present a H_0 value always a little bigger than 0. Increasing the number of the odd nodes in the "chain tree," this squared value decreases asymptotically to zero. The *H* index, in any case, displays a structural difference between trees composed of an even vs. an odd number of nodes (Fig. 11.12).

11.5.1 Graph and MST Complexity

The *H* indicator (11.32) represents the *global hubness* of graph. When $H = 0$, the tree is a one-dimensional line and its complexity is minimal. When $H = 1$, the tree presents only one hub and its complexity is the maximum that a tree can attain. The complexity of a graph, in fact, is connected to its entropy. The quantity of information in a graph is linked to the graph diameter and to the connectivity of the vertices: given the number of vertices, the shorter the diameter, the bigger the entropy. Starting from the classical notion of entropy we can thus write

$$E = -K \cdot \sum_{i}^{N} p_i \cdot \ln(p_i) \tag{11.36}$$

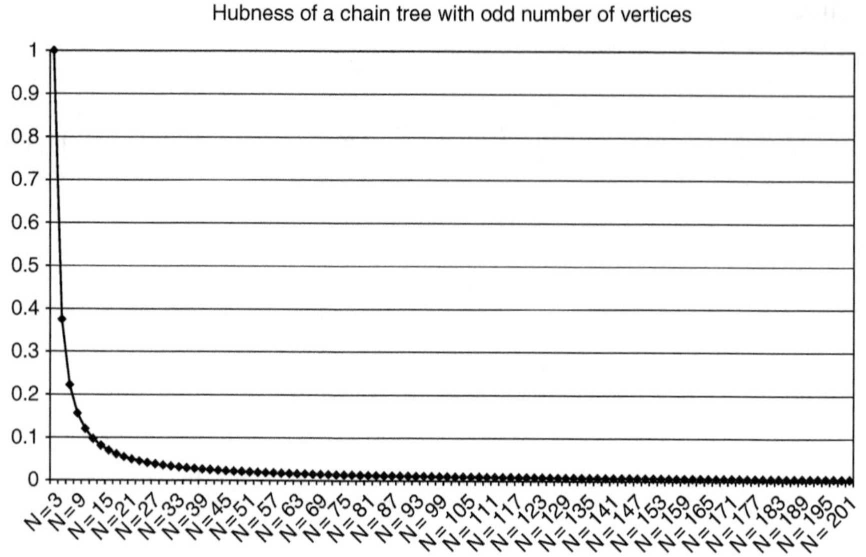

Fig. 11.12 Equation (11.34)

If we name $E(G)$ the topological entropy of a generic tree graph, we can write

$$E(G) = -\frac{A}{M} \cdot \sum_{i}^{N} \frac{C_i}{A} \cdot \ln\left(\frac{C_i}{A}\right), \; 0 < E(G) < \infty \qquad (11.37)$$

where A is the number of graph edges ($N-1$, when the graph is a tree); N the number of graph vertices; M the number of pruning cycles necessary to deconnect the graph completely; and C_i the degree of connectivity of each vertex.

The quantity C_i/A measures the probability that a generic node C_j, where $j \neq i$, has to be directly linked to the node C_i. This means that the entropy of a graph, $E(G)$, will increase when the number of vertices with a large number of links increases. Accordingly, the probability to arrange the links of N vertices, using a random process, into a linear chain is the lowest. Therefore, the higher the number of pruning cycles, M, needed for a graph, the smaller the graph entropy. Equation (11.37) shows clearly that a "hub tree" has more entropy than a "chain tree." Consequently, when the H index of a tree increases, its redundancy increases as well.

At this point, it is necessary to illustrate how the H function and the corresponding topological entropy work for any generic a-directed graph. According to the H function, the complexity of any graph is ruled by (11.32); in particular, we have $0 < H_0 < 2$.

More specifically, $0 < H_0 < \frac{1}{2}$ for trees (with the exception of "star trees" for which $H_0 = 1$). For a regular graph, the corresponding H function lies in the interval $1.\overline{6} \leq H_0 < 2$.

For any other kind of graph (except trees), the H function can take any value of the feasible interval, depending on its degree of symmetry: the more symmetric the graph, the higher the corresponding H value. For the sake of clarity, let us now consider in detail how to compute the H function and the topological entropy of a generic graph. We begin by introducing the concept of the *pruning table* as a useful presentational tool:

$$\begin{vmatrix} M & G & L & N \\ 1 & g_1 & l_1 & n_1 \\ \vdots & \vdots & \vdots & \vdots \\ k & g_k & l_k & n_k \end{vmatrix}$$

where M is the counter of the pruning cycles; G is the gradient of the Mth pruning cycle; L is the number of deleted links at the Mth pruning cycle; and N is the number of deleted nodes at the Mth pruning cycle.

Take as an example the graph

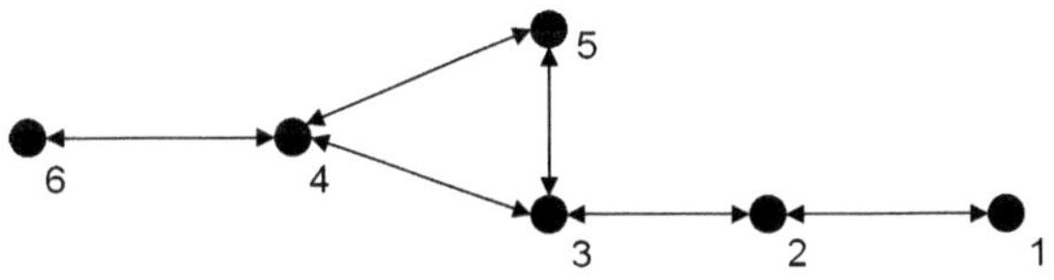

The corresponding pruning table will be

M	G	L	N
1	1	2	2
2	1	1	1
3	2	3	3

At this point, applying (11.32) and (11.37), it is possible to compute the H function and the topological entropy of this specific graph as follows:

$$\varphi = \frac{1}{P}\sum_j^P S_{TGj} = \frac{1}{2}\sum_j^2 S_{TGj} = \frac{1}{2}(1+2) = \frac{3}{2} = 1.5$$

$$\mu = \frac{A}{M} = \frac{6}{3} = 2$$

$$H_0 = \frac{\mu \cdot \varphi - 1}{A} = \frac{2 \times 1.5 - 1}{6} = \frac{1}{3} = 0.33$$

$$E(G) = -\frac{A}{M} \cdot \sum_i^N \frac{c_i}{A} \ln\left(\frac{c_i}{A}\right) = 4.04561706$$

To help the reader familiarize with these computations, we report as an example values of the H function and of the topological entropy for different graphs, each of which is made of only six nodes:

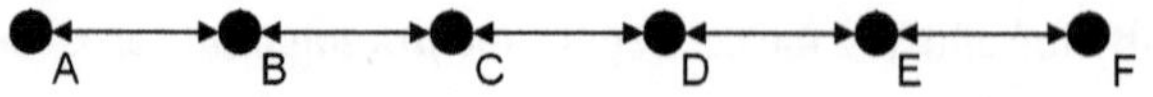

Chain: $H = 0.2$; $E(G) = 3.5116$

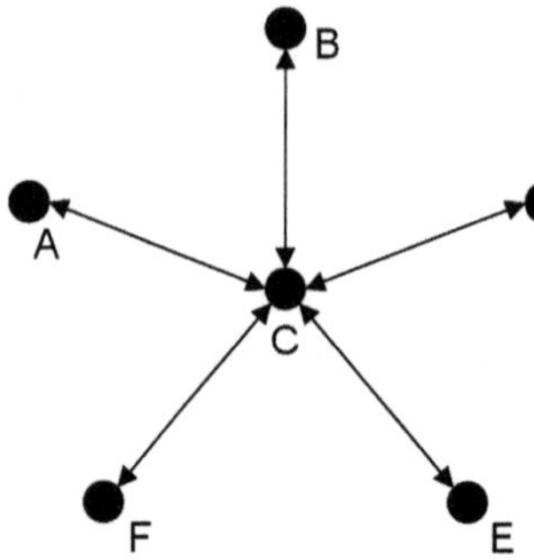

Star: $H = 1$; $E(G) = 8.0471$

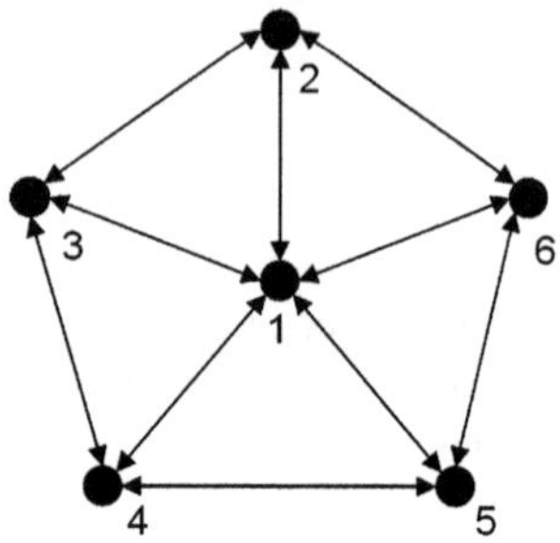

Closed star: $H = 1.7$; $E(G) = 21.5253$

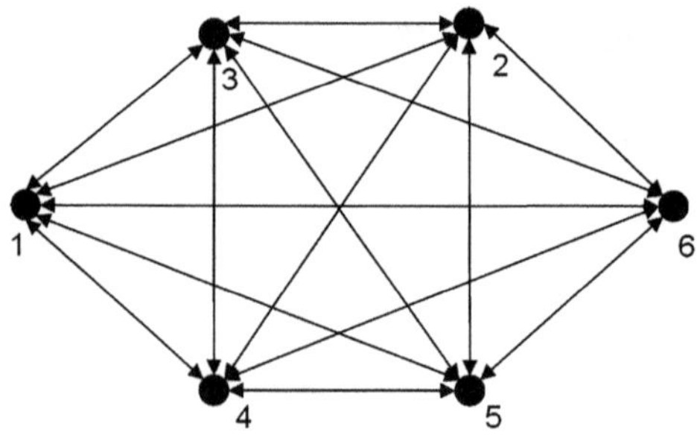

Complete graph: $H = 1.93$; $E(G) = 32.9583$

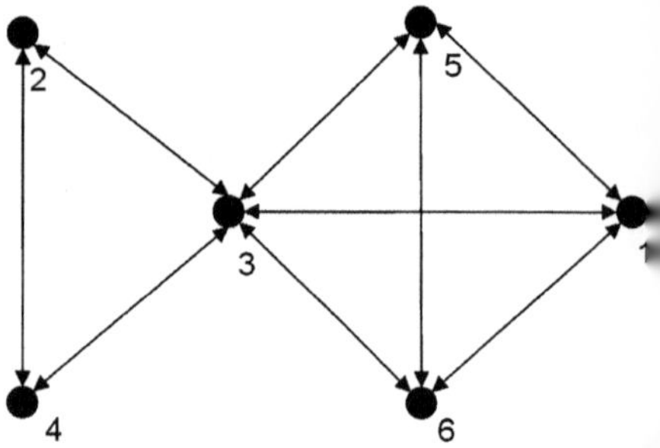

R-graph (**a**): $H = 0.72$; $E(G)$=9.4213

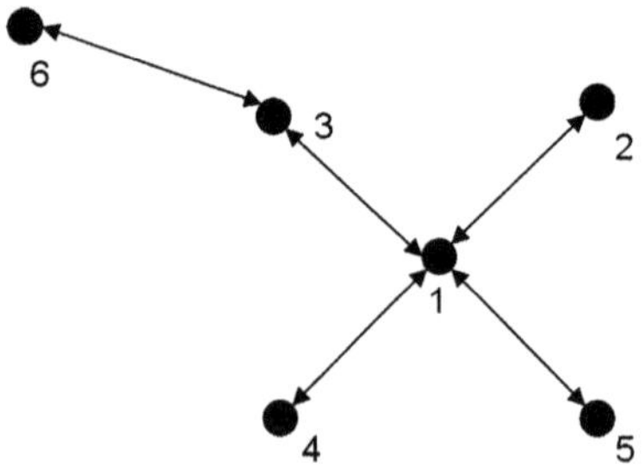

R-graph (**b**): $H = 0.5$; $E(G) = 7.1214$

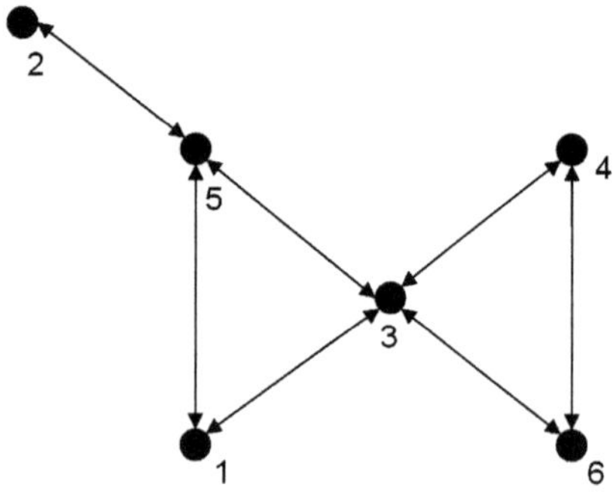

R-tree: $H = 0.4$; $E(G) = 4.5814$

It is easy to check how hubness and topological entropy, in the examples above, vary in ways that reflect, respectively, the graph's depth of connectivity layers and the occurrence of nodes with a large number of connections. Notice also that the two measures need not always be concordant (compare, e.g., the "star" graph and the R-graph (**a**)).

11.6 The Delta *H* Function

Considering how the structure of a given graph is changed by a pruning process, it becomes natural to think of what happens to graphs, and in particular to MSTs, as one or more of their nodes are deleted. In which way will the graph have to be organized to continue to reflect as best as possible the underlying structure of relationships once one or more nodes are taken away? How will the other nodes rearrange their links on the basis of the underlying metric and constraints, to connect each other once again?

Define a H index for each one of N different MSTs, generated from the original distance matrix by deleting one different vertex at each step:

$$H_i = \frac{\mu_i \cdot \varphi_i - 1}{A - 1}, \quad 0 \leq H_i < 2 \tag{11.38}$$

where as above

$$\mu_i = \frac{1}{M}\sum_{j}^{M} Nd_j = \frac{N}{M}, \; \varphi = \frac{1}{P}\sum_{k}^{P} S_{TG\,k}$$

A is the number of links of the graph ($N - 1$ for tree graphs); M the number of cycles of the pruning algorithm; P the number of pruning classes; Nd_j the number of nodes without link at the jth iteration; and $S_{TG\,k}$ the class k pruning gradient.

Each H_i represents the tree complexity of the same, original distance matrix when the ith vertex is deleted. Consequently, the difference between the complexity of the whole MST (i.e., H_0) and the complexity of any of the MSTs that are obtained by deleting one of the graph vertices (H_i) is the measure of the contribution of that specific (i) vertex of the graph to the original graph's global complexity:

$$\delta H_i = H_0 - H_i \tag{11.39}$$

This new index measures to what extent each vertex of a graph contributes to increase ($\delta H_i < 0$) or to decrease ($\delta H_i > 0$) the redundancy of the original, overall graph. We have named this function *delta H function*; it can be applied to any kind of graph.

11.6.1 Auto-CM, MST, and the Delta H Function: An Example

Let us now consider a toy data set to test how the previous formalism works in practice and what kind of insight it yields for a given problem. In what follows, we will guide the reader along a thorough illustration of the techniques introduced so far. We will work on the gang data set, a small, very well-known and widely used data set, made of 27 records and 5 variables, and clearly modeled on the *West Side Story* musical (Table 11.4):

Table 11.4 Gang data set

Name	Gang	Age	Education	Status	Profession
Art	Jets	40'	Junior school	Single	Pusher
Al	Jets	30'	Junior school	Married	Burglar
Sam	Jets	20'	College	Single	Bookie
Clyde	Jets	40'	Junior school	Single	Bookie
Mike	Jets	30'	Junior school	Single	Bookie
Jim	Jets	20'	Junior school	Divorced	Burglar
Greg	Jets	20'	High school	Married	Pusher
John	Jets	20'	Junior school	Married	Burglar
Doug	Jets	30'	High school	Single	Bookie
Lance	Jets	20'	Junior school	Married	Burglar
George	Jets	20'	Junior school	Divorced	Burglar
Pete	Jets	20'	High school	Single	Bookie
Fred	Jets	20'	High school	Single	Pusher
Gene	Jets	20'	College	Single	Pusher
Ralph	Jets	30'	Junior school	Single	Pusher
Phil	Sharks	30'	College	Married	Pusher
Ike	Sharks	30'	Junior school	Single	Bookie
Nick	Sharks	30'	High school	Single	Pusher
Don	Sharks	30'	College	Married	Burglar
Ned	Sharks	30'	College	Married	Bookie
Karl	Sharks	40'	High school	Married	Bookie
Ken	Sharks	20'	High school	Single	Burglar
Earl	Sharks	40'	High school	Married	Burglar
Rick	Sharks	30'	High school	Divorced	Burglar
Ol	Sharks	30'	College	Married	Pusher
Neal	Sharks	30'	High school	Single	Bookie
Dave	Sharks	30'	High school	Divorced	Pusher

The structure of the data set is the following:

- Gang = {Jets, Sharks};
- Age = {20s, 30s, 40s};
- Education = {Junior school, high school, college};
- Status = {Married, single, divorced};
- Profession = {Pusher, Bookie, Burglar}.

First of all, it is necessary to transform each string variable into a Boolean one (Table 11.5):

Table 11.5 Binary gang data set

	Jets	Sharks	20'	30'	40'	JH	Col	HS	Single	Married	Divorced	Pusher	Burglar	Bookie
Art	1	0	0	0	1	1	0	0	1	0	0	1	0	0
Al	1	0	0	1	0	1	0	0	0	1	0	0	0	1
Sam	1	0	1	0	0	0	1	0	1	0	0	0	1	0
Clyde	1	0	0	0	1	1	0	0	1	0	0	0	1	0
Mike	1	0	0	1	0	1	0	0	1	0	0	0	1	0
Jim	1	0	1	0	0	1	0	0	0	0	1	0	0	1
Greg	1	0	1	0	0	0	0	1	0	1	0	1	0	0
John	1	0	1	0	0	1	0	0	0	1	0	0	0	1
Doug	1	0	0	1	0	0	0	1	1	0	0	0	1	0
Lance	1	0	1	0	0	1	0	0	0	1	0	0	0	1
George	1	0	1	0	0	1	0	0	0	0	1	0	0	1
Pete	1	0	1	0	0	0	0	1	1	0	0	0	1	0
Fred	1	0	1	0	0	0	0	1	1	0	0	1	0	0
Gene	1	0	1	0	0	0	1	0	1	0	0	1	0	0
Ralph	1	0	0	1	0	1	0	0	1	0	0	1	0	0
Phil	0	1	0	1	0	0	1	0	0	1	0	1	0	0
Ike	0	1	0	1	0	1	0	0	1	0	0	0	1	0
Nick	0	1	0	1	0	0	0	1	1	0	0	1	0	0
Don	0	1	0	1	0	0	1	0	0	1	0	0	0	1
Ned	0	1	0	1	0	0	1	0	0	1	0	0	1	0
Karl	0	1	0	0	1	0	0	1	0	1	0	0	1	0
Ken	0	1	1	0	0	0	0	1	1	0	0	0	0	1
Earl	0	1	0	0	1	0	0	1	0	1	0	0	0	1
Rick	0	1	0	1	0	0	0	1	0	0	1	0	0	1
Ol	0	1	0	1	0	0	1	0	0	1	0	1	0	0
Neal	0	1	0	1	0	0	0	1	1	0	0	0	1	0
Dave	0	1	0	1	0	0	0	1	0	0	1	1	0	0

The new data set is now made of 14 binary variables, most of which orthogonal to each other. As we want to use an auto-CM ANN to process the records, we must, as remarked above, transpose this matrix (Table 11.6).

The data set is then submitted to the auto-CM ANN for the learning session. The set is structured such that the variables are the hyperpoints and the records are the hyperpoint coordinates. After about 30 epochs, the auto-CM, with a contractive factor of 6.19615221, is completely trained (RMSE = 0.00000000) and the weights matrix reads as in Table 11.7.

Applying (11.12), we transform the weights matrix into a distance matrix (Table 11.8).

We can therefore now compute the MST of the data set that turns out to be as in Fig. 11.13.

What does the MST tell us? It provides a ready-to-access spatialization of the complex pattern of associations among the variables that characterize each one of the gang members, as well as their belonging to a specific gang. In particular, notice how the MST perfectly separates the two gangs into sub-trees whose boundaries are marked, respectively, by Ike and Mike. Close-by subjects in the networks

Table 11.6 Gang data set transposed

	Art	Al	Sam	Clyde	Mike	Jim	Greg	John	Doug	Lance	George	Pete	Fred	Gene	Ralph	Phil	Ike	Nick	Don	Ned	Karl	Ken	Earl	Rick	Ol	Neal	Dave
Jets	1	1	1	1	1	1	1	1	1	1	1	1	1	1	1	0	0	0	0	0	0	0	0	0	0	0	0
Sharks	0	0	0	0	0	0	0	0	0	0	0	0	0	0	0	1	1	1	1	1	1	1	1	1	1	1	1
20'	0	0	1	0	0	1	1	1	0	1	1	1	1	1	0	0	0	0	0	0	0	1	0	0	0	0	0
30'	0	1	0	0	1	0	0	0	1	0	0	0	0	0	1	1	1	1	1	1	0	0	0	1	1	1	1
40'	1	0	0	1	0	0	0	0	0	0	0	0	0	0	0	0	0	0	0	0	1	0	1	0	0	0	0
JH	1	1	0	1	1	1	0	1	0	1	1	0	0	0	1	0	1	0	0	0	0	0	0	0	0	0	0
Col	0	0	1	0	0	0	0	0	0	0	0	0	0	1	0	1	0	0	1	1	0	0	0	0	1	0	0
HS	0	0	0	0	0	0	1	0	1	0	0	1	1	0	0	0	0	1	0	0	1	1	1	1	0	1	1
Single	1	0	1	1	1	0	0	0	1	0	0	1	1	1	1	0	1	1	0	0	0	1	0	0	0	1	0
Married	0	1	0	0	0	0	1	1	0	1	0	0	0	0	0	1	0	0	1	1	1	0	1	0	1	0	0
Divorced	0	0	0	0	0	1	0	0	0	0	1	0	0	0	0	0	0	0	0	0	0	0	0	1	0	0	1
Pusher	1	0	0	0	0	0	1	0	0	0	0	0	1	1	1	1	0	1	0	0	0	0	0	0	1	0	1
Burglar	0	0	1	1	1	0	0	0	1	0	0	1	0	0	0	0	1	0	0	1	1	0	0	0	0	1	0
Bookie	0	1	0	0	0	1	0	1	0	1	1	0	0	0	0	0	0	0	1	0	0	1	1	1	0	0	0

Table 11.7 Auto-CM weights matrix

	Art	Al	Sam	Clyde	Mike	Jim	Greg	John	Doug	Lance	George	Pete	Fred	Gene	Ralph	Phil	Ike	Nick	Don	Ned	Karl	Ken	Earl	Rick	Ol	Neal	Dave
Art	0.00	102.83	119.92	165.02	148.80	105.24	111.43	103.89	117.11	103.89	105.24	114.94	154.44	156.81	167.02	31.70	108.60	102.58	1.00	1.00	11.01	46.86	13.07	1.00	31.70	42.05	30.91
Al	102.83	0.00	52.30	103.38	157.46	147.54	122.17	168.08	135.95	168.08	147.54	51.76	51.39	51.94	156.25	113.35	104.77	42.03	150.80	113.24	33.01	24.15	88.16	112.03	113.35	42.87	47.70
Sam	119.92	52.30	0.00	153.46	148.72	105.00	104.28	103.25	147.55	103.25	105.00	166.47	148.99	169.14	114.74	17.26	92.51	40.03	20.26	77.74	27.95	104.27	1.00	1.00	17.26	92.00	1.00
Clyde	165.02	103.38	153.46	0.00	165.81	105.80	50.72	104.44	147.95	104.44	105.80	150.01	117.16	122.03	148.53	1.00	143.32	41.18	1.00	26.59	62.47	45.40	11.29	1.00	1.00	92.77	1.00
Mike	148.80	157.46	148.72	165.81	0.00	103.04	49.93	101.71	170.65	101.71	103.04	145.38	112.34	117.02	171.26	47.82	166.98	116.33	50.50	105.68	23.67	39.40	1.00	49.82	47.82	146.38	48.50
Jim	105.24	147.54	105.00	105.80	103.04	0.00	106.05	166.10	54.29	166.10	173.10	102.37	101.48	103.64	102.16	1.00	31.09	1.00	30.22	1.00	1.00	88.42	29.96	62.25	1.00	1.00	10.99
Greg	111.43	122.17	104.28	50.72	49.93	106.05	0.00	153.87	124.99	153.87	106.05	152.99	168.79	144.17	101.02	96.92	1.00	83.74	30.53	36.13	114.08	89.11	110.91	40.01	96.92	32.77	99.14
John	103.89	168.08	103.25	104.44	101.71	166.10	153.87	0.00	52.90	175.97	166.10	100.66	99.79	101.91	100.85	37.30	30.76	1.00	96.50	38.95	41.49	81.93	97.61	27.09	37.30	1.00	1.00
Doug	117.11	135.95	147.55	147.95	170.65	54.29	124.99	52.90	0.00	52.90	54.29	168.13	155.77	118.15	160.01	44.66	139.56	150.84	47.17	98.80	88.45	99.17	36.21	117.38	44.66	165.25	114.30
Lance	103.89	168.08	103.25	104.44	101.71	166.10	153.87	175.97	52.90	0.00	166.10	100.66	99.79	101.91	100.85	37.30	30.76	1.00	96.50	38.95	41.49	81.93	97.61	27.09	37.30	1.00	1.00
George	105.24	147.54	105.00	105.80	103.04	173.10	106.05	166.10	54.29	166.10	0.00	102.37	101.48	103.64	102.16	1.00	31.09	1.00	30.22	1.00	1.00	88.42	29.96	62.25	1.00	1.00	10.99
Pete	114.94	51.76	166.47	150.01	145.38	102.37	152.99	100.66	168.13	100.66	102.37	0.00	169.39	148.66	109.97	1.00	85.27	103.91	1.00	25.28	101.29	146.15	41.01	39.20	1.00	140.72	36.64
Fred	154.44	51.39	148.99	117.16	112.34	101.48	168.79	99.79	155.77	99.79	101.48	169.39	0.00	167.88	147.39	27.47	36.30	144.16	1.00	1.00	37.38	146.99	40.64	38.85	27.47	106.63	100.30
Gene	156.81	51.94	169.14	122.03	117.02	103.64	144.17	101.91	118.15	101.91	103.64	148.66	167.88	0.00	149.65	75.22	41.83	98.44	18.67	16.13	1.00	105.88	1.00	1.00	75.22	42.20	26.62
Ralph	167.02	156.25	114.74	148.53	171.26	102.16	101.02	100.85	160.01	100.85	102.16	109.97	147.39	149.65	0.00	104.64	152.59	146.99	48.22	43.80	1.00	40.44	1.00	47.57	104.64	115.44	104.42
Phil	31.70	113.35	17.26	1.00	47.82	1.00	96.92	37.30	44.66	37.30	1.00	1.00	27.47	75.22	104.64	0.00	108.98	144.39	165.75	165.72	106.45	38.36	101.82	109.50	175.41	104.60	151.98
Ike	108.60	104.77	92.51	143.32	166.98	31.09	1.00	30.76	139.56	30.76	31.09	85.27	36.30	41.83	152.59	108.98	0.00	154.28	109.00	145.74	95.37	124.23	37.85	107.32	108.98	167.22	107.45
Nick	102.58	42.03	40.03	41.18	116.33	1.00	83.74	1.00	150.84	1.00	1.00	103.91	144.16	98.44	146.99	144.39	154.28	0.00	103.99	101.95	95.76	152.93	99.62	148.30	144.39	169.39	166.05
Don	1.00	150.80	20.26	1.00	50.50	30.22	30.53	96.50	47.17	96.50	30.22	1.00	1.00	18.67	48.22	165.75	109.00	103.99	0.00	165.64	99.47	103.86	145.64	153.54	165.75	104.63	109.67
Ned	1.00	113.24	77.74	26.59	105.68	1.00	36.13	38.95	98.80	38.95	1.00	25.28	1.00	16.13	43.80	165.72	145.74	101.95	165.64	0.00	152.28	37.63	102.68	107.38	165.72	142.30	107.51
Karl	11.01	33.01	27.95	62.47	23.67	1.00	114.08	41.49	88.45	41.49	1.00	101.29	37.38	1.00	1.00	106.45	95.37	95.76	99.47	152.28	0.00	105.50	166.13	104.26	106.45	139.10	102.99
Ken	46.86	24.15	104.27	45.40	39.40	88.42	89.11	81.93	99.17	81.93	88.42	146.15	146.99	105.88	40.44	38.36	124.23	152.93	103.86	37.63	105.50	0.00	152.02	149.55	38.36	153.34	101.38
Earl	13.07	88.16	1.00	11.29	1.00	29.96	110.91	97.61	36.21	97.61	29.96	41.01	40.64	1.00	1.00	101.82	37.85	99.62	145.64	102.68	166.13	152.02	0.00	153.01	101.82	101.15	107.15
Rick	1.00	112.03	1.00	1.00	49.82	62.25	40.01	27.09	117.38	27.09	62.25	39.20	38.85	1.00	47.57	109.50	107.32	148.30	153.54	107.38	104.26	149.55	153.01	0.00	109.50	149.44	164.74
Ol	31.70	113.35	17.26	1.00	47.82	1.00	96.92	37.30	44.66	37.30	1.00	1.00	27.47	75.22	104.64	175.41	108.98	144.39	165.75	165.72	106.45	38.36	101.82	109.50	0.00	104.60	151.98
Neal	42.05	42.87	92.00	92.77	146.38	1.00	32.77	1.00	165.25	1.00	1.00	140.72	106.63	42.20	115.44	104.60	167.22	169.39	104.63	142.30	139.10	153.34	101.15	149.44	104.60	0.00	148.50
Dave	30.91	47.70	1.00	1.00	48.50	10.99	99.14	1.00	114.30	1.00	10.99	36.64	100.30	26.62	104.42	151.98	107.45	166.05	109.67	107.51	102.99	101.38	107.15	164.74	151.98	148.50	0.00

Table 11.8 Auto-CM distance matrix

	Art	Al	Sam	Clyde	Mike	Jim	Greg	John	Doug	Lance	George	Pete	Fred	Gene	Ralph	Phil	Ike	Nick	Don	Ned	Karl	Ken	Earl	Rick	Ol	Neal	Dave
Art	0	0.5695	0.6641	0.9139	0.8240	0.5828	0.6171	0.5753	0.6485	0.5753	0.5828	0.6365	0.8553	0.8684	0.9249	0.1755	0.6014	0.5681	0.0055	0.0055	0.0610	0.2595	0.0724	0.0055	0.1755	0.2329	0.1712
Al	0.5695	0	0.2897	0.5725	0.8720	0.8170	0.6766	0.9308	0.7529	0.9308	0.8170	0.2866	0.2846	0.2877	0.8653	0.6277	0.5802	0.2328	0.8351	0.6271	0.1828	0.1337	0.4882	0.6204	0.6277	0.2374	0.2641
Sam	0.6641	0.2897	0	0.8498	0.8236	0.5815	0.5775	0.5718	0.8171	0.5718	0.5815	0.9219	0.8251	0.9367	0.6354	0.0956	0.5123	0.2217	0.1122	0.4305	0.1548	0.5775	0.0055	0.0055	0.0956	0.5095	0.0055
Clyde	0.9139	0.5725	0.8498	0	0.9182	0.5859	0.2809	0.5784	0.8193	0.5784	0.5859	0.8307	0.6488	0.6758	0.8226	0.0055	0.7937	0.2280	0.0055	0.1473	0.3459	0.2514	0.0625	0.0055	0.0055	0.5137	0.0055
Mike	0.8240	0.8720	0.8236	0.9182	0	0.5706	0.2765	0.5633	0.9450	0.5633	0.5706	0.8051	0.6221	0.6480	0.9484	0.2648	0.9247	0.6442	0.2797	0.5853	0.1311	0.2182	0.0055	0.2759	0.2648	0.8106	0.2686
Jim	0.5828	0.8170	0.5815	0.5859	0.5706	0	0.5873	0.9198	0.3006	0.9198	0.9586	0.5669	0.5620	0.5740	0.5658	0.0055	0.1722	0.0055	0.1674	0.0055	0.0055	0.4897	0.1659	0.3448	0.0055	0.0055	0.0609
Greg	0.6171	0.6766	0.5775	0.2809	0.2765	0.5873	0	0.8521	0.6922	0.8521	0.5873	0.8472	0.9347	0.7984	0.5594	0.5367	0.0055	0.4637	0.1691	0.2001	0.6317	0.4935	0.6142	0.2216	0.5367	0.1815	0.5490
John	0.5753	0.9308	0.5718	0.5784	0.5633	0.9198	0.8521	0	0.2930	0.9745	0.9198	0.5574	0.5526	0.5644	0.5585	0.2066	0.1704	0.0055	0.5344	0.2157	0.2297	0.4537	0.5405	0.1500	0.2066	0.0055	0.0055
Doug	0.6485	0.7529	0.8171	0.8193	0.9450	0.3006	0.6922	0.2930	0	0.2930	0.3006	0.9311	0.8626	0.6543	0.8861	0.2473	0.7729	0.8353	0.2612	0.5472	0.4898	0.5492	0.2005	0.6500	0.2473	0.9151	0.6330
Lance	0.5753	0.9308	0.5718	0.5784	0.5633	0.9198	0.8521	0.9745	0.2930	0	0.9198	0.5574	0.5526	0.5644	0.5585	0.2066	0.1704	0.0055	0.5344	0.2157	0.2297	0.4537	0.5405	0.1500	0.2066	0.0055	0.0055
George	0.5828	0.8170	0.5815	0.5859	0.5706	0.9586	0.5873	0.9198	0.3006	0.9198	0	0.5669	0.5620	0.5740	0.5658	0.0055	0.1722	0.0055	0.1674	0.0055	0.0055	0.4897	0.1659	0.3448	0.0055	0.0055	0.0609
Pete	0.6365	0.2866	0.9219	0.8307	0.8051	0.5669	0.8472	0.5574	0.9311	0.5574	0.5669	0	0.9381	0.8233	0.6090	0.0055	0.4722	0.5754	0.0055	0.1400	0.5610	0.8094	0.2271	0.2171	0.0055	0.7793	0.2029
Fred	0.8553	0.2846	0.8251	0.6488	0.6221	0.5620	0.9347	0.5526	0.8626	0.5526	0.5620	0.9381	0	0.9297	0.8162	0.1521	0.2010	0.7983	0.0055	0.0055	0.2070	0.8140	0.2251	0.2152	0.1521	0.5905	0.5554
Gene	0.8684	0.2877	0.9367	0.6758	0.6480	0.5740	0.7984	0.5644	0.6543	0.5644	0.5740	0.8233	0.9297	0	0.8287	0.4165	0.2316	0.5451	0.1034	0.0893	0.0055	0.5863	0.0055	0.0055	0.4165	0.2337	0.1474
Ralph	0.9249	0.8653	0.6354	0.8226	0.9484	0.5658	0.5594	0.5585	0.8861	0.5585	0.5658	0.6090	0.8162	0.8287	0	0.5795	0.8450	0.8140	0.2671	0.2425	0.0055	0.2239	0.0055	0.2634	0.5795	0.6393	0.5783
Phil	0.1755	0.6277	0.0956	0.0055	0.2648	0.0055	0.5367	0.2066	0.2473	0.2066	0.0055	0.0055	0.1521	0.4165	0.5795	0	0.6035	0.7996	0.9179	0.9177	0.5895	0.2124	0.5639	0.6064	0.9714	0.5793	0.8417
Ike	0.6014	0.5802	0.5123	0.7937	0.9247	0.1722	0.0055	0.1704	0.7729	0.1704	0.1722	0.4722	0.2010	0.2316	0.8450	0.6035	0	0.8544	0.6036	0.8071	0.5281	0.6880	0.2096	0.5943	0.6035	0.9261	0.5951
Nick	0.5681	0.2328	0.2217	0.2280	0.6442	0.0055	0.4637	0.0055	0.8353	0.0055	0.0055	0.5754	0.7983	0.5451	0.8140	0.7996	0.8544	0	0.5759	0.5646	0.5303	0.8469	0.5517	0.8213	0.7996	0.9381	0.9195
Don	0.0055	0.8351	0.1122	0.0055	0.2797	0.1674	0.1691	0.5344	0.2612	0.5344	0.1674	0.0055	0.0055	0.1034	0.2671	0.9179	0.6036	0.5759	0	0.9173	0.5508	0.5752	0.8065	0.8503	0.9179	0.5794	0.6073
Ned	0.0055	0.6271	0.4305	0.1473	0.5853	0.0055	0.2001	0.2157	0.5472	0.2157	0.0055	0.1400	0.0055	0.0893	0.2425	0.9177	0.8071	0.5646	0.9173	0	0.8433	0.2084	0.5686	0.5946	0.9177	0.7880	0.5954
Karl	0.0610	0.1828	0.1548	0.3459	0.1311	0.0055	0.6317	0.2297	0.4898	0.2297	0.0055	0.5610	0.2070	0.0055	0.0055	0.5895	0.5281	0.5303	0.5508	0.8433	0	0.5842	0.9200	0.5774	0.5895	0.7703	0.5704
Ken	0.2595	0.1337	0.5775	0.2514	0.2182	0.4897	0.4935	0.4537	0.5492	0.4537	0.4897	0.8094	0.8140	0.5863	0.2239	0.2124	0.6880	0.8469	0.5752	0.2084	0.5842	0	0.8419	0.8282	0.2124	0.8492	0.5614
Earl	0.0724	0.4882	0.0055	0.0625	0.0055	0.1659	0.6142	0.5405	0.2005	0.5405	0.1659	0.2271	0.2251	0.0055	0.0055	0.5639	0.2096	0.5517	0.8065	0.5686	0.9200	0.8419	0	0.8473	0.5639	0.5602	0.5934
Rick	0.0055	0.6204	0.0055	0.0055	0.2759	0.3448	0.2216	0.1500	0.6500	0.1500	0.3448	0.2171	0.2152	0.0055	0.2634	0.6064	0.5943	0.8213	0.8503	0.5946	0.5774	0.8282	0.8473	0	0.6064	0.8276	0.9123
Ol	0.1755	0.6277	0.0956	0.0055	0.2648	0.0055	0.5367	0.2066	0.2473	0.2066	0.0055	0.0055	0.1521	0.4165	0.5795	0.9714	0.6035	0.7996	0.9179	0.9177	0.5895	0.2124	0.5639	0.6064	0	0.5793	0.8417
Neal	0.2329	0.2374	0.5095	0.5137	0.8106	0.0055	0.1815	0.0055	0.9151	0.0055	0.0055	0.7793	0.5905	0.2337	0.6393	0.5793	0.9261	0.9381	0.5794	0.7880	0.7703	0.8492	0.5602	0.8276	0.5793	0	0.8224
Dave	0.1712	0.2641	0.0055	0.0055	0.2686	0.0609	0.5490	0.0055	0.6330	0.0055	0.0609	0.2029	0.5554	0.1474	0.5783	0.8417	0.5951	0.9195	0.6073	0.5954	0.5704	0.5614	0.5934	0.9123	0.8417	0.8224	0

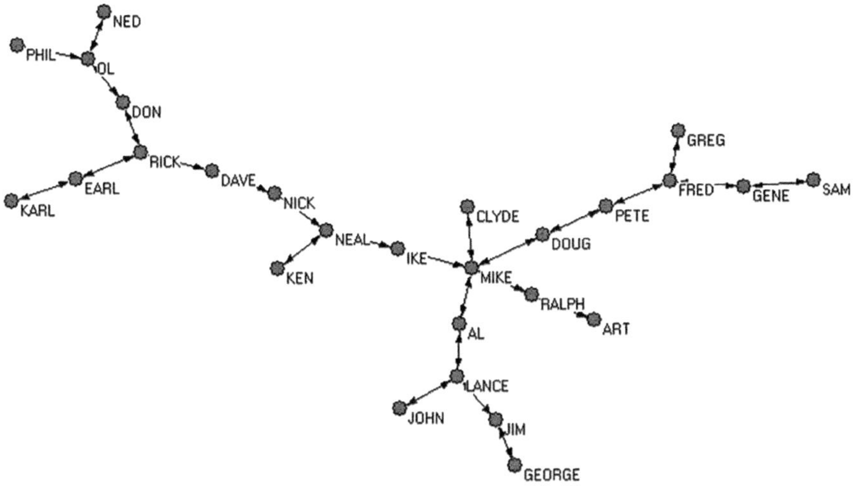

Fig. 11.13 The MST of the global network ($H_0 = 0.10989$)

correspond to subjects that basically present close-by personal characteristics; moreover, the tree structure clearly points out how specific subsets of subjects constitute sub-families of common traits within the large gang family. Nothing like this neat, hands-on representation of variables association can be obtained by means of the classic techniques today; moreover, no one of such techniques may properly take into account the contribution that each variable or subject provides to the database's overall variation. We will elaborate on this point below.

Coming to the technical details, the local indices for this tree are shown in Table 11.9.

As to the global indices for global hubness (H_0, H_1) and for graph entropy (E_0, E_1), they are shown in Table 11.10.

From the hubness point of view and from the entropy point of view, if we remove from the graph Rick, or Mike, or Neal, or Don, the complexity of the graph, and consequently its entropy, increases; whereas if we remove from the global graph Al, the complexity of the graph, and consequently its entropy, decreases. That is absolutely not evident if we analyze the same graph by comparing the local indices. A naïve point of view could suggest exactly the opposite: since Mike is a large hub (as many as five links), if he is removed from the graph, then the global network has to become simpler. But this is not necessarily the case, in fact. What happens when Mike is removed does not depend simply on how connected Mike is, but more generally on whether or not Mike's hubness may be taken over by someone else, depending on the whole relational structure lying in the database. From the global viewpoint, the rearrangement of the network as some of its vertices are removed may lead to extremely complex, hard to anticipate results (Fig. 11.14).

Table 11.9 MST local indices

Vertex degree equation (11.28)	
Art	1
Clyde	1
George	1
Greg	1
John	1
Karl	1
Ken	1
Ned	1
Phil	1
Sam	1
Al	2
Dave	2
Don	2
Doug	2
Earl	2
Gene	2
Ike	2
Jim	2
Nick	2
Pete	2
Ralph	2
Fred	3
Lance	3
Neal	3
Ol	3
Rick	3
Mike	5

Clustering strength equation (11.30)	
Clyde	0.2
Greg	0.3333
John	0.3333
Ken	0.3333
Ned	0.3333
Phil	0.3333
Art	0.5
George	0.5
Karl	0.5
Sam	0.5
Al	0.5
Ike	0.5
Doug	0.5714
Don	0.6667
Ralph	0.6667
Dave	0.8
Nick	0.8
Pete	0.8
Earl	1
Gene	1
Jim	1
Rick	1.5
Fred	1.8
Lance	1.8
Neal	1.8
Ol	1.8
Mike	2.7778

Pruning rank equation (11.31)	
Art	1
Clyde	1
George	1
Greg	1
John	1
Karl	1
Ken	1
Ned	1
Phil	1
Sam	1
Earl	2
Gene	2
Jim	2
Ralph	2
Ol	2
Don	3
Fred	3
Lance	3
Al	4
Pete	4
Rick	4
Dave	5
Doug	5
Nick	6
Mike	6
Ike	7
Neal	7

As already anticipated, if we remove from Fig. 11.14 the vertices Don, Rick, Neal and Mike the new MST will show a more complex structure, whereas if we remove the vertex Al the new MST will be simpler (Fig. 11.15). Notice how Al (two links), whose removal makes the MST simpler, is exactly as connected as, say, Don, whose removal makes the MST more complex: it is simply impossible to deduce what the final outcome of the removal will be by looking at the nodes' connectedness, let alone establish any general relationship between the degree of connectedness and the after-removal structure of the graph (Fig. 11.16).

These surprising "nonlinear" properties of the MST adaptation to the removal of some of its entries is a clear illustration of the "global" character of the auto-CM computation. Local changes in the MST structure therefore bring about possibly vast global changes. This is unlikely to happen with methods that are based on couple-by-couple computations of strengths of association: in these cases, the subtraction of an entry simply destroys information, in particular all and only that information that is related to the local interaction of that specific entry with all of the other ones.

Table 11.10 MST indices for global hubness and for graph entropy

Global hubness equations (11.32)–(11.38)	
H(0) =	**0.10989**
H(Al) =	0.09
H(Art) =	0.108571
H(Sam) =	0.108571
H(Clyde) =	0.108571
H(Jim) =	0.108571
H(Greg) =	0.108571
H(John) =	0.108571
H(Doug) =	0.108571
H(Lance) =	0.108571
H(George) =	0.108571
H(Pete) =	0.108571
H(Fred) =	0.108571
H(Gene) =	0.108571
H(Ralph) =	0.108571
H(Phil) =	0.108571
H(Ike) =	0.108571
H(Nick) =	0.108571
H(Ned) =	0.108571
H(Karl) =	0.108571
H(Ken) =	0.108571
H(Earl) =	0.108571
H(Ol) =	0.108571
H(Dave) =	0.108571
H(Rick) =	0.133333
H(Mike) =	0.133333
H(Neal) =	0.133333
H(Don) =	0.133333

Graph entropy equation (11.37)	
E(0) =	**18.52077**
E(Al) =	15.42418
E(Art) =	17.50778
E(Jim) =	17.50778
E(Nick) =	17.50778
E(Karl) =	17.50778
E(John) =	17.58254
E(Lance) =	17.58254
E(George) =	17.58254
E(Pete) =	17.58254
E(Fred) =	17.58254
E(Gene) =	17.58254
E(Phil) =	17.58254
E(Sam) =	17.58254
E(Ned) =	17.58254
E(Greg) =	17.58254
E(Ken) =	17.58254
E(Earl) =	17.58254
E(Ol) =	17.58254
E(Dave) =	17.58254
E(Doug) =	17.66717
E(Ike) =	17.66717
E(Clyde) =	17.66717
E(Ralph) =	17.74192
E(Neal) =	20.42575
E(Rick) =	20.51296
E(Don) =	20.51296
E(Mike) =	20.52449

11.7 Auto-CM and Maximally Regular Graph (MRG)

The MST represents what we could call the "nervous system" of any data set. In fact, summing up all of the connection strengths among all the variables, we get the total energy of that system. The MST selects only the connections *that minimize this energy*, i.e., the only ones that are really necessary to keep the system coherent. Consequently, all the links included in the MST are fundamental, but, on the contrary, not every "fundamental" link of the data set needs to be in the MST. Such a limit is intrinsic to the nature of MST itself: every link that gives rise to a cycle into the graph (viz., that destroys the graph's "treeness") is eliminated, whatever its strength and meaningfulness. To fix this shortcoming and to better capture the

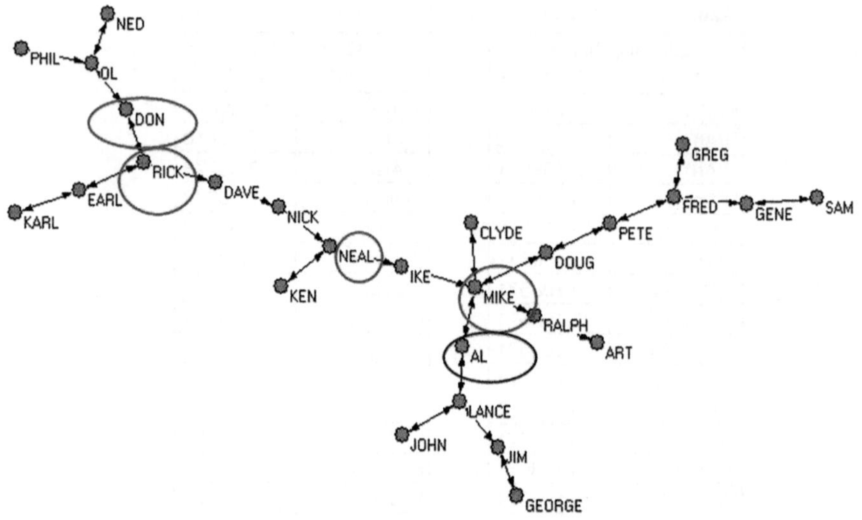

Fig. 11.14 The marked MST of the global network ($H_0 = 0.10989$)

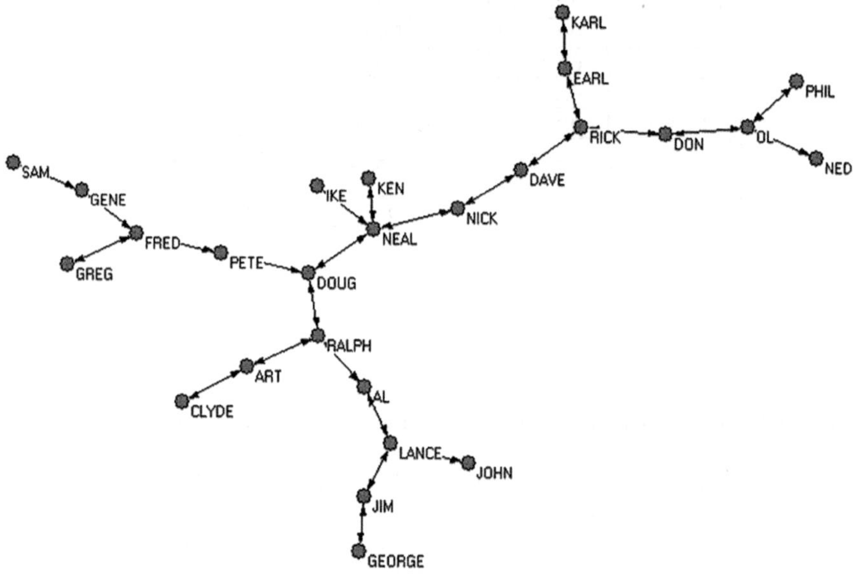

Fig. 11.15 New MST without Mike ($H_0 = 0.13333$)

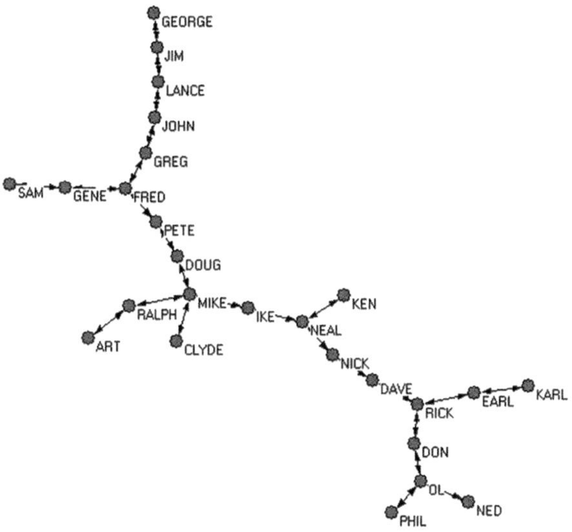

Fig. 11.16 New MST without Al ($H_0 = 0.09$)

intrinsic complexity of a data set, it is necessary to add more links to the MST, according to two criteria:

- The new links have to be *relevant* from a quantitative point of view.
- The new links have to be able to generate new *cyclic regular microstructures* from a qualitative point of view.

Consequently, the MST tree graph is transformed into an undirected graph with cycles. Because of the cycles, the new graph is a dynamic system, involving in its structure the *time* dimension. This is the reason why this new graph should provide information not only about the structure but also about the *functions* of the variables of the data set.

To build the new graph, we need to proceed as follows:

- Assume the MST structure as the starting point of the new graph.
- Consider the sorted list of the connections skipped during the derivation of the MST.
- Estimate the *H* function of the new graph each time that you add a new connection to the MST basic structure, to monitor the variation of the complexity of the new graph at every step.

We will call *maximally regular graph* (MRG) the graph whose *H* function attains the highest value among all the graphs generated by adding back to the original MST, one by one, the missing connections previously skipped during the computation of the MST itself. Starting from (11.32), the MRG may be characterized as follows:

$$
\begin{aligned}
&H_i = f(G(A_p,N))/^{*} \text{ generic function on a graph with } A_p \text{ arcs and } M\text{nodes}^{*}/\\
&H_i = \frac{\mu_p \cdot \varphi_p - 1}{A_p}/^{*} \text{ calculation of } H \text{ function, where } H_0 \text{ represents MST complexity }^{*}/\\
&MRG = Max\{H_i\}/^{*} \text{ graph with highest } H^{*}/\\
&i \in [0,1,2,\ldots R]/^{*}\text{index of } H \text{ function}^{*}/\\
&p \in [N-1,N,N+1,\ldots,N-1+R]/^{*} \text{ index for the number of graph arcs}^{*}/\\
&R \in \left[0,1,..,\frac{(N-1)\cdot(N-2)}{2}\right]/^{*} \text{ number of the skipped arcs during the MST generation}^{*}/
\end{aligned}
\tag{11.40}
$$

The R number is a key variable during the computation of the MRG. R could in fact be also null, when the computation of the MST calls for no connections to be skipped. In this case, there is no MRG for that data set.

R, moreover, makes sure that the last – and consequently the weakest – connection added to generate the MRG is always more relevant than the weakest connection of the MST. The MRG, finally, generates, starting from the MST, the graph presenting the *highest number of regular microstructures that make use of the most important connections* of the data set. The higher the value of the H function at the connections selected to generate the MRG, the more meaningful the microstructures of the MRG.

11.7.1 Maximally Regular Graph: An Example

Let us consider again the gang data set (Table 11.4) to compute its MRG (Fig. 11.17).

In this example, the H function reaches its peak when the seventh of the connections skipped during the MST generation is added back. So the MRG needs seven extra connections to be added to the MST and, consequently, the H function value is almost 50% higher with respect to its value at the original MST ($H(0) = 10.99$ vs. $H(7) = 15.38$). It is then not surprising that the structure of the two graphs turns out to be very different (Figs. 11.18 and 11.19).

The MRG carries a richer amount of information than the MST. The boundary between the two gangs, i.e., between Jets and Sharks members, is now represented no longer by a couple of subjects, but rather by a cycle of four subjects: Neal and Ken are Sharks, while Doug and Mike are Jets. So, looking at the MRG, the edges between Jets and Sharks seem apparently to be fuzzy and negotiable, and in particular less clear-cut than in the MST case. But this appearance is very misleading. In fact, the four subjects lying on the border are all outliers in their respective gangs: by placing them all on the border, this feature becomes much clearer and provides a better insight of what makes a “typical” Jet or Shark. Furthermore, Al, a member of the Jets gang, is placed at the top of an autonomous circuit of links among four Jets members, as he is the head of a new virtual gang hidden into the Jets gang. Looking at the MRG, moreover, we also receive more information about the internal structure of the two gangs: because of the bigger number of cycles, the Jets gang reveals itself as more complex and articulated that the Sharks gang. Finally, the cycle including

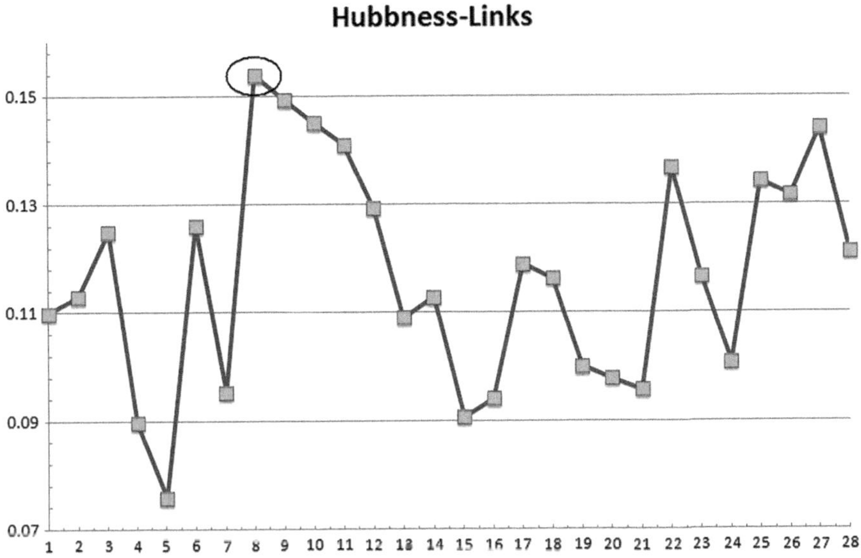

Fig. 11.17 Computing the MRG hubness of the gang data set

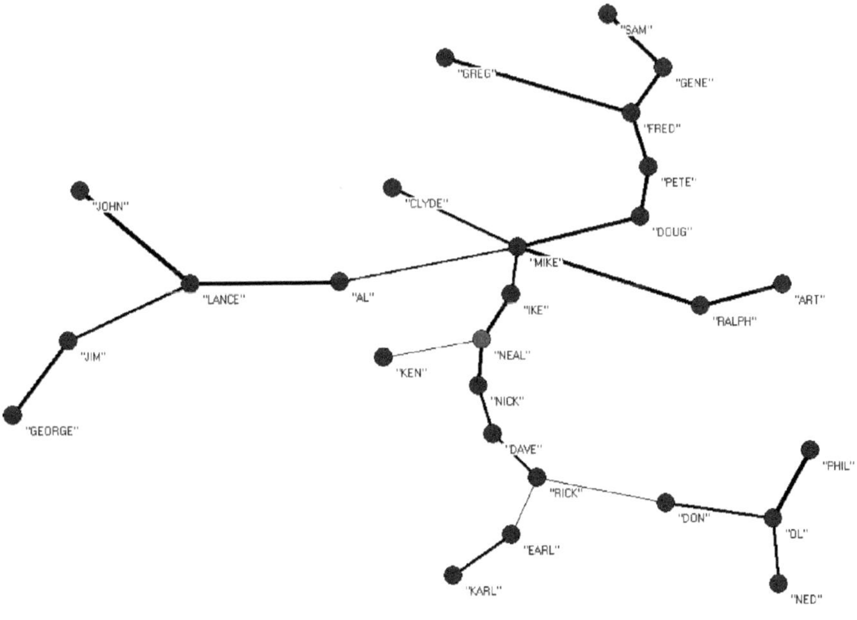

Fig. 11.18 MST of the gang data set

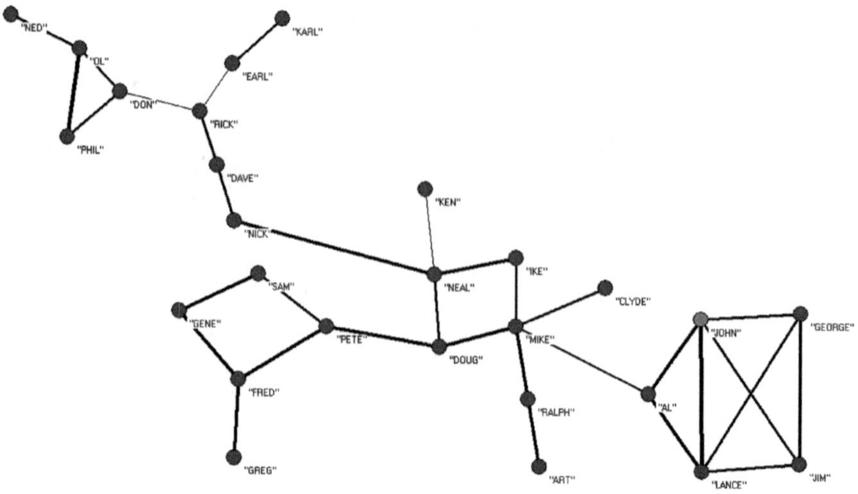

Fig. 11.19 MRG of the gang data set

Don, Ol, and Phil represents a prototype of the Sharks member, whose features are very different from Jets subjects. In the same way, Jets show two different prototypes; the first is represented by the cycle including Gene, Sam, Fred, and Pete; the second by the cycle including John, George, Lance, and Jim.

According to the MRG, the structural features of each prototype may be stated as follows:

- Prototype of gang hybridization:

$$\left[\frac{\text{Jets}}{\text{Sharks}}\right] + 30' + \left[\frac{\text{Junior school}}{\text{High school}}\right] + \text{Single} + \text{Bookie}$$

- Prototype of Sharks member:

$$30' + \text{College} + \text{Married} + \left[\frac{\text{Pusher}}{\text{Burglar}}\right]$$

- First prototype of Jets member:

$$20' + \left[\frac{\text{College}}{\text{High school}}\right] + \text{Single} + \left[\frac{\text{Bookie}}{\text{Pusher}}\right]$$

- Second prototype of Jets member:

$$20' + \text{Junior school} + \left[\frac{\text{Married}}{\text{Divorced}}\right] + \text{Burglar}$$

Compared to the MST, therefore, the MRG adds all and only those extra features that are really useful in understanding the prototypes that are hidden into the database: in other words, it adds the optimal amount of complexity that is necessary to read the phenomenon. Dropping any information from the MRG would amount to oversimplifying the representation; adding more information would amount to messing it up with irrelevant details.

11.8 Conclusions

In this chapter we have presented original new material in a variety of respects: new theoretical hypotheses, new mathematical algorithms, and new criteria to measure the complexity of the networks. In particular we have presented the following.

We have presented the math, the topology, and the algorithm of a new ANN, called *auto-contractive map* (auto-CM). The auto-CM system reshapes the distances among variables or records of any data set, considering their global vectorial similarities, and consequently drawing out the specific warped space in which such variables or records live, thereby providing a proper theoretical representation of their actual variability.

We have shown how a known filter as the *MST* can be used to cluster a distance matrix, generated from a data set, in a very useful and effective way. In particular, we have shown how the MST can be regarded as the minimal representation that takes into account the basic level of information below which the structure of the independence among variables loses its coherence.

We have presented a new index, called *H function*, to evaluate the topological complexity of any kind of graph, and we have shown its mathematical consistency and provided hints about its applications.

We have furthermore created, starting from the *H* function, a new index to measure the relevance and the contribution of any node within a semantic graph (a graph generated by a data set). We have named this new index *delta H function*.

Finally, we have defined a new type of semantic graph, using the *H* function, and named it *maximally regular graph* (MRG). From an MST, generated from any metric, the MRG reshapes the links among nodes in order to maximize the fundamental and the most regular structures implicated in any data set.

We are aware that this new approach, although very promising, leaves many questions open and needs further scrutiny to investigate its properties and potential shortcomings. In forthcoming research, we plan to develop it from both the theoretical and the empirical sides, by better exploring and characterizing the structural features of the auto-CM and the mathematical properties of the *H* and delta *H* functions, and of the MRG. On the empirical side, we plan to apply this methodology to state-of-the art problems that are relevant in specific disciplinary literatures. It is of course of particular interest to evaluate how our approach performs against traditional methods in the analysis of networks, be them of a physical or social nature. We look forward to this exciting prospect.

Bibliography

Contractive Maps

Arcidiacono, G. (1984). The De Sitter universe and projective relativity. In V. De Sabbata and T. M. Karade (Eds.), *Relativistic astrophisies and cosmology* (pp. 64–88). Singapore: World Scientific.

Arcidiacono, G. (1986). *Projective relativity, cosmology and gravitation*. Cambridge, USA: Hadronic Press.

Beckman, B. (2006). Special relativity with geometry expression. *J Symbolic Geometry* 1, 51–56.

Buscema, M. (2006). *Sistemi ACM e imaging diagnostico. Le immagini mediche come matrici attive di connessioni*. Italia, Milano: Springer-Verlag. [ACM Systems and Diagnostic Imaging. Medical Images as Active Connections Matrixes].

Buscema, M. (1994). Self-reflexive networks. Theory, topology, applications. *Quality & Quantity*, n.29 (pp. 339–403). Dordrecht, The Netherlands: Kluwer Academic Publishers.

Buscema, M., Didoné, D., and Pandin, M. (1994). Reti Neurali AutoRiflessive, Teoria, Metodi, Applicazioni e Confronti. *Quaderni di Ricerca*, Armando Editore, n.1. [Self-Reflexive Networks: Theory, Methods, Applications and Comparison, Semeion Research-book by Armando Publisher, Rome, n.1].

Davies, P. (1989). *The cosmic blueprint*. New York: Simon and Schuster.

Fantappiè, L. (1954). *Su una Nuova Teoria di Relatività Finale*, Rend. Accademia dei Lincei, Rome, November, 1954. [On a New Theory of Final Relativity].

Fantappiè, L. (1991). *Principi di una Teoria Unitaria del Mondo Fisico e Biologico*, (1944, original), Di Rienzo, Rome, 1991. [Principles for an Unified Theory of the Physical and Biological World].

Flandern, T. van. (2003). Lorentz contraction. *Apeiron* 10(4), 152–158, October.

Hawking. S. W. and Hartle, J. B. (1983). Wave function of the universe. *Phys. Rev. D* XXVIII, 2960.

Licata, I. (1991). Minkowski's space-time and Dirac's vacuum as ultrareferential fundamental reference frame. *Hadronic J.* 14, 225–250.

Pardy, M. (1997). Cerenkov effect and the Lorentz contraction. *Phys. Rev. A* 55(3), 1647–1652, March.

MST, Graphs, and Physical Networks

Barabasi, A-L. (2007). Network medicine – from obesity to the "diseasome". *N Engl J Med* 357, 4 July 26.

Bratislava, P. K. (2000). Graphs with same peripherical and center eccentric vertices. *Mathematica Bohemica* 3, 331–339, 125.

Costa, L. da F., Rodriguez, F. A., Travieso, G., and Villas Boas, P. R. (2006). *Characterization of complex networks. A survey of measurements*. Istituto de Fisica de Sao Carlos, Universidade de Sao Paulo, May 17.

Cormen, T. H., Leiserson, C. E., Rivest, R. L., and Stein, C. (2001). *Introduction to algorithms*. MIT Press and McGraw-Hill (pp. 567–574). 2nd edition. ISBN 0-262-03293-7. Section 23.2: The algorithms of Kruskal and Prim.

Fredman, M. L. and Willard, D. E. (1990). *Trans-dichotomous algorithms for minimum spanning trees and shortest paths* (pp. 719–725). 31st IEEE Symp. Foundations of Comp. Sci.

Gabow, H. N., Galil, Z., Spencer, T., and Tarjan, R. E. (1986). Efficient algorithms for finding minimum spanning trees in undirected and directed graphs. *Combinatorica* 6, 109–122.

Goodrich, M. T. and Tamassia, R. (2006). *Data structures and algorithms in Java* (p. 632). John Wiley & Sons Inc. 4th Edition. ISBN 0-471-73884-0. Section 13.7.1: Kruskal's Algorithm.
Karger, D. R., Klein, P. N., and Tarjan, R. E. (1995). A randomized linear-time algorithm to find minimum spanning trees. *J. ACM.* 42, 321–328.
Kruskal. J. B. (1956). On the shortest spanning subtree of a graph and the traveling salesman problem. *Proc. Am. Math. Soc.* 7(1) (Feb), 48–50.
Reka Zsuzsanna, A. (2001). *Statistical mechanics of complex networks*. Dissertation, Department of Physics, Notre Dame Un, Indiana.

Theory of Probability and Bayesian Networks

Berger, J. O. (1985). *Statistical decision theory and Bayesian analysis*. Springer-Verlag. 2nd edition. ISBN 0-387-96098-8.
Berger, J. O. and Strawderman, W. E. (1996). Choice of hierarchical priors: admissibility in estimation of normal means. *Ann. Stat.* 24, 931–995.
Bernardo, J. M. (1979). Reference posterior distributions for Bayesian inference. *J. Royal Stat. Soc.* Series B 41, 113–147.
Gelman, A., Carlin, J. B., Stern, H. S., and Rubin, D. B. (2003). *Bayesian data analysis*. CRC Press. 2nd edition. . ISBN 1-58488-388-X.
Jaynes, E. T. (1968). "Prior probabilities". IEEE transactions on systems science and cybernetics. SSC-4, 227–241, Sept. Reprinted In Roger D. Rosenkrantz, Compiler, E. T. Jaynes: Papers on Probability, Statistics and Statistical Physics. Dordrecht, Holland: Reidel Publishing Company, (pp. 116–130), 1983. ISBN 90-277-1448-7.

Euclidean Distance

Abdi, H. (1990). Additive-tree representations. Lecture Notes in Biomathematics, 84, 43–59.
Abdi, H. (2003). Multivariate analysis. In M. Lewis-Beck, A. Bryman, and T. Futing (Eds.), *Encyclopedia for research methods for the social sciences*. Thousand Oaks: Sage.
Abdi, H. (2007). Distance. In N. J. Salkind (Ed.), *Encyclopedia of measurement*.
Greenacre, M. J. (1984). *Theory and applications of correspondence analysis*. London: Academic Press.
Rao, C. R. (1995). Use of Hellinger distance in graphical displays. In E.-M. Tiit, T. Kollo, and H. Niemi (Ed.), *Multivariate statistics and matrices in statistics* (pp. 143–161). Leiden, The Netherlands: Brill Academic Publisher.

Back-Propagation Networks

AA.VV. (1991). *Advanced in neural information processing*. (Vol. 3). San Mateo, CA: Morgan Kaufman.
Anderson, J. A. and Rosenfeld, E. (Eds.) (1988). *Neurocomputing foundations of research*. Cambridge, Massachusetts, London, England: The MIT Press.
Bridle, J. S. (1989). Probabilistic interpretation of feed forward classification network outputs, with relationships to statistical pattern recognition. In F. Fogelman-Soulié and J. Hérault (Eds.), *Neuro-computing: Algorithms, architectures* (pp. 227–236). New York: Springer-Verlag.

Buscema, M. and Massini, G. (1993). *Il Modello MQ*. Armando, Rome: Collana Semeion. [The MQ Model: Neural Networks and Interpersonal Perception, Semeion Collection by Armando Publisher].

Buscema, M. (1994). *Squashing theory. Modello a Reti Neurali per la Previsione dei Sistemi Complessi*, Collana Semeion, Rome: Armando. [Squashing Theory: A Neural Network Model for Prediction of Complex Systems, Semeion Collection by Armando Publisher].

Buscema, M., Matera, F., Nocentini, T., and Sacco, P. L. (1997). Reti Neurali e Finanza. Esercizi, Idee, Metodi, Applicazioni. *Quaderni di Ricerca*, Rome: Armando. n. 2 [Neural networks and finance. Exercises, ideas, methods, applications, semeion research-book by Armando Publisher, n.2].

Chauvin, Y. and Rumelhart, D. E. (Eds.) (1995). *Backpropagation: Theory, architectures, and applications*. Hillsdale, New Jersey: Lawrence Erlbaum Associates, Inc. Publishers, 365 Brodway.

Fahlman, S. E. (1988). An empirical study of learning speed in back-propagation networks. CMV Technical Report, CMV-CS-88-162.

Freeman, J. A. and Skapura, D. M. (1991). *Neural networks, algorithms, application and programming techniques*. Addison Wesley, CNV Series.

Gorman, R. and Sejnowski, T. J. (1988). Analysis of hidden units in layered networks trained to classify sonar targets. *Neural Networks* 1, 76–90.

Jacobs, R. A. (1988). Increased rates of convergence through learning rate adaptation. *Neural Network* 1, 295–307.

Lapedes, A. and Farber, R. (1987). Nonlinear Signal Processing Using Neural Networks: Prediction and System Modeling, Los Alamos National Laboratory Report LA-UR-87-2662.

Liu, Q., Hirono, S., and Moriguchi, I. (1992). Application of functional-link net in QSAR. 1. QSAR for activity data given by continuous variate. *Quant. Struct. -Act. Relat. //* 135–141, School of Pharmaceutical Sciences, Kitasato University, Shirokane, Minato-ku, Tokyo 108, Japan.

Liu, Q., Hirono, S., and Moriguchi, I. (1992). Application of functional-link net in QSAR. 2. QUSAR for Activity Data Given by Continuous Variate. *Quant. Struct. -Act. Relat. //* 318–324, School of Pharmaceutical Sciences, Kitasato University, Shirokane, Minato-ku, Tokyo 108, Japan.

McClelland, J. L. and Rumelhart, D. E., (1988). *Explorations in parallel distributed processing*. Cambridge MA: The MIT Press.

Metzger, Y and Lehmann, D. (1990). Learning Temporal Sequence by Local Synaptic Changes. *Network 1*, 169–188.

Minai, A. A. and Williams, R. D. (1990). Acceleration of Backpropagation Through Learning Rate and Momentum Adaptation, International Joint Conference on Neural Networks, vol. 1, January, 676–679.

Minsky, M. (1954). *Neural nets and the brain-model problem*. Doctoral Dissertation, Princeton University.

Minsky, M and Papert, S. (1988). *Perceptrons*. Cambridge MA: MIT Press. (Expanded edition 1988).

Mulsant, B. H. (1990). A neural network as an approach to clinical diagnosis. *Neural Modeling* 7(1), 25–36.

McCord Nelson, M. and Illingworth, W. T. (1991). *A practical guide to neural network*. New York: Addison Wesley.

NeuralWare.(1993). *Neural computing*. Pittsburgh, PA: NeuralWare Inc.

NeuralWare (1995). *Neural computing*. Pittsburgh, PA: NeuralWare Inc.

Rosenblatt, F. (1962). *Principles of neurodynamics*. New York: Spartan.

Rumelhart, D. E and McClelland, J. L. (Eds.) (1986). *Parallel distributed processing, Vol. 1 foundations, explorations in the microstructure of cognition, Vol. 2 psychological and biological models*. Cambridge MA, London: The MIT Press, England..

Rumelhart, D. E., Hinton, G. E., and Williams, R. J. (1986). Learning internal representations by error propagation. In Rumelhart D. E. and McClelland J. L. (eds.), *Parallel distributed processing* (Vol. 1, Appendix 2), Cambridge, MA: MIT Press.

Rumelhart, D. E., Hinton, G. E., and Williams, R. J. (1988). Learning internal representations by back propagating errors, *Nature* 323, 533–536. In Anderson (1988).
Samad, T. (1988). Back-propagation is significantly. *International Neural Network Society Conference Abstracts*.
Samad, T (1989). *Back-propagation extension*. Honeywell SSDC Technical Report, 1000 Bane Ave, N., Golden Valley, NN 55427, 1989.
Smith, M. (1993). *Neural networks for statistical modeling*. New York: Van Nostrand Reihnold.
Tawel, R. (1989). Does neuron learn like the synapse? In Touretzky D. S (ed). *Neural information processing systems (NIPS) 1988*, 169–176, SanMateo, CA, Morgan Kaufmann.
Touretzky, D. S (Ed.) (1989). *Advances in neural information processing systems*. (Vol. 1). San Mateo CA: Morgan Kaufman.
Touretzky, D. S (Ed.) (1990). *Advances in neural information processing systems*. (Vol. 2). San Mateo CA: Morgan Kaufman.
Touretzky, D. S (Ed.) (1990). *Connectionist models*. Proceedings of the 1990 Summer School, San Mateo CA: Morgan Kaufman.
Touretzky, D.S., Elman, J. L., Sejnowski, T. J., and Hinton, G. E. (1990). *Connectionist models*. Proceedings of the 1990 Summer School. San Mateo CA: Morgan Kaufmann.
Weigend, A. S., Rumelhart, D. E., and Huberman, B. A. (1991). Back-propagation, weight-elimination and time series prediction. *AA.VV*, 857–882.
Werbos, P. (1974). *Beyond regression: new tools for prediction and analysis in behavioral sciences*. Phd Thesis, Cambridge MA: Harvard.
Widrow, B. and Steams, S. D. (1985). *Adaptive signal processing*. Signal Processing Series. Englewood Cliffs, NJ: Prentice-Hall.

Research Software

Buscema (2002): M Buscema, Contractive Maps, Ver 1.0, Semeion Software #15, Rome, 2000–2002.
Buscema (2007): M Buscema, Constraints Satisfaction Networks, Ver 10.0, Semeion Software #14, Rome, 2001–2007.
Buscema (2008): M Buscema, MST, Ver 5.0, Semeion Software #38, Rome, 2006–2008.
Massini (2007a): G Massini, Trees Visualizer, Ver 3.0, Semeion Software #40, Rome, 2007.
Massini (2007b): G Massini, Semantic Connection Map, Ver 1.0, Semeion Software #45, Rome, 2007.

Chapter 12
An Artificial Intelligent Systems Approach to Unscrambling Power Networks in Italy's Business Environment

Massimo Buscema and Pier L. Sacco

Abstract The role of interlocking directorates in the creation and maintenance of business power elites in the United States and elsewhere, and more generally their role in the corporate governance structures of mature capitalist economies, is a widely researched and debated subject. Results on this matter would be likely to carry substantial implications in a variety of fields, from industrial organization to policy, from corporate finance to governance itself. But in spite of a massive and long-lasting research effort, the literature so far yielded relatively controversial results over the majority of the issues at stake. The starting point of our work is the hypothesis that the impasse is due to the fact that so far researchers have looked at the wrong pieces of evidence, i.e. direct relational links among people sitting in specific boards. Corporate elites are connected in much more complex ways, and power networks depend much more on members' degrees of embeddedness in the *whole* network than on the *local* structure of board affiliations. We therefore develop an alternative approach, that we call the reverse approach, which *derives* interlock structures starting from actual affiliation data but exploring hidden relationships between members and constructing an alternative network representing *fundamental* rather than *apparent* interlocks, i.e. the real nature of the connection among corporations on the basis of the level of embeddedness of their board members. To construct this alternative, more fundamental network structure, we make use of AutoCM artificial neural networks (ANNs) (see Buscema and Sacco, Chapter 11, this volume) and explain how they can be used to develop an alternative kind of network analysis that may deliver more conclusive evidence about interlock causes, characteristics and dynamics, while at the same time avoiding the main pitfalls pointed out by the institutionalist criticism of traditional approaches.

M. Buscema (✉)
Semeion Research Center, Via Sersale, Rome, Italy
e-mail: m.buscema@semeion.it

V. Capecchi (eds.), *Applications of Mathematics in Models, Artificial Neural Networks and Arts*, DOI 10.1007/978-90-481-8581-8_12,

12.1 Introduction

The role of interlocking directorates in the creation and maintenance of business power elites in the United States and elsewhere, and more generally their role in the corporate governance structures of mature capitalist economies, is a widely researched and debated subject. Results on this matter would be likely to carry substantial implications in a variety of fields, from industrial organization to policy, from corporate finance to governance itself. But in spite of a massive and long-lasting research effort, the literature so far yielded relatively controversial results over the majority of the issues at stake.

There are of course conflicting explanations about the reasons for this impasse. Not only there is a sharp contraposition between scholars who believe that the research produced so far makes sense and others who reject it altogether, but also within the field of the supporters, there are different parties maintaining rival explanations for the same phenomena in the absence of conclusive evidence on either side. Mark Mizruchi (1996), a much distinguished contributor to this literature, sorts out no less than six different possible reasons explaining interlocks. The existing schools of thought contributing to the literature differ as to the relative importance they attribute to such reasons. However, the basic controversy has to do with whether one accepts or not the idea that certain economic and social factors drive the emergence of interlocks without specific reference to the historical, cultural and institutional context. The institutionalist critique of this literature maintains that existing analyses are fundamentally flawed by this theoretical fallacy and that the varieties of existing forms of capitalism bring about quite different results in terms of causes, structure and dynamics of interlocks, also starting from relatively similar economic and social fundamentals.

The current status quo provides some ground for both positions, and there seems to be little margin for reaching a wide consensus. The available evidence looks too mixed and complex to allow clear-cut conclusions. The starting point of our work is the hypothesis that the impasse is due to the fact that so far researchers have looked at the wrong pieces of evidence, i.e. direct relational links among people sitting in specific boards. Corporate elites are connected in much more complex ways, and power networks depend much more on members' degrees of embeddedness in the *whole* network than on the *local* structure of board affiliations. We therefore develop an alternative approach, that we call the reverse approach, which *derives* interlock structures starting from actual affiliation data but exploring hidden relationships between members and constructing an alternative network representing *fundamental* rather than *apparent* interlocks, i.e. the real nature of the connection among corporations on the basis of the level of embeddedness of their board members. To construct this alternative, more fundamental network structure, we make use of AutoCM artificial neural networks (ANNs) (see Buscema and Sacco, this volume) and explain how they can be used to develop an alternative kind of network analysis that may deliver more conclusive evidence about interlock causes, characteristics and dynamics, while at the same time avoiding the main pitfalls pointed out by the institutionalist criticism of traditional approaches. We therefore apply this methodology to the analysis of interlocks in the Italian business environment and find its hidden power network structure, which is totally unintelligible from the analysis of apparent connections among businesses. We moreover show how such network adapts dynamically to incoming news and events. Although our methodology calls for further scrutiny and for deeper empirical analysis before it can be regarded as a viable alternative to more traditional approaches to the explanation and analysis of interlocks, we feel that it may be regarded as a promising first step.

The structure of the rest of the chapter is as follows. In Section 12.2, we provide a concise review of the most relevant literature on interlocks. In Section 12.3, we discuss its basic shortcomings and argue about our proposed alternative, the so-called reverse approach. Section 12.4 briefly reviews the basic methodology of AutoCM ANNs and their implications in the present context. Section 12.5 presents the database and the basic results, namely the hidden interlock structure for the Italian case. Section 12.6 provides some interpretations and discussions of the results. Section 12.7 concludes.

12.2 Interlocking Directorates: A Tentative (Partial) Chronology of the Literature

The issue of interlocking directorates has been extensively addressed in the sociological literature of the past decades. Its origin can be found in the long-lasting querelle on the role of interest groups in corporate governance, which finds its classical topoi in Mills (1956) and Galbraith (1971). As Dooley (1969) points out in his seminal paper, the practice of interlocking directorates has a long tradition (see, e.g., Roy, 1983 for a historical account of its dynamics in early 20th-century US, and Mizruchi, 1982 for its later developments; see also Pennings 1980) and is relatively robust against attempts at reform. Pfeffer (1972) points out that the size and the composition of the US boards are modelled by an optimal adaptation to (i.e. by an optimal cooptation of) the business environment, and therefore if interlocks are a systematic feature of the current practice, they must have an economic rationale and will persist over time (see also Pfeffer and Salancik, 2003 for an up-to-date formulation). Allen (1974) elaborates on the point by observing that interlocks amount to a cooperative strategy among firms that try to keep business environment uncertainty under control, and in fact the nature of the interlocks reflects the firm's market focus (i.e. local firms tend to participate in local interlocks), although a general trend towards more far-reaching interlock structures can be extrapolated. Useem (1979) draws attention on the inner group of American business elite members that sit in several major company boards and on the positive feedback dynamics that implies that their identification with multiple interests makes them more palatable candidates to sit in public and non-profit institutional boards than peers that are strictly linked to a specific corporate entity. The nature of the inner group corporate and non-corporate relationships assigns to its members a key role in the advocacy and promotion of the interests of the overall business elite. Useem and Mccormack

(1981) find similar results for the inner group of the British business elite. Clawson and Neustadtl (1989) find that the interlocked American business elite tends to adopt politically conservative attitudes that are felt to better defend their class interests. More systematic results in this vein are found in Mizruchi (1989, 1990).

Whereas this early body of literature seems to converge on a somewhat functional view of the role of interlocking directorates in ensuring the business environment's overall stability, the pathbreaking paper by Mintz and Schwartz (1981) and their subsequent book (Mintz and Schwartz 1985) argue that the logic of interlocking in the United States does not obey system-wide functional imperatives but is rather shaped by the power and centrality of a dominant, finance-based interest group. On the other hand, building on earlier graph-theoretic contributions such as Sonquist and Koenig (1975), Burt (1979, 1980, 1983) and Burt et al. (1980) proposes a structural theory of interlocking directorate formation according to which interlocks are created in economic sectors where profitability is threatened and tend to develop towards those sectors that constrain or impede it. In fact, successful interlocking in such contexts proves to be substantially rewarding in terms of profitability and is a distinctive, specific component of the interest group's wider strategy of cooptive relationality. This thesis is strengthened by the results of Koenig et al. (1979), who find that the maintenance of interlock ties is controlled by personal acquaintance and belonging to the inner circle rather than by corporate affiliation. Koenig and Gogel (1981) go on to develop a business elite-focused class hegemony theory that challenges the by then conventional wisdom of management control theory. Moving from the results of Koenig et al. (1979), Palmer (1983) develops a more comprehensive view of the relational structure that underlies interlock ties and finds that the empirical evidence only partially supports their role as formal coordination devices and therefore questions the claim that they can be regarded as the backbone of the power structure of the US business environment. On the other hand, in his analysis of the Canadian post-war business environment, Ornstein (1984) finds support for the relevance of interlock ties both from the inter-corporate and from the power elite perspectives, arguing that their relative relevance depends on specific cases. More specifically, Galaskiewicz et al. (1985), working on a US metropolitan area case study, argue that it is the *interaction* of individual and corporate dimensions that predicts the development of interlock ties. Palmer et al. (1986) provide particularly sharp results, showing that the effective channels for interlocking maintenance are basically two: interindustry coordination between financial and nonfinancial firms, and common belonging of business elite members to the same *local* class segment. Stearns and Mizruchi (1986), however, question the validity of the previous literature in that it focuses on the analysis of interlock maintenance in terms of likelihood of reconstitution of broken ties between given couple of firms, whereas, they argue, the essential aspect is the maintenance of functional ties between a given firm and other firms operating in a given strategically complementary sector, and not between that firm and a specific firm of the complementary sector. They argue that factors that warrant the maintenance of functional ties are independent or even negatively correlated with the ones that warrant direct reconstruction of broken ties. These results, according to the authors, make a strong case for the organizational explanation of interlock structure and dynamics. Richardson (1987) goes on with the analysis of direct reconstruction of broken ties on a Canadian database, finding that such kinds of ties are the only ones meaningfully related to corporate profitability. Financial control-motivated and cooptive interlocks are found irrelevant for corporate profitability, whereas the other way round makes sense: financial control- and cooptation-based interlocks are more easily found when a given corporation is profitable. On the other hand, Mizruchi and Stearns (1988) find that the cooptation of finance-related directors in industrial boards becomes more likely during phases of business cycle downturns, when corporate profitability is under pressure. An alternative approach is proposed by Zajac (1988), who treats interlocks formation from the viewpoint of business elite members who are regarded as optimizing self-interested agents. Stokman et al. (1988) provide evidence from a Dutch database that somewhat supports Zajac's approach in that it shows that cooptation of business elite members is basically determined by individual characteristics.

Overall, the results of this first wave of research have been mixed and somewhat inconclusive. Mizruchi (1996) carries out a systematic review of the literature and addresses the basic criticisms that are mounting against it, restating its relevance and meaningfulness while admitting that initial enthusiasm was probably overstated and that new methodological approaches, integrating personal narratives with hard data, are called for to settle the open issues. New impulse to the literature arrives from works that propose somewhat fresh approaches such as those of Palmer et al. (1995), Geletkanycz and Hambrick (1997), Uzzi (1996, 1997), Kono et al. (1998), Haunschild (1993), and Haunschild and Beckman (1998). Geletkanycz and Hambrick work on industry multilayered databases and find new arguments for the existence of interlocking directorates as part of an interorganizational strategy of coordination and uncertainty reduction. Uzzi advocates the Granovetter (1985) embeddedness notion to argue that embedded networking may ensure firms a definite competitive advantage, at least under a certain critical threshold of networking (beyond which the network becomes too self-referential to react optimally to external shocks). Palmer et al. also make reference to the embeddedness perspective to evaluate the relative role of ownership structures vs. social ties in determining predatory vs. friendly acquisition in the United States during the 1960s and find that, although social relationship factors are important, economic factors have been dominant. Kono et al. argue that interlocks must be seen as spatially situated phenomena and therefore differ markedly according to their local vs. non-local nature; moreover, the structure of interlocks itself depends heavily on the spatial attributes of corporate assets such as headquarter location in the national geography of corporate headquarters, the location of the firm's factories and plants, and the spatial distribution of the firm's shareholder participations. Haunschild suggests that directors tend to imitate the acquisition strategies of the companies on whose boards they sit, and therefore interlocks favour waves of acquisition. Haunschild and Beckman test the informational value of interlocks by evaluating the effect that the availability of alternative informational channels produces on the relationship between interlocks and corporate acquisitions, finding substantial support for the informational role of interlocks and therefore making a further case for the interorganizational approach.

In his comment to the Palmer et al. paper, however, Fligstein (1995) makes a radical case against the meaningfulness and explanatory power of the network approach altogether, and of the literature on interlocking directorates in particular, arguing in favour of an institutionalist approach that focuses on the historical, legal and cultural determinants of specific business environments, which differ widely across time and space (his approach is systematically presented and discussed in Fligstein, 1996).

In spite of this criticism, and partly also thanks to it, the new wave of research on corporate interlocks has spurred inquiry in several new, promising directions and has encouraged more context-sensitive theoretical approaches. Palmer and Barber (2001) emphasize how the strategy of corporate acquisitions may reflect the quest for social status and the recognition of well-networked but under-reputed challengers. This explanation of acquisition dynamics finds support in the data against more traditional ones such as resource dependence, institutional pressure or agency problems. Beckman and Haunschild (2002) show that the performance of corporate acquisition depends on the presence of tied partners with heterogeneous experience, and performance is further increased by multiplex relationships with tied partners (see, e.g., Wasserman and Faust 1994), thus making a case for ties as channels of networked learning. In a somewhat complementary way, Carpenter and Westphal (2001) in turn suggest that although the extent of interlocking per se does not imply effective support of strategic decision making by a given corporate board, those interlocks that provide significant knowledge inputs actually do. Westphal and Frederickson (2001) go further to suggest that the informational and experience linkages that characterize a given corporate board can promote substantial strategic change and that the extent of such effect can even be masked by the greater visibility of executive decision making. In fact, new CEOs tend to be chosen by virtue of their familiarity with the strategies that characterize the board members' home companies. Although the link between relational ties and information dynamics clearly emerges in some of the studies just cited above, the logic of cooptation displays an overall complexity that challenges simple explanations; for instance, on the one side, experience heterogeneity matters for certain reasons, whereas experience homogeneity matters for other reasons, and conclusions are hardly extendable beyond the database under scrutiny. Beckman et al. (2004) put forward a new attempt at a general theory by arguing that choice of alliance and interlock partners, and in particular choice between network expansion and stabilization, rests on a trade-off between different forms of uncertainty: firm specific vs. market level.

Research in the latest years has progressively expanded from analysis of the causes and consequences of interlock ties to increasingly refined typologies of ties, and social network structures. Results, however, remain somewhat inconclusive and a great deal of caution and attention has to be devoted to isolate logically and empirically the various concurring effects. One of the latest examples of this state of things is the results obtained by Mizruchi et al. (2008) as they find that neither bonus achievement among commercial bankers is clearly associated with one's social network density nor tie strength produces similar effects in networks serving different functional tasks: an analytically accurate statement, but also an admission of the problematic nature of the relationship between social ties and actor performance as it has been framed by the research conducted so far. Although the literature is clearly dealing with important and relevant topics, its accomplishments do not seem to match the enormous amount of research effort poured into it and the overwhelming amount of processed data.

12.3 Context Matters: Dealing with Complexity Through the "Reverse Approach"

The sceptical remarks of Fligstein about the meaningfulness of interlock research and his call for a deeply rooted institutional analysis of the different business environments, recently restated in Fligstein and Choo (2005), seem to find some legitimation in the relative inconclusiveness of such literature. Analysis of specific cases outside the familiar North American environments, such as Kogut and Walker (2001) for Germany, shows that, in such contexts, the small world properties of the inner circle of the business elite reveal a resilience against outside perturbations that seems to stem from specific cultural conditions. Fligstein and Merand (2002) explicitly analyze the impact of EU market integration on the economic globalization trends and the self-referential effect that they have brought about on the development of European economies. The EU market paradigm seems to be the expression of a different notion of a post-industrial market economy rather than the US one. In the former, the state still plays an outstanding role and careful economic regulation remains the rule. In the latter, as noted, e.g., by Mizruchi (2007), we witness an increasing fragmentation of isolated, self-concerned corporate interests in the absence of real external disciplining forces. The over-regulated EU model therefore presents radical differences with respect to the possibly under-regulated US one, and such differences arise from basically different notions of what is, or should be, a market economy, as maintained by Orr (1997a). The comparative analysis of Scott (1987, 1991) further stresses the differences between the United States, the east Asian and European contexts with respect to the causes and structures of corporate power networks; on the peculiarities of the east Asian case, see also Zang (2001). Biggart and Beamish (2003) make a formidable attempt at the synthesis of the different theoretical traditions and approaches on the two sides of the Atlantic, comparing the network theory approach of North American research with the sociology of conventions approach typical of the European literature, and call for a theoretical synthesis that combines the advantages of both in an expanded institutional approach.

The proposal of Biggart and Beamish casts a different light on our reconstruction of the debate of interlocking directorates in that it provides a possible explanation of the limitations of a theoretical perspective too much focused on the meso-analytic level of social networking and therefore biased by its lack of concern for contextual factors of a cultural, historical, institutional nature. On the other hand, dismissing the possibility of a social network analysis altogether would be an equally biased choice, as it is clearly the case from the literature results that social ties in general, and interlocks in particular, do matter, although in a very complex way.

An ideal test bed for this encompassing perspective would in principle be the Italian case. Like Germany, Italy is characterized by a distinctive and highly idiosyncratic form of capitalism that is centred on family connections (see, e.g., Orr 1997b). In the Italian case, then, the primary source of interlocks is evident and not at all mysterious: They reflect (extended) family ties, within a complex social exchange network where different entrepreneurial or shareholder families make alliances, posit reciprocal vetoes, and so on. On the other hand, also in Italy the story is not as simple as that. Time and space conditions may make a lot of difference. For instance, parts of the country that are characterized by a long-lasting tradition of large corporations express a corporate culture that is quite different from those that are characterized by most recent small- and medium-size firm-based economic development. Also, different generations of the corporate elite manifest different propensities to stabilize or widen their relational networks, as a response to various cultural or economic conditions and even contingencies. The literature on interlock ties in the Italian context is small and heterogeneous. Early examples are Chiesi (1982), Brioschi et al. (1990), Bianco and Pagnoni (1997), Ferri and Trento (1997), Corrado (2000), whereas more recent ones are Brunello et al. (2003), Murgia (2006) and Farina (2007). A thorough historical account of the early 20th-century phase can be found in Vasta and Baccini (1997). The Italian scholarly evidence on the extent and relevance of interlocking practices is partial, but there seem to be substantial enough favourable clues (see, e.g., Murgia, 2006), especially in those sectors of the economy where large corporations play a leading role. In the absence of a body of literature that can be compared in size and depth of analysis to the one developed around the North American cases, however, and even on the basis of such strong theoretical presumptions on the peculiarities of Italian corporate networks, it is hard to make sharp statements about the structure and dynamics of interlocks in the Italian context, and it is far from unlikely that even in the presence of an equally ample body of evidence, its analytical interpretation would still be partly inconclusive at best. For this reason, in this chapter we develop what we could call a *reverse*approach to the issue, taking the Italian case as an acid test, with a view of generalizing it subsequently to other European cases, as well as to North American and east Asian ones.

The basic motivation behind our reverse approach is the following. We argue that if so far the large, empirically based analytical research on interlocking directorates has delivered somewhat disappointing results, this may have to do with some basic methodological flaw. We maintain that such a flaw may be the excess of emphasis that has been given so far to interlocks based on direct relational links, i.e. on the structure of *visible* connections between specific corporate boards. The inconclusive evidence might be the consequence of the fact that such relational structure fails to capture the real, inherent structure of corporate power networks, whose accurate tracing calls for more sophisticated analytical tools rather than state-of-the-art social network theory. What is missing from the current theoretical framework is the idea that what is more relevant in defining business power networks is not who actually talks to whom in which board but rather what are the companies that share the same *relational patterns* across boards. In other words, it is not the geography of affiliation per se which is important but rather the level of embeddedness in the *whole* (i.e. global) network. By focusing on affiliation, previous analyses have therefore introduced a possibly serious bias that might be responsible for the inconclusiveness of the research conducted so far.

Focusing on the Italian case as an acid test seems to be a promising starting point in that the relatively small size of the business community (if compared to the US one) and the weight of family-oriented corporate governance strategies might suggest that interlocking patterns should be especially visible even using traditional techniques. If such techniques fail to single out a clear-cut structure even in these conditions, and if on the contrary it can be cut out neatly using alternative techniques, then there is room to maintain that a new theoretical approach is called for and that the successful techniques could be a good starting ground to build it. This is exactly what we will try to demonstrate in the current chapter.

We will proceed as follows. In the first place, one should ask why should we speak of a "reverse" approach. The reason is simple and intuitive: whereas in the traditional approach one takes for granted the definition of what interlocks are (e.g. common affiliation of two or more persons to one or more boards) and explores to what extent they are correlated with relevant economic and social variables, in the reverse approach we *derive and identify* a certain interlock pattern (if any) from data on boards affiliation only, and then infer from its characteristics its nature, causes and implications, to be checked through interpretation and analysis of available economic and social data. In the reverse approach, therefore, we do not try to apply a given, standardized notion of interlock to widely differing business environments, forcing them all into the same relational logic. This is the basic criticism addressed to the traditional approach by institutionalist scholars and is invoked to dismiss the overall relevance of interlock research. Rather, we find out a certain interlock pattern that in some cases may be deeply related to actual common affiliation to the same boards, but in other cases may relate corporations that basically share very little or no affiliation to their boards, while displaying similar patterns of embeddedness in that particular power network that makes them part of a common elite. Therefore, the definition of what an interlock *literally* is is strongly dependent on the institutional context. What becomes relevant is, instead, a *substantialist* definition of interlocks as common belonging to a cohesive and coherent subgroup that spans and controls the whole network. The reverse approach entirely addresses the criticisms of the institutionalist scholars by making the *formal* structure of interlocks entirely context dependent, while at the same time pointing out that in every given context an idiosyncratic form of interlock-based power elite may emerge and rule.

To develop our reverse approach, we need new and different analytical tools with respect to those commonly employed in social network analysis. Whereas the latter explores the structure and regularities of *observable* social links, we need tools that are able to extract regularities based on non-observable (i.e. hidden) social links, by analyzing the complex, non-linear pattern of co-variation among the set of variables that characterize the sample population. In particular, we will make use of an innovative kind of artificial neural networks (ANNs) called AutoCM (see Buscema and Sacco, this volume) and will use them to construct a new type of graph-theoretic representation of social networks that deals with the hidden, rather than directly observable, social relationships among players. We will show that, in the case of the Italian business network, whereas the analysis of the structure of direct relational links reveals very little or no evidence of an embedded power elite, the analysis of the structure of hidden links provides neatly shaped evidence in this respect. Moreover, the structure of this power elite changes in reasonable and traceable ways as incoming news and events introduce novel elements into the picture.

12.4 AutoCM: A New Methodological Foundation for "Fundamental" Network Analysis

A comprehensive introduction to AutoCM structure and properties is provided in Chapter 11 (Buscema and Sacco, this volume). Therefore, in this section we simply and briefly discuss the proprieties of AutoCM that are relevant for our purposes, referring the reader to the relevant chapter for a more thorough presentation.

The specificity of the AutoCM ANN architecture is that of being able to compute the *global* statistics of the association between variables belonging to a given data set. In other words, the AutoCM does not proceed by building on the measures of associations between couple of variables but directly works on the whole pattern and on all possible reciprocal influences between variables of every order. In this way, AutoCM is able to trace regularities which do not simply have to do with "common occurrences" among variables in certain ways but entail the analogies in the ways such variables tend to relate to the whole set of variables. In principle, the co-occurrence of a given couple of variables could exhibit no significant property, but at the same time the two could be deeply related in terms of the way they "wrap up" the entire data set. In other words, their relationship turns out to be "functional" rather than "formal".

The strategy used by the AutoCM to learn global patterns is somewhat surprising and can be reconstructed by analyzing the training phase of suitable test problems, as in Buscema and Sacco (this volume). During the training process, the AutoCM looks in turn for common traits among inputs, then reconstructs the overall variability of the sample to look then, in turn, for the specific characteristics of each single input and for differential traits, and finally becomes unresponsive to further presentations of the inputs once they carry no extra informational gain. The very same geometry of the AutoCM weights seems to reflect an idiosyncratic, complex representation of the knowledge built during the training phase which in the example developed in the cited chapter can be made especially apparent and readable.

This particular learning strategy seems especially appropriate for the problem of reconstructing actual "functional" interlock patterns between parties belonging to the same business network but not necessarily sharing a substantial number of board members. And it is even more appropriate when one considers how the analysis of the database carried out by the AutoCM can be suitably "spatialized". The matrix of weights that represents the AutoCM's "knowledge" acquired through the training process of analysis of the global pattern of associations among variables can be, in fact, transformed into a matrix of distances among nodes, i.e. it admits a graph-theoretic representation. In particular, one can build an optimal graph-theoretic representation by means of the so-called minimum spanning tree (MST), i.e. the tree that, given the distance matrix, provides an arrangement of the nodes such that it minimizes total distance. The MST then represents the most "economical" way to spatially arrange (i.e. to relate) variables in such a way so as to maintain their mutual coherence in the global pattern of associations. In this visual representation, physical proximity reflects strength of association.

Once this graph-theoretic representation is obtained, it can be explored by means of all of the customary tools of network analysis, and in particular it is possible to study the structure and degree of connectivity of each single node or properly chosen subset of nodes. In our specific example, the MST computed for the data set of board affiliations gives us a tree connecting in complex ways corporations that do not necessarily share board members to a significant degree. Moreover, this representation allows us to evaluate each company's role in determining the structure of the overall graph. To do this, we can simply compute how the MST is reorganized once we delete that specific company from the data set. In some cases the effect is almost negligible, in others it may be spectacular. The result does not depend not on how a specific company is connected within the overall business environment but also on whether its contribution to the tree's overall complexity can be "taken over" by some other company or not. This feature can by no means be deducted by simply looking at the local connectivity structures of the graph. It is very difficult, if not impossible, to deduce a priori what will be the consequences of the rearrangement, at the global and local level, of deleting each given node. The contribution of each node to the graph's overall complexity can be computed by means of a new measure that we call "hubness" (*H*) (see Buscema and Sacco, this volume). Hubness measures the "complexity" of each given graph. The deletion of a node from the graph can then be evaluated in terms of its consequences on the resulting graph's hubness. When we evaluate single nodes in terms of their contribution to the graph's overall hubness, it may turn out that relatively "marginal" ones (when evaluated through conventional criteria) have great importance, whereas more "central" ones are not so crucial. In terms of our specific example under study, it may happen that relatively "well-connected" companies which appear to play a central role in the overall pattern may result much less relevant than expected (in the sense that their going out of business would not prompt radical changes in the actual power network), whereas some other less connected ones could, once stepped out of the picture, command massive changes and would therefore be much more relevant in sustaining a given power network in its actual form. This is clearly the most apparent effect of the "global" representation of the pattern of associations provided by the AutoCM as opposed to more traditional techniques. The often underplayed non-linear properties of the network dynamics, which are very hard to trace by means of the conventional approaches, become much clearer and open to analysis and interpretation. Reasoning in terms of direct links, the deletion of each given node does not make any sense in that it simply destroys information, and very little can be learned from it. In our approach, on the contrary, most of the relevant deductions come from learning the "functional" contribution of each given node to the overall architecture of connections.

The MST representation, however, in spite of being the most "economical" representation of the AutoCM's knowledge (i.e. the one that employs the least possible number of connections between nodes), is not necessarily the most accurate one in that it could overlook some further connections which, although unnecessary to generate the MST, could be practically very relevant to understand the global pattern of associations. In other words, whereas all of the connections included in the MST are certainly relevant to the reconstruction of the backbone of the sample's connectivity pattern, it need not be the case that all of the relevant connections will be found in the MST. Inclusion of these further relevant connections would introduce the possibility of cycles, i.e. of closed paths, that would turn the original MST into a graph. Is there a way to complicate the "optimal" MST by introducing all and only those extra connections that are essential to understand the global pattern in all of its complexity? The answer is affirmative, and to construct this new graph we must once again refer to the hubness measure H. In particular, we proceed as follows: Starting from the MST, we introduce back all of the links between nodes that have been omitted from the optimal tree representation and evaluate to what extent they have an impact on the resulting graph's hubness (i.e. measure of complexity). The "appropriate" graph, that we call maximally regular graph (MRG), is obtained when we have introduced back into the graph those links that maximize the overall graph's hubness H. Once the maximal value of H is attained, the introduction of further, previously omitted connections causes graph complexity to diminish, i.e. destroys information and therefore proves to be unnecessary to the appropriate representation of the underlying networking pattern.

The re-introduction of previously deleted connections may be of extreme importance for the interpretation of the actual networking pattern, and all the more so, the higher their contribution to the graph's hubness H. In particular, such connections will typically give rise to characteristic regular microstructures (loops) that represent hubs of various importance in the global architecture of the network. Even visual inspection of the network will generally easily allow to isolate "diamond-like" structures (in particular, regular sub-graphs) which constitute the graph's "functional kernels". Among such diamond-like structures, there will typically be one which, for its centrality and dimension, clearly represents the functional core ("the" kernel) of the network, its most deeply rooted relational hub.

In terms of our specific object of study, then, the MRG represents an alternative graph-theoretic representation of the underlying business power network with respect to the one obtained by simply reconstructing the geography of common board affiliation. Whereas the latter depicts what we could call the formal dimension of interlocking, the former is more focused on the functional dimension and is likely to exhibit clearer, more stable and more traceable properties that allow to characterize more firmly the nature and features of the inter-corporate connectivity within a given business environment. In particular, the central "diamond" of the MRG representation of the Italian business environment will correspond, according to our approach, to the core of the underlying power network: a statement with clear empirical implications that can be properly tested on the basis of further pieces of evidence from various sources.

It is therefore our contention that, once a certain business environment has been properly represented in terms of the corresponding MRG, we start from the correct premises to be able to evaluate the nature and properties of the corresponding power network and that more traditional representations fail to deliver clear-cut results in this respect because the background theoretical representation is ill-posed and fails to point out the relevant connection structure. This claim must of course be subject to careful and detailed scrutiny. In the present chapter we want to make a first step in this direction by analyzing the recent evolution of interlocking patterns in the Italian business environment, as announced above. It is our intention, in future research, to carry out more detailed and systematic analysis on this specific case study, as well as on data coming from different business environments with different characteristics, including European, North American and Far Eastern cases.

12.5 Power Structure Dynamics in the Italian Business Environment

Although there is generally a strong and understandable bias that leads outside observers, and often even sophisticated analysts, to personalize power relationships, focusing on the position of specific individuals within the network, rather than on the overall structure of the network itself, this temptation is particularly compelling in the Italian case, where the overly familistic character of business power relationships causes an almost compulsory tendency to read business events in the light of the dynamics of personal (or, more generally, extended "family") relationships. A consequence of this, however, is the difficulty to properly understand the actual structure of power network by over-emphasizing the role of more "visible" and well-known individuals, families, corporations and groups, and by underscoring that of the players that prefer to work away from the spotlights. On the other hand, an excessive emphasis on personalization may be read as an indirect signal of the difficulty to have a grasp of the real, underlying power dynamics that fails to emerge from the apparent properties of the network and therefore leads many to conclude that there is little more to be understood beyond the personal level.

To investigate the existence of an underlying, complex power structure for the Italian case, we have built two distinct databases relating to different but close moments in time. The first one contains the 226 listed companies in the Italian stock exchange as of March 2006 and the respective 1873 members sitting in one or more boards. The second one contains the 240 listed companies in the Italian stock exchange as of November 2007 and the respective 1973 members sitting in one or more boards. The reason for this double but temporally close sampling is to check to what extent the actual structure of the underlying power network has been modified, if any, by incoming events and to trace such modifications to specific events, in order to get a first understanding of the dynamic properties of the network.

In the first place, we start from the March 2006 database and begin by drawing the actual mapping of the "apparent" connections between companies in order to see to what extent a "visible" structure emerges. We consider two possibilities: first, the structure of the connections between companies which have at least one board member in common and second, the structure of the connections between companies that have at least two board members in common. The results are shown in Figs. 12.1 and 12.2 below.

Inspection of Figs. 12.1 and 12.2 gives a few interesting insights. First of all, in terms of the structure of "apparent" links, the Italian business environment is not wholly connected. Second, one notices the existence of a diamond-like, complete subgraph in a relatively marginal position, but its role in the overall structure is quite vague. Specifically, looking at the structure of connections in terms of at least one board member in common, it is very difficult to sort out any clear structural regularity apart from a somewhat fuzzy core–periphery relation (a more dense pattern of connections among a certain number of companies, a more sparse pattern for some more marginal companies, and a small number of isolated satellite components). Passing to the structure of connections with at least two members in common, the network structure almost entirely evaporates, and the whole business environment gets broken into a constellation of mostly small or very small components. On the basis of this evidence, it is not particularly surprising that analysts do not pay special attention to the possibility of existence of an underlying power structure and focus attention on personalizations and on intelligence of local connections of apparently outstanding importance as proxies for the understanding of the whole.

But what happens when we analyze the same database on the basis of a totally different kind of network representation, namely the MRG? The following result emerges (Fig. 12.3).

By means of the MRG representation, a totally different picture results. In particular, the Italian business environment turns out to be much more connected than one could expect from the analysis of "apparent" links, and in most cases, connections appear relatively strong even in peripheral regions of the graph. The central "diamond-like" kernel is perfectly recognizable, and the whole of the remaining network can be entirely characterized in terms of branches departing from one of the nodes of the central kernel (see Fig. 12.4 below). Also, a few more peripheral kernels can be found, most of which are complete. We leave a closer inspection of this graph for the following section and go on examining the results of the November 2007 database.

In the case of the second database, it is hardly surprising at this point that the same structural regularities occur. But it is somewhat more surprising that at a few months' distance from the first database, the inherent power structure has undergone some nontrivial changes. Memberships in the central kernel have changed to some extent, and the corresponding structure of branches has been modified accordingly.

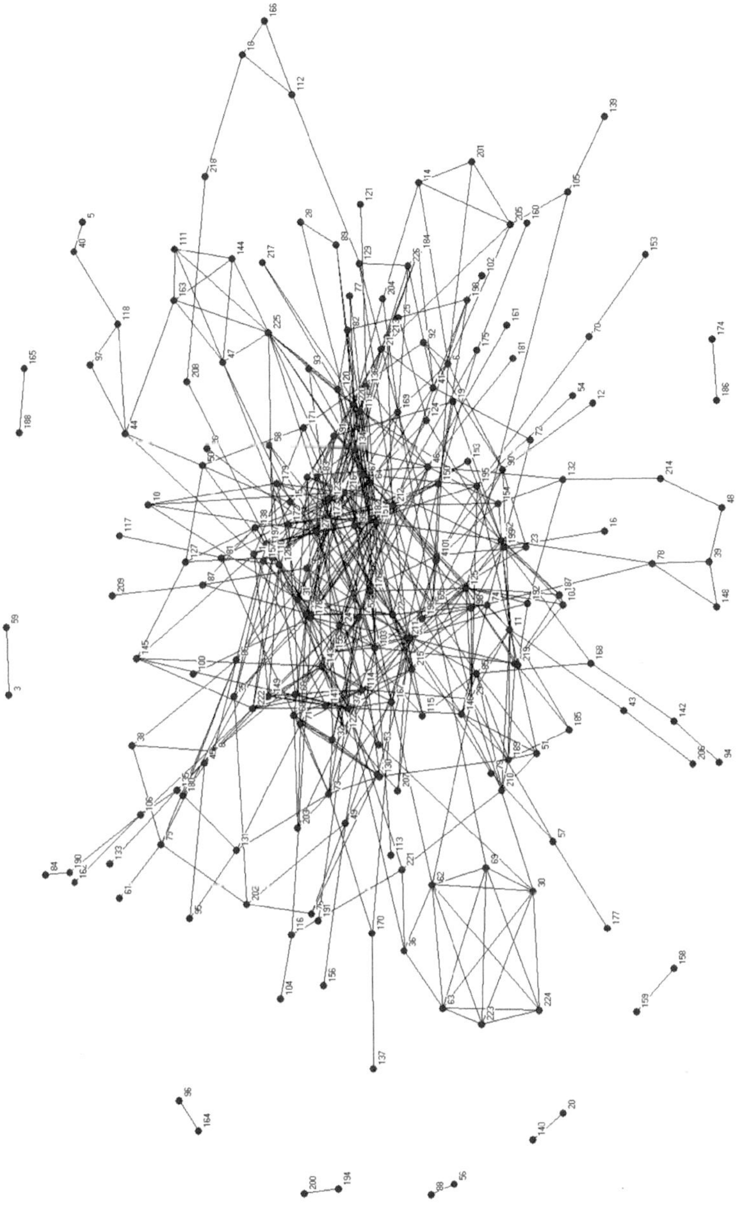

Fig. 12.1 March 2006 database: explicit links among companies with at least one common board member

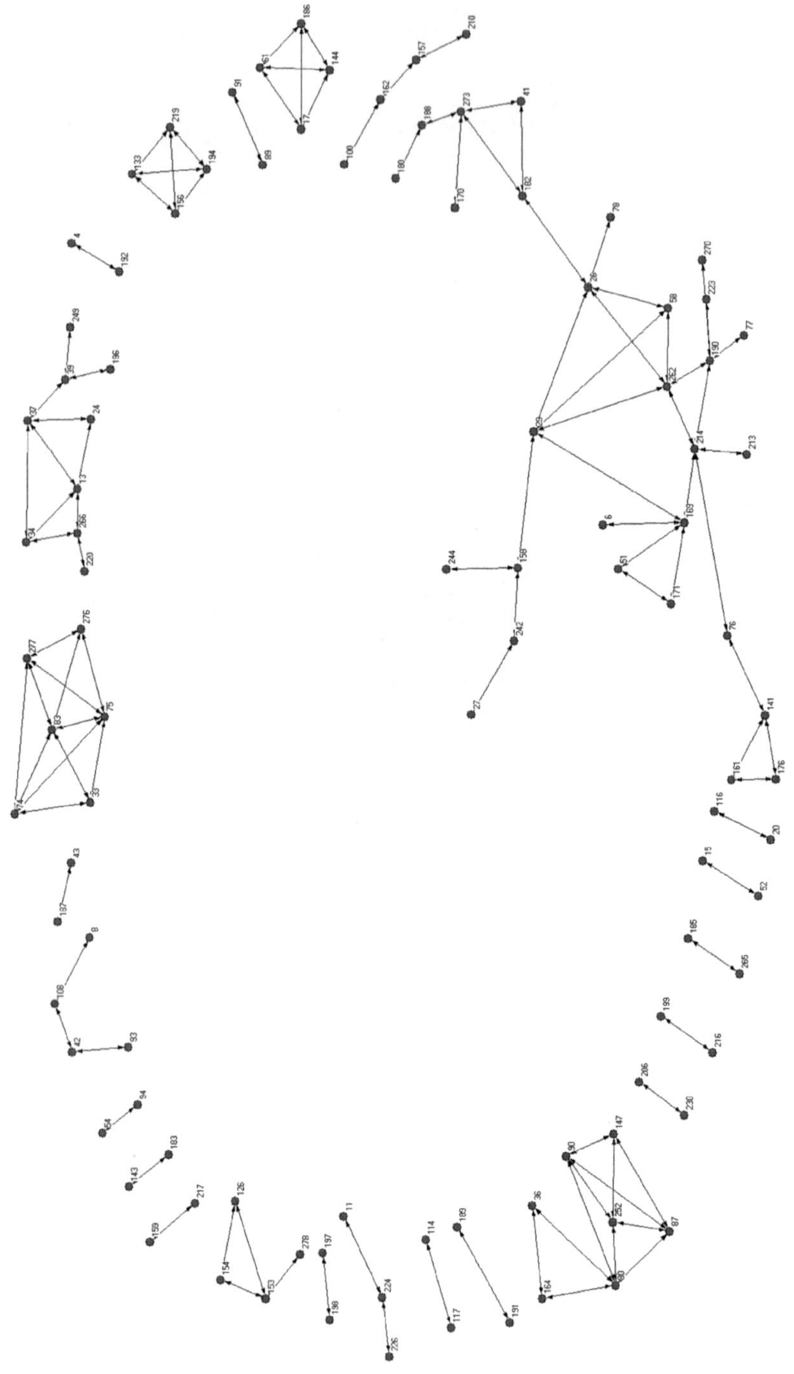

Fig. 12.2 March 2006 database: explicit links among companies with at least two common board members

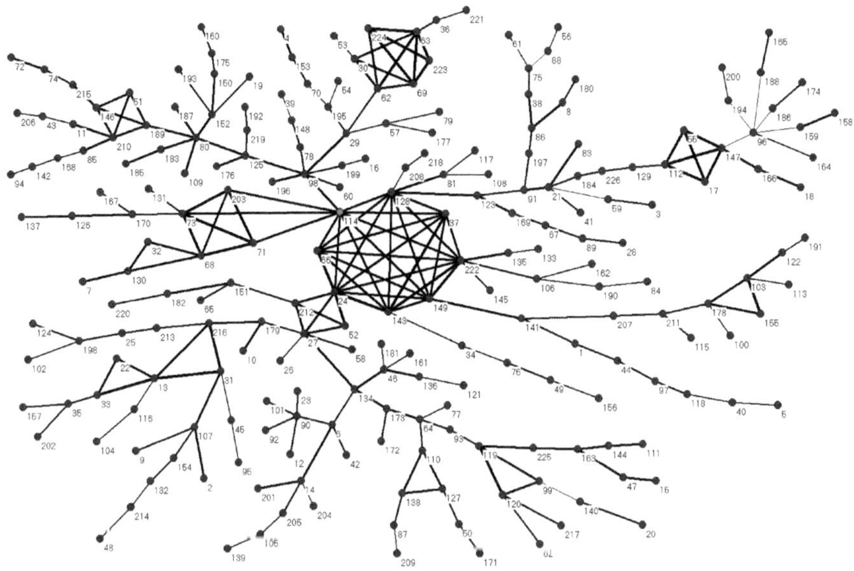

Fig. 12.3 March 2006 database: MRG representation

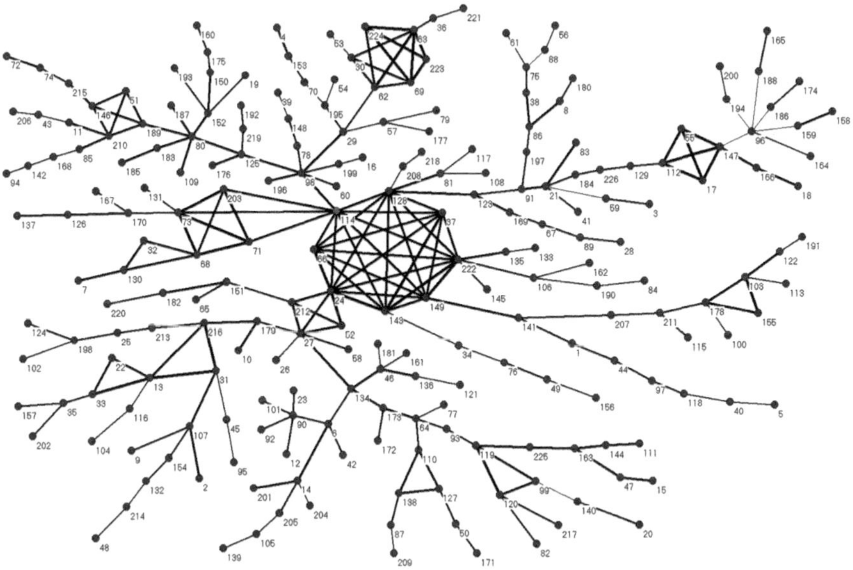

Fig. 12.4 March 2006 database: partition of the Italian business environment into branches of the central kernel

This surprisingly quick-paced dynamic response provides us with an interesting opportunity to test the meaningfulness of the MRG network representation of the Italian business network, checking whether it is possible to trace the changes back

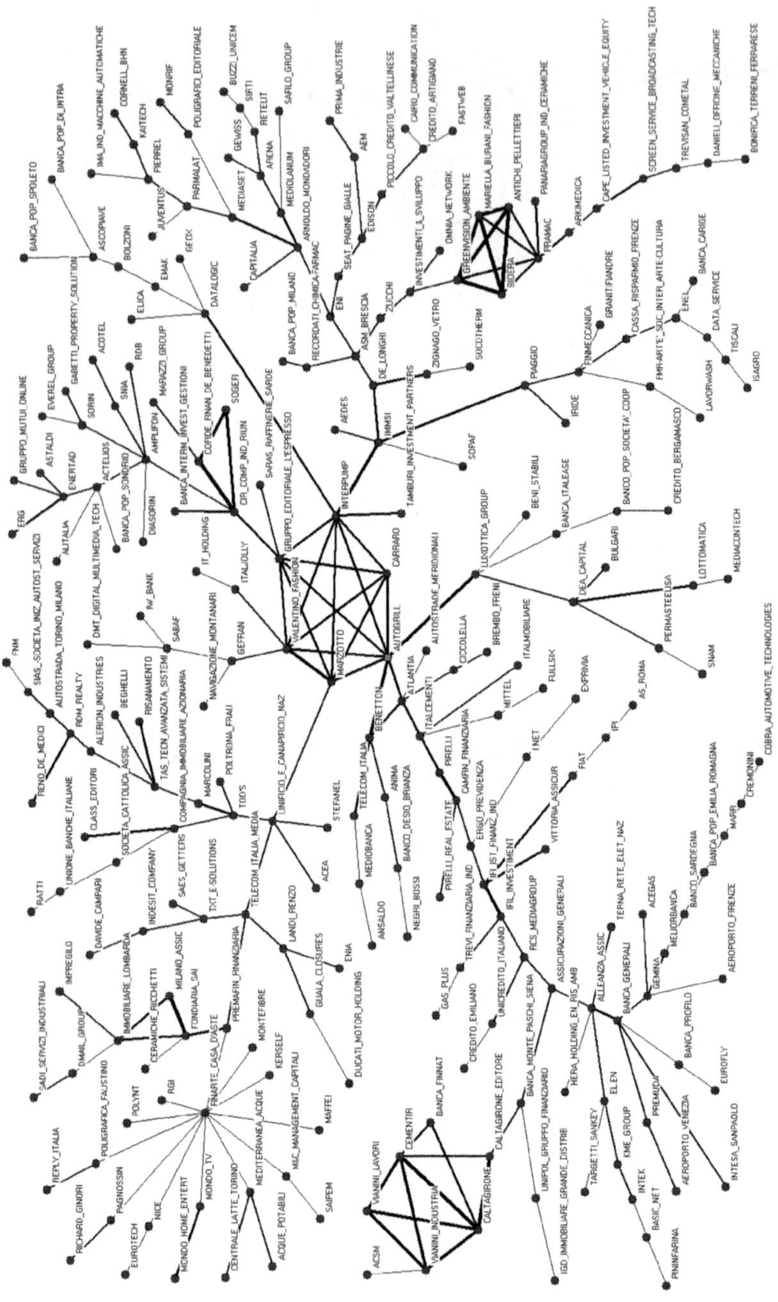

Fig. 12.5 November 2007 database: MRG representation

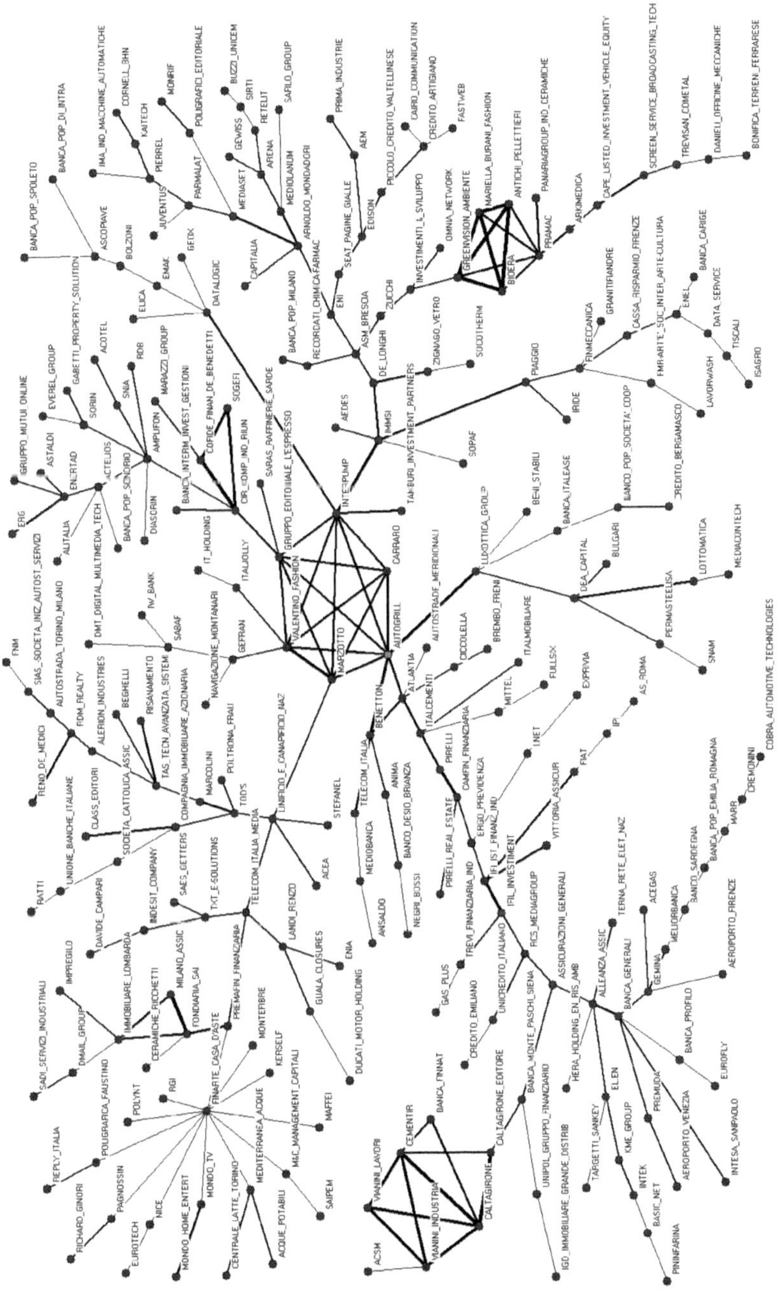

Fig. 12.6 November 2007 database: partition of the Italian business environment into branches of the central kernel

to specific events that have occurred meanwhile in a sensible way and to study how the overall structure of the network has adjusted to such changes (in terms of the "functional" rather than formal and apparent connectivity of the various companies in the overall business environment) (Figs. 12.5 and 12.6).

12.6 Power Structure Dynamics in the Italian Business Environment: March 2006–November 2007

In this section we analyze and interpret the findings obtained through the MRG network representation in the previous section. Again, we start from the March 2006 database and investigate the structure of the central kernel for this case more closely (Fig 12.7).

To begin with, it is interesting to note that, as of March 2006, the central kernel is made of companies which are mostly controlled by outstanding Italian entrepreneurial families. Specifically, "L'Espresso" group refers to the D Benedetti Family, "Autogrill SpA" to Benetton, "Carraro" to the homonymous family, both "Marzotto Manifattura" and "Valentino Fashion SpA" to the Marzotto family, "Luxottica" to Del Vecchio. The "Interpump" group, a world leader in its sector (high-pressure pumps), has still its founder (Fulvio MontipÚ) as CEO but is less characterized in terms of a leading entrepreneurial family. Interpump is therefore the classical example of a corporation that would be easily overlooked by "personalistic" reconstructions of the power network of Italy's business environment. Finally, "Banca Nazionale del Lavoro" (BNL) is the notable exception. At that time, BNL has been the object of a controversial attempt at takeover and, after the failure of

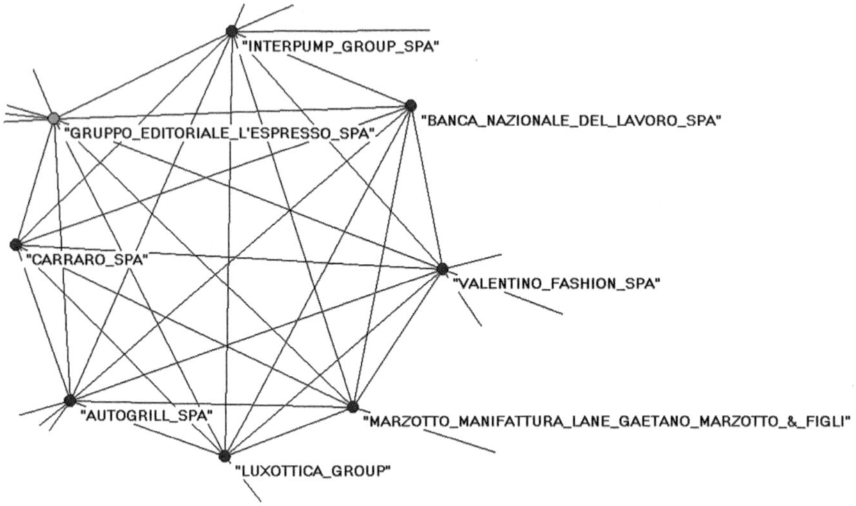

Fig. 12.7 March 2006 database: the central kernel

the latter due to a complex series of economic and political reasons, is about to be acquired by the French banking group BNP Paribas. It is the only company in the kernel whose governance cannot be traced back to an entrepreneurial family and, together with "Carraro", is the only member of the kernel without branches. The condition of being part of the kernel without generating branches seems to signal a centrality in the power network that is not determined by the functional relationship to more complex aggregations of corporate interests, but rather to "power balance" kind of factors. In particular, the presence of BNL in the central kernel is especially meaningful in the light of its crucial role in one of the most critical passages of the recent history of corporate governance in Italy; if the failed takeover attempt would have been successful, the structure of the Italian power network would have changed radically. It is also quite remarkable that two different companies referring to the same family, namely "Marzotto" and "Valentino", are both distinct components of the kernel and generate two distinct branches. This somewhat anomalous situation, however, deserves specific clarification (see below).

To gain further insight, it may be useful at this point to have a closer look at the various branches.

The "L'Espresso" branch, for instance, is one of the most extended and complex. Not surprisingly, it includes companies referring to the "root" family such as "Sogefi", "Cir", "Cofide" and "CDB", not incidentally forming a secondary kernel that generates a significant sub-branch including among others "Parmalat SpA" (in whose board sits a member of the family). But the other sub-branch, which articulates around "Fastweb SpA" (no common board members with "L'Espresso"), spans a quite complex and heterogeneous galaxy of firms which includes several major Italian family groups such as Caltagirone, Cremonini and Berlusconi and major banking and insurance groups such as "Monte dei Paschi" and "Unipol". The presence of companies controlled by the Berlusconi family in this branch may look particularly surprising if one notices that the publications of "L'Espresso" group probably represent one of the most extreme opponents of Mr. Silvio Berlusconi's political project, but it is to be remarked at the same time that the De Benedetti and Berlusconi families, in spite of the dissonance in political views, have ongoing business partnerships. It is however beyond doubt that, if the centrality of "L'Espresso" group would be no surprise for several business analysts, the relative "marginality" of groups such as the ones related to the Berlusconi and Caltagirone families would certainly challenge the views of anyone maintaining a "personalized" approach to the unscrambling of the Italian business power network (Fig. 12.8).

Also the "Autogrill" branch, referring to the Benetton family, spans some of the most important Italian corporations. The secondary diamond rooted in the central kernel comprises companies such as "Benetton Group SpA" and "Autostrade SpA", which clearly refer to the family, but also "Telecom Italia SpA", one of the giants of Italian IT, whose board does not include members of the family and only has one common member with the board of "Autogrill" (firmly linked to the family; he is the CEO of a family holding). From the secondary diamond, basically three different branches depart: one, small but extremely significant, that comprises major players of the banking sectors, such as "Mediobanca", "Unicredito" and "Capitalia"

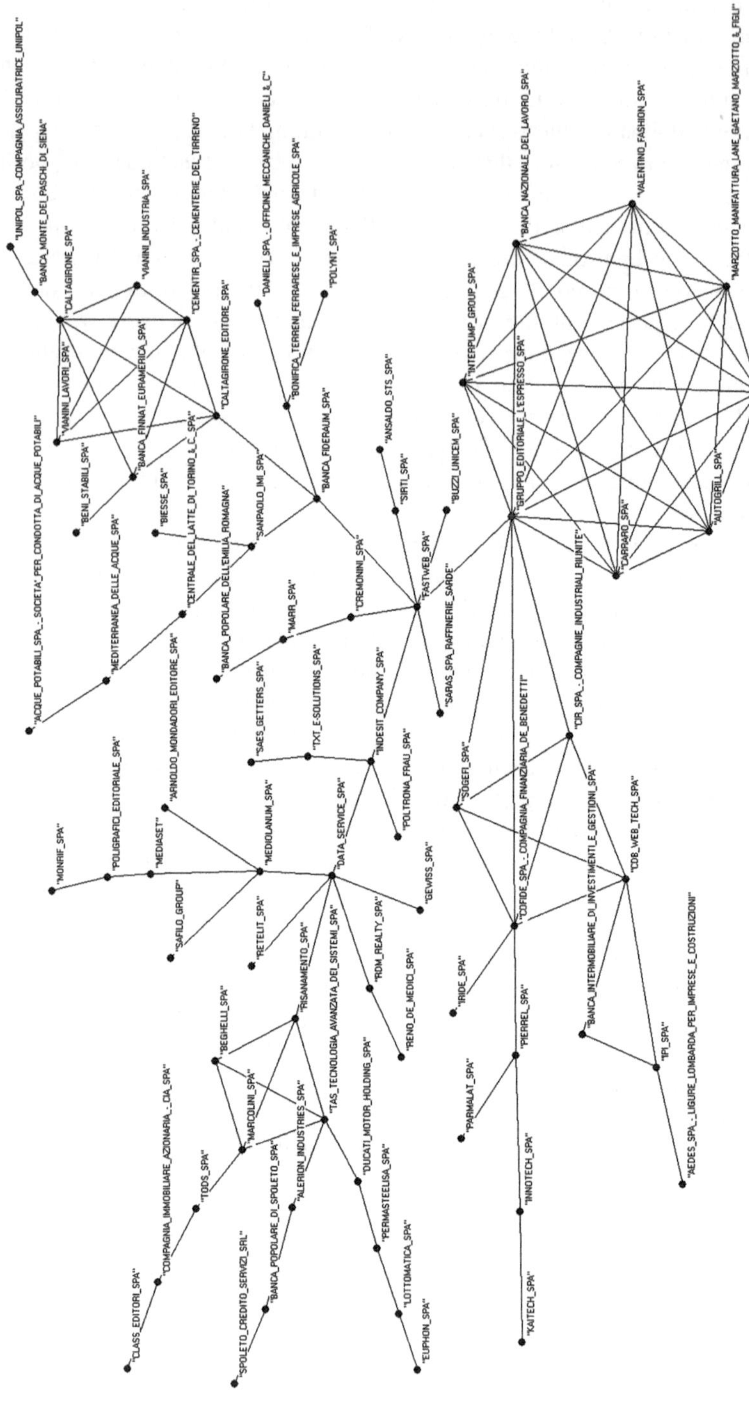

Fig. 12.8 March 2006 database: "L'Espresso" branch

(the two latter having subsequently merged in May 2008), and one of the country's most important publishing groups, "RCS". The second branch includes huge utility companies such as "Terna", major banks and insurance companies such as "Banca Intesa" and "Generali", respectively, huge general contractors such as "Impregilo" and big IT players such as Tiscali. Finally, the third, vast and highly composite sub-branch includes corporations such as FIAT, Pirelli, Erg, as well as Italy's public airplane carrier "Alitalia" and the huge defence and aerospace holding "Finmeccanica", among others. Again, the "functional" affiliation within the whole power network of this heterogeneous collection of major country players from the Benetton group is likely to appear surprising to most analysts to say the least. It is interesting to stress that the network here relates companies without any link, however transitive and indirect, among board members, such as "FIAT SpA" and "Lavorwash SpA", a multinational group producing high-pressure cleaning systems (Fig. 12.9).

We now come to one of the most puzzling and controversial features of the MRG, namely the fact that two distinct companies referring to a same family (Marzotto) are both part of the central kernel, each one at the root of a branch of its own. First of all, it is interesting to note that such branch has a relatively modest development if compared to the ones examined so far and that they are characterized by a lower incidence of major players – in the "Marzotto" branch, "Fondiaria-Sai", an insurance company of premier importance, and "Telecom Italia Media" (which controls the La7 and MTV Italy TV channels) on one sub-branch and "ACEA", Rome's utility corporation, on the other. The "Valentino" branch, which is particularly small, does not contain major players. "Valentino Fashion Group" has been listed relatively recently, in 2005, after a restructuring of the Marzotto group to manage the group's brands in the fashion industry, whereas the "Marzotto" company had to focus on the traditional core business of the group, i.e. the manufacturing of high-quality textile fibres. In July 2007, however, the situation of the group underwent an important change with the acquisition of the "Valentino Fashion Group" by the private equity fund Permira, thereby getting out from the Marzotto main radius of influence. One might conjecture that this significant change in the company's control and governance would cause a major shift of "Valentino" in the global power network structure. This has not been the case, however, at least in the short run; in the new scenario designed by the November 2007 database, in which major changes will be registered, both the "Marzotto" and "Valentino" components are still included in the central kernel, and the relevance of the "Marzotto" branch is significantly increased. This aspect further confirms that the presence of "Valentino" in the kernel is not simply related to matters of family control but to its specific role in the global architecture of the power network (Figs. 12.10 and 12.11).

Let us now consider the "Interpump" branch, which is highly articulate and rooted, as already emphasized, in a corporation that analysts would hardly include in the central kernel on the basis of their common sense judgment. This branch includes huge energy multinationals such as "Eni" and important utilities such as "AEM", "Edison", "Snam", world leaders in packaging machines such as "IMA" and in luxury such as "Bulgari", world leaders in shoes such as "GEOX" as well

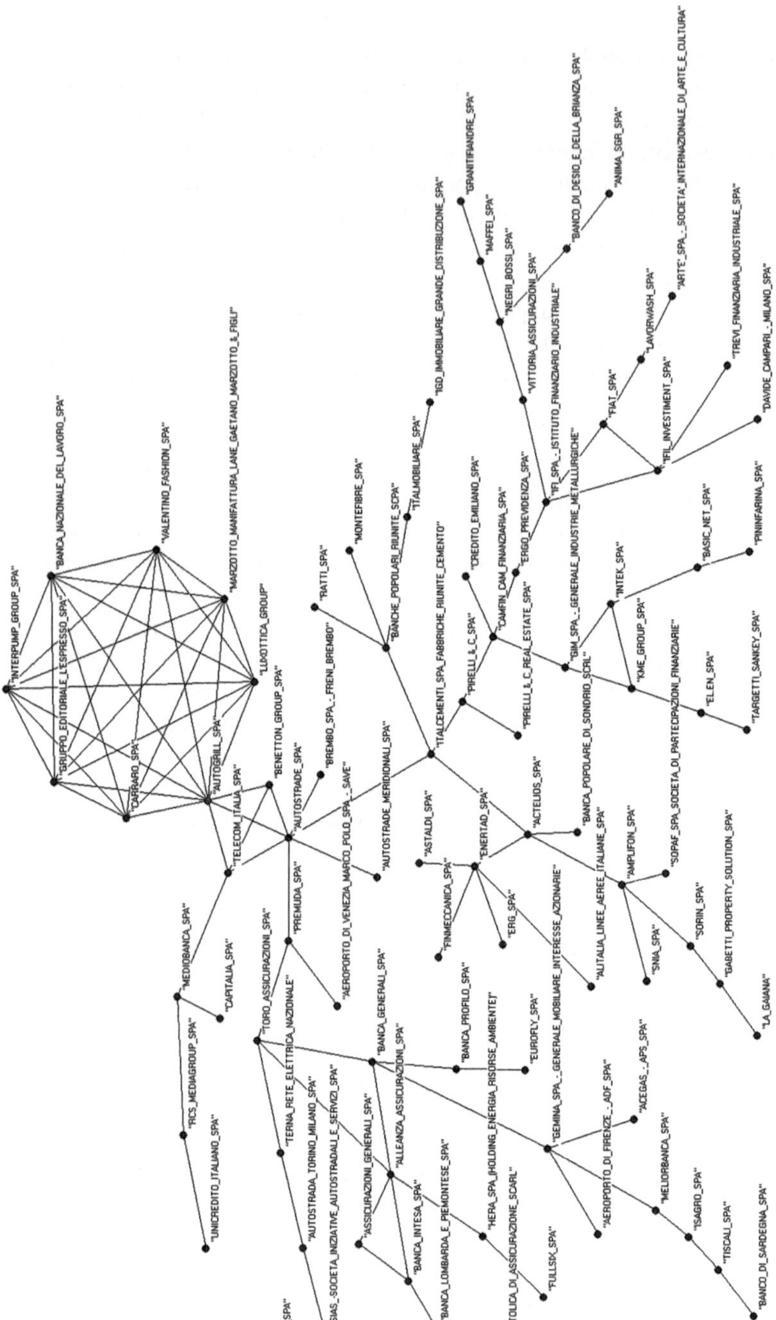

Fig. 12.9 March 2006 database: "Autogrill" branch

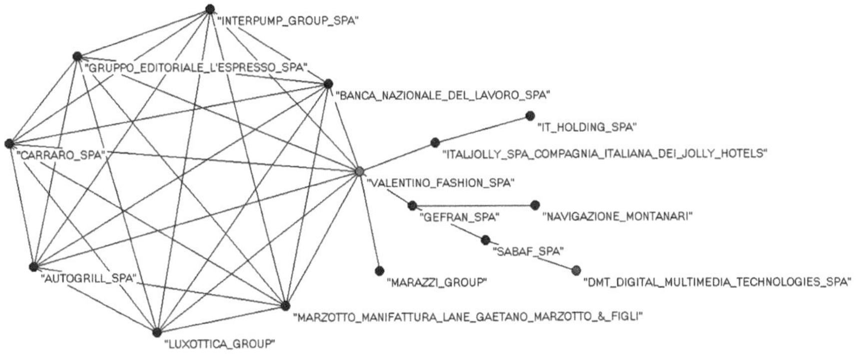

Fig. 12.10 March 2006 database: "Valentino" branch

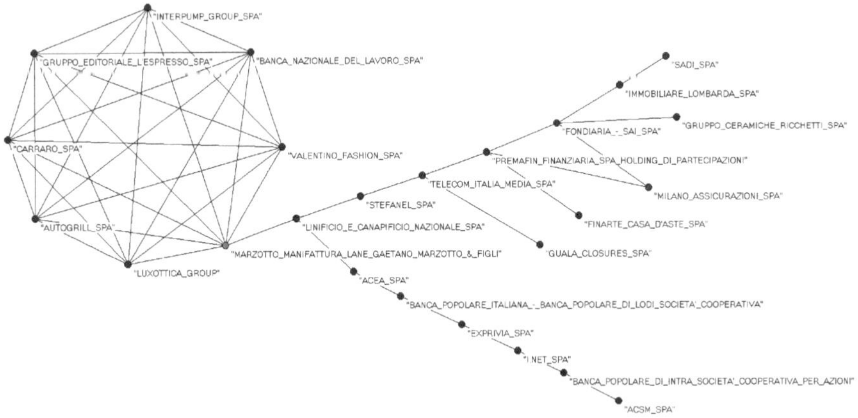

Fig. 12.11 March 2006 database: "Marzotto" branch

as pharmaceutical companies like "Recordati" and multimedia companies such as "SEAT Pagine Gialle". There are also a few medium-sized banking groups such as "Banca Popolare di Milano", "Banca Carige", "Cassa di Risparmio di Firenze" (the latter will become part of the "Intesa Sanpaolo" group at the beginning of 2008). It is interesting to note that, overall, the "Interpump" branch, although quite well developed, is less prominent than the two big ones associated with major entrepreneurial families such as "L'Espresso" and "Autogrill". Also, it is remarkable that this branch concentrates the bulk of Italy's energy and utility sector and some of the most dynamic up-and-coming "new" Italian entrepreneurs such as Moretti Polegato's "GEOX". Finally, in this branch there are significant sub-branches that have been built by the MRG in spite of the fact that there is not even an indirect, transitive link between the respective boards (Fig. 12.12).

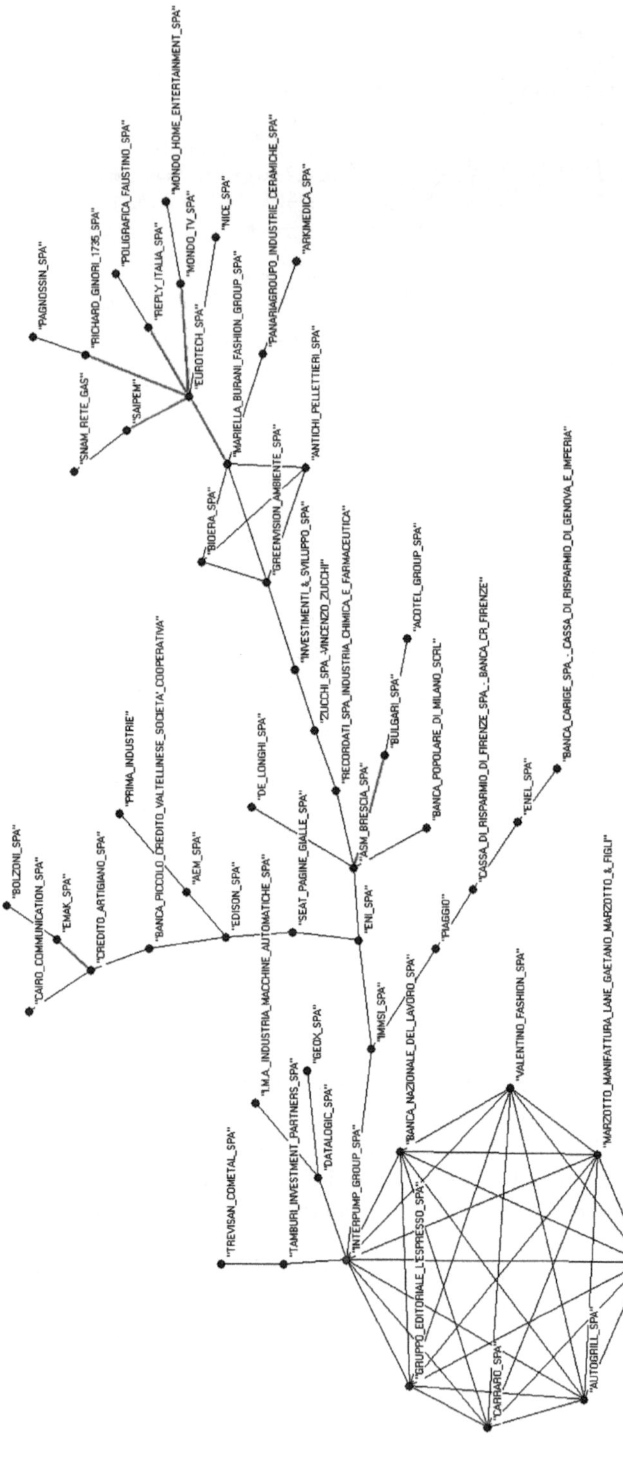

Fig. 12.12 March 2006 database: "Interpump" branch

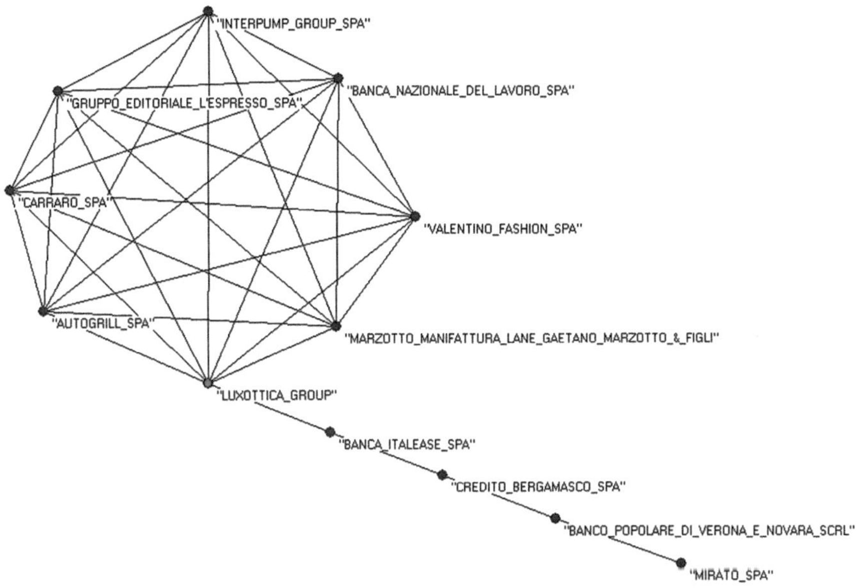

Fig. 12.13 March 2006 database: "Luxottica" branch

Finally, we have the "Luxottica" branch that, although corresponding to a primary entrepreneurial family (Del Vecchio), is tiny and very simple in structure – actually, linear, basically centred on the medium-sized "Banco Popolare" banking group (Fig. 12.13).

The two remaining nodes of the central kernel "BNL" and "Carraro" have no branches. As of March 2006, then, we can say that the structure of the power network of the Italian business environment is organized around four basic hubs: "L'Espresso", "Autogrill", "Marzotto" and "Interpump". It is important, however, not to overlook the role of those nodes in the central kernel that seem to play a secondary role; they may not be as important as the former in terms of hubs, but they may be of crucial importance in keeping together the global architecture of the network. For instance, some of the board members of "Luxottica" play a crucial role in the establishment of indirect links among the whole network: Leonardo Del Vecchio, founder and CEO, also sits in two key boards, those of "Generali" ("Autogrill" branch) and "Beni Stabili" ("L'Espresso" branch), whereas Gianni Mion and Sergio Erede sit, respectively, in the boards of (among others) "Autogrill" and "Telecom", and "L'Espresso", "Interpump" and "Carraro"; that is to say, they together span the whole of the central kernel. Accordingly, board members of "Carraro" also sit in the boards of "Autogrill", "L'Espresso", "Interpump" and "Luxottica". The central kernel thus acts as a sort of cohesive "distributional" channel that guarantees more or less direct connections between branches of the Italian economy.

To what extent does the global architecture of the network change from early 2006 to late 2007? The most important event that occurred meanwhile is the acquisition of BNL by BNP Paribas, which thus takes away one of the elements of the central kernel, albeit one that did not have any branch at all. But again confirming the non-linear structure of the network where each element of the kernel, whatever be the extension of its respective branch, plays a key "functional" role in sustaining the whole architecture, it turns out that this event brings about important consequences, at just a few months' distance from the previous picture (see Fig. 12.5; we report the MST also in Fig. 12.14 for completeness).

We report the central kernel and its immediate vicinities as of November 2007 in Fig. 12.15 for the reader's convenience.

A few important novelties are easily noted: the (obvious) disappearance of "BNL" but also the disappearance of "Luxottica". The rest of the kernel is stable and carries over from March 2006. In the new situation, "Luxottica" is still very close to the central kernel but as a direct neighbour of "Autogrill", at the very root of the respective branch.

The "L'Espresso" group has undergone a radical reshaping and a significant downsizing, losing all of the "big players" branching from it in early 2006 and accessing "Erg" and "Alitalia", which were previously in the "Autogrill" branch. "Interpump", on the contrary, expands significantly, and its branch now includes players such as "Fastweb" (previously at the core of "L'Espresso" branch), "Finmeccanica" (previously "Autogrill"), "Mediaset" and "Cremonini" (again, both previously "L'Espresso"), "Tiscali" (previously "Autogrill"). "Autogrill" itself, in spite of the "loss" of various big players, still maintains a high development as a branch, including "Unipol", "Monte dei Paschi" and "Caltagirone" (from "L'Espresso"). The new outstanding banking group "Intesa Sanpaolo" is also in this branch; previously "Banca Intesa" was in the "Autogrill" branch, whereas "Sanpaolo IMI" in "L'Espresso". As already noted, "Luxottica" becomes integrated in the "Autogrill" branch as well. Other key players such as "Pirelli", "Unicredito", "RCS" and "Mediobanca" remain within the "Autogrill" branch. Another branch that witnesses a significant development is "Marzotto", although no new major players enter the branch. Finally, "Valentino" confirms its relatively marginal standing and "Carraro" remains the only node in the kernel without branches.

Overall, the new scenario described by the November 2007 database seems to signal a shift of influence from "L'Espresso" to "Interpump", with "Autogrill" maintaining its central role and "Marzotto" playing a more active complementary role. These deductions, however, must be taken with a grain of salt because of the complex non-linear interdependencies among the various portions of the network. There seems to be, however, evidence of a major shift in the structure of the underlying power network between the two periods of observation, partly as an adjustment caused by the acquisition of BNL by BNP-Paribas (Figs. 12.16, 12.17 and 12.18).

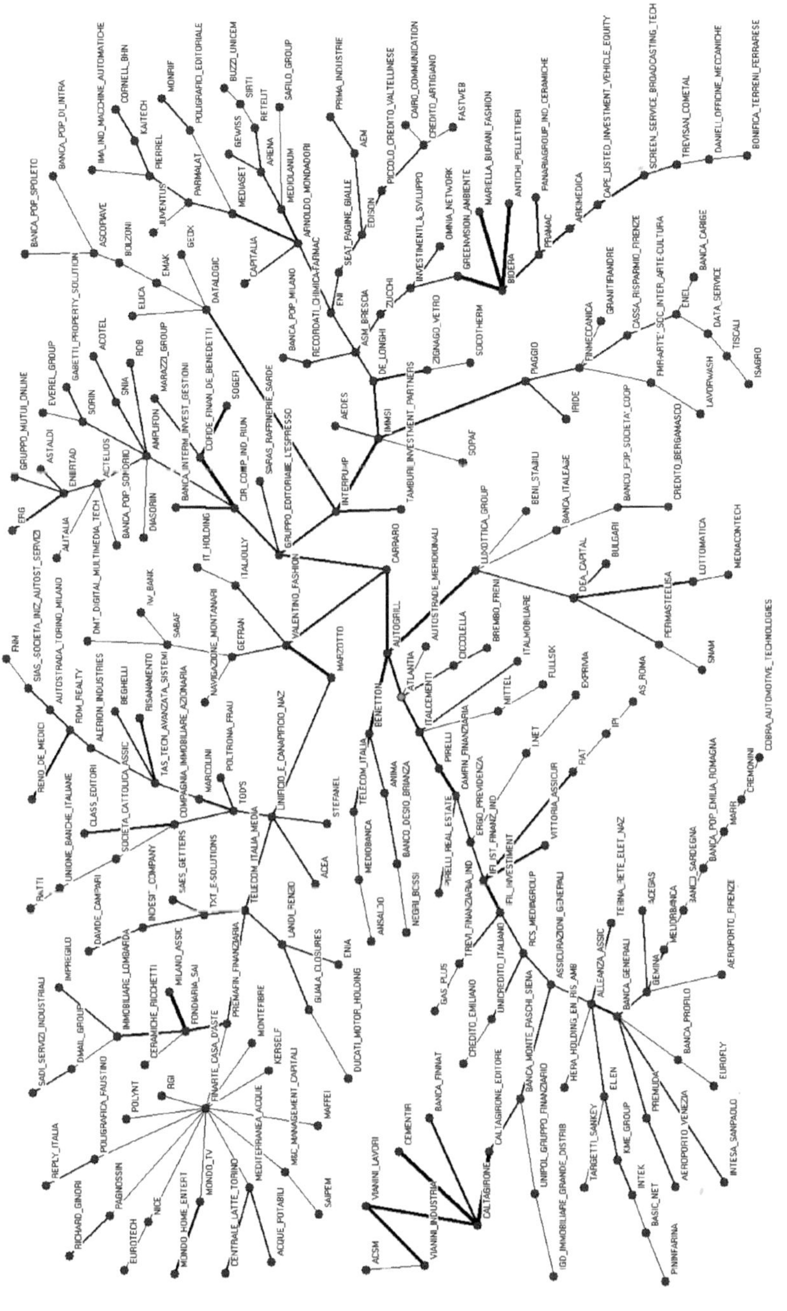

Fig. 12.14 November 2007 database: MST representation

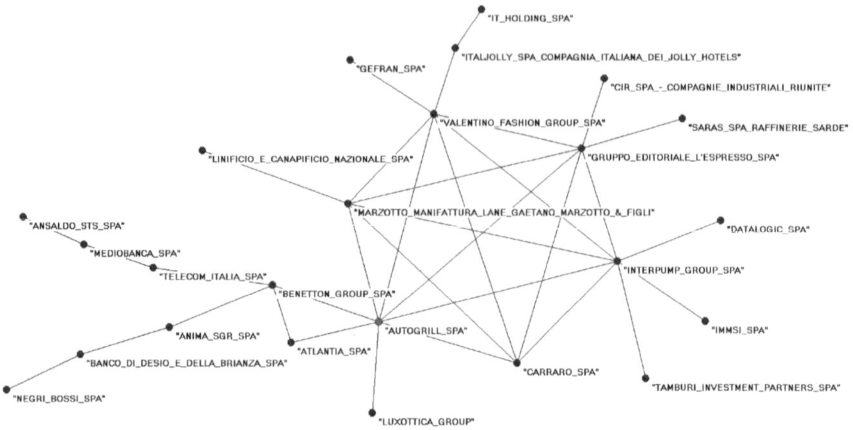

Fig. 12.15 November 2007 database: central kernel

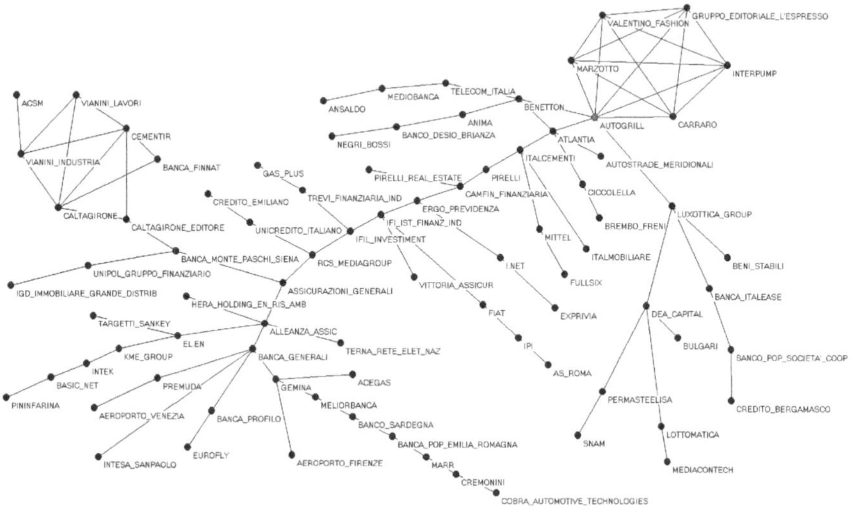

Fig. 12.16 November 2007 database: Autogrill branch

12.7 Conclusions

In this chapter we have proposed an alternative approach to the issue of analysis of interlocking directorates and the structure of power networks in business environments. We have maintained that the difficulty encountered in the previous literature in demonstrating the existence and relevance of such network may have been caused by an improper choice of the method of representation and analysis of such networks. Rather than working on the structure of apparent connections (i.e. actual overlaps of member affiliations across the various boards), we have developed an

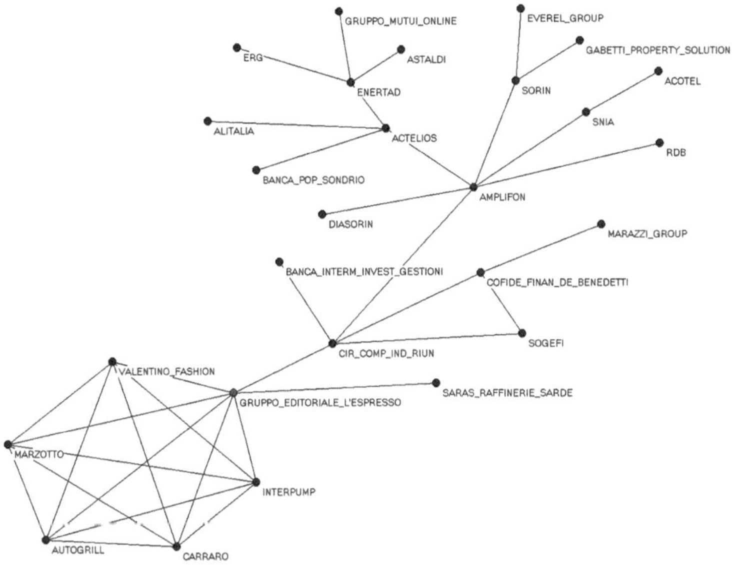

Fig. 12.17 November 2007 database: L'Espresso branch

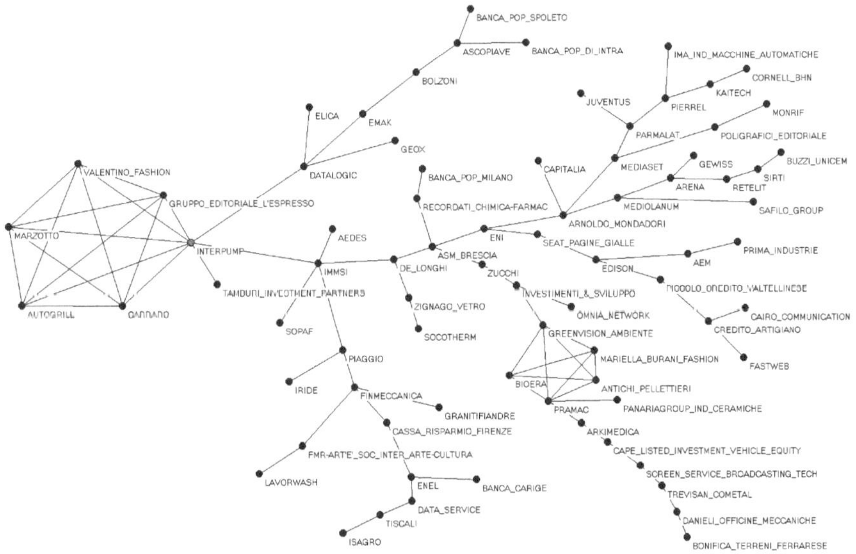

Fig. 12.18 November 2007 database: Interpump branch

approach that explores the global structure of the network in terms of functional regularities (i.e. the contribution of each corporation to the construction of the actual network). As a result, in the Italian case study 2006–2007, a clear-cut power network structure has emerged and its evolution has been tracked during the period of observation. Unlike the traditional approach, which tries to find evidence of *some* form of power network from the available data, here we therefore construct a *specific* power network that is amenable to direct scrutiny and analysis though a variety of independent information sources and viewpoints.

It is clear that the present chapter can at best be considered a very preliminary step in the construction to a full-fledged alternative approach. Many open points remain and call for extensive further research and development. The analysis conducted here on the actual power network resulting from the MRG representation is extremely crude and preliminary. The findings about the structure and content of the various branches have to be conducted in much greater detail and need to draw from a variety of different sources. An analogous MRG representation for board members rather than companies may also be carried out, in spite of the computational burden that it will entail. Moreover, there is the need to construct a theoretical framework that allows to interpret this specific network structure and dynamics in a meaningful and consistent way.

In short, then, most of the work is still to be done. But we are convinced that the approach presented in this chapter may be an interesting step towards the rejuvenation of a literature that, following the already beaten path, seems to have arrived at something of a cul-de-sac. Here we provide an approach to empirical analysis that allows to work on a specific hypothesis to be tested and explored in its highest level of detail, providing insights that can be of direct interest and use also to practitioners, including financial, economic and political analysts. We hope that this will attract fresh interest and energy on the research topic, which we still feel of interest and quite important to understand the dynamics and characteristic of the current phase of post-industrial, global capitalism.

Bibliography

Allen, M. P. (1974). The structure of interorganizational elite cooptation: interlocking corporate directorates. *Am. Sociol. Rev.* 39, 393–406.

Beckman, C. M. and Haunschild, P. R. (2002). Network learning: the effects of partners' heterogeneity of experience on corporate acquisitions. *Adm. Sci. Q.* 46, 92–124.

Beckman, C. M., Haunschild, P. R., and Phillips, D. J. (2004). Friends or strangers? firm-specific uncertainty, market uncertainty, and network partner selection. *Organ. Sci.* 15, 259–275.

Bianco, M. and Pagnoni, E. (1997). Interlocking directorates across listed companies in Italy: the case of banks. *Banca Nazionale del Lavoro Quart. Rev.* Special Issue, 215–144.

Biggart, N. W. and Beamish, T. D. (2003). The economic sociology of conventions: habit, custom, practice, and routine in market order. *Ann. Rev. Sociol.* 29, 443–464.

Brioschi, F., Buzzachi, L., and Colombo, M. G. (1990). *Gruppi di imprese e mercato finanziario. La struttura del potere nell'industria italiana.* Rome, Italy: Nuova Italia Scientifica.

Brunello, G., Graziano, C., and Parigi, B. M. (2003). CEO turnover in insider-dominated boards: the Italian case. *J. Banking Fin.* 27, 1027–1051.

Burt, R. S. (1979). A structural theory of interlocking corporate directorates. *Soc. Networks* 1, 415–435.

Burt, R. S. (1980). Cooptive corporate actor networks: a reconsideration of interlocking directorates involving American manufacturing. *Adm. Sci. Q.* 25, 557–582.

Burt, R. S. (1983). *Corporate profits and cooptation. Networks of market constraints an directorate ties in the American economy*. New York: Academic Press.

Burt, R. S., Christman, K. P., and Kilburn, Jr. H. C. (1980). Testing a structural theory of corporate cooptation: interorganizational directorate ties as a strategy for avoiding market constraints on profits. *Am. Sociol. Rev.* 45, 821–841.

Buscema, M. and Sacco, P. L. (2008). *Auto-contractive maps, the h function and the maximally regular graph (MRG): a new methodology for data mining*. This volume.

Carpenter, M. A. and Westphal, J. D. (2001). The strategic context of external network ties: examining the impact of director appointments on board involvement in strategic decision making. *Acad. Manage. J.* 4, 639–660.

Chiesi, A. M. (1982). L'Èlite finanziaria italiana. *Rassegna Italiana di Sociologia* 23, 571–595.

Clawson, D. and Neustadtl, A. (1989). Interlocks, PACs, and corporate conservatism. *Am. J. Sociol.* 94, 749–773.

Corrado, R. (2000). Interlocking directorates and the dynamics of intercorporate shareholdings among large Italian firms. *Working Paper Series 146*, University of Bologna.

Dooley, P. C. (1969). The interlocking directorate. *Am. Econ. Rev.* 59, 314–323.

Farina, V. (2007). Potere istituzionale e performane degli intermediari finanziari: analisi del caso italiano. *Working Paper*, Universit‡ Tor Vergata, Rome.

Ferri, F. and Trento, S. (1997). La dirigenza delle grandi banche e delle grandi imprese: ricambio e legami. In Barca, F. (Ed.), *Storia del capitalismo italiano dal dopoguerra ad oggi* (pp. 405–427). Roma: Donzelli.

Fligstein, N. (1995). Networks of power of the finance conception of control? comment on palmer, Barber, Zhou and Soysal. *Am. Soc. Rev.* 60, 500–503.

Fligstein, N. (1996). Markets as politics: a political–cultural approach to market institutions. *Am. Soc. Rev.* 61, 656–673.

Fligstein, N. and Merand, F. (2002). Globalization or Europeanization? evidence on the European economy since 1980. *Acta Sociologica* 45, 7–22.

Fligstein, N. and Choo, J. (2005). Law and corporate governance. *Ann. Rev. Law Soc. Sci.* 1, 61–84.

Galaskiewicz, J., Wasserman, S., Rauschenbach, B., Bielefeld, W., and Mullaney, P. (1985). The influence of corporate power, social status and market position on corporate interlocks in a regional network. *Soc Forces* 64, 403–431.

Galbraith, J. K. (1971). *The new industrial state*. Boston, MA: Houghton Mifflin.

Geletkanycz, M. A. and Hambrick, D. C. (1997). The external ties of top executives: implications for strategic choice and performance. *Adm. Sci. Q.* 42, 654–681.

Granovetter, M. (1985). Economic action and social structure: the problem of embeddedness. *Am. J. Sociol.* 91, 481–510.

Haunschild, P. R. (1993). Interorganizational imitation: the impact of interlocks on corporate acquisition activity. *Adm. Sci. Q.* 38, 564–592.

Haunschild, P. R. and Beckman, C. M. (1998). When do interlocks matter? alternate sources of information and interlock influence. *Adm. Sci. Q.* 43, 815–844.

Koenig, T., Gogel, R., and Sonquist, J. (1979). Models of the significance of interlocking corporate directorates. *Am. J. Econ. Sociol.* 38, 173–186.

Koenig, T. and Gogel, R. (1981). Interlocking corporate directorships as a social network. *Am. J. Econ. Sociol.* 40, 37–50.

Kogut, B. and Walker, G. (2001). The small world of Germany and the durability of national networks. *Am. Sociol. Rev.* 66, 317–335.

Kono, C., Palmer, D., Friedland, R., and Zafonte, M. (1988). Lost in space: the geography of corporate interlocking directorates. *Am. J. Sociol.* 103, 863–911.

Mills, C. W. (1956). *The power elite*. Oxford, UK: Oxford University Press.

Mintz, B. A. and Schwartz, M. (1981). Interlocking directorates and interest group formation. *Am. Sociol. Rev.* 46, 851–869.

Mintz, B. A. and Schwartz, M. (1985). *The power structure of American business*. Chicago, IL: The University of Chicago Press.

Mizruchi, M. S. (1982). *The American corporate network: 1904–1974*. Beverly Hills, CA: Sage.

Mizruchi, M. S. (1989). Similarity of political behavior among large American corporations. *Am. J. Sociol.* 95, 401–424.

Mizruchi, M. S. (1990). Determinants of political opposition among large American corporations. *Soc. Forces* 68, 1065–1088.

Mizruchi, M. S. (1996). What do interlocks do? an analysis, critique, and assessment of research on interlocking directorates. *Ann. Rev. Sociol.* 22, 271–298.

Mizruchi, M. S. (2007). *Power without efficacy: the decline of the American corporate elite*. Working paper, University of Michigan, Ann Arbor.

Mizruchi, M. S. and Stearns L. B. (1988). A longitudinal study of the formation of interlocking directorates. *Adm. Sci. Q.* 33,194–210.

Mizruchi, M. S., Stearns L. B., and Fleischer A. (2008). *Getting a bonus: performance, social networks, and reward among commercial bankers*. Working paper, University of Michigan, Ann Arbor.

Murgia, G. (1986). L'impatto dell'interlocking sulle imprese del settore IT del Lazio: uno studio basato sulla social network analysis. Working Paper, Universita Tor Vergata, Rome.

Ornstein, M. (1984). Interlocking directorates in Canada: intercorporate or class alliance?". *Adm. Sci. Q.* 29, 210–231.

Orr, M. (1997a). The institutional analysis of capitalist economies. In Orr, M., Biggart, N.W., Hamilton, G.G. (Eds.), *The economic organization of East Asian capitalism* (pp. 297–310). Tousand Oaks, CA: Sage.

Orr, M. (1997b). The institutional logic of small-firm economies in Italy and Taiwan. In Orr, M., Biggart, N. W., and Hamilton, G. G. (Eds.), *The economic organization of East Asian capitalism* (pp. 340–367). Tousand Oaks, CA: Sage.

Palmer, D. (1983). Broken ties: interlocking directorates and intercorporate coordination. *Adm. Sci. Q.* 28, 40–55.

Palmer, D. and Barber, B. M. (2001). Challengers, elites, and owning families: a social class theory of corporate acquisitions in the 1960s. *Adm. Sci. Q.* 46, 87–120.

Palmer, D., Friedland, R., and Singh, J. V. (1986). The ties that bind: organizational and class bases of stability in a corporate interlock network. *Am. Sociol. Rev.* 51, 781–796.

Palmer, D., Barber, B. M., Zhou, X., and Soysal, Y. (1995). The friendly and predatory acquisition of large U.S. corporations in the 1960s: the other contested terrain. *Am. Sociol. Rev.* 60, 469–499.

Pennings, J. M. (1980). *Interlocking directorates*. San Francisco, CA: Jossey-Bass.

Pfeffer, J. (1972). Size and composition of corporate boards of directors: the organization and its environment. *Adm. Sci. Q.* 17, 218–228.

Pfeffer, J. and Salancik, G. R. (2003). *The external control of organizations: a resource dependence perspective*. New York: Harper and Row.

Richardson, R. J. (1987). Directorship interlocks and corporate profitability. *Adm. Sci. Q.* 32, 367–386.

Roy, W. G. (1983). Interlocking directorates and the corporate revolution. *Social Sci. History* 7, 143–164.

Scott, J. (1987). Intercorporate structures in Western Europe: a comparative historical analysis. In Mizruchi, M. S. and Schwartz, M. (Eds.), *Intercorporate relations* (pp. 208–232). New York: Cambridge University Press.

Scott, J. (1991). Networks of corporate power: a comparative assessment. *Ann. Rev. Sociol.* 17, 181–203.

Sonquist, J. A. and Koenig, T. (1975). Interlocking directorates in the top US corporations: a graph theory approach. *Critical Sociol.* 5, 196–229.

Stearns, L. B. and Mizruchi, M. S. (1986). Broken-tie reconstitution and the functions of interorganizational interlocks: a reexamination. *Adm. Sci. Q.* 31, 522–538.

Stokman, F. N., Van Der Knoop, J., and Wasseur, F. W. (1988). Interlocks in the Netherlands: stability and careers in the period 1960–1980. *Soc. Networks* 10, 183–208.

Useem, M. (1979). The social organization of the American business elite and participation of corporation directors in the governance of American institutions. *Am. Sociol. Rev.* 44, 553–572.
Useem, M. and Mccormack, A. (1981). The dominant segment of the British business elite. *Sociology* 15, 381–406.
Uzzi, B. (1996). The sources and consequences of embeddedness for the economic performance of organizations: the network effect. *Am. Sociol. Rev.* 61, 674–698.
Uzzi, B. (1997). Social structure and competition in interfirm networks: the paradox of embeddedness. *Adm. Sci. Q.* 42, 35–67.
Vasta, M. and Baccini, A. (1997). Bank and industry in Italy, 1911–1936: new evidence using the interlocking directorates technique. *Financ. Hist. Rev.* 4, 139–159.
Wasserman, S. and Faust, K. (1994). *Social network analysis. methods and applications*. New York: Cambridge University Press.
Westphal, J. D. and Frederickson, J. W. (2001). Who directs strategic change? director experience, the selection of new CEOs, and change in corporate strategy. *Strat. Manage. J.* 22, 1113–1137.
Zajac, E. J. (1988). Interlocking directorates as an interorganizational strategy: a test of critical assumptions. *Acad. Manag. J.* 31, 428–438.
Zang, X. (2001). Resource dependency, Chinese capitalism, and intercorporate ties in Singapore. Working Paper Series no. 6, City University of Hong Kong.

Chapter 13
Multi–Meta-SOM

Giulia Massini

Abstract The Multi-SOM–Meta-SOM system is a supervised ANN model able to create *future maps* of the input. Therefore, it not only is able to correctly classify the input basing on an external target but can also provide information concerning the articulation of classes and their relationships with each other. The Multi-SOM–Meta-SOM system is composed of two different nets: the first one (Multi-SOM) is supervised, while the second one (Meta-SOM), which is not supervised, processes the weights of the first one and reproduces a classificatory output. The Multi-SOMs are influenced by the SOM networks, but they upset their structure, transforming them into supervised networks; the Meta-SOM networks maintain the structure and purposes of the SOMs, but their input is constituted by the models of the input classes created by the Multi-SOMs.

13.1 The Multi-SOM–Meta-SOM System

The Multi-SOM–Meta-SOM system is a supervised RNA model able to create *future maps* of the input. Therefore, it not only is able to correctly classify the input basing on an external target but can also provide information concerning the articulation of classes and their relationships with each other. The Multi-SOM–Meta-SOM system is composed of two different nets: the first one (Multi-SOM) is supervised, while the second one (Meta-SOM), which is not supervised, processes the weights of the first one and reproduces a classificatory output. The Multi-SOMs are influenced by the SOM networks, but they upset their structure, transforming them into supervised networks; the Meta-SOM networks maintain the structure and purposes of the SOMs, but their input is constituted by the models of the input classes created by the Multi-SOMs.

G. Massini (✉)
Semeion Research Center, Via Sersale, Rome, Italy
e-mail: g.massini@semeion.it

V. Capecchi (eds.), *Applications of Mathematics in Models, Artificial Neural Networks and Arts*, DOI 10.1007/978-90-481-8581-8_13,

13.1.1 The SOM Networks

The self-organizing map (SOM) is a neural network attributed to Teuvo Kohonen (Kohonen 1982, 1984, 1990, 1995), who developed it between 1979 and 1982. It is an unsupervised type of network which offers a classification of the input vectors creating a prototype of the classes and a projection of the prototypes on a two-dimensional map (but n-dimensional maps are also possible) that is able to record the relative proximity (or neighbourhood) between the classes.

Therefore, the network offers the following important synthetic information on the input:

1. It operates a classification of the input vectors on the basis of their vector similarity and assigns them to a class.
2. It creates a prototypical model of the classes with the same cardinality (number of variables) as the input vector.
3. It provides a measurement, expressed as a numerical value, of the distance/proximity of the various classes.
4. It creates a relational map of the various classes, placing each class on the map itself.
5. It provides a measurement of the distance/proximity existing between the input vectors from the class they belong to and between the input vectors and other classes.

The relative simplicity of the network architecture allowed its dissemination in terms of how successfully its implementation could be replicated.

13.1.2 SOM: Architecture

A typical SOM network is made up of two layers of units: a one-dimensional input (n-cardinality vector) and a two-dimensional output layer [lines (r) $\times$ columns (c)], also known as Kohonen's map (M matrix of $mr \times mc$ dimensions). A matrix of the weights records the relation between each unit of the output layer and each unit of the input layer [W matrix of ($mr \times mc \times n$) dimensions]. The weight vector connecting each output unit to an input unit is called a "codebook" (vector **wrc** of n-cardinality) (Fig. 13.1). Within the SOM network, each output unit can be interpreted as a class whose codebook represents the prototype.

13.1.3 SOM: Base Algorithm

The SOM algorithm is based on a competitive algorithm founded on the vector quantification principle: at each cycle of life in the network, the unit from Kohonen's layer whose codebook is most similar to the input wins. This unit is given the name of Winner Unit (WU). Consequently, the WU codebook is modified to get it even

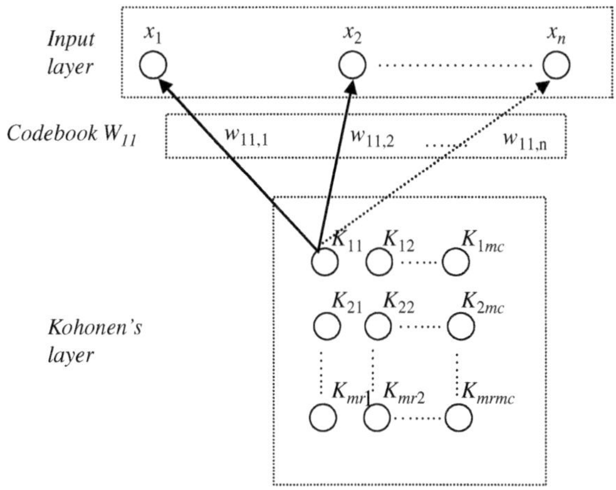

Fig. 13.1 SOM with n-nodes of input, with $(m_r \cdot m_c)$ units of Kohonen's layer. This architecture allows the inputs to be classified into m^2 classes, each being a sub-class represented by a codebook

closer to the input. The codebooks belonging to the units that are physically near the WU (which are part of the neighbourhood) are also put closer to the input of a given delta.

The algorithm calculates a first stage during which the parameters of neighbourhood and corrections of weights are set and the codebook initialization is carried out; this stage is followed by the cyclic stage of codebook adjustment. In this stage the codebooks are modified for the network to classify the input records. In short, the SOM algorithm is organized as follows.

13.1.3.1 Initialization Stage

- Layering of the input vectors;
- Definition of the dimensions (rows × columns) of the matrix which, in its turn, determines the number of classes and therefore of prototypes (codebook);
- Initialization of the codebooks: the value of the vectors of each codebook are random;
- Definition of the function (Gaussian, Mexican hat, etc.) and of the parameters regulating the neighbourhood of the Winner Unit and of the weight correction delta.

13.1.3.2 Cyclic Calibration Stage

- Presentation of the input vectors (pattern) in a random and cyclic way.
- Calculation of the d-activation of the K units of Kohonen's layer: the activation is calculated as vector distance between the input vector X and the weight vector W_j (m_j codebook) which links the K unit to the input nodes.

The classic way to calculate the Euclidean distance between the vectors is as follows:

$$d_j = \|X - W_j\| = \sqrt{\sum_{i=1}^{N} (x_i - w_{ij})^2}$$

- Determination of the winning unit WU: the node of the K layer whose activation is less:

$$\mathrm{WU}{:}d_w = \min_{j \in [1 \ldots M]} \left\{ d_j \; \|X - W_j\| = \sqrt{\sum_{i=1}^{N} (x_i - w_{ij})^2} \right\}$$

- Correction of the codebook (matrix of the W_{ij} weights) of the winning unit and the units adjacent to the winning unit in relation to the function set to determine the level of weight correction according to the input and the proximity to the WU.
- Updating of the factors determining the proximity and layering of the delta correction of the codebooks.

The distinctive characteristic of the SOM is mainly related to the updating of the weights, carried out not only on those related to the WU but also, according to the chosen function, on the weights belonging to the units which are physically close to it. This characteristic also allows the SOM to show the position occupied by the class within the matrix in relation to the position occupied by the other classes. This type of topological mapping, able to organize the classes through spatial relations, has been given the name of *feature mapping*. As will be shown later, this important topological feature was lost when a supervised network which uses, just like the SOMs, a competitive algorithm in the same way of the learning vector quantization (*LVQ*) networks (Kohonen 1988) was tried to be created.

13.1.3.3 Topology of Neighbourhood

The neighbourhood of a WU is defined by the degree of physical proximity (v) existing between the WU and the other K units. Each unit of Kohonen's layer occupies a position on the matrix of the coordinates (r, c) for which the neighbourhood is indexed with a scalar degree from 1 to the maximum line and column dimension:

$$v_i = \pm r \text{ or } v_i = \pm c$$

where max i = max r or max c.

Function $h(v)$ regulates the size of the neighbourhood and the extent of the corrections which need to be made on the codebooks of the units close to the WU. With the passing of time (cycles during which all the training set models are viewed) the neighbourhood is reduced until it disappears; in this case the only unit to which the codebook is corrected is the WU. Since the codebooks are set during the initialization stage with random values within the layering range, the proximity of the WU at the beginning of the learning stage is regulated with a maximum size in order to allow for all the codebooks to be modified and put closer to the input vectors. The reduced proximity with wide matrices can determine the fact that some areas of the K matrix remain isolated because the codebooks are too different from the input vectors. Function $h(v)$ must also allow for the extent of the correction to be bigger for the units close to the WU and therefore to decrease when v is larger. The Gaussian function has been shown to meet these needs remarkably well:

$$h\,(v) = \mathrm{e}^{\frac{v^2}{\sigma}}$$

$$h(v) = \exp(-(\mathrm{SQR}(v)/\sigma))$$

where d is the physical proximity of the unit to the WU and σ is a parameter which linearly decreases by Δ as time increases, thereby modifying the width of the curve (bell) and thus the extent of the neighbourhood. Figures 13.2 and 13.3 show examples of neighbourhood space topologies.

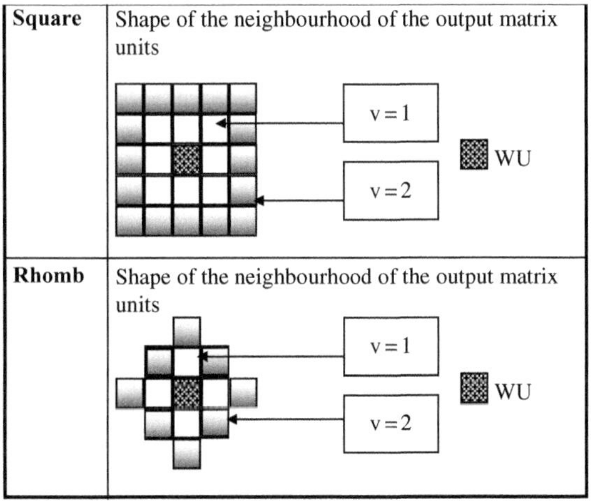

Fig. 13.2 Topology of the neighbourhood space of a Winner Unit in a square and in a rhomb; in the illustration, v is the degree of proximity of the K units to the WU

13.1.4 Correction of the Codebook

The rate of correction a codebook undergoes is determined by various factors:

1. Difference (d) existing between the vector codebook and the input vector;
2. Physical distance to the WU (v);

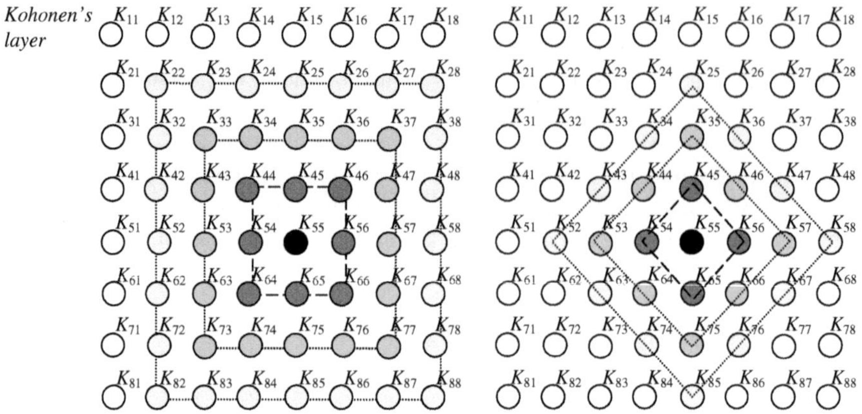

Fig. 13.3 Example of the topology of the neighbourhood space with matrix K ($8r \times 8c$), where the WU is the K_{55} unit. The first matrix shows a neighbourhood in a square, while the second shows a neighbourhood in a rhomb. We can notice from the illustration that, for example, while in the matrix to the left the v distance of the K_{66} unit to the WU is 1, in the matrix to the right the v distance of the K_{66} unit to the WU is 2

3. Function of the neighbourhood $h(v)$ which determines a $\Delta\sigma$; and
4. Function of weight layering in relation to the period of life of the network which determines a $\Delta\alpha$.

In a SOM the *codebooks* are moved closer to the input vector, therefore for each generic *codebook* W, the distance existing between the corresponding weights w_{ij} and the variables x_i of the generic input vector X is calculated as follows:

$$d_j = \left\| X - W_j \right\| = \sqrt{\sum_{i=1}^{N} \left(x_i - w_{ij}\right)^2}$$

On the basis of the function $h(v)$ of the neighbourhood, $\Delta\sigma$ is therefore calculated in relation to the value of the parameter σ and the proximity (v) of the unit K to the WU. $\Delta\sigma$ is the measure which assumes y in the function $h(v)$ when $x = v$. In the case in which function $h(v)$ is the *Gaussian curve*, $\Delta\sigma$ is calculated in the following way (Fig. 13.4):

$$\Delta\sigma = e^{\frac{v^2}{\sigma}}$$

The $\Delta\alpha$ is calculated as a factor of a linear function decreasing in relation to the time the network is alive. Therefore, the function of correction of the *codebooks* is as follows:

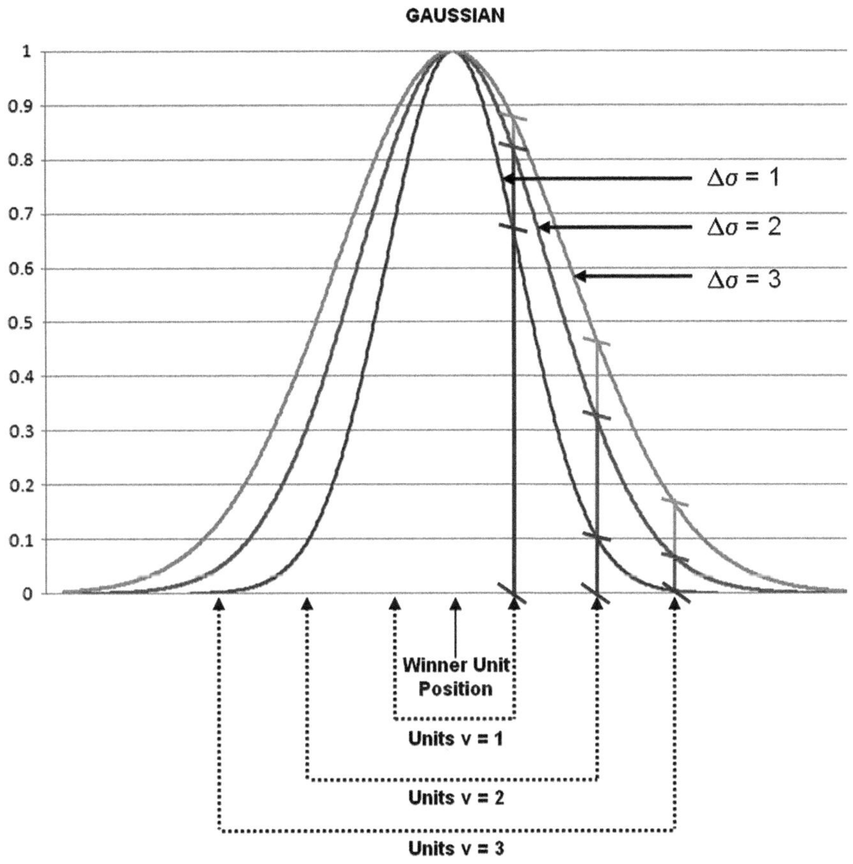

Fig. 13.4 The illustration shows how when the parameter σ (1, 2, 3) changes – parameter that determines the correction curve of the neighbourhood function – the number of units that are part of the neighbourhood and the extent of the correction ($\Delta\sigma$) made on the weights also change

$$f(w) = \alpha \cdot e^{\frac{v^2}{\sigma}} \sqrt{\sum_{i=1}^{N} \left(x_i - w_{ij}\right)^2}$$

$$wij = wij + \alpha(x_i - w_{ij})$$

13.2 The LVQ – Learning Vector Quantization

Teuvo Kohonen worked on the *learning vector quantization* (LVQ) since 1988, drawing on part of the principles of the SOMs: the *vector quantization* and the *construction of prototypes of classes* (*codebook*). However, he created a supervised architecture showing a monodimensional classification layer (it is a vector, not a matrix), contrary to the SOMs. Moreover, the units are regulated by the "winner-take-all" (WTA) competitive principle, allowing the correction only to the codebook, which is most similar to the input. In this way, the very important concept of good neighbourhood of the SOMs is lost in the LVQs and the same happens to the capacity of a faded articulation of spatially contiguous classes.

13.2.1 LVQ: Architecture

An LVQ network is composed of three one-dimensional layers of unit: 1) an input layer (cardinality vector *n*) X_i, *where* $i = (1, 2,\ldots, N)$; 2) a layer of intermediate *K*, also called *Kohonen's* layer [cardinality vector $m = m_c \times m_p$, where *c* is the number of classes, or target, through which the input vectors are articulated and *p* is a multiple through which it is possible to multiply the units that are ready to record the classes; 3) a layer of output O. The units of the *K* layer are indicated as K_j, where $j = (1, 2, \ldots, M)$.

The *K* layer is the effective network layer. The activation of each one of its nodes is calculated, for each cycle, like the vectorial distance (Euclidean, in the most common formation) between the weights vector connected to that unit K_j (codebook V_{ij}) and the pattern vector with input X_i.

The output *O* layer has a number *C* of units, corresponding to the number of classes (cardinality vector *c*). The generic node of the *O* node will be indicated as O_z, where $z = (1, 2, \ldots, C)$. According to the basic formulation, only the unit of the output layer connected with the K_j node is activated for each cycle. Its function is less important, that is, its *codebook* is more similar to the input vector.

It is possible to have connections only between contiguous layers. The input layer is completely connected to the intermediate layer; therefore, the weights matrix W_{ij} is composed of $n \times m$ values. The intermediate layer has specific connections to the output layer: each unit group of the *K* layer belonging to a *C* class is connected to a single output unit. For this reason the weights matrix W_{jz} will record the values of the $c \times (c \times p)$ connections (Figs. 13.5 and 13.6).

13.2.2 LVQ: Base Algorithm

Since the LVQ is a supervised network, it will have a training phase where the network gets skilled to correctly recognize and classify the input vectors. The network will have to be able to assign the input to the nodes of the Kohonen's layer designed for a specific class. In the initialization phase it is decided *how many* and *which* nodes of the intermediate layer are designed for each class and the *codebooks* are initialized with random values. Briefly, the LVQ algorithm is articulated as follows.

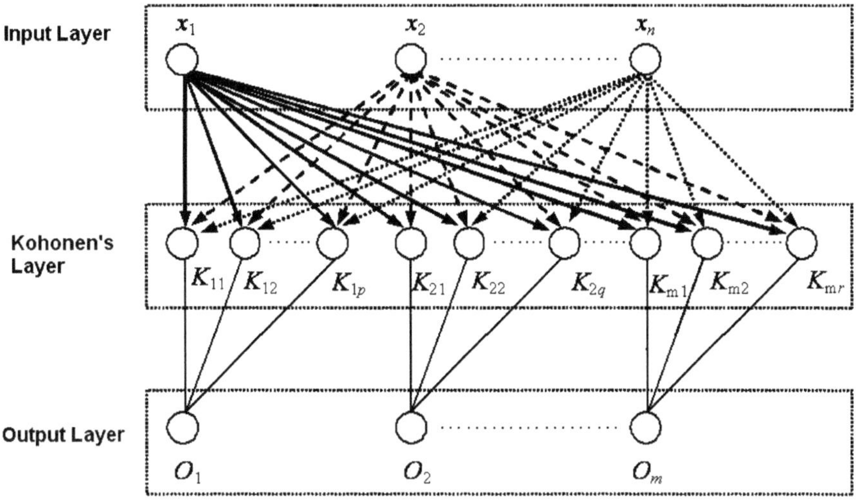

Fig. 13.5 LVQ with n input nodes, having $(p + q + \cdots + r)$ units of the Kohonen's layer with m output nodes. This architecture allows to classify the n inputs into m classes, each class being respectively articulated in $(p, q, \ldots, r)$ sub-classes and each sub-class being represented by a codebook

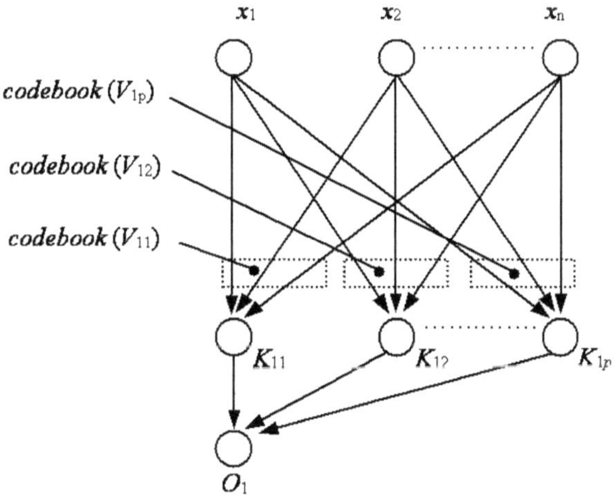

Fig. 13.6 LVQ: representation of the articulation of an O_1 class through vector codebooks $V_1, V_2, \ldots, V_p$

13.2.2.1 Initialization Phase

- Scaling the input vectors;
- Defining the number of units for each class and assigning the class for each unit (intermediate layer);

- Initializing the *codebooks* with random values within a specific range (as shown by the scaling of the input vector).

13.2.2.2 Learning Cyclic Phase

- Presenting the input vector (*pattern*);
- Calculating the activation of K units of the intermediate layer;
- Determining the WU winning unit: node of the intermediate layer K, whose activation is less important;
- Calculating the activation of the output layer units;
- Checking the congruence between the WU class of belonging and the input vector class of belonging;
- Correcting the *codebook* (weights vector w_{ij}) according to the congruence between the input and the output class of belonging.

13.2.2.3 Correction of the Codebook (Matrix of the W_{ij} Weights)

According to the Winner Takes All (WTA) logic, only the weights connecting the Winner Unit to the input layer are corrected, according to the following two alternative modalities:

Right classification: approaching of the weights vector, *codebook* m_c, of the WU to the input vector:

$$m_c(t+1) = m_c(t) + \alpha(t)\,[x(t) - m_c(t)]$$

Wrong classification: detachment of the weights vector, *codebook* m_c, of the WU from the input vector:

$$m_c(t+1) = m_c(t) - \alpha(t)\,[x(t) - m_c(t)]$$

where x is the input vector; m_c is the WU vector; t represents how many times all patterns were exposed to the cycle of the network learning phase (epochs).

The parameter α (*learning rate*) can be steady or decreasing with respect to t: $0 > \alpha(t) < 1$.

13.3 The Multi-SOM–Meta-SOM System

The system is a supervised network not only providing input classifications but also creating its local *feature map* on the classes and the global *feature map* on the phenomenology.

In the study of a phenomenology articulable in classes, the system's aim is to answer to the needs of studying the complex, not linear, relations existing between the classes and the variables characterizing the same classes. In the study of an instance, it wants to give an answer to the need to identify the class of belonging and the relations that this instance has with the other elements of the same and the other classes. The system is particularly useful when the classes are not linearly separable and when it is necessary to understand the relations between classes.

13.3.1 Multi-SOM: Classification and Mapping of the Input in Separate Classes

The Multi-SOM begins from the attempt of the author to create a supervised network that is not only able to correctly classify the input but also able to sub-articulate the classes through the creation of prototypes. The Multi-SOM is a supervised classificator able to classify inputs on the basis of external targets and is a spontaneous classificator of the sub-classifications of these classes.

This last important feature, which is a direct heritage of the SOMs, allows to have important information about the classes and it permits to study their implicit logic.

This is very useful when the classes are not separated in a linear way and then in each class there can be complex input articulations involving more factors.

13.3.2 Architecture

A Multi-SOM network is composed of a one-dimensional input layer (cardinality vector *n*) X_i, *where* $i = (1, 2, \ldots, N)$, and a two-dimensional multi-layer M having classificatory and output function, composed of Q (number of classes or targets) square matrices having dimensions $M = m_r \times m_c$ indicated as M_l, $l = (1, 2, \ldots, Q)$. Each K cell (or unit) of this multi-layer is detected by K_j^{Ml}, where the apex Ml represents the matrix of belonging, and by $j = (1, 2, \ldots, C)$, where C is the product of the matrix dimensions ($m_r\ m_c$). Each matrix is associated with a single target.

It is possible to find connections only between layers: the input layer is totally connected to the output layer. The vector registering the connections between each unit of the output layer and all units of the input layer is called codebook $(m_j)^{Ml}$. The codebooks have the same cardinality of the input and their function is to create prototypes of the input. Instead, the cells composing the different matrices of the output layer classify the inputs through the codebooks (Fig. 13.7).

13.3.3 Basic Facts

In a Multi-SOM, each matrix is associated with a single target (or class) and a target is associated with just one matrix. Consequently, there are as many matrices as the targets.

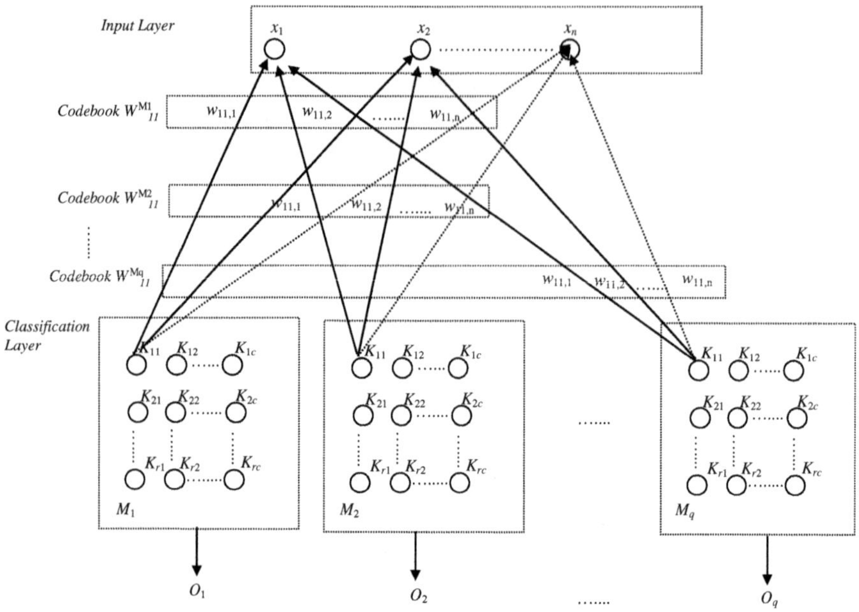

Fig. 13.7 Multi-SOM with n input nodes, with $(r \times c \times q)$ units of the Kohonen's layer organized as q matrices $(r \times c)$ and with q output. This architecture allows to classify the records (composed of n inputs) into q classes, each class being, respectively, articulated on a matrix of $r \times c$ sub-classes and each sub-class being represented by a codebook

Therefore, given the Q classification matrices, some basic facts concerning the Multi-SOM networks have to be considered:

- Winner Matrix (WM)
  - *Virtual Winner Matrix* (WM^V)
- Winner Unit (WU)
  - *Global Winner Unit* (WU^G)
  - *Local Winner Unit* (WU^L)

In the SOM networks, a *Winner Unit* indicates the output unit having the least activation value (d_{min}) for each cycle and with respect to the model of input; its codebook is, in fact, most similar to the input vector. In the Multi-SOMs the concept of *Winner Unit* is replaced with that of *Local Winner Unit* (WU^L), when it is referred to the unit having globally the least activation in each matrix (*M*), and that of *Global Winner Unit* (WU^G), when it is referred to the unit having globally the least activation of all the *Local Winner Units* (WU^L).

Moreover, at each training cycle, given an input vector, the matrix whose class or target of belonging corresponds to the input class or the target of belonging is

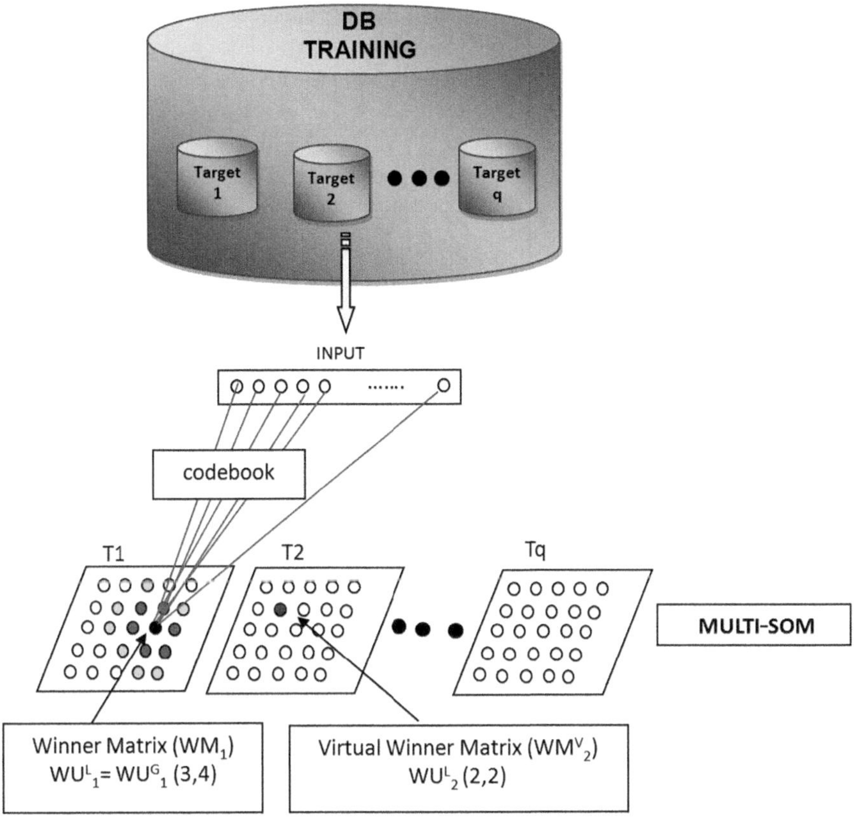

Fig. 13.8 Multi-SOM: the figure shows an example of wrong classification, where a target 2 vector in input finds a more similar codebook in the target 1 matrix

defined as *virtual Winner Matrix* (WM). Instead, the *Winner Matrix* (WM) is the matrix containing the *Global Winner Unit* (regardless of being the right matrix or not). In the training phase, if the indexes i of the WM^V and WM correspond, then this means that the input model is classified correctly. As a consequence, the correction feature of the codebooks will be different, depending on whether the matrix is the right or the wrong one (Fig. 13.8).

13.3.4 Base Algorithm

13.3.4.1 Initialization Phase

- Scaling the input vectors;
- Defining the dimensions of each matrix and creating the Q matrices in a number equal to the Q classes to which the input vectors belong;

- Pre-assigning each matrix to only one of the Q classes;
- Initializing the *codebooks*;
- Defining the function (*Gaussian, Mexican hat, etc.*) and the parameters regulating the correction of the WU weights (*codebook*) and of the unit weights composing their neighbourhood, respectively.

13.3.4.2 Training Cyclic Phase

- Presenting the input vectors (*patterns*) in a random and cyclic way;
- Calculating the d-activation of the units K_j of the Q matrices (M_l): the activation is calculated, as in the SOMs and in the LVQs, on the basis of the vectorial distance between the input vector X_i and the weights vector W_j^{Ml}(*codebook*$_{ji}$) connecting that unit K_j^{Ml} to the input units.

  A possible way to calculate the *Euclidean distance* between the vectors is as follows:

$$d_j = \left\| X - W_j^{Ml} \right\| = \sqrt{\sum_{i=1}^{N} \left(x_i - w_{ji}^{Ml} \right)^2}$$

  When d is equal to zero, the input vector and the codebook have the same values; when d increases, the difference between both vectors also increases.
- Determining the winning $\mathrm{WU^L}$ unit for each matrix and then the $\mathrm{WU^G}$, with the $\mathrm{WU^L}$ having d with less value:

$$\mathrm{WU^L}{:}d_w = \min_{j\in[1..C]} \left\{ d_j \left\| X - W_j \right\| = \sqrt{\sum_{i=1}^{N} \left(x_i - w_{ji} \right)^2} \right\}$$

where C = number of codebooks in a matrix

$$\mathrm{WU^G}{:}d_w = \min_{l\in[1..Q]} (WU_l^L)$$

where Q = number of matrices = number of targets.

- Checking the congruence between the class of belonging of the $\mathrm{WU^G}$ and of the input vector;
- Correcting the *codebooks* according to the congruence between input and output class of belonging:
- *Right classification:* $\mathrm{WU^G} = \mathrm{WU^v}$.

  Approach of the $\mathrm{WU^G}$ weights vector (*codebook* m_j^{Ml}) and the codebooks belonging to its neighbourhood to the input vector:

$$w_{ji}^{M_l}(t+1) = w_{ji}^{M_l}(t) + \Delta w_{ji}^{M_l}$$

$$\Delta w_{ji}^{M_l} = \alpha \cdot e^{\frac{v^2}{\sigma}} \cdot \left(x_i - w_{ji}^{M_L}\right)$$

Since v indicates the distance from the WU^G, v will be 1 when the w values refer to the WU^G codebook, while it will increase depending on the distance from the WU^G. Consequently, the correction delta will decrease. This means that the correction is greater for the WU^G codebook and it will decrease more and more as the units go far from the WU^G.

- *Wrong classification*: WU^G <> WU^V.

  If the classification is wrong, then the weights of two matrices will be modified: the one where there is the WU^G and the one which was supposed to win. However, the correction is made with opposed modality. If in the first case the weights of the WU^G and its neighbourhood are pushed far from the model of the quantity Δw, in the second case the weights of the WM^V will be approached in the same quantity.

  Therefore, there will be two situations:

  (a) *Detachment* of the WU^G weights vector (*codebook* m_j^{Ml}) and of the codebook belonging to its neighbourhood from the input vector:

$$w_{ji}^{M_L}(t+1) = w_{ji}^{M_L}(t) - \Delta w_{ji}^{M_l}$$

  (b) *Approaching* of the WM^V weights vector (*codebook* m_j^{Ml}) and of the codebook belonging to its neighbourhood to the input vector:

$$w_{ji}^{M_L}(t+1) = w_{ji}^{M_l}(t) + \Delta w_{ji}^{M_l}$$

13.3.4.3 Testing Phase

The testing phase of the network is similar to that concerning the most known supervised networks; a sample of pattern, which was never visualized by the network, is set and the ability of the network to classify on the basis of the percentage of correctly classified pattern with respect to the sample is evaluated.

In the Multi-SOM network the different input vectors are visualized one by one and the distance from the codebooks of all Q matrices with the same vectorial distance function d, used in the training phase, is calculated. Since in the training phase a target was assigned to each matrix, the input vector is classified on the basis of the matrix containing the codebook with the minor distance (*min* activation of the unitK_j^{Ml}). The output of each matrix is therefore the value of activation of its own WU^L. The global output is the matrix index whose WU^L has the minor activation.

13.3.5 Conclusions

The network provides the following important brief information about the input of the training phase:

a. Ability to provide a supervised classification of the input, dividing it into classes based on the vectorial similarity;
b. Ability to provide more than a prototypical model of each class having the same input cardinality (codebook);
c. Ability to provide a brief value of the distance/proximity between the different sub-classes;
d. Ability to provide a relational map of the different sub-classes, positioning them on the maps itself (indexes on the matrices);
e. Ability to provide a brief value of the distance/proximity between the inputs from the class of belonging and from the other classes.

   Moreover, for each pattern of the testing or recall sample, it provides the following information:

f. Classification of the input, assigning it to the unit which has, within all matrices, the most similar codebook. The input is therefore associated with the matrix class containing the WU^G.
g. The WU^G activation value *d* measures the similarity of that pattern to the sub-class of belonging.
h. The position of the WU^G in its matrix provides information concerning the relation between that pattern and the other sub-classes.
i. The WU^L generated by that pattern in the other matrices, as their respective activation value *d*, indicates how that pattern is different from the models of each sub-class.
j. The exact analysis, that is, a value assumed by each variable in the pattern vector of input, with respect to the values of the same variables in the codebook of both the WU^G and the WU^L, like potentially any other codebook, gives information about the quantity of the difference.

13.4 From the Multi-SOM to the Meta-SOM

In the Multi–Meta-SOM system, the Multi-SOM is able to sub-articulate the classes used to set up the phenomenon to be observed and it can also create a prototype (codebook) for each one of these classes.

At the end of the training phase it is possible to detect important information about the relation between the different sub-classifications and about the sample by analysing the following factors:

- The vectorial difference between prototypes (codebooks): brief measurement of the similarity between prototypes.
- The physical distance between prototypes: brief measurement resulting from the corresponding position of the matrix cells, each one of them bound to a single codebook.
- The difference between the variable values in the prototypes: it is possible to compare the value assumed by a single variable in a prototype with the same variable in the other prototypes.
- The analysis of the sub-samples concerning a codebook as its own prototype: each sub-sample can be analysed with statistical measurements such as average, variation.
- The comparison between different sub-samples.

The Multi-SOM capacity to sub-articulate a class into prototypes, maintaining the same vectorial format of the input (cardinality), allows to newly encode these prototypes as inputs for a new network.

The Multi-SOM is able to compress the initial information from a qualitative point of view, representing in the diversification of the codebooks the implicit variety in the initial macro-classes.

In the Meta–Multi-SOM system, it is possible to find a very important process occurring in the initialization phase: the *dimensioning of the matrices*. According to the functions and parameters regulating the neighbourhood of a unit and to the function regulating the weights correction rate, this process must be aimed to articulate the sub-samples so that there will be no empty sub-samples, but rather samples tending to be greater than the two units. This bond suggests that if the initial inputs were equally distributed on the matrices in order to have Q matrices of the same dimensions, then these matrices should be at least a half of the class having less numerousness than the Q initial classes. It is clear that the internal inconsistent distribution of each class and the need not to have cells unable to encode any input compel to find matrices having shortened dimensions.

Each one of the new inputs composed of prototypes, resulting from the qualitative compression made by the Multi-SOM, is associated with a target based on the Multi-SOM matrix of belonging. Therefore, they are organized in Q samples having the same numerousness of the dimensions of a Multi-SOM matrix $(m_r \cdots m_c)$. This group of Multi-SOM prototypes is called a Meta sample.

Therefore, given Q initial classes and Q Multi-SOM matrices having dimensions $c = m_r \cdot \cdot m_c$, the Meta sample composed of Multi-SOMs codebooks will be formed by $C \cdot Q$ input pattern and articulated in Q classes, each one composed of C vectors.

13.5 Meta-SOM

The term Meta-SOM indicates a SOM network where inputs are composed of the codebooks resulting from a Multi-SOM and associated with a target: the Multi-SOM matrix of belonging. The Meta-SOM matrix is set with a number of units equal at least to the number of correlated Multi-SOM codebooks. In the last epoch, at the end of the training phase, the target is assigned to each Meta-SOM matrix unit, letting flow all inputs (that is, the Multi-SOM codebooks); the input target is associated with each WU Meta-SOM cycle.

At the end, it is possible to find three kinds of output units Km_rm_c depending on how the network classified the inputs:

- *Classificatory units*: matrix cells where inputs coming from a single target are placed.
- *Non-classificatory units*: it is possible to find them every time the number of Meta-SOM matrix cells is greater than the number of Multi-SOM codebooks. In these cells, no training sample input is placed.
- *Ambiguous units*: cells where inputs coming from different targets are placed.

Therefore, each Meta-SOM Km_rm_c cell is associated with two percentage vectors, both composed of as many fields as the targets:

1. Percentage of subjects classified by the Km_rm_c cell belonging to the target l with respect to the total number of subjects concerning that target l traceable in the training sample;
2. Percentage of subjects classified by the Km_rm_c cell belonging to the target l with respect to all subjects registered in that cell j (Figs. 13.9 and 13.10).

13.6 An Example: The Classification of Digits

13.6.1 The DB

The DB is composed of 1593 digits [0, 1, 2, ..., 9] originally handwritten by adult people and then transformed into binary value digital pictures; the value "1" was used to mark the form of the picture and the value "0" was used to show the background (the DB was created by the Tattile company of Brescia). People had to write the 10 digits twice on a sheet of paper: the first time slowly and the second time quickly.

The digits obtained were scanned and then normalized in a 16×16 pixel format, having as a result 256 pixels for each picture (Figs. 13.11 and 13.12).

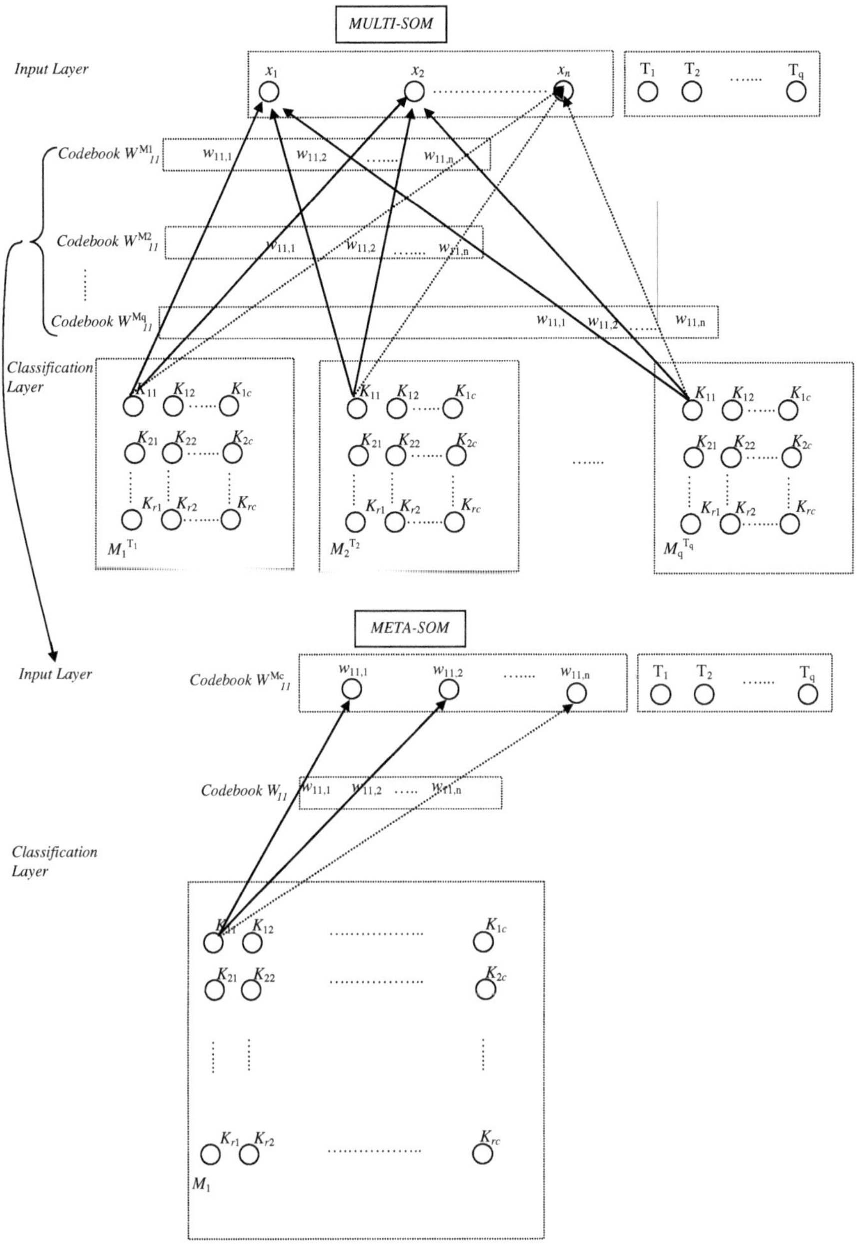

Fig. 13.9 Architecture of the Multi–Meta-SOM system

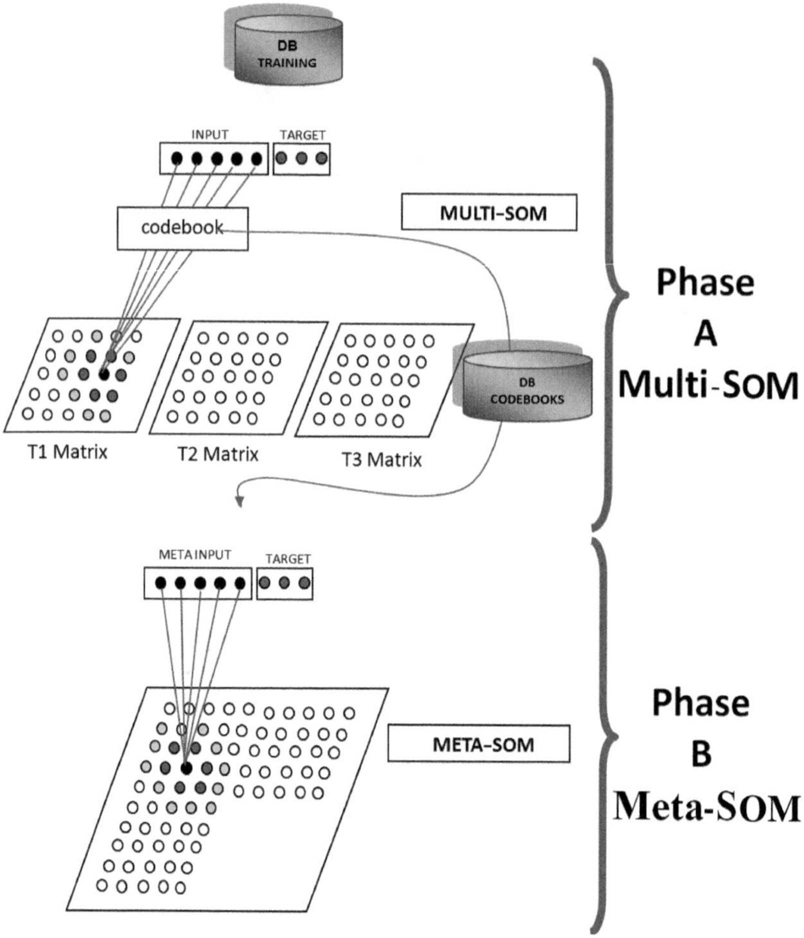

Fig. 13.10 Training process in the Multi–Meta-SOM system: the input of the Multi-SOMs is composed of the DB record values, while the input of the Meta-SOMs is composed of the so-called Multi-SOM codebook values. In phase A, it gets skilled with the Multi-SOM network and it is possible to define its codebooks. In phase B, it will be the Meta-SOM input

13.6.2 The Training–Testing Samples

In order to proceed with the experiment, the DB was divided at random into two sub-samples: the *training* sample composed of 797 digits and the *recall* sample composed of the remaining 796 digits (Figs. 13.13 and 13.14).

The following tableshows the composition of both samples divided with respect to the target typology.

Each input pattern is a record composed of 256 values forming a number (value 1 for the form, value 0 for the background) and of 10 values defining the target; only

0	0	0	0	0	1	1	1	1	1	1	1	1	0	0	0
0	0	0	0	0	1	1	0	0	0	0	1	1	1	0	0
0	0	0	0	1	1	0	0	0	0	0	0	1	1	1	0
0	0	0	0	1	1	0	0	0	0	0	0	0	1	1	0
0	1	1	0	1	1	0	0	0	0	0	0	0	0	1	1
1	1	0	0	0	0	0	0	0	0	0	0	0	0	1	1
1	1	0	0	0	0	0	0	0	0	0	0	0	0	1	1
1	1	0	0	0	0	0	0	0	0	0	0	0	0	1	1
1	1	0	0	0	0	0	0	0	0	0	0	0	0	1	1
1	1	0	0	0	0	0	0	0	0	0	0	0	0	1	0
1	1	0	0	0	0	0	0	0	0	0	0	0	1	1	0
1	1	0	0	0	0	0	0	0	0	0	0	1	1	1	0
1	1	1	0	0	0	0	0	0	0	0	0	1	1	0	0
0	1	1	1	0	0	0	0	0	1	1	1	1	0	0	0
0	0	1	1	1	1	1	0	1	1	1	1	0	0	0	0
0	0	0	1	1	1	1	1	1	1	0	0	0	0	0	0

Fig. 13.11 Model of the first record of the digit DB reproducing a zero: the values "1" represent the picture and the values "0" represent the background

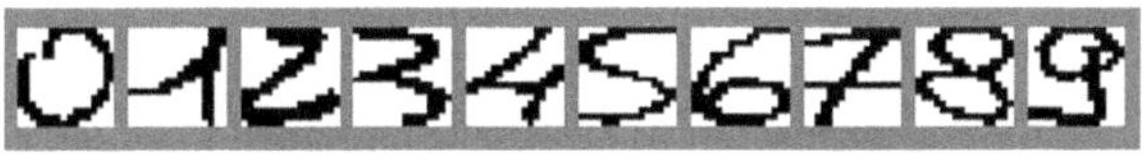

Fig. 13.12 Example of the 10 input typologies of the digit DB

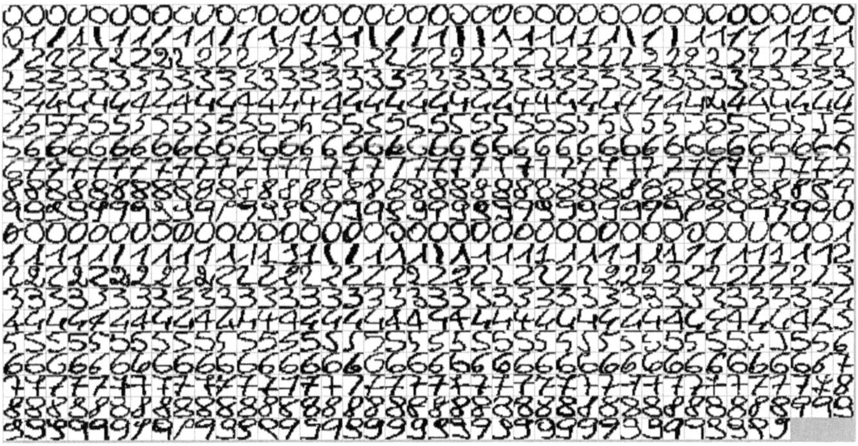

Fig. 13.13 The 797 digits of the training sample

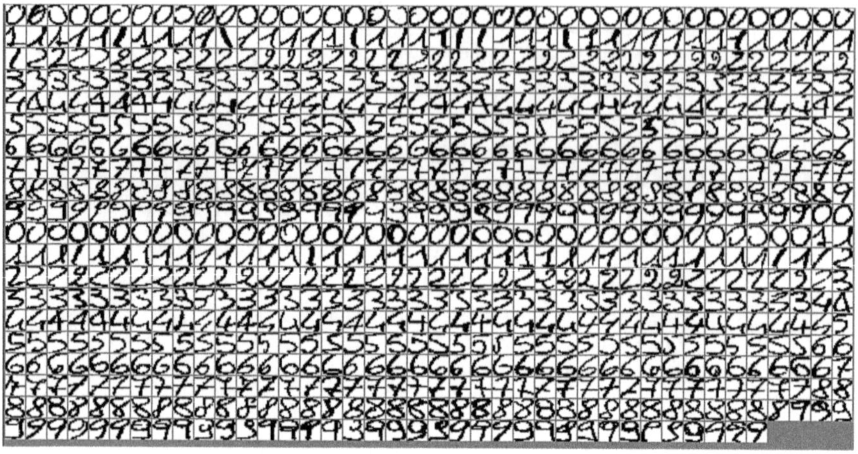

Fig. 13.14 The 796 digits of the recall sample

Models	Training	Testing	Sample
Zero	81	80	161
One	80	82	162
Two	80	79	159
Three	80	79	159
Four	80	81	161
Five	80	79	159
Six	80	81	161
Seven	79	79	158
Eight	77	78	155
Nine	80	78	158
TOT	797	796	1593

one of them is set as 1 (picture belonging to the target), while the other nine values are set as 0.

13.6.3 Structure of the Multi-SOM

In order to proceed with the training, 10 matrices were created, each one of them having dimensions equal to 5×5. The codebooks concerning each matrix cell are composed of 256 unit vector, encoding the 16×16 pictures, which represent the numbers.

For the correction of the WU codebooks and its neighbourhood, it was outlined the Gaussian function, where σ, initially equal to 1, at each epoch decreases of 0.01. The square form was chosen as the topology of the neighbourhood. The codebooks correction Δw was scaled of a factor α; when it was initialized to 1, it decreased of 0.01 at each epoch:

$$w_{ji}^{M_l}(t+1) = w_{ji}^{M_l}(t) \pm \Delta w_{ji}^{M_l} \tag{13.1}$$

$$\Delta w_{ji}^{M_l} = \alpha \cdot e^{\frac{v^2}{\sigma}} \cdot \left(x_i - w_{ji}^{M_l}\right) \tag{13.2}$$

where

$$\sigma(t+1) = \sigma(t) - 0.01 \ \ (\text{per } \sigma > 0)$$

$$\alpha(t+1) = \alpha(t) - 0.01 \ \ (\text{per } \alpha > 0)$$

In the initialization phase, random weights were assigned to the codebooks.

13.6.4 The Multi-SOM Training

The training lasted 100 epochs. At the end, the 250 codebooks of the 10 matrices were as shown in Fig 13.15.

The figure allows seeing that each matrix is specialized for the encoding of a number and that within it the spatial distribution of the different codebooks is appropriate; the prototypes of the numbers are assigned to the matrix cells so that it is possible to put the most similar ones after another. In Fig. 13.16, for example, it is important to remark that the first codebook of the first matrix represents a zero (cell 1,1 of the matrix 1 placed at the upper left corner of the figure). It is possible to see the values effectively constituting that codebook, as a descriptive example, in the figure.

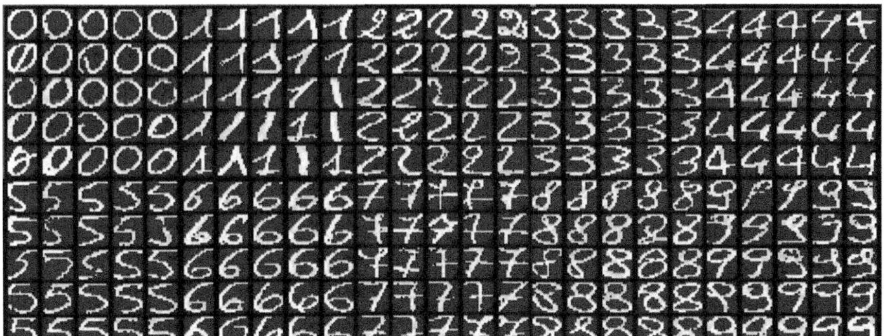

Fig. 13.15 Configuration of the 256 codebooks belonging to the 10 Multi-SOM matrices, using colours. In the picture, the side-by-side distribution of the 10 matrices is arbitrary, as they are spatially independent of each other; instead, the spatial disposition of the 25 codebooks of each matrix is not arbitrary

	1	2	3	4	5	6	7	8	9	10	11	12	13	14	15	16
1	0.00	0.00	0.00	0.28	1.00	1.00	1.00	1.00	1.00	1.00	1.00	1.00	0.85	0.71	0.00	0.00
2	0.00	0.00	0.62	1.00	1.00	0.86	0.66	0.28	0.14	0.00	0.15	0.29	1.00	1.00	0.28	0.00
3	0.00	0.49	1.00	1.00	0.64	0.28	0.36	0.00	0.00	0.00	0.00	0.00	0.44	1.00	1.00	0.28
4	0.20	1.00	1.00	0.77	0.00	0.14	0.00	0.00	0.00	0.00	0.00	0.00	0.00	0.64	1.00	0.80
5	0.64	1.00	1.00	0.00	0.00	0.00	0.00	0.00	0.00	0.00	0.00	0.00	0.00	0.29	1.00	1.00
6	1.00	1.00	0.62	0.00	0.00	0.00	0.00	0.00	0.00	0.00	0.00	0.00	0.00	0.00	1.00	1.00
7	1.00	0.77	0.14	0.00	0.00	0.00	0.00	0.00	0.00	0.00	0.00	0.00	0.00	0.00	0.77	1.00
8	1.00	0.77	0.00	0.00	0.00	0.00	0.00	0.00	0.00	0.00	0.00	0.00	0.00	0.00	1.00	1.00
9	1.00	0.77	0.20	0.00	0.00	0.00	0.00	0.00	0.00	0.00	0.00	0.00	0.00	0.29	1.00	1.00
10	1.00	0.77	0.34	0.20	0.00	0.00	0.00	0.00	0.00	0.00	0.00	0.00	0.14	0.67	1.00	0.57
11	1.00	1.00	0.29	0.00	0.00	0.00	0.00	0.00	0.00	0.00	0.00	0.00	0.52	1.00	1.00	0.00
12	0.86	1.00	0.80	0.14	0.00	0.00	0.00	0.00	0.00	0.00	0.00	0.52	0.80	1.00	0.49	0.00
13	0.35	1.00	1.00	0.64	0.00	0.00	0.00	0.00	0.00	0.38	0.80	1.00	1.00	0.49	0.00	0.00
14	0.00	0.28	1.00	1.00	0.64	0.44	0.44	0.67	0.67	0.80	1.00	0.77	0.49	0.00	0.00	0.00
15	0.00	0.00	0.14	0.80	1.00	1.00	1.00	1.00	1.00	1.00	0.77	0.00	0.00	0.00	0.00	0.00
16	0.00	0.00	0.00	0.14	0.51	0.65	1.00	0.58	1.00	0.28	0.00	0.00	0.00	0.00	0.00	0.00

Fig. 13.16 Values of the Multi-SOM codebook $m_{1,1}{}^{Ml}$ (cell 1,1 of the matrix 1). The values are rounded to two decimals. Moreover, in order to make the reading easier, the cells with value 1 are shown in white, the cells with values between 0 and 1 in light grey and the cells with value 0 in *dark grey*

13.6.5 The Multi-SOM Testing

The testing was made on the remaining 796 sample digits. The codebooks obtained at the end of the training phase were determined and the records of the 796 testing sample digits were inserted one by one. For each record the Winner Matrix was registered; it was compared with the target of the record itself and the faults were counted. When the Winner Matrix did not coincide with the input vector target, it means that there is a fault.

FF_Bp24.nnr													
Conf Mat	Out 1	Out 2	Out 3	Out 4	Out 5	Out 6	Out 7	Out 8	Out 9	Out 10	Row Total	Errors	Accuracy
Target 0	75	0	1	0	2	0	0	0	2	0	80	5	93.75%
Target 1	0	69	4	1	3	0	1	4	0	0	82	13	84.15%
Target 2	0	3	64	4	0	1	1	0	5	1	79	15	81.01%
Target 3	0	0	0	67	1	3	0	1	1	6	79	12	84.81%
Target 4	1	5	0	0	72	2	1	0	0	0	81	9	88.89%
Target 5	0	0	2	2	0	71	1	1	1	1	79	8	89.87%
Target 6	1	0	1	0	0	0	78	1	0	0	81	3	96.30%
Target 7	0	3	1	4	4	0	0	66	0	1	79	13	83.54%
Target 8	0	3	7	2	1	0	3	0	60	2	78	18	76.92%
Target 9	3	0	1	3	1	1	0	2	1	66	78	12	84.62%
Col Total	80	83	81	83	84	78	85	75	70	77	796	108	

A.Mean Acc 86.39%
W.Mean Acc 86.43%

FF_Sn24.nnr													
Conf Mat	Out 1	Out 2	Out 3	Out 4	Out 5	Out 6	Out 7	Out 8	Out 9	Out 10	Row Total	Errors	Accuracy
Target 0	75	0	0	0	2	1	0	0	2	0	80	5	93.75%
Target 1	0	80	1	0	1	0	0	0	0	0	82	2	97.56%
Target 2	0	3	70	1	0	2	1	0	1	1	79	9	88.61%
Target 3	0	1	0	73	0	1	0	1	1	2	79	6	92.41%
Target 4	0	5	0	0	73	1	1	0	1	0	81	8	90.12%
Target 5	0	0	2	3	1	72	0	0	1	0	79	7	91.14%
Target 6	0	0	0	0	3	2	74	0	2	0	81	7	91.36%
Target 7	0	5	2	2	1	0	1	67	1	0	79	12	84.81%
Target 8	1	1	5	1	0	0	1	0	67	2	78	11	85.90%
Target 9	1	1	0	3	1	2	0	1	2	67	78	11	85.90%
Col Total	77	96	80	83	82	81	78	69	78	72	796	78	

A.Mean Acc 90.15%
W.Mean Acc 90.20%

Fig. 13.17 Testing results with classical feedforward backpropagation networks

Similarly, training and testing were made on the two samples using classical feedforward backpropagation networks. Later, there was a comparison of the performances of both networks (Figs. 13.17 and 13.18).

As it is possible to see, the values resulting from the testing can be compared in both kinds of network.

Multi-SOM 5x5x10

	0	1	2	3	4	5	6	7	8	9	Row Total	Errors	Accuracy
Target 0	76	0	1	0	1	0	1	0	1	0	80	4	95%
Target 1	0	75	2	0	0	2	0	3	0	0	82	7	91.46%
Target 2	0	2	73	1	0	1	0	0	1	1	79	6	92.41%
Target 3	0	0	0	75	0	1	0	0	1	2	79	4	94.94%
Target 4	0	5	3	0	72	0	0	0	0	1	81	9	88.89%
Target 5	0	0	1	4	0	67	0	0	1	6	79	12	84.81%
Target 6	2	0	0	0	0	2	76	1	0	0	81	5	93.83%
Target 7	0	8	1	0	2	0	0	67	1	0	79	12	84.81%
Target 8	0	2	6	2	0	1	1	1	63	2	78	15	80.77%
Target 9	1	0	0	6	1	2	0	0	5	63	78	15	80.77%
Col Total	79	92	87	88	76	76	78	72	73	75	796	89	88.77%

A.Mean Acc. 88.77%
W.Mean 88.82%

Fig. 13.18 Testing results with the Multi-SOM having 10 matrices, each one composed of 5 × 5 codebooks

13.7 From the Multi-SOM Codebooks to the Meta-SOM Training

The Multi-SOM codebooks are used as sample of training for the Multi-SOMs. The training sample will therefore be composed of 250 digits (the Multi-SOM codebooks) split for the 10 targets, each one with 25 records. The following table shows the composition of the sample divided with respect to its target typology.

Models	Training
Zero	25
One	25
Two	25
Three	25
Four	25
Five	25
Six	25
Seven	25
Eight	25
Nine	25
TOT	250

Each input pattern (codebook) is a record composed of 256 values defining a number (values between 1 and 0) and of 10 values defining the target. Only 1 of these 10 values is set as 1 (picture belonging to the target), while the other 9 values are set as 0.

13.7.1 Set-Up of the Meta-SOM Network

As was already explained, the Meta-SOM network is a normal SOM network, but its initially random codebook values are modified during the training of a Multi-SOM codebook vision.

The dimensions of the matrix are decided according to the number of codebooks coming from the Multi-SOM, which will have to be checked by the Meta-SOM network. The number of cells must be preferentially equal or greater than the number of Multi-SOM codebooks.

Since there are 250 codebooks in the Multi-SOM, in this case a Meta-SOM matrix with dimensions equal to 16×16, composed of 256 codebooks, was created. If each one of these 250 initial codebooks was on a cell of the new Meta-SOM network, six cells would remain outside and it would be impossible to assign them a target.

Each one of the new codebooks of each matrix cell in turn is composed of 256 unit vector, encoding a 16×16 picture.

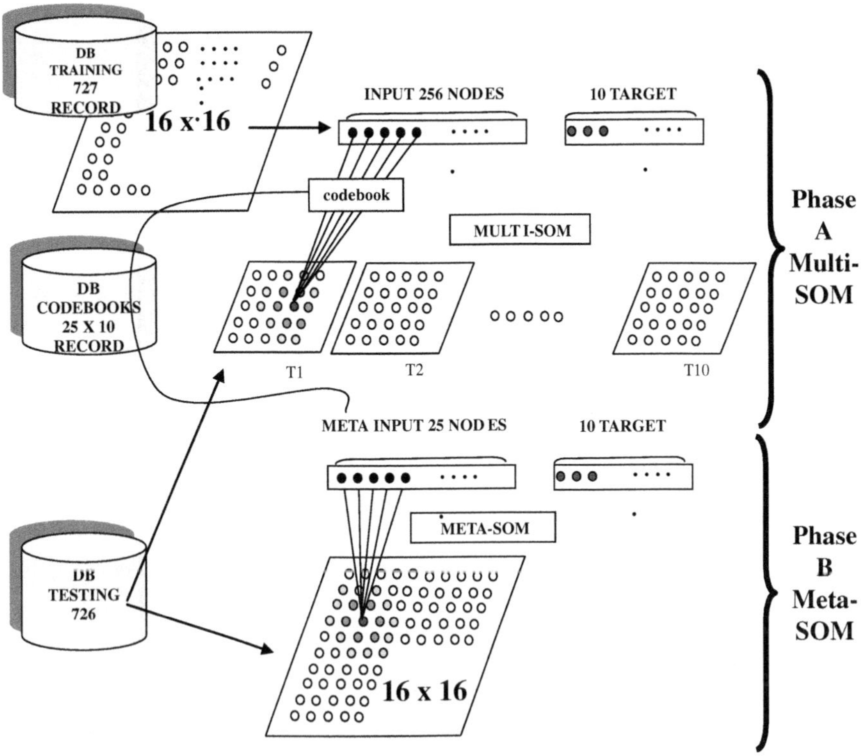

Fig. 13.19 Training process in the Multi–Meta-SOM system within the experiment on the digit DB

The correction parameters of the weights and the neighbourhood were set up as those of the Multi-SOMs (Fig. 13.19).

13.7.1.1 Training of the Meta-SOM Network

The Meta-SOM training lasted 100 epochs; at each epoch the 250 codebooks of the 10 Multi-SOM matrices were visualized at random (Fig. 13.20).

At the end of the training phase, a target is associated with each matrix cell of the Meta-SOM, letting flow the 250 input patterns one by one (the 250 codebooks of the 10 Multi-SOM matrices) and registering which cell is more representative for them (Winner Unit) (Figs. 13.21 and 13.22).

13.7.2 Recall in Multi–Meta-SOM System

When both Multi and Meta-SOM networks have learned and both completed the training phase, testing consisted of the following phases:

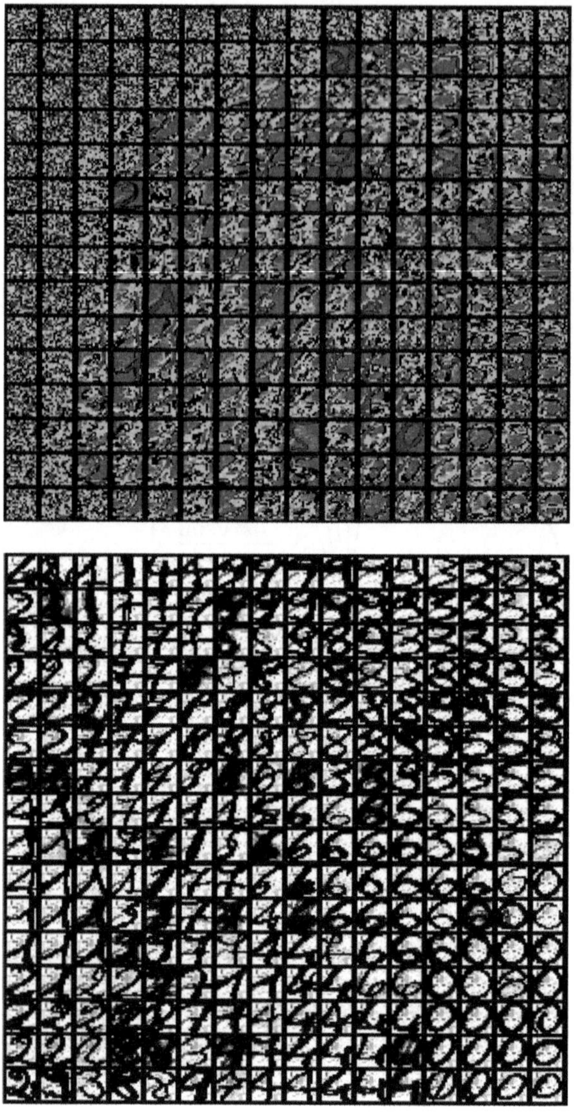

Fig. 13.20 The picture on the left shows a moment of the Meta-SOM training phase, when the codebooks are going to be formed on the model of the codebooks coming from the Multi-SOM, while the picture on the right indicates the end of the Meta-SOM training phase (duration 100 epochs)

1. Processing the records of the 796 testing digits with Multi-SOM network and recording the output:
    a. Winner Matrix index,
    b. bar and column position of Winner Unit in Winner Matrix,
    c. distance from Winner Unit;

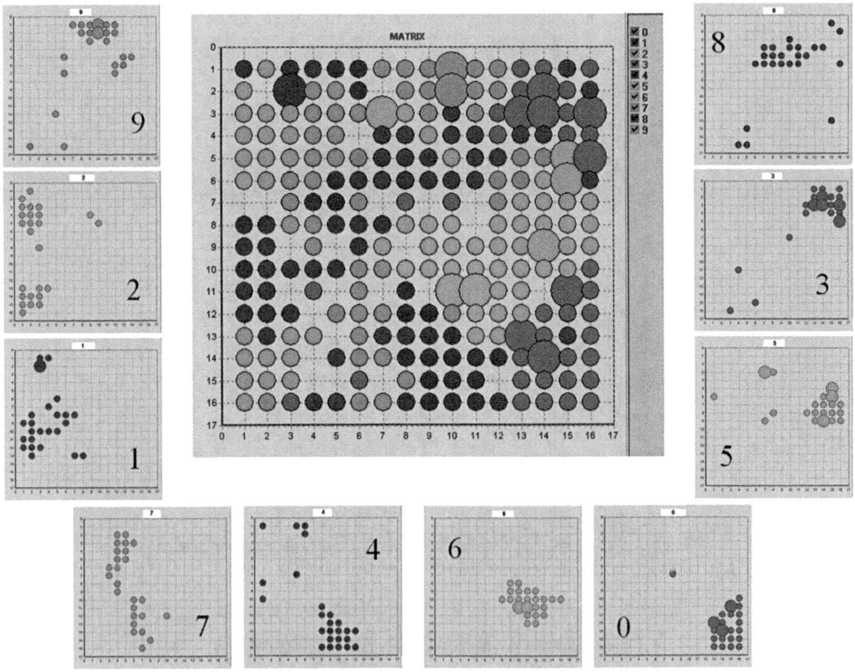

Fig. 13.21 Distribution with respect to the frequency of the Multi-SOM matrix codebooks on the Meta-SOM matrix 16 × 16

2. Processing the records of the 796 testing digits with Meta-SOM network and recording the output:

   d. bar and column position of Winner Unit,
   e. distance from the Winner Unit;

3. Processing the Multi-SOM Winner Unit codebook with Meta-SOM network and recording the output:

   f. bar and column position of the Winner Unit,
   g. distance from the Winner Unit;

4. Compare if the three outputs coincide referring to the target (Fig. 13.23).

We show two examples in which all three outputs agree in assigning the target to input vector.

Fig. 13.24 shows an example of exact recall of digit Db:

- The Multi-SOM classifies correctly the input vector (record 86) that represents the digit 2 in W_3 matrix cell (2,1).

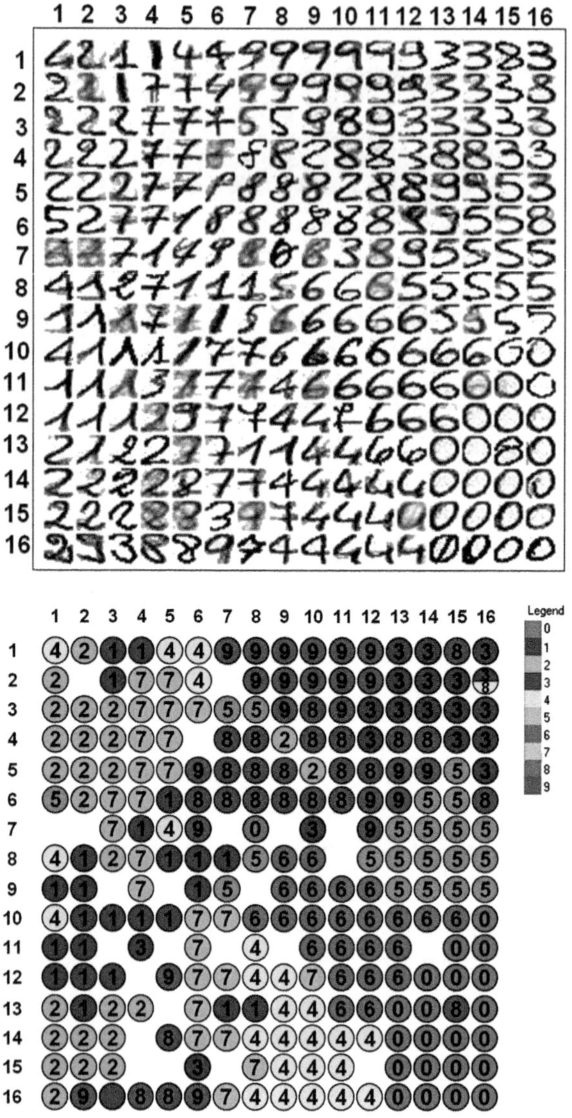

Fig. 13.22 *Left*: Meta-SOM codebook. *Right*: assigning of the target to Meta-SOM matrix codebooks; blank spaces refer to non-codified cells, to which it was not possible to assign a target in a direct way. 2,16 cell has an ambiguous target (3/8)

- The Meta-SOM classifies correctly the same input vector (record 86) in cell (14,2) (compare Fig. 13.22 for target assignment to Meta-SOM cells).
- The Meta-SOM classifies correctly $W_{3(2,1)}$ codebook (Winner Unit of Multi-SOM) in cell (14,2).

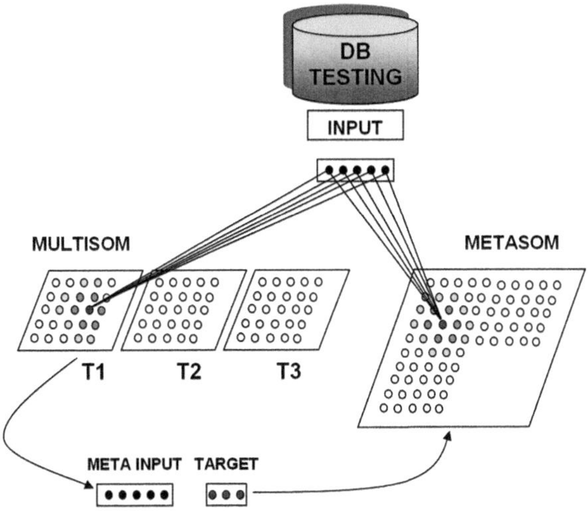

Fig. 13.23 Testing/recall processing in a Multi–Meta-SOM system: Multi-SOM and Meta-SOM inputs are constituted by a DB values record. However, the Meta-SOMs are able to receive, as input, the codebook of Multi-SOM Winner Unit also

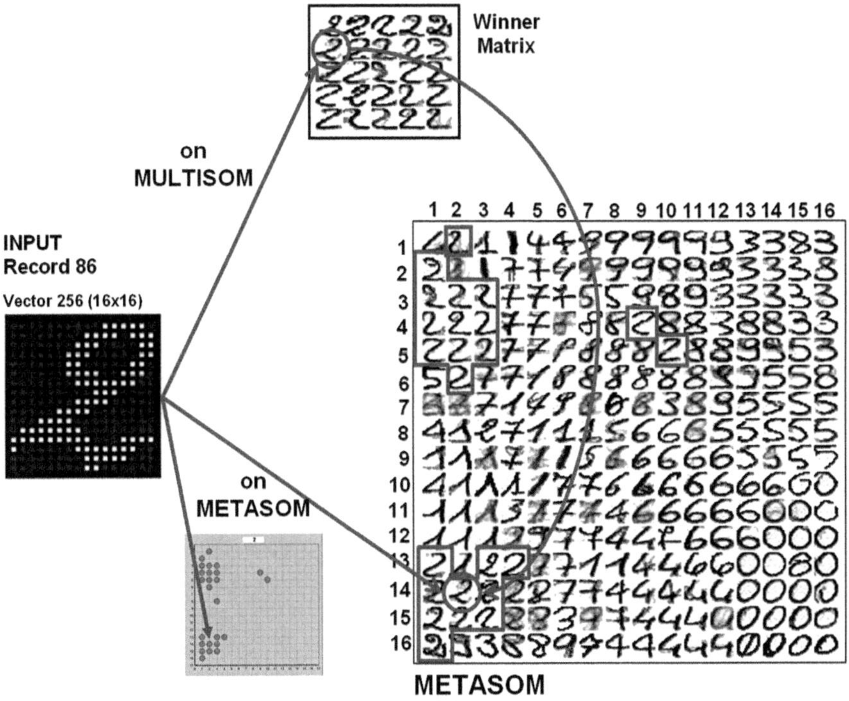

Fig. 13.24 Example of testing/recall processing in Multi–Meta-SOM system

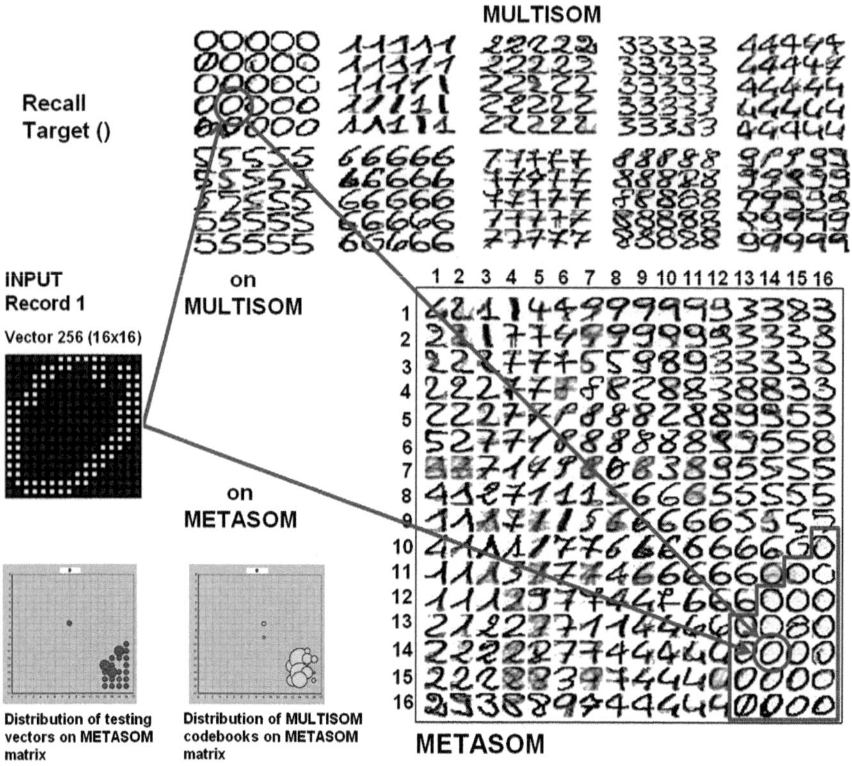

Fig. 13.25 Example of testing/recall processing in Multi–Meta-SOM system

Fig. 13.25 shows an example of exact recall of digit DB:

- The Multi-SOM classifies correctly the input vector (record 1) that represents the digit 0 in W_1 matrix cell (4,2).
- The Meta-SOM classifies correctly the same input vector (record 1) in cell (14,14) (compare Fig. 13.22 for target assignment to Meta-SOM cells).
- The Meta-SOM classifies correctly $W_{1(4,2)}$codebook (Winner Unit of Multi-SOM) in cell (14,14).

Here we show an example in which there is no concordance between the three outputs in target assignment to input vector. In this case, the Multi-SOM makes a mistake in classifying the input, while the Meta-SOM is not able to classify it, placing it on a non-codifying cell.

In Fig. 13.26

- The Multi-SOM classifies in a wrong way the input vector (record 2) that represents 0 digit in W_9 matrix cell (2,2).

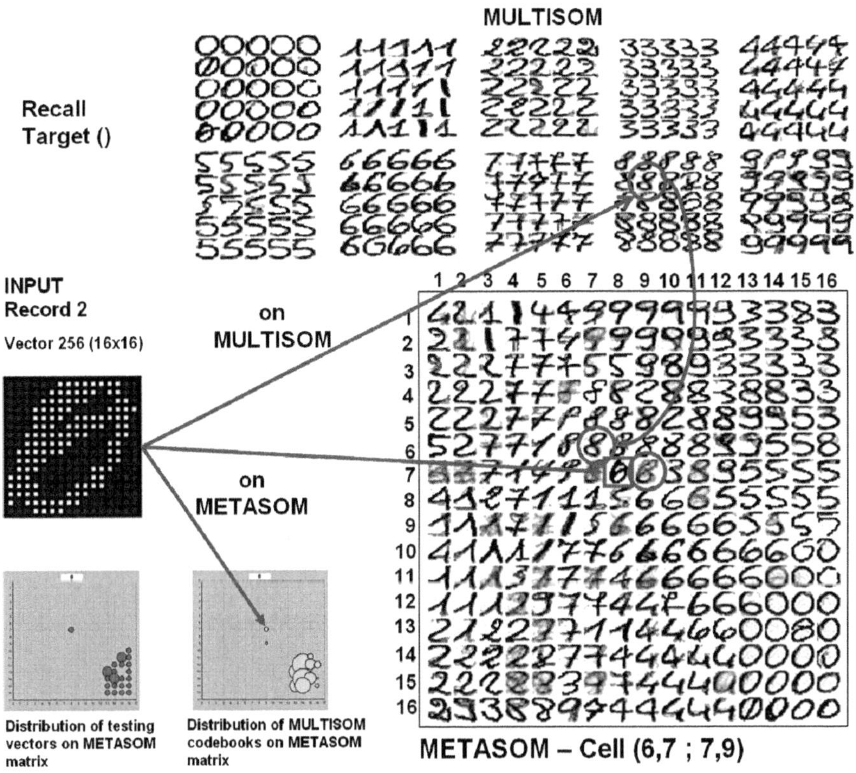

Fig. 13.26 Example of testing/recall processing in Multi–Meta-SOM system

- The Meta-SOM is not able to classify the input vector (record 2) as it refers to cell (7,9) which does not codify a target.
- The Meta-SOM classifies in a wrong way $W_{9(2,2)}$ codebook (Winner Unit of Multi-SOM) in cell (6,7) which has a wrong target compared to the input.

This discordance of classification can be useful in detecting an error. The process of immission of input and codebooks can be repeated till we define the stability, that is, the repetition of the output or of the output sequence (Fig. 13.27).

An input vector in time $t_1$is submitted both to Multi-SOM and to Meta-SOM. In time t_2 the Meta-SOM Winner Unit codebook is submitted to Multi-SOM and the Multi-SOM Winner Unit codebook is submitted to Meta-SOM. This last instance is repeated till the stabilization of Meta-SOM and Multi-SOM Winner Units.

In the following figure (Fig. 13.28) we show the iterative process starting from the input record 1 (already shown in Fig. 13.25 example) immediately stable.

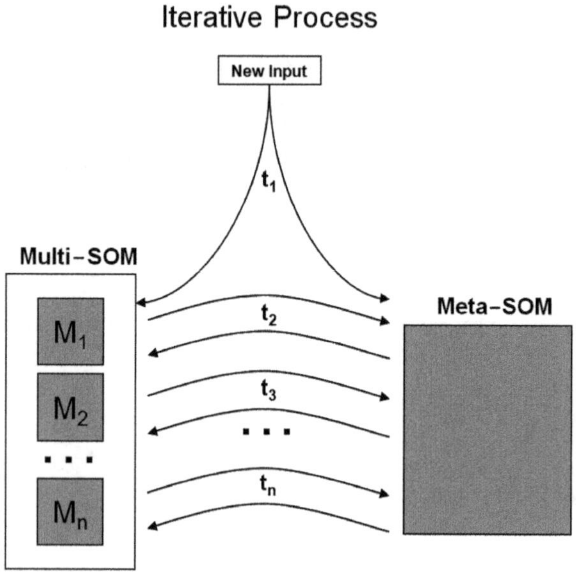

Fig. 13.27 Iterative process of recall/testing in Multi–Meta-SOM system

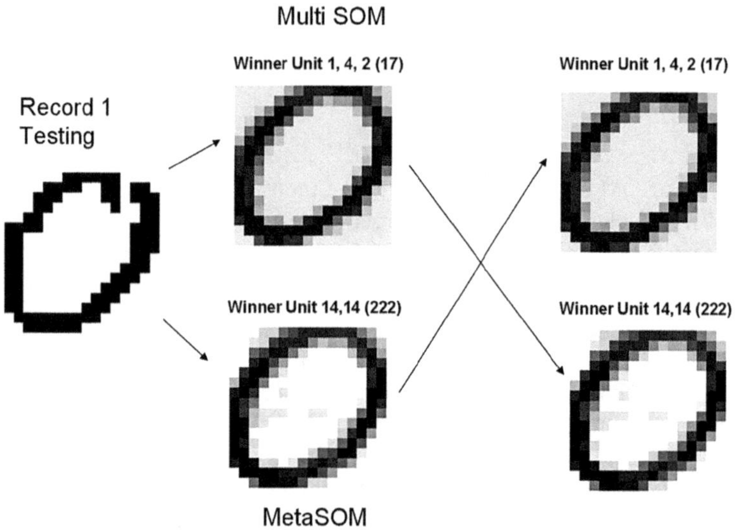

Fig. 13.28 Iterative process of testing/recall in Multi–Meta-SOM system

Bibliography

Kohonen, T. (1982). Self-organized formation of topologically correct feature maps. *Biological Cybernetics*, 43, 59–69.

Anderson, J. A. and Rosenfeld, E. (Eds.) (1988). *Neurocomputing foundations of research.* Cambridge, MA, The MIT Press.

Kohonen, T. (1984). *Self-Organization and associative memories*. Vol. 8: Springer series in information sciences. Berlin: Springer-Verlag.

Kohonen, T. (1988). Learning vector quantization, *Neural Networks* 1, 303.

Kohonen, T. (1990). The Self-organizing map. *Proceedings IEEE*, 78, 1464–1480.

Kohonen, T. (1995). *Self-organizing maps*. Berlin, Heidelberg: Springer-Verlag.

Chapter 14
How to Perform Data Mining: The "Persons Arrested" Dataset

Massimo Buscema

Abstract This paper presents an example of how to apply nonlinear auto-associative systems to data analysis. For this reason we have presented data and equations in a style that is unusual for such a paper.

Nonlinear auto-associative systems often fall under the generic name of non-supervised Artificial Neural Networks (ANNs). These systems, however, represent a powerful set of techniques for data mining and they do not deserve simply a generic name. We propose to name this set of ANNs "Auto-poietic ANNs" (that is, systems that organize their behaviors by themselves).

Auto-poietic ANNs are a complex mix of different topologies, learning rules, signal dynamics, and cost functions. So, their mathematics can be very different from one to another and their capability to discover hidden connections within the same dataset can be very different too. This represents both the strength and the weakness of these algorithms.

All the Auto-poietic ANNs, in fact, can determine within a dataset how each (independent) variable is associated with the others, also considering nonlinear associations involved in parallel many-to-many relationships. But, because of the specific mathematics of each one of these algorithms, the final findings of their application to the same dataset can be different. Consequently, when we apply different Auto-poietic ANNs to the same sample of data, we can find as the result of their learning process different frames of associations among the same set of variables. The problem, at this point, is: which of these frames is more grounded? If the dataset represents a real situation, which of the resulting frames should we follow to organize a productive strategy of manipulation in the real world?

At the end of this paper we propose a new method to create a complex fusion of different Auto-poietic ANNs and we name this the Models Fusion Methodology (MFM).

M. Buscema (✉)
Semeion Research Center, Via Sersale, Rome, Italy
e-mail: m.buscema@semeion.it

V. Capecchi (eds.), *Applications of Mathematics in Models, Artificial Neural Networks and Arts*, DOI 10.1007/978-90-481-8581-8_14,

14.1 Data Description

From 2004 the London Metropolitan Police in partnership with the Semeion Research Center for Science and Communication (Rome, Italy) activated the Central Drugs Trafficking Database (CDTD). The main aim of this project was to organize all the data concerning drugs trafficking in London within a relational database to allow for superior intelligence on drug trafficking, using a new set of artificial intelligence algorithms, patented by Semeion in the last few years.

The results of this project were included in a special report published in March 2006. The report was evaluated enthusiastically in May 2006 by independent British academics. The CDTD project is presently waiting to be managed and continued by the new MET Intelligence Bureau (MIB) (source: MPS Drugs Strategy 2007–2010 and Delivery Plan, Chapters 6.1, 6.2, 6.3, 6.4, 6.5, 6.6, 6.7, 6.8, 6.9, 9.10, 6.11, 6.12, and 6.13).

We extracted from the CDTD relational database a dataset of 1117 persons arrested in the last four months of 2006 in London, according to the following variables and areas:

Areas	Variables
Places	Home_Boroughs
	Borough_of_Arrest
Anagraphic_Data	Gender
	Nation_Group
	Ethnic_Group
	Age
Past_Criminal_Curriculum	Convictions_Number
	Offences_Number
	Age_at_first_Conviction
	Years_From_Last_Conviction
	Drug_Offences
	TheftKindred_Offences
	Offences_vs_Persons
	Weapons_Offences
	Sexual_Offences
	Offences_VS_Police
	Fraud_Offences
	Offences_VS_Property
	Drug_Trafficking
	Other_Offences
	Total_Offences
Findings_of_the_Arrest	Number_of_Arrests
	Number_of_Drug_Seizures
	Cash_Seizures
	Pounds_Seizures
	Type_of_Drugs_Seizures
Organization_and_Modalities_of_the_Arrest	Tactic
	Arrest_Mode

We further articulated each variable into micro-variables:

A. Places:

1. Home boroughs:

Micro-Variables	Cases	%	Micro-Variables	Cases	%
Barking_and_Dagenham	8	0.72%	Hounslow	23	2.06%
Barnet	18	1.61%	Islington	54	4.83%
Bexley	10	0.90%	Kensington_and_Chelsea	37	3.31%
Brent	45	4.03%	Kingston_upon_Thames	3	0.27%
Bromley	32	2.86%	Lambeth	71	6.36%
Camden	43	3.85%	Lewisham	65	5.82%
Croydon	40	3.58%	Merton	20	1.79%
Ealing	40	3.58%	Newham	46	4.12%
Enfield	27	2.42%	Redbridge	13	1.16%
Greenwich	18	1.61%	Richmond_upon_Thames	5	0.45%
Hackney	50	4.48%	Southwark	73	6.54%
Hammersmith_and_Fulham	22	1.97%	Sutton	13	1.16%
Haringey	40	3.58%	Tower_Hamlets	39	3.49%
Harrow	13	1.16%	Waltham_Forest	34	3.04%
Havering	12	1.07%	Wandsworth	20	1.79%
Hillingdon	19	1.70%	Westminster	22	1.97%
Total	975		Borough not avalable	142	12.71%

2. Borough of Arrest:

Micro-Variables	Cases	%	Micro-Variables	Cases	%
Arr_Barking_and_Dagenham	8	0.36%	Arr_Hounslow	43	1.94%
Arr_Barnet	44	1.98%	Arr_Islington	116	5.23%
Arr_Bexley	23	1.04%	Arr_Kensington_and_Chelsea	180	8.12%
Arr_Brent	76	3.43%	Arr_Kingston_upon_Thames	10	0.45%
Arr_Bromley	128	5.77%	Arr_Lambeth	130	5.86%
Arr_Camden	168	7.57%	Arr_Lewisham	120	5.41%
Arr_Croydon	32	1.44%	Arr_Merton	39	1.76%
Arr_Ealing	76	3.43%	Arr_Newham	65	2.93%
Arr_Enfield	25	1.13%	Arr_Redbridge	16	0.72%
Arr_Greenwich	41	1.85%	Arr_Richmond_upon_Thames	8	0.36%
Arr_Hackney	162	7.30%	Arr_Southwark	130	5.86%
Arr_Hammersmith_and_Fulham	24	1.08%	Arr_Sutton	39	1.76%
Arr_Haringey	94	4.24%	Arr_TowerHamlets	56	2.52%
Arr_Harrow	16	0.72%	Arr_WalthamForest	40	1.80%
Arr_Havering	21	0.95%	Arr_Wandsworth	54	2.43%
Arr_Hillingdon	29	1.31%	Arr_Westminster	114	5.14%
Total*	2127		Borough not avalable	91	4.10%
* same persons can be arrested more times in the same borough					

B. Anagraphic Data

1. Gender:

Micro-Variables	Cases	%
Sex_Male	985	88.18%
Sex_Female	111	9.94%
Sex_notknown	21	1.88%
Total	1117	

2. Nation Group:

Micro-Variables	Code	Cases	%
Africans	AFR	49	4.39%
Asiatic	ASIA	10	0.90%
People from east of Europe	EASTEU	14	1.25%
European	EU	34	3.04%
Irish	IRE	7	0.63%
Jamaicans	JAM	128	11.46%
People from Middel-East	ME	10	0.90%
Non UK citizens	NK	91	8.15%
People from South America	SAME	14	1.25%
Turkish and Cypriots	TU-CY	16	1.43%
UK citizens	UK	721	64.55%
People from Vietnam	VTN	23	2.06%
	Total	1117	

3. Ethnic Group:

Micro-Variables	Code	Cases	%
White_European	EA1	374	33.48%
Dark_European	EA2	86	7.70%
Afro-Caribbean	EA3	531	47.54%
Asia	EA4	80	7.16%
Oriental	EA5	32	2.86%
Arab	EA6	13	1.16%
Not avalable		1	0.09%
Total	1117		

4. Age:

Micro-Variables	Cases	%
Age(UpTo18)	17	1.52%
Age(18-21)	144	12.89%
Age(21-25)	272	24.35%
Age(25-35)	355	31.78%
Age(35-45)	226	20.23%
Age(Over45)	103	9.22%
Total	1117	

C. Past Criminal Curriculum

1. Convictions Number:

Micro-Variables	Cases	%
ConvictionsNumber(0)	177	15.85%
ConvictionsNumber(1)	271	24.26%
ConvictionsNumber(2)	120	10.74%
ConvictionsNumber(3)	96	8.59%
ConvictionsNumber(4)	78	6.98%
ConvictionsNumber(5-10)	215	19.25%
ConvictionsNumber(11-20)	107	9.58%
ConvictionsNumber(over-20)	53	4.74%
Total	1117	

2. Offences Number:

Micro-Variables	Cases	%
OffencesNumber(0)	175	15.67%
OffencesNumber(1)	145	12.98%
OffencesNumber(2)	114	10.21%
OffencesNumber(3–5)	202	18.08%
OffencesNumber(6–10)	184	16.47%
OffencesNumber(11–20)	160	14.32%
OffencesNumber(20–50)	106	9.49%
OffencesNumber(over–50)	31	2.78%
Total	1117	

3. Age at first Conviction:

Micro-Variables	Cases	%
FirstConvAge(up-to-18)	415	37.15%
FirstConvAge(19-21)	221	19.79%
FirstConvAge(22-27)	217	19.43%
FirstConvAge(28-33)	122	10.92%
FirstConvAge(34-39)	75	6.71%
FirstConvAge(40-45)	38	3.40%
FirstConvAge(46-51)	20	1.79%
FirstConvAge(over-51)	9	0.81%
Total	1117	

4. Years from last Conviction:

Micro-Variables	Cases	%
Off_LastConvAge(0)	218	19.52%
Off_LastConvAge(1)	466	41.72%
Off_LastConvAge(2)	353	31.60%
Off_LastConvAge(3-5)	45	4.03%
Off_LastConvAge(6-10)	24	2.15%
Off_LastConvAge(11-20)	6	0.54%
Off_LastConvAge(over20)	5	0.45%
Total	1117	

D. Type and Number of Offences

1. Drug offences:

Micro-Variables	Cases	%
Drug_Possession_Offences	194	14.76%
AR_OFF_Other_Drug_Offences	38	2.89%
Off_Drug(0)	250	19.03%
Off_Drug(1)	277	21.08%
Off_Drug(2)	189	14.38%
Off_Drug(3-5)	232	17.66%
Off_Drug(6-10)	134	10.20%
Off_Drug(over-10)	35	2.66%
Total*	1314	
* One person can be present in more items		

2. Theft and Kindred Offences:

Micro-Variables	Cases	%
Only Theft_and_Kindred_Offences	86	7.15%
Off_TheftKindred(0)	659	54.78%
Off_TheftKindred(1-5)	301	25.02%
Off_TheftKindred(6-10)	74	6.15%
Off_TheftKindred(11-20)	48	3.99%
Off_TheftKindred(over-20)	35	2.91%
Total*	1203	
* One person can be present in		
more items		

3. Offences against Person:

Micro-Variables	Cases	%
OffencesAgainstPerson(only)	9	0.80%
Off_AgainstPerson(0)	927	82.33%
Off_AgainstPerson(1)	91	8.08%
Off_AgainstPerson(2)	54	4.80%
Off_AgainstPerson(3-5)	37	3.29%
Off_AgainstPerson(over-5)	8	0.71%
Total*	1126	
* One person can be present in		
more items		

4. Weapons Offences

Micro-Variables	Cases	%
Offensive_Weapon_Offences(Only)	41	3.47%
Firearms_Offences	23	1.95%
Off_OffensiveWeapons(0)	895	75.78%
Off_OffensiveWeapons(1)	127	10.75%
Off_OffensiveWeapons(2)	52	4.40%
Off_OffensiveWeapons(over-2)	43	3.64%
Total*	1181	
* One person can be present in		
more items		

5. Sexual Offences:

Micro-Variables	Cases	%
Off_Sexual(0)	1091	97.67%
Off_Sexual(1)	12	1.07%
Off_Sexual(2)	5	0.45%
Off_Sexual(over-2)	9	0.81%
Total	1117	

6. Offences against Police:

Micro-Variables	Cases	%
Off_RelatedToPolice(0)	812	72.69%
Off_RelatedToPolice(1)	131	11.73%
Off_RelatedToPolice(2-5)	128	11.46%
Off_RelatedToPolice(over-5)	46	4.12%
Total	1117	

7. Fraud Offences:

Micro-Variables	Cases	%
Off_Fraud(0)	969	86.75%
Off_Fraud(1)	76	6.80%
Off_Fraud(2-5)	54	4.83%
Off_Fraud(over-5)	18	1.61%
Total	1117	

8. Offences against Property:

Micro-Variables	Cases	%
Off_AgainstProperty(0)	966	86.48%
Off_AgainstProperty(1)	89	7.97%
Off_AgainstProperty(2)	28	2.51%
Off_AgainstProperty(more)	34	3.04%
Total	1117	

9. Drug Trafficking Offences:

Micro-Variables	Cases	%
Drug_trafficking_Offences(0)	211	18.89%
Drug_trafficking_Offences(1)	725	64.91%
Drug_trafficking_Offences(2-5)	137	12.26%
Drug_trafficking_Offences(over-5)	44	3.94%
Total	1117	

10. Other Offences:

Micro-Variables	Cases	%
AR_OFF_Kidnapping_and_Abduction_offences	8	5.84%
Other_violent_offences	74	54.01%
Other_offences	55	40.15%
Total	137	

11. Total Number of Offences:

Micro-Variables	Cases	%
Off_Total(0)	178	15.94%
Off_Total(1)	148	13.25%
Off_Total(2)	111	9.94%
Off_Total(3-5)	199	17.82%
Off_Total(6-10)	185	16.56%
Off_Total(11-20)	161	14.41%
Off_Total(20-50)	104	9.31%
Off_Total(over-50)	31	2.78%
Total	1117	

E. Findings of the Arrest

1. Total Number of Arrests:

Micro-Variables	Cases	%
NumOfArrests(1)	600	53.72%
NumOfArrests(2)	302	27.04%
NumOfArrests(3)	113	10.12%
NumOfArrests(over-3)	102	9.13%
Total	1117	

2. Number of Drug Seizures:

Micro-Variables	Cases	%
NumOfDrugSeizures(0)	123	11.01%
NumOfDrugSeizures(1)	360	32.23%
NumOfDrugSeizures(2)	285	25.51%
NumOfDrugSeizures(3-5)	241	21.58%
NumOfDrugSeizures(over-5)	108	9.67%
Total	1117	

3. Number of Cash Seizures:

Micro-Variables	Cases	%
NumOfCashSeizures(0)	807	72.25%
NumOfCashSeizures(1)	260	23.28%
NumOfCashSeizures(over-1)	50	4.48%
Total	1117	

4. Number of Pounds Seizures:

Micro-Variables	Cases	%
Pounds(0)	840	75.20%
Pounds(up100)	58	5.19%
Pounds(up500)	118	10.56%
Pounds(up1000)	47	4.21%
Pounds(up5000)	39	3.49%
Pounds(over-5000)	15	1.34%
Total	1117	

5. Type of Drugs Found:

Micro-Variables	Cases	%
Cannabis	1019	36.43%
Cocaine	471	16.84%
Crack	591	21.13%
Heroin	588	21.02%
MDMA	128	4.58%
Total	2797	

F. Organization and Modalities of the Arrest

1. Number of Tactics, Type of Tactics, Number of Sequences, Type of Action:

Micro-Variables	Cases	%
NumOfTactics(1)	409	6.87%
NumOfTactics(2)	358	6.01%
NumOfTactics(3)	190	3.19%
NumOfTactics(over-3)	160	2.69%
GenericTactic_Search_of_Object	61	1.02%
GenericTactic_Search_of_Person	873	14.66%
GenericTactic_Search_of_Premises	973	16.34%
GenericTactic_Covert_Purchase	534	8.97%
GenericTactic_Controlled_Delivery	11	0.18%
GenericTactic_Other	153	2.57%
NumOfTacticSequences(1)	986	16.55%
NumOfTacticSequences(2)	54	0.91%
NumOfTacticSequences(3-5)	34	0.57%
NumOfTacticSequences(over-5)	43	0.72%
InOperation(0)	935	15.70%
InOperation(1)	82	1.38%
InOperation(2-5)	57	0.96%
InOperation(over-5)	43	0.72%
Total	5956	

2. Arrest Mode:

Micro-Variables	Cases	%
Non-Law_Enforcement_Agent	49	0.86%
Other_Law_Enforcement_Agent	25	0.44%
ViolentOnArrest(0)	1068	18.76%
ViolentOnArrest(1)	33	0.58%
ViolentOnArrest(more-1)	16	0.28%
ArrMode_NA	6	0.11%
ArrMode_Direct(0)	304	5.34%
ArrMode_Direct(1)	517	9.00%
ArrMode_Direct(2)	187	3.29%
ArrMode_Direct(3-5)	78	1.37%
ArrMode_Direct(over-5)	31	0.54%
ArrMode_Result_of_Enquiries(0)	1035	18.18%
ArrMode_Result_of_Enquiries(1)	44	0.77%
ArrMode_Result_of_Enquiries(2)	19	0.33%
ArrMode_Result_of_Enquiries(over-2)	19	0.33%
ArrMode_Given_into_custody	27	0.47%
ArrMode_Other(0)	1002	17.60%
ArrMode_Other(1)	83	1.46%
ArrMode_Other(2)	16	0.28%
ArrMode_Other(over-2)	16	0.28%
OnBailAtTimeOfOffence(0)	1047	18.39%
OnBailAtTimeOfOffence(1)	42	0.74%
OnBailAtTimeOfOffence(2)	17	0.30%
OnBailAtTimeOfOffence(over-2)	11	0.19%
Total	5692	

14.2 Explorative Analysis Using Self-Organizing Maps

The "Persons Arrested" dataset seems to be very rich in information. But to explore this information any bivariate analysis from cross-tabulation to the Chi-squared test is useless.

The "Persons Arrested" dataset, in fact, is formed of 1117 records and 28 variables, further articulated into 246 micro-variables. Any analysis of this dataset, to provide useful information, has to consider the interaction of all the 246 atomic variables together among each record and the others. Any other reduction, without a valid motivation, may lead to deep misunderstandings.

So we need to approach this dataset using only *multivariate* analysis.

But we cannot process this dataset simply using a *linear multivariate* technique. The assumption of linearity, when analyzing human activity, is completely arbitrary. The reduction of the number of variables, for example, according to the explained variance criterion, is rough. Nobody can know a priori whether marginal differences between a couple of variables represents noise or key information.

To undertake a first serious exploration of the "Persons Arrested" dataset we need to process these data using a *non highly linear multivariate* technique such as the Self-organizing map (SOM) (Kohonen 1990; 1995a; 1995b).

SOMs, in fact, present many suitable features:

a. SOMs are not sensitive to the variables cardinality.
b. The SOM processes all the records and all the variables simultaneously.
c. The SOM is an Artificial Neural Network (ANN) and consequently it provides its best organization of the data, processing the same data many times over time. This is a fundamental method for considering nonlinear relationships among data.
d. The SOM clusters the whole data according to global similarities.
e. The SOM squashes variables and records of the dataset into two dimensions, and during this multidimensional scaling, it selects only the most important features of the dataset.
f. The SOM results in tables and maps that are very easy to understand.

During our experimentation we used two versions of Semeion research software[1]. We experimented with different SOM configurations with different map formats: 15×15, 20×20, 30×30.

Because the results were seen to be stable in all experimentation we selected the SOM map 30×30 which produces the minimum Topographic Error:

[1] M. Buscema, Mos: Maps Organizing System, version 2.0, Semeion Software #26, Rome 2002–2007; G Massini, SOM, Shell for programming Self-organizing maps, Version 7.0, Semeion Software#19, Rome 2000–2007.

SOM 30x30					
Data File	Codebook File	Topographic Error	Quantization Error	Map Compactness Error	Codebook Error
Persons(246x1117)	Persons30x30_Sigmoid	0.00%	9.61%	1.12%	0.13%

We considered topographic error as relevant to evaluating SOM performance, only because this cost function, along with the quantization error, is very well known in SOM literature. But we think that the codebook error and the map compactness error are more consistent cost functions, very suitable to defining the SOM codebook, after the training phase.

At this point it is useful to define these concepts:

Topographic Error: after the SOM training, the two nearest codebooks for each record are considered. If the two codebooks are adjacent, the projection is considered right, if the two codebooks do not belong to the same cell neighborhood, a topographic error is counted (in a SOM squared grid each cell has a neighborhood composed of the eight nearest cells).

Quantization Error: This index is not really an error. It is simply the mean of the variance that the SOM has collected inside each codebook. This index is zero when the SOM puts every record in a different cell. But in this case the SOM ANN has not executed its task, that is, to cluster the dataset.

So quantization error can work only as a clustering index of SOM training.

Codebook Error: This index, ideated by M. Buscema in 2006 at Semeion, is very useful to measure the compactness of each codebook, after the SOM training phase.

The codebook error traces for each cell (codebook) the circle of minimal radius, whose center is the codebook itself, able to include all the records belonging to that cell. All the other records included in that circle are considered a compactness error of that codebook.

Codebook Error Equations

- Distance between the k-th record clustered into the i-th cell and the codebook of the same cell:

$$d_{i,i_k} = \sqrt{\sum_s \left(C_{i_s} - R_{i_{k_s}}\right)^2}$$

- $R_{i\text{Max}}$ is the record clustered into the i-th cell, whose distance from its codebook is the highest:

$$d_{i,i\text{Max}} = \operatorname*{Max}_k \left\{d_{i,i_k}\right\}$$

- Distance between the k-th record, clustered into the j-th cell, and the codebook of the i-th cell:

$$d_{i,j_k} = \sqrt{\sum_s \left(C_{i_s} - R_{j_{k_s}}\right)^2};$$

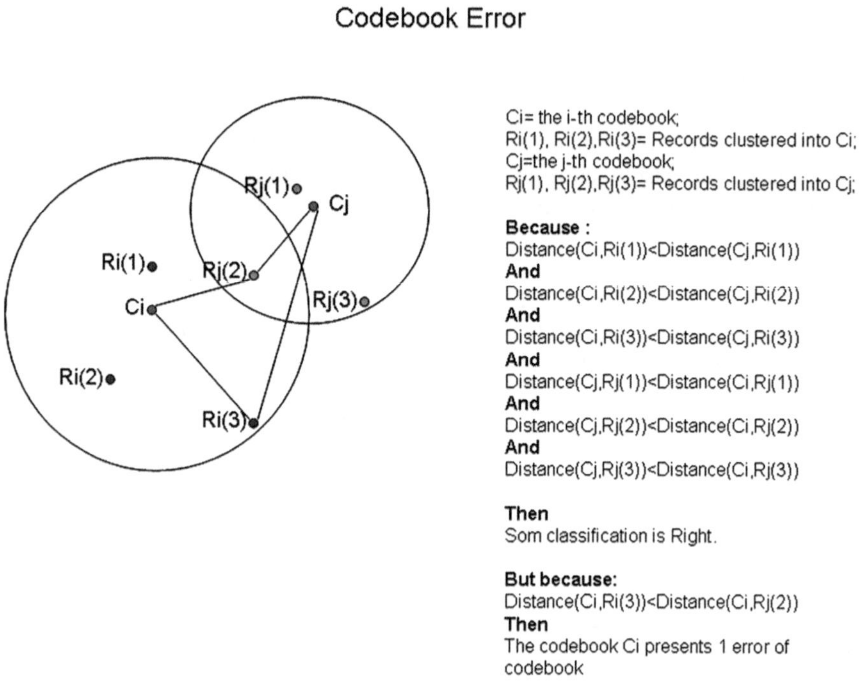

- if $\left(d_{i,j_k} < d_{i,i_{\text{Max}}}\right)$ $\text{error}_{i,j}++$;

$$E_i = \frac{1}{T-N_i} \cdot \sum_{j \neq i}^{C} \text{error}_{i,j};$$

$$N_i = \text{Total Records in Cell i-th}; T = \text{TotalRecords};$$

$$E^* = \frac{1}{C} \cdot \sum_{i}^{C} E_i; C = \text{Total Number of Cells}.$$

Map Compactness Error: is a more restrictive form of the codebook error. For each cell the minimal circle including all the records clustered in that cell is centered each time on every record of the codebook. All the records clustered in other cells, included in one of the circles are considered an error of map compactness.

Map Compactness Error Equations

R_{i_k} is the k-th record clustered into the i-th cell.

Distance between the k-th record and the z-th record, clustered into the same cell:

$$d_{i,\,i_{k,z}} = \sqrt{\sum_{s} \left(R_{i_{ks}} - R_{i_{zs}}\right)^2};$$

Max distance into the i-th cell from the k-th record:

$$d_{i,\,i_{k,\mathrm{Max}}} = \operatorname*{Max}_{z}\left\{d_{i,\,i_{k,z}}\right\}$$

Distance between the k-th record clustered into the i-th cell and z-th record clustered into the j-th cell:

$$d_{i,\,j_{k,z}} = \sqrt{\sum_{s}\left(R_{i_{k_s}} - R_{j_{z_s}}\right)^2}$$

$$\text{if}\left(d_{i,j_{k,z}} < d_{i,i_{k,\mathrm{Max}}}\right)\ \mathrm{error}_{i,j}++;$$

$$E_i = \frac{1}{N_i \cdot (T - N_i)} \sum_{j \neq i}^{C} \mathrm{error}_{i,j};$$

$$E^* = \frac{1}{C} \cdot \sum_{i}^{C} E_i.$$

N_i = Total Records in Cell i-th;T = TotalRecords; C = Total Number of Cells. The SOM trained matrix was composed of 900 codebooks organized in a topology of 30 × 30 cells (see Fig. 14.1).

Each codebook of the trained SOM is an ideal prototype for the similar records clustered in that cell. Consequently, each codebook is a vector of 246 features, where

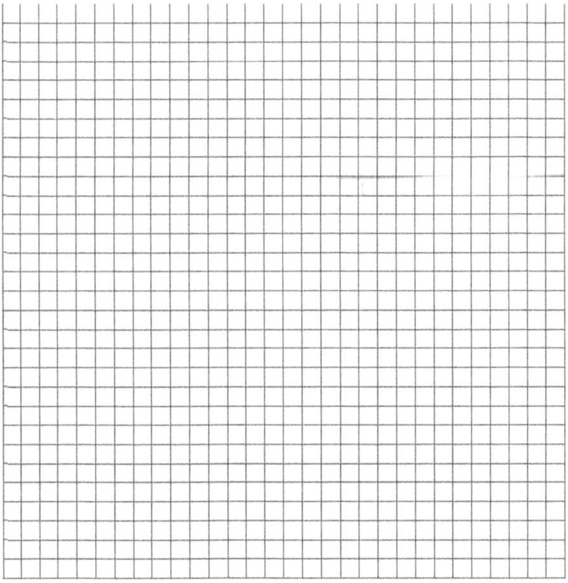

Fig. 14.1 The 30× 30 SOM matrix grid

every vector component (variable) can be more or less active, according to the prototype that the SOM selects for that cell: close cells have similar prototypes, fairway cells have different prototypes.

So, the double task of the SOM during the training phase is:

1. to distribute all the records of the sample in the same cell, or in close cells or in fairway cells, according to their global similarities;
2. and, simultaneously, to generate dynamically for each cell its specific codebook (prototype of the records clustered together).

   After 100 epochs of training, the SOM clustering was ended.

Figure 14.2 shows that data were clearly clustered into the grid: many cells remained empty and others attracted many records. This is methodologically relevant: the number of the available cells is 900, and the number of records to be projected into the grid is 1117. Consequently, a random distribution of the records into the cell should have been possible: quite a record for one cell. All the same, the SOM concentrates similar records only in the closer cells and creates a big cell distance among different records. This is a qualitative feature showing the consistency of the SOM clustering.

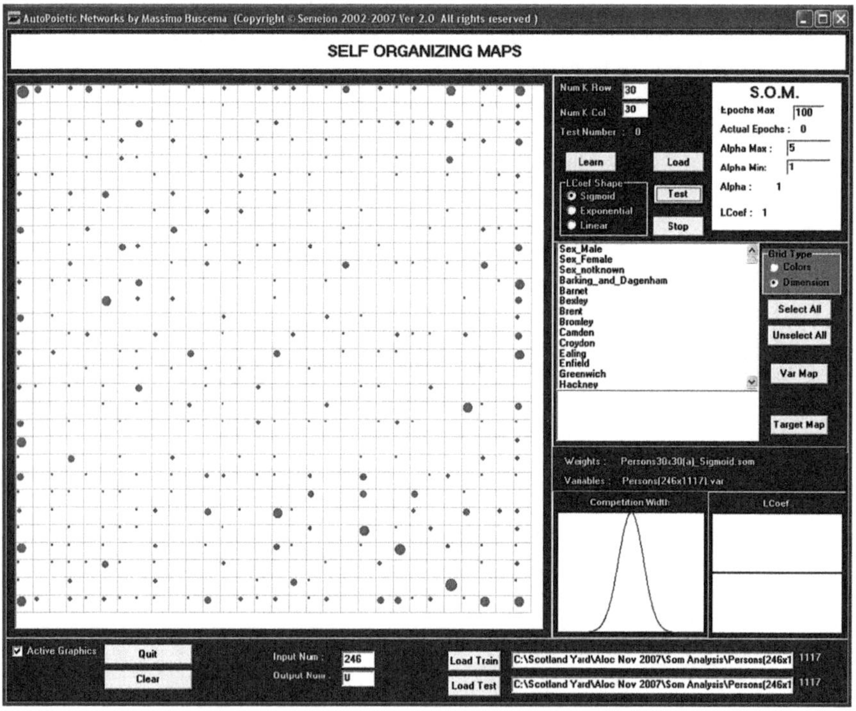

Fig. 14.2 One of the SOM software sets after the training phase: the bigger the circle, the more records clustered into a cell

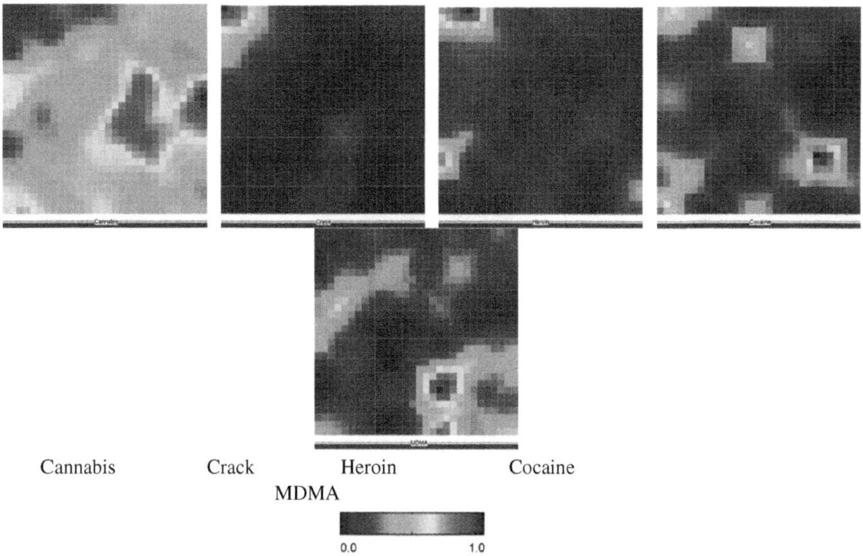

Fig. 14.3 An effective example could be the slices generated by the SOM about the type of drugs found during the arrest

The SOM also generates a different codebook for every cell: each cell of the trained SOM, in fact, presents a prototype of all dataset variables in its specific location. We have to figure out a cube of 246 slices, where each slice represents the distribution of the activation value of each variable in the 30×30 grid.

An effective example could be the slices generated by the SOM about the type of drugs found during the arrest (see Fig. 14.3):

Comparing these maps we observe:

1. Cannabis distribution is extensive and quite spread out, with two big concentrations:
    a. The first one in the center of the map;
    b. the second on the east side of the map.
2. Crack and heroin have a similar and specific distribution, but heroin has also two other small clusters:
    c. The first in the south-west of the map;
    d. the second, smaller cluster, in the south-east of the map.
3. Cocaine has a complex distribution, clustered into at least four groups:
    e. The biggest, in the east-south-east of the map, close to the main cannabis distribution group;
    f. the second one, in the south-west of the map, overlapped some cannabis activities;

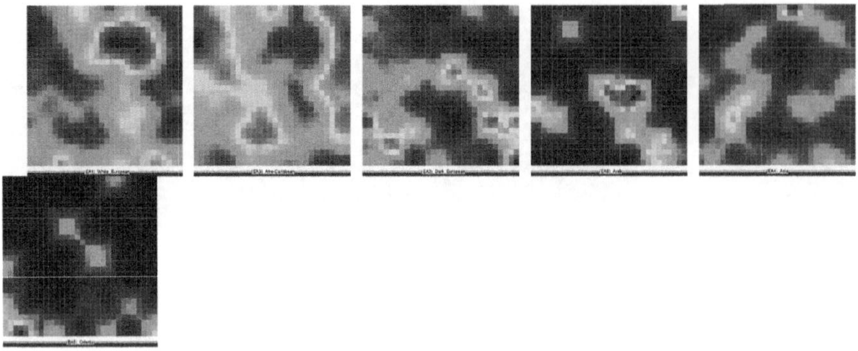

White Euro Afro-Caribbean Dark Euro Arabs Asiatic Oriental

Fig. 14.4 The slices representing the distribution of ethnic groups

g. the third one, in the north-west of the map, overlapped with the main distribution of crack and heroin;
h. the fourth, toward the north of the map, is a free space, not particularly frequented by the other three drugs.

4. MDMA distribution seems to be similar to that of cocaine, with the exception that MDMA prefers to be distributed with cannabis, but not with heroin and crack.

The next problem is to identify which ethnic group and/or nation group are eventually associated with this map of types of drugs.

The slices representing the distribution of ethnic groups can provide some answers to our question (Fig. 14.4):

White Europeans seem to be specialized in cocaine and partially in cannabis, while Dark Europeans seem divided into two groups:

1. The first one managing most of the cocaine trafficking, MDMA included;
2. the second implied in heroin and other drugs.

Arabs appear concentrated in cannabis and MDMA, while Orientals have a strong niche in a small and separate market of cocaine.

The Asiatic ethnic group seems to be weakly linked to cannabis, but another group (in the north of the map) appears to work as a "generic dealer."

The Afro-Caribbean ethnic group is divided into three big clusters:

1. The first one completely dedicated to crack and heroin trafficking (north-east of the map);
2. the second one in a more generic trafficking setting, working and/or competing also with Asiatic and Dark European ethnic groups (the east side of the map);

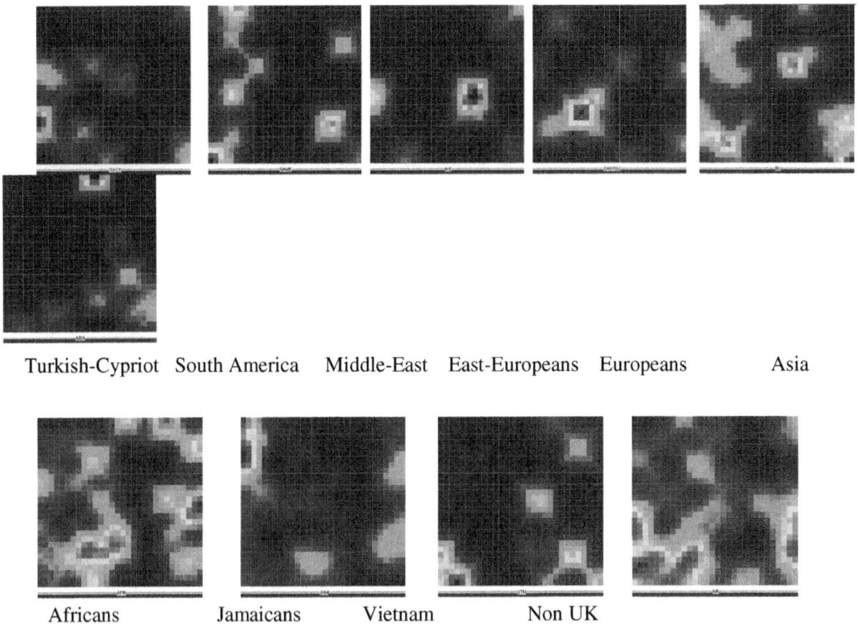

Fig. 14.5 Clustering of the nation group variable

3. the third one, linked to the first group, more dedicated to the cannabis market.

The nation groups variables are also clustered by SOM in a very informative way (Fig. 14.5):

The Turkish-Cypriot nations group is one of the dark European groups that have built a monolithic niche for heroin.

South Americans, instead, seem articulated into two groups: one specialized in cannabis and the other specialized in the most important cocaine trafficking.

People from the Middle East are concentrated in MDMA, while the East European group does not have a specific drug profile. The same is the case for people from Asia and for the three groups of Africans.

European people are spread out on the map, in many small clusters, while Jamaicans represent a strong group specialized in crack and heroin, two generic groups and one group more orientated towards cocaine.

Another novelty is represented by the distribution on the SOM map of the females arrested (Fig. 14.6):

Females are concentrated into four groups:

1. The first group in the north-west of the map: these females are Jamaican and are specialized in crack (not necessary in heroin);

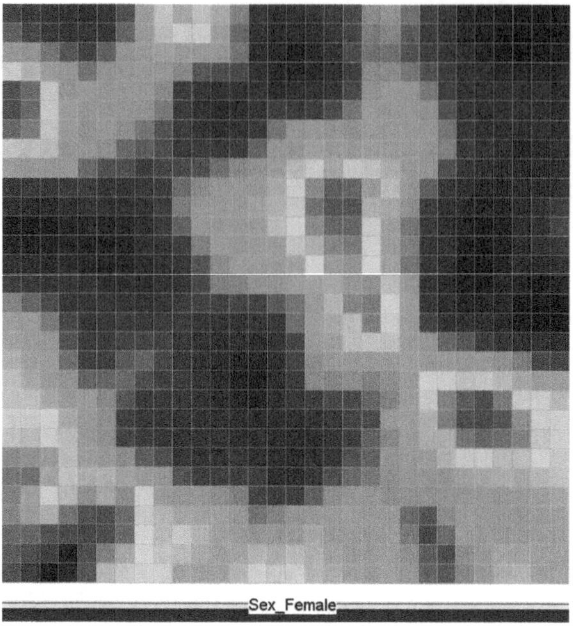

Fig. 14.6 Gender: Female

2. the second group positioned in the south-west of the map is fundamentally cocaine- and cannabis-oriented and is composed of White and Dark Europeans ;
3. the third group, in more or less the center of the map, is also specialized in cannabis, but is completely different from the second one, because also Arab and Asiatic women can belong to this group;
4. the fourth group in the south-east of the map seems to be composed only of Dark European women completely dedicated to cocaine and MDMA.

Obviously, this analysis could go on in a more detailed way. For this reason we prefer to show a series of tables, where each variable is shown with its most associated variables. The association index is the linear correlation of each variable with all the others in any specific codebook trained by the SOM. Naturally, all the SOM codebooks are generated in a nonlinear way (see the SOM features mentioned earlier) and the linear correlation of the codebooks preserves the absolute nonlinearity of these findings. It is like saying that we want to establish which kind of linear correlation exists among a group of nonlinear dynamics.

Below are shown the SOM prototypes by means of some of the key variables (Tables 14.1a–b, 14.2a–j, 14.3a–f, 14.4a–e):

UK citizens and people coming from Africa seem to segment the drug market of the prototypical male dealer. The prevalent male ethnic groups are Afro-Caribbean and Asiatic and Tower Hamlet and Harrow are the boroughs where they work most of the time and where they are arrested. Typically they are young persons with an intensive criminal curriculum. At the moment of the arrest they use to have a lot of

Table 14.1a Male prototype

Male			
Places	Home borough	Tower_Hamlets	0.28
		Ealing	0.24
		Islington	0.22
	Borough of Arrest	Arr_TowerHamlets	0.33
		Arr_Harrow	0.28
Anagraphic Data	Gender		
	Nation Group	UK	0.37
		AFR	0.34
	Ethnic Group	(EA3)_Afro-Caribbean	0.40
		(EA4)_Asia	0.28
	Age	Age(21-25)	0.47
Past Criminal Curriculum	Convictions	ConvictionsNumber(5-10)	0.44
		ConvictionsNumber(4)	0.34
	Offences	OffencesNumber(6-10)	0.30
		OffencesNumber(11-20)	0.24
	Age at the first Conviction	Off_FirstConvAge(19-21)	0.36
		Off_FirstConvAge(up-to-18)	0.30
	Offences at the last Conviction	Off_LastConvAge(1)	0.34
		Off_LastConvAge(2)	0.31
	Types and Number of Offences	Off_Drug(3-5)	0.63
		Off_AgainstPerson(2)	0.52
		Off_OffensiveWeapons(1)	0.43
		Other_violent_offences	0.41
		Offensive_Weapon_Offences	0.40
		Off_Fraud(1)	0.39
		Off_RelatedToPolice(1)	0.38
		Off_OffensiveWeapons(2)	0.35
		Off_RelatedToPolice(2-5)	0.33
		Off_Sexual(1)	0.33
		Off_Total(6-10)	0.30
		Off_TheftKindred(1-5)	0.30
		NumOfArrests(3)	0.28
		Off_Drug(6-10)	0.27
		Off_Total(11-20)	0.24
		Off_AgainstProperty(1)	0.24
		Off_Fraud(2-5)	0.24
		Drug_trafficking_Offences(1)	0.23
		Firearms_Offences	0.23
		OffencesAgainstPerson	0.22
Findings of the Arrest	Type of Seizure	Pounds(up5000)	0.32
		NumOfCashSeizures(1)	0.32
		Pounds(up500)	0.30
		Pounds(over-5000)	0.23
		Pounds(up1000)	0.23
	Drugs Associated		
Tactics and Arrest Mode	Type of Tactics	GenericTactic_Search_of_Person	0.53
		InOperation(0)	0.22
	Arrest Mode	OnBailAtTimeOfOffence(1)	0.36
		OnBailAtTimeOfOffence(2)	0.30
		AR_OFF_Kidnapping_and_Abduction_offences	0.28
		ArrMode_Other(1)	0.25

cash and they result to be on bail. There is not a specific type of drug for the male prototype.

The female prototype is more complex. The females are preferentially Orientals or Dark Europeans. They are usually elderly (also more than 51 years old), very often they are "clean" and cocaine is their favorite drug. Generally they are not from the UK. They usually come from Europe, Vietnam, and South America.

Table 14.1b Female prototype

Female			
Places	Home borough	Bexley	0.37
		Lambeth	0.30
		Croydon	0.27
	Borough of Arrest	Arr_Bexley	0.39
		Arr_Kingston_upon_Thames	0.35
Anagraphic Data	Gender		
	Nation Group	EU	0.51
		VTN	0.49
		NK	0.44
		SAME	0.30
	Ethnic Group	(EA5)_Oriental	0.61
		(EA2)_Dark_European	0.46
		(EA1)_White_European	0.25
	Age	Age(UpTo18)	0.25
Past Criminal Curriculum	Convictions	ConvictionsNumber(0)	0.47
		ConvictionsNumber(1)	0.30
	Offences	OffencesNumber(0)	0.48
		OffencesNumber(1)	0.28
		OffencesNumber(2)	0.27
	Age at the first Conviction	Off_FirstConvAge(over-51)	0.60
		Off_FirstConvAge(34-39)	0.47
		Off_FirstConvAge(28-33)	0.44
		Off_FirstConvAge(40-45)	0.41
		Off_FirstConvAge(46-51)	0.39
		Off_FirstConvAge(22-27)	0.30
	Offences at the last Conviction	Off_LastConvAge(0)	0.47
	Types and Number of Offences	Off_OffensiveWeapons(0)	0.52
		Other_offences	0.51
		Off_Drug(0)	0.50
		Off_Total(0)	0.47
		Off_RelatedToPolice(0)	0.40
		Off_AgainstPerson(0)	0.34
		Off_TheftKindred(0)	0.32
		Off_Fraud(0)	0.31
		Off_Total(1)	0.28
		Off_Total(2)	0.26
		Off_Drug(1)	0.22
Findings of the Arrest	Type of Seizure	NumOfCashSeizures(0)	0.25
		NumOfDrugSeizures(0)	0.23
	Drugs Associated	Cocaine	0.40
Tactics and Arrest Mode	Type of Tactics	GenericTactic_Controlled_Delivery	0.28
		Non-Law_Enforcement_Agent	0.26
		InOperation(1)	0.25
		NumOfTactics(1)	0.21
	Arrest Mode	OnBailAtTimeOfOffence(0)	0.47
		ViolentOnArrest(0)	0.33
		ArrMode_Given_into_custody	0.26
		ArrMode_Result_of_Enquiries(2)	0.23
		ArrMode_Direct(0)	0.22

People coming from African countries are usually associated with one of the Afro-Caribbean groups expert in cannabis. People coming from Asia are too few to allow some inference, but in any case they seem to be slightly MDMA oriented.

People coming from the East of Europe are a nonspecific drug oriented group, probably small and recent, whose unique common feature is to live in two boroughs: Ealing and Harrow.

The group named "Europeans" is in fact a group of Dark Europeans, mainly young females, strongly linked with persons from Turkey and Cyprus with a strong inclination towards heroin trafficking.

Table 14.2a Africa nation group

AFRICA			
Places	Home borough	Newham	0.39
		Redbridge	0.29
		Hammersmith_and_Fulham	0.28
		Waltham_Forest	0.26
	Borough of Arrest		
Anagraphic Data	Gender	Sex_Male	0.34
	Nation Group	NK	0.32
	Ethnic Group	(EA3)_Afro-Caribbean	0.42
	Age		
Past Criminal Curriculum	Convictions		
	Offences		
	Age at the first Conviction		
	Offences at the last Conviction	Off_LastConvAge(2)	0.28
	Types and Number of Offences	NumOfDrugSeizures(2)	0.36
Findings of the Arrest	Type of Seizure		
	Drugs Associated	Cannabis	0.25
Tactics and Arrest Mode	Type of Tactics		
	Arrest Mode	ArrMode_Other(1)	0.34

Table 14.2b Asia nation group

ASIA			
Places	Home borough	Hammersmith_and_Fulham	0.45
		Hounslow	0.37
	Borough of Arrest	Arr_Hammersmith_and_Fulham	0.56
		Arr_Hounslow	0.40
Anagraphic Data	Gender		
	Nation Group		
	Ethnic Group		
	Age	Age(25-35)	0.31
Past Criminal Curriculum	Convictions	ConvictionsNumber(1)	0.36
	Offences	OffencesNumber(1)	0.45
	Age at the first Conviction		
	Offences at the last Conviction		
	Types and Number of Offences	Off_Total(1)	0.45
		Off_Drug(1)	0.39
Findings of the Arrest	Type of Seizure	NumOfCashSeizures(0)	0.25
	Drugs Associated	MDMA	0.14
Tactics and Arrest Mode	Type of Tactics		
	Arrest Mode		

Irish people are too few to allow some grounded inference. In any case, the few Irish persons arrested present a very compact prototype: experienced delinquents, expert in different types of crimes, on bail at the time of the offence and inclined to deal with MDMA.

Table 14.2c East Europe nation group

EST EUROPE			
Places	Home borough	Ealing	0.48
		Harrow	0.43
	Borough of Arrest		
Anagraphic Data	Gender		
	Nation Group		
	Ethnic Group		
	Age		
Past Criminal Curriculum	Convictions	ConvictionsNumber(3)	0.33
	Offences	OffencesNumber(3-5)	0.52
	Age at the first Conviction	Off_FirstConvAge(19-21)	0.42
	Offences at the last Conviction		
	Types and Number of Offences	NumOfArrests(1)	0.38
		Off_RelatedToPolice(0)	0.34
		Off_Total(3-5)	0.52
Findings of the Arrest	Type of Seizure		
	Drugs Associated	Heroin	0.01
Tactics and Arrest Mode	Type of Tactics	InOperation(1)	0.37
	Arrest Mode	ArrMode_Direct(1)	0.43

Table 14.2d Europe nation group

EUROPE			
Places	Home borough		
	Borough of Arrest		
Anagraphic Data	Gender	Sex_Female	0.51
	Nation Group	TU-CY	0.39
	Ethnic Group	(EA2)_Dark_European	0.64
	Age	Age(UpTo18)	0.44
Past Criminal Curriculum	Convictions		
	Offences	OffencesNumber(1)	0.43
	Age at the first Conviction	Off_FirstConvAge(28-33)	0.43
		Off_FirstConvAge(34-39)	0.34
	Offences at the last Conviction		
	Types and Number of Offences	Off_Drug(1)	0.32
		Off_Total(1)	0.43
		Off_OffensiveWeapons(0)	0.41
Findings of the Arrest	Type of Seizure		
	Drugs Associated	Heroin	0.26
Tactics and Arrest Mode	Type of Tactics		
	Arrest Mode		

People coming from the Middle East, usually Arabs, are few and seem to have an inclination to hide their sex. Usually they were arrested, because of cannabis possession, for the first time when they were already older (from 34 to 39 years old).

Table 14.2e Ireland nation group

IRELAND			
Places	Home borough		
	Borough of Arrest		
Anagraphic Data	Gender		
	Nation Group		
	Ethnic Group	(EA1)_White_European	0.42
	Age		
Past Criminal Curriculum	Convictions		
	Offences	OffencesNumber(20-50)	0.46
	Age at the first Conviction		
	Offences at the last Conviction	ConvictionsNumber(11-20)	0.49
	Types and Number of Offences	Off_TheftKindred(6-10)	0.59
		Off_Total(20-50)	0.47
		Off_RelatedToPolice(2-5)	0.42
		Off_TheftKindred(11-20)	0.40
		Off_AgainstProperty(1)	0.42
		Off_Fraud(1)	0.47
Findings of the Arrest	Type of Seizure		
	Drugs Associated	MDMA	0.24
Tactics and Arrest Mode	Type of Tactics		
	Arrest Mode	OnBailAtTimeOfOffence(1)	0.43

Table 14.2f Jamaica nation group

JAMAICA			
Places	Home borough	Haringey	0.65
	Borough of Arrest	Arr_Hackney	0.68
		Arr_Lewisham	0.57
Anagraphic Data	Gender		
	Nation Group		
	Ethnic Group	(EA3)_Afro-Caribbean	0.58
	Age		
Past Criminal Curriculum	Convictions		
	Offences		
	Age at the first Conviction	Of_FirstConvAge(28-33)	0.63
	Offences at the last Conviction		
	Types and Number of Offences	NumOfArrests(over-3)	0.58
Findings of the Arrest	Type of Seizure		
	Drugs Associated	Crack	0.60
		Heroin	0.32
Tactics and Arrest Mode	Type of Tactics	ArrMode_Result_of_Enquiries(over-2)	0.60
		NumOfTactics(over-3)	0.60
		NumOfTacticSequences(3-5)	0.57
	Arrest Mode		

Table 14.2g Middle East nation group

ME			
Places	Home borough	Kingston_upon_Thames	0.45
		Sutton	0.31
		Brent	0.32
	Borough of Arrest		
Anagraphic Data	Gender	Sex_notknown	0.33
	Nation Group		
	Ethnic Group	(EA6)_Arab	0.59
	Age		
Past Criminal Curriculum	Convictions		
	Offences		
	Age at the first Conviction	Off_FirstConvAge(34-39)	0.37
	Offences at the last Conviction		
	Types and Number of Offences	Drug_Possession_Offences	0.39
		NumOfArrests(2)	0.28
Findings of the Arrest	Type of Seizure		
	Drugs Associated	Cannabis	0.29
		MDMA	0.09
Tactics and Arrest Mode	Type of Tactics		
	Arrest Mode	ArrMode_Direct(2)	0.31

Table 14.2h South America nation group

SAME			
Places	Home borough	Kensington_and_Chelsea	0.33
	Borough of Arrest	Arr_Greenwich	0.44
		Arr_Bexley	0.43
		Arr_Kensington_and_Chelsea	0.39
		Arr_PL_NA	0.33
Anagraphic Data	Gender		
	Nation Group	VTN	0.43
	Ethnic Group		
	Age		
Past Criminal Curriculum	Convictions		
	Offences		
	Age at the first Conviction		
	Offences at the last Conviction		
	Types and Number of Offences	Off_FirstConvAge(40-45)	0.30
Findings of the Arrest	Type of Seizure	NumOfDrugSeizures(over-5)	0.31
	Drugs Associated	Cocaine	0.53
		Heroin	0.27
Tactics and Arrest Mode	Type of Tactics	IrOperation(1)	0.37
	Arrest Mode		

Table 14.2i Turkey and Cyprus nation group

TU-CY			
Places	Home borough		
	Borough of Arrest		
Anagraphic Data	Gender		
	Nation Group	EU	0.39
		NK	0.38
	Ethnic Group	(EA2)_Dark_European	0.55
	Age		
Past Criminal Curriculum	Convictions	ConvictionsNumber(0)	0.43
	Offences	OffencesNumber(0)	0.43
	Age at the first Conviction	Off_FirstConvAge(over-51)	0.48
		Off_FirstConvAge(34-39)	0.43
	Offences at the last Conviction	Off_LastConvAge(0)	0.40
	Types and Number of Offences	Off_Drug(0)	0.44
		Off_Total(0)	0.43
Findings of the Arrest	Type of Seizure		
	Drugs Associated	Heroin	0.29
Tactics and Arrest Mode	Type of Tactics		
	Arrest Mode		

South American persons are more defined: usually they live in Kensington, but very often they are arrested outside of Kensington. They are strongly associated with a Vietnamese group and they are specialized in large quantities of cocaine, also their first conviction was when they were quite aged (around 40–45 years old). Sometimes they are also involved in heroin trafficking.

Table 14.2j Vietnam nation group

VTN			
Places	Home borough	Bexley	0.50
	Borough of Arrest	Arr_Bexley	0.64
Anagraphic Data	Gender	Sex_Female	0.49
	Nation Group		
	Ethnic Group	(EA5)_Oriental	0.75
	Age		
Past Criminal Curriculum	Convictions		
	Offences		
	Age at the first Conviction	Off_FirstConvAge(over-51)	0.57
		Off_FirstConvAge(40-45)	0.53
		Off_FirstConvAge(46-51)	0.45
		Off_FirstConvAge(34-39)	0.44
	Offences at the last Conviction		
	Types and Number of Offences	Other_offences	0.62
		Off_Drug(0)	0.44
Findings of the Arrest	Type of Seizure		
	Drugs Associated	Cocaine	0.29
Tactics and Arrest Mode	Type of Tactics		
	Arrest Mode		

Table 14.3a White European ethnic group

(EA1)_White_European

Places	Home borough	Sutton	0.46
		Barking_and_Dagenham	0.44
	Borough of Arrest		
Anagraphic Data	Gender		
	Nation Group	UK	0.53
	Ethnic Group		
	Age		
Past Criminal Curriculum	Convictions	ConvictionsNumber(11-20)	0.43
	Offences		
	Age at the first Conviction		
	Offences at the last Conviction		
	Types and Number of Offences	Off_AgainstProperty(1)	0.54
		Off_TheftKindred(6-10)	0.46
		Off_AgainstProperty(2)	0.45
		Other_offences	0.45
Findings of the Arrest	Type of Seizure		
	Drugs Associated	MDMA	0.27
		Cocaine	0.13
		Cannabis	0.10
		Heroin	-0.19
		Crack	-0.24
Tactics and Arrest Mode	Type of Tactics	Other_Law_Enforcement_Agent	0.55
	Arrest Mode		

Aged Turkish and Cypriot persons seem to be the head of the young European female group trafficking in heroin.

The Vietnamese group is represented by aged women working in cocaine trafficking associated with a group of South American persons (see above).

Most of the White Europeans arrested live in Sutton and in Barking and Dagenham, and they are mainly UK citizens with a high number of convictions. Typically, they have committed one or more offences against property. Their favorite drug is MDMA, and cocaine may be their second choice.

Dark Europeans are clustered as European females, typically coming from Turkey and Cyprus, without a criminal curriculum and dedicated to cocaine and sometimes to heroin and cannabis trafficking.

The Afro-Caribbean group are described as Jamaican and African males, often arrested in Camden and Hackney. Most of them are persons with over three arrests, mainly because of crack, but also because of heroin. They are reluctant to deal in cannabis, cocaine, and MDMA. Police need more than three tactics to catch them and each arrest typically occurs in a direct and violent way.

Asian persons are arrested generally in two boroughs, Tower Hamlets and Ealing, where they also live. The age of their first conviction is when they are between 19

Table 14.3b Dark European ethnic group

(EA2)_Dark_European			
Places	Home borough		
	Borough of Arrest		
Anagraphic Data	Gender	Sex_Female	0.46
	Nation Group	EU	0.64
		TU-CY	0.55
	Ethnic Group		
	Age		
Past Criminal Curriculum	Convictions		
	Offences		
	Age at the first Conviction		
	Offences at the last Conviction		
	Types and Number of Offences	Off_Fraud(0)	0.52
		Off_AgainstPerson(0)	0.51
		Off_RelatedToPolice(0)	0.46
		Off_Sexual(0)	0.46
		Off_OffensiveWeapons(0)	0.46
		Off_AgainstProperty(0)	0.46
Findings of the Arrest	Type of Seizure		
	Drugs Associated	Cocaine	0.27
		Heroin	0.18
		Cannabis	0.18
		MDMA	0.04
		Crack	-0.01
Tactics and Arrest Mode	Type of Tactics		
	Arrest Mode		

and 21 years old. They usually deal in cannabis. A couple of police tactics (typically "Search a Person") are needed to catch them.

The "Oriental" ethnic group is composed mainly of old Vietnamese females implied in cocaine traffic, with also some inclination towards cannabis and MDMA.

The Arabs arrested have the same profile as the people coming from the Middle East, described earlier.

It could be useful to organize the SOM results from the Types of Drugs point of view. This view will show the main profile of any drug in terms of:

1. Places where the persons are arrested and/or where they live;
2. basic Anagraphic data of the arrested persons;
3. their fundamental criminal curriculum;
4. findings of their arrest;
5. organization and modalities of their arrest.

The following tables, consequently, should make explicit the *prototype* of the persons arrested in London from the *type of drug* viewpoint.

Table 14.3c Afro-Caribbean ethnic group

(EA3)_Afro-Caribbean			
Places	Home borough		
	Borough of Arrest	Arr_Camden	0.39
		Arr_Hackney	0.38
Anagraphic Data	Gender	Sex_Male	0.40
	Nation Group	JAM	0.58
		AFR	0.42
	Ethnic Group		
	Age		
Past Criminal Curriculum	Convictions		
	Offences		
	Age at the first Conviction		
	Offences at the last Conviction		
	Types and Number of Offences	NumOfArrests(over-3)	0.40
Findings of the Arrest	Type of Seizure		
	Drugs Associated	Crack	0.37
		Heroin	0.20
		Cannabis	-0.19
		Cocaine	-0.21
		MDMA	-0.28
Tactics and Arrest Mode	Type of Tactics	NumOfTactics(over-3)	0.43
	Arrest Mode	ViolentOnArrest(1)	0.45
		ArrMode_Direct(3-5)	0.38

Persons arrested because of cannabis: Table 14.4a synthesizes the profile of persons arrested because of *cannabis* (but not only). Many of these people generally live in *Sutton* and *Richmond Upon Thames* and they are usually arrested in these boroughs. Gender is not meaningful, but many of them are persons coming from the *Middle East and Africa*. From the ethnic point of view they are often *Asiatic and Arabs*. Most of them are young (*from 21 to 25 years old*), with a *robust curriculum in offences and convictions*, not only linked to drug problems. During the arrest more seizures very often are executed and sometimes cannabis is associated with MDMA. The more effective tactics for this arrest are a "generic search of premises," a "generic search of person," and a "generic controlled delivery." And these tactics often have to be activated more than once as a result of many *enquiries*.

Persons arrested because of cocaine: Table 14.4b synthesizes the profile of persons arrested because of *cocaine* (but not only). Mainly these persons live in *Bexley*, *Bromley*, *Haringey*, and *Croydon*. Most of them are arrested in their home borough, but with some exceptions: many persons are arrested in *Kingston Upon Thames*, but many of them come from elsewhere. There is a specific link between *women* and cocaine. The same specific link is present with people coming from *South America*, *Vietnam*, and *Jamaica*. The main ethnic groups of the persons arrested because of

Table 14.3d Asiatic ethnic group

(EA4)_Asia

Places	Home borough	Ealing	0.52
		Tower_Hamlets	0.47
		Hounslow	0.46
	Borough of Arrest	Arr_TowerHamlets	0.46
		Arr_Ealing	0.40
Anagraphic Data	Gender		
	Nation Group		
	Ethnic Group		
	Age		
Past Criminal Curriculum	Convictions		
	Offences		
	Age at the first Conviction	Off_FirstConvAge(19-21)	0.41
	Offences at the last Conviction		
	Types and Number of Offences		
Findings of the Arrest	Type of Seizure		
	Drugs Associated	Cannabis	0.18
		MDMA	0.03
		Cocaine	-0.15
		Heroin	-0.23
		Crack	-0.28
Tactics and Arrest Mode	Type of Tactics	GenericTactic_Search_of_Person	0.41
		NumOfTactics(2)	0.39
	Arrest Mode	ArrMode_Result_of_Enquiries(0)	0.39

cocaine seem to be *Dark Europeans*, *Oriental*, and *White European*. Their age is between *25 and over 45* and their criminal *curriculum tends to be clean*. They sometimes have *one offence in elderly age* (beyond the 40s). Their arrest is correlated to *many drug seizures and cash seizures. Heroin, crack, and MDMA* are associated with cocaine seizures. *Many tactics and tactics sequences* are needed to find cocaine, and very often they are the result of many *enquiries*. "Controlled Delivery" and "Covert Purchase" are shown to be the more effective tactics to find cocaine.

Persons arrested because of heroin: Table 14.4c synthesizes the profile of persons arrested because of *heroin* (but not only). There is not a specific borough where they are arrested. Typically the ethnic groups are *Jamaican*, *Turkish*, and *Cypriots*.

These persons seem to be clustered into two sub-groups: the first one is composed of very *young people*, without relevant past offences, while the second group is composed of *adult and very expert delinquents* with an impressive curriculum in the field, collecting every kind of crime in robust quantity. In fact, their arrest is always associated with significant seizures of drugs.

These people associate *heroin* trafficking with *crack* and also with *cocaine*. Many tactics and tactics sequences, such as *Covert Purchase*, are needed to arrest these persons, often in violent mode, at the end of many enquiries.

Table 14.3e Oriental ethnic group

(EA5)_Oriental			
Places	Home borough		
	Borough of Arrest		
Anagraphic Data	Gender	Sex_Female	0.61
	Nation Group	VTN	0.75
	Ethnic Group		
	Age		
Past Criminal Curriculum	Convictions	ConvictionsNumber(0)	0.55
	Offences	OffencesNumber(0)	0.55
	Age at the first Conviction	Off_FirstConvAge(over-51)	0.67
	Offences at the last Conviction	Off_LastConvAge(0)	0.52
	Types and Number of Offences	Other_offences	0.59
		Off_Drug(0)	0.56
		Off_Total(0)	0.54
Findings of the Arrest	Type of Seizure		
	Drugs Associated	Cocaine	0.24
		Cannabis	0.13
		MDMA	0.12
		Heroin	-0.04
		Crack	-0.21
Tactics and Arrest Mode	Type of Tactics		
	Arrest Mode		

Persons arrested because of crack: Table 14.4d synthesizes the profile of persons mainly arrested because of *crack*. The crack prototype seems to be very defined: *Afro Caribbean* and *Jamaican, aged between 25 and 35 years old* (sometimes between 35 and 45 years old). These people seem to be divided into two sub-groups: the first one whose individuals generally have collected *more than 20 convictions* and the second one with persons who have typically two convictions. The first group has also *committed more than 50 offences, in every kind of known crime*. The *average age* of their first crime is often late: *between 25 and 33 years old*. Most of them were found with more *than three and/or five doses* of crack, often associated with heroin, and only sometimes with cocaine. *Covert purchase* is the most effective tactic used by the police with this kind of drug crime and *direct arrest* is a common way to capture these persons, very often in *violent mode*.

Persons arrested because of MDMA: Table 14.4e synthesizes the profile of persons mainly arrested because of *MDMA*. Most of these persons were arrested in the *South of London*. They are *white Europeans*, composed of a small group of *Irish* and more generally of *UK citizens with one or two offences* in their curricula. These persons are sometimes *young (22–27 years old) and sometimes old (46–51 years old)*. Typically they are expert in *drug offences and theft and kindred offences*.

Table 14.3f Arab ethnic group

(EA6)_Arab

Places	Home borough	Kingston_upon_Thames	0.36
		Harrow	0.34
	Borough of Arrest	Arr_Richmond_upon_Thames	0.33
		Arr_Kingston_upon_Thames	0.33
Anagraphic Data	Gender		
	Nation Group	ME	0.59
	Ethnic Group		
	Age	Age(18-21)	0.39
Past Criminal Curriculum	Convictions	ConvictionsNumber(3)	0.35
	Offences		
	Age at the first Conviction	Off_FirstConvAge(34-39)	0.33
	Offences at the last Conviction		
	Types and Number of Offences		
Findings of the Arrest	Type of Seizure		
	Drugs Associated	Cannabis	0.17
		MDMA	0.10
		Cocaine	0.04
		Heroin	-0.03
		Crack	-0.07
Tactics and Arrest Mode	Type of Tactics	Non-Law_Enforcement_Agent	0.32
	Arrest Mode		

During the seizures moderate quantities of *cash are found, generally in pounds.* Sometimes other drugs are associated including cocaine and cannabis. They are arrested usually *in a violent and direct way by non Law-Enforcement Agents.*

14.3 Explorative Analysis Using Auto-Contractive Maps

The SOM is a very well known and effective ANN suitable for data mining. But it is not the only one. The Auto-contractive map (Auto-CM), for instance, was recently shown to be a very robust and powerful ANN to discover hidden links within large datasets.

14.3.1 Learning Equations

The CM presents a three-layered architecture: an Input layer, where the signal is captured from the environment, a Hidden layer, where the signal is modulated inside the CM, and an Output layer by which the CM influences the environment according to the stimuli previously received (Fig. 14.7) (Buscema 2007a, 2007b; Buscema et al. 2008c; Buscema and Grossi. 2008a; Licastro et al. 2010)

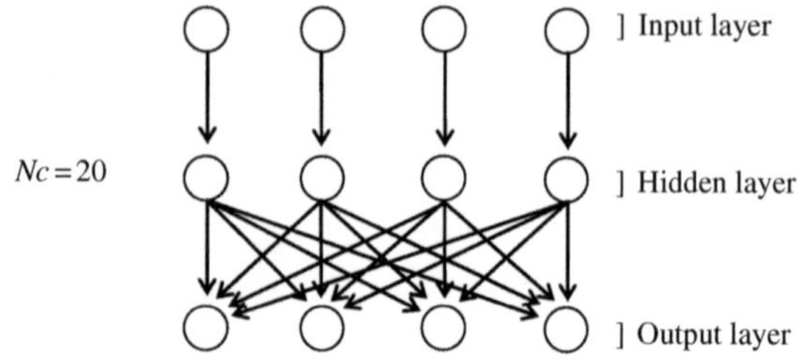

Fig. 14.7 The figure gives an example of an Auto-CM with $N = 4$

Each layer is composed of *N* units. Then the whole CM is composed of *3 N* units. The connections between the Input layer and the Hidden layer are mono-dedicated, whereas the ones between the Hidden layer and the Output layer are at maximum gradient. Therefore, in relation to the units the number of the connections Nc, is given by: $Nc = N\,(N + 1)$.

All the connections of the CM may be initialized both by equal values and by values at random. The best practice is to initialize all the connections with the same positive value, close to zero.

The learning algorithm of the CM may be summarized in four orderly steps:

Signal transfer from the Input into the Hidden layer;
Adaptation of the connections value between the Input layer and the Hidden layer; *
Signal transfer from the Hidden layer into the Output layer; *
Adaptation of the connections value between the Hidden layer and the Output layer.
*Step 2 and 3 may take place in parallel.

We define as $m^{[s]}$ the units of the Input layer (sensors), scaled between 0 and 1, as $m^{[h]}$ the ones of the Hidden layer, and as $m^{[t]}$ the ones of the Output layer (system target). We define **v** the vector of monodedicated connections, **w** the matrix of the connections between the Hidden layer and the Output layer, and n the discrete time of the weights evolution, or rather n is the number of cycles of elaboration that, starting from zero increases itself by a unit at each successive cycle: $n \in N$.

The signal forward transfer equations and the learning ones are:

a. Signal transfer from the Input to the Hidden:

$$m_{i_{(n)}}^{[h]} = m_i^{[s]} \left(1 - \frac{v_{i_{(n)}}}{C} \right) \tag{14.1}$$

where C = a positive real number not lower than 1, named the Contractive Factor, and where *(n)* subscript has been omitted from Input layer units, these being constant at every elaboration cycle.

Table 14.4a Cannabis key variable prototype

Cannabis			
Places	Home borough	Sutton	0.43
		Richmond_upon_Thames	0.41
		Hounslow	0.26
		Bexley	0.25
		Waltham_Forest	0.24
		Hammersmith_and_Fulham	0.22
		Barking_and_Dagenham	0.21
		Newham	0.19
		Barnet	0.18
		Brent	0.18
		Havering	0.17
		Ealing	0.16
		Lewisham	0.14
		Harrow	0.11
	Borough of Arrest	Arr_Richmond_upon_Thames	0.43
		Arr_Sutton	0.33
		Arr_Place_Not Avalable	0.31
		Arr_Harrow	0.23
		Arr_Newham	0.22
		Arr_Redbridge	0.21
		Arr_Hammersmith_and_Fulham	0.18
		Arr_Bexley	0.15
		Arr_Kingston_upon_Thames	0.12
		Arr_WalthamForest	0.12
		Arr_Merton	0.12
Anagraphic Data	Gender	Sex_Male	0.01
		Sex_Female	-0.03
	Nation Group	ME	0.29
		AFR	0.25
		VTN	0.13
		NK	0.10
	Ethnic Group	(EA4)_Asia	0.18
		(EA6)_Arab	0.17
		(EA5)_Oriental	0.13
		(EA1)_White_European	0.10
	Age	Age(21-25)	0.29
		Age(18-21)	0.13
Past Criminal Curriculum	Convictions	ConvictionsNumber(3)	0.39
		ConvictionsNumber(4)	0.36
		ConvictionsNumber(2)	0.13
	Offences	OffencesNumber(6-10)	0.30
		OffencesNumber(3-5)	0.25
	Age at the first Conviction	Off_FirstConvAge(19-21)	0.12
		Off_FirstConvAge(over-51)	0.10
	Years From the last Conviction	Off_LastConvAge(6-10)	0.27
		Off_LastConvAge(2)	0.21
	Types and Number of Offences	AR_OFF_Other_Drug_Offences	0.55
		Other_offences	0.48
		Drug_Possession_Offences	0.36
		OffencesAgainstPerson	0.26
		Off_Total(3-5)	0.25
		Drug_trafficking_Offences(1)	0.25
		Theft_and_Kindred_Offences	0.24
		Off_RelatedToPolice(0)	0.24
		Firearms_Offences	0.22
		Off_Drug(2)	0.22
		Off_TheftKindred(1-5)	0.20
		Offensive_Weapon_Offences	0.16
		Off_Drug(1)	0.14
Findings of the Arrest	Arrests	NumOfArrests(2)	0.34
		NumOfArrests(3)	0.15
	Type of Seizure	NumOfDrugSeizures(2)	0.47
		NumOfCashSeizures(over-1)	0.17
		NumOfDrugSeizures(3-5)	0.12
	Drugs Associated	MDMA	0.18
Tactics and Arrest Mode	Type of Tactics	GenericTactic_Search_of_Premises	0.52
		NumOfTacticSequences(1)	0.47
		GenericTactic_Search_of_Person	0.35
		ArrMode_Result_of_Enquiries(2)	0.29
		GenericTactic_Controlled_Delivery	0.21
		NumOfTactics(2)	0.21
		NumOfTactics(3)	0.16
		ArrMode_Result_of_Enquiries(1)	0.15
		NumOfTactics(1)	0.14
	Arrest Mode	ArrMode_Other(1)	0.18
		ArrMode_Other(2)	0.18
		OnBailAtTimeOfOffence(2)	0.17
		AR_OFF_Kidnapping_and_Abduction_offences	0.16
		ViolentOnArrest(more-1)	0.14
		ArrMode_Direct(2)	0.37

b. Adaptation of the connections $v_{i_{(n)}}$ through $\Delta v_{i_{(n)}}$ trapping the energy difference generated by Eq. (14.1):

$$\Delta v_{i_{(n)}} = \left(m_i^{[s]} - m_{i_{(n)}}^{[h]}\right) \cdot \left(1 - \frac{v_{i_{(n)}}}{C}\right); \tag{14.2}$$

$$v_{i_{(n+1)}} = v_{i_{(n)}} + \Delta v_{i_{(n)}}. \tag{14.3}$$

Table 14.4b Cocaine key variable prototype

Cocaine			
Places	Home borough	Bexley	0.35
		Bromley	0.23
		Haringey	0.22
		Croydon	0.21
		Lambeth	0.18
		Kensington_and_Chelsea	0.16
		Borough not avalable	0.15
		Sutton	0.10
	Borough of Arrest	Arr_Bexley	0.46
		Arr_Kingston_upon_Thames	0.39
		Arr_Bromley	0.35
		Arr_Haringey	0.33
		Arr_Kensington_and_Chelsea	0.32
		Arrest borough not avalable	0.30
		Arr_Hammersmith_and_Fulham	0.27
		Arr_Islington	0.25
		Arr_Westminster	0.25
		Arr_Southwark	0.21
		Arr_Lambeth	0.19
		Arr_Sutton	0.18
		Arr_Greenwich	0.17
		Arr_Brent	0.17
		Arr_Barnet	0.14
		Arr_WalthamForest	0.13
		Arr_Hackney	0.12
		Arr_Lewisham	0.11
Anagraphic Data	Gender	Sex_Female	0.40
		Sex_Male	-0.39
	Nation Group	SAME	0.53
		VTN	0.29
		JAM	0.21
		EU	0.19
	Ethnic Group	(EA2)_Dark_European	0.27
		(EA5)_Oriental	0.24
		(EA1)_White_European	0.13
	Age	Age(25-35)	0.24
		Age(35-45)	0.20
		Age(Over45)	0.17
Past Criminal Curriculum	Convictions	ConvictionsNumber(1)	0.28
		No_ConvictionsNumber	0.18
	Offences	OffencesNumber(1)	0.28
		No_OffencesNumber	0.19
		OffencesNumber(20-50)	0.15
	Age at the first Conviction	Off_FirstConvAge(40-45)	0.39
		Off_FirstConvAge(46-51)	0.34
		Off_FirstConvAge(over-51)	0.30
		Off_FirstConvAge(34-39)	0.25
		Off_FirstConvAge(28-33)	0.19
		Off_FirstConvAge(22-27)	0.17
	Years From the last Conviction	No_YearsFrom_LastConvAge	0.16
	Types and Number of Offences	Drug_trafficking_Offences(over-5)	0.33
		NumOfArrests(2)	0.28
		Other_offences	0.28
		Off_Total(1)	0.28
		NumOfArrests(over-3)	0.25
		Drug_Possession_Offences	0.25
		No_OffensiveWeapons	0.23
		Off_Drug(over-10)	0.21
		Theft_and_Kindred_Offences	0.19
		Off_Total(20-50)	0.14
		Off_Drug(1)	0.13
		Off_TheftKindred(11-20)	0.12
		Off_Fraud(over-5)	0.12
		Off_AgainstProperty(more)	0.11
		Drug_trafficking_Offences(2-5)	0.10
Findings of the Arrest	Type of Seizure	NumOfDrugSeizures(over-5)	0.44
		NumOfCashSeizures(over-1)	0.14
		Pounds(up1000)	0.12
	Drugs Associated	Heroin	0.32
		Crack	0.25
		MDMA	0.20
Tactics and Arrest Mode	Type of Tactics	GenericTactic_Controlled_Delivery	0.36
		NumOfTacticSequences(over-5)	0.34
		InOperation(over-5)	0.34
		GenericTactic_Covert_Purchase	0.29
		InOperation(1)	0.28
		NumOfTactics(over-3)	0.27
		ArrMode_Result_of_Enquiries(2)	0.22
		ArrMode_Result_of_Enquiries(over-2)	0.15
	Arrest Mode	ArrMode_Direct(over-5)	0.33
		ArrMode_Direct(2)	0.29
		ArrMode_Other(over-2)	0.24
		ArrMode_Other(2)	0.19
		ViolentOnArrest(more-1)	0.12

c. Signal transfer from the Hidden to the Output:

$$Net_{i_{(n)}} = \sum_{j}^{N} m_{j_{(n)}}^{[h]} \cdot \left(1 - \frac{w_{i,j_{(n)}}}{C}\right); \tag{14.4}$$

$$m_{i_{(n)}}^{[t]} = m_{i_{(n)}}^{[h]} \left(1 - \frac{Net_{i_{(n)}}}{C}\right). \tag{14.5}$$

Table 14.4c Heroin key variable prototype

Heroin			
Places	Home borough	Kensington_and_Chelsea	0.64
		Haringey	0.51
		Bromley	0.35
		Southwark	0.17
		Camden	0.12
	Borough of Arrest	Arr_Kensington_and_Chelsea	0.79
		Arr_Bromley	0.78
		Arr_Haringey	0.76
		Arr_Westminster	0.54
		Arr_Greenwich	0.52
		Arr_Lewisham	0.46
		Arr_Southwark	0.45
		Arr_Islington	0.40
		Arr_Barnet	0.38
		Arr_Hackney	0.33
		Arr_Camden	0.32
		Arr_Brent	0.28
Anagraphic Data	Gender	Sex_notknown	0.16
		Sex_Female	0.08
		Sex_Male	-0.13
	Nation Group	JAM	0.32
		TU-CY	0.29
		SAME	0.27
		EU	0.26
	Ethnic Group	(EA3)_Afro-Caribbean	0.20
		(EA2)_Dark_European	0.18
	Age	Age(35-45)	0.27
		Age(25-35)	0.13
		Age(UpTo18)	0.13
Past Criminal Curriculum	Convictions	ConvictionsNumber(0)	0.17
		ConvictionsNumber(over-20)	0.17
	Offences	OffencesNumber(over-50)	0.22
		OffencesNumber(0)	0.17
	Age at the first Conviction	Off_FirstConvAge(34-39)	0.29
		Off_FirstConvAge(28-33)	0.23
		Off_FirstConvAge(over-51)	0.15
	Offences at the last Conviction	No_YearsFrom_LastConvAge	0.17
	Types and Number of Offences	Drug_trafficking_Offences(over-5)	0.79
		Off_Drug(over-10)	0.57
		Off_Drug(6 10)	0.27
		Off_OffensiveWeapons(over-2)	0.24
		Off_Total(over-50)	0.22
		Off_RelatedToPolice(over-5)	0.22
		Off_AgainstProperty(more)	0.21
		Drug_trafficking_Offences(2-5)	0.21
		Off_TheftKindred(over-20)	0.19
		Off_AgainstPerson(1)	0.19
		Off_AgainstPerson(3-5)	0.16
		Off_Sexual(over-2)	0.10
Findings of the Arrest	Type of Seizure	NumOfDrugSeizures(over-5)	0.81
		NumOfDrugSeizures(3-5)	0.14
	Drugs Associated	Crack	0.73
		Cocaine	0.32
Tactics and Arrest Mode	Type of Tactics	InOperation(over-5)	0.79
		NumOfTacticSequences(over-5)	0.79
		GenericTactic_Covert_Purchase	0.79
		NumOfArrests(over-3)	0.73
		NumOfTactics(over-3)	0.66
		ArrMode_Result_of_Enquiries(over-2)	0.55
		InOperation(2-5)	0.32
		NumOfTacticSequences(3-5)	0.28
		NumOfTacticSequences(2)	0.24
		GenericTactic_Other	0.23
	Arrest Mode	ArrMode_Direct(over-5)	0.78
		ArrMode_Other(over-2)	0.71
		OnBailAtTimeOfOffence(over-2)	0.25
		ViolentOnArrest(1)	0.18
		ArrMode_Direct(3-5)	0.13

d. Adaptation of the connections $w_{i,j_{(n)}}$ through $\Delta w_{i,j_{(n)}}$ trapping the energy differences generated by Eq. (14.5):

$$\Delta w_{i,j_{(n)}} = \left(m_{i_{(n)}}^{[h]} - m_{i_{(n)}}^{[t]}\right) \cdot \left(1 - \frac{w_{i,j_{(n)}}}{C}\right) \cdot m_{j_{(n)}}^{[h]}; \tag{14.6}$$

$$w_{i,j_{(n+1)}} = w_{i,j_{(n)}} + \Delta w_{i,j_{(n)}}. \tag{14.7}$$

The value $m_{j_{(n)}}^{[h]}$ of Eq. (14.6) is used for proportioning the change of the connection $w_{i,j_{(n)}}$ to the quantity of energy liberated by the node $m_{j_{(n)}}^{[h]}$ in favor of node $m_{i_{(n)}}^{[t]}$.

Table 14.4d Crack key variable prototype

Crack			
Places	Home borough	Kensington_and_Chelsea	0.64
		Haringey	0.59
		Eromley	0.34
		Barnet	0.29
		Scuthwark	0.13
		Kingston_upon_Thames	0.10
		Borough not avalable	0.10
	Borough of Arrest	Arr_Bromley	0.90
		Arr_Haringey	0.87
		Arr_Kensington_and_Chelsea	0.82
		Arr_Lewisham	0.77
		Arr_Hackney	0.73
		Ar_Barnet	0.64
		Arr_Islington	0.64
		Arr_Westminster	0.59
		Arr_Southwark	0.54
		Arr_Camden	0.46
		Arr_Greenwich	0.41
		Arr_Brent	0.23
		Arr_Croydon	0.17
		Arrest borcugh not avalable	0.16
		Arr_Lambeth	0.11
Anagraphic Data	Gender	Sex_notknown	0.16
		Sex_Female	0.00
		Sex_Male	-0.05
	Nation Group	JAM	0.60
		SAME	0.14
	Ethnic Group	(EA3)_Afro-Caribbean	0.37
	Age	Age(25-35)	0.17
		Age(35-45)	0.13
Past Criminal Curriculum	Convictions	ConvictionsNumber(2)	0.13
		ConvictionsNumber(over-20)	0.13
	Offences	OffencesNumber(over-50)	0.17
	Age at the first Conviction	Off_FirstConvAge(28-33)	0.25
		Off_FirstConvAge(34-39)	0.13
	Offences at the last Conviction	Off_LastConvAge(1)	0.26
	Types and Number of Offences	Drug_trafficking_Offences(over-5)	0.91
		Off_Drug(over-10)	0.51
		Off_Drug(6-10)	0.44
		Drug_trafficking_Offences(2-5)	0.40
		Off_AgainstPerson(1)	0.22
		Off_OffensiveWeapons(over-2)	0.20
		Off_Total(over-50)	0.17
		Off_RelatedToPolice(over-5)	0.17
		Off_AgainstProperty(more)	0.16
		Off_AgainstPerson(3-5)	0.14
		Off_TheftKindred(over-20)	0.14
		Off_Sexual(over-2)	0.12
		Off_Total(11-20)	0.11
Findings of the Arrest	Type of Seizure	NumOfDrugSeizures(over-5)	0.90
		NumOfDrugSeizures(3-5)	0.26
	Drugs Associated	Heroin	0.73
		Cocaine	0.25
Tactics and Arrest Mode	Type of Tactics	NumOfArrests(over-3)	0.96
		GenericTactic_Covert_Purchase	0.96
		NumOfTactics(over-3)	0.91
		InOperation(over-5)	0.90
		NumOfTacticSequences(over-5)	0.90
		ArrMode_Result_of_Enquiries(over-2)	0.81
		NumOfTacticSequences(3-5)	0.57
		InOperation(2-5)	0.54
		GenericTactic_Other	0.38
		NumOfTacticSequences(2)	0.28
	Arrest Mode	ArrMode_Direct(over-5)	0.91
		ArrMode_Other(over-2)	0.85
		OnBailAtTimeOfOffence(over-2)	0.39
		ViolentOnArrest(1)	0.32
		ArrMode_Direct(3-5)	0.28

With the CM the learning process, conceived as an adjustment of the connections in relation to the minimization of Energy, corresponds to the continuous acceleration and deceleration of velocities of the learning signals (corrections $\Delta w_{i,j_{(n)}}$ and $\Delta v_{i_{(n)}}$) inside the ANN connection matrix.

14.3.2 Auto-CM: Theoretical Consideration

Auto-contractive maps do not behave as a regular ANN:

In addition they learn starting from all connections set up with the same values; therefore they do not suffer the problem of symmetric connections.

Table 14.4e

MDMA			
Places	Home borough	Sutton	0.45
		Bexley	0.38
		Brent	0.33
		Borough not avalable	0.32
		Hounslow	0.29
		Merton	0.24
		Croydon	0.16
	Borough of Arrest	Arr_Sutton	0.47
		Arr_Merton	0.44
		Arrest borough not avaiable	0.37
		Arr_Wardsworth	0.33
		Arr_Bexley	0.29
		Arr_Kingston_upon_Thames	0.29
		Arr_Ealing	0.28
		Arr_Brent	0.26
		Arr_Enfield	0.25
		Arr_Lambeth	0.23
		Arr_Hounslow	0.18
		Arr_WalthamForest	0.17
		Arr_Hammersmith_and_Fulham	0.15
		Arr_Croydon	0.14
		Arr_Newham	0.11
Anagraphic Data	Gender	Sex_notknown	0.30
		Sex_Female	0.06
		Sex_Male	-0.15
	Nation Group	IRE	0.24
		UK	0.15
		ASIA	0.14
		VTN	0.10
	Ethnic Group	(EA1)_White_European	0.27
		(EA5)_Oriental	0.12
		(EA6)_Arab	0.10
	Age	Age(25-35)	0.22
Past Criminal Curriculum	Convictions	ConvictionsNumber(1)	0.34
	Offences	OffencesNumber(1)	0.27
		OffencesNumber(2)	0.12
	Age at the first Conviction	Off_FirstConvAge(22-27)	0.29
		Off_FirstConvAge(46-51)	0.28
	Offences at the last Conviction	Off_LastConvAge(1)	0.14
	Types and Number of Offences	Drug_Possession_Offences	0.58
		Theft_and_Kindred_Offences	0.45
		Off_Total(1)	0.26
		Off_Drug(1)	0.23
		Offensive_Wespon_Offences	0.22
		Drug_trafficking_Offences(2-5)	0.19
		No_OffensiveWeapons	0.19
		AR_OFF_Kidnapping_and_Abduction_offences	0.16
		AR_OFF_Other_Drug_Offences	0.15
		No_TheftKindred	0.15
		Off_Total(2)	0.12
		Firearms_Offences	0.12
		Other_offences	0.12
		No_RelatedToPolice	0.12
		No_AgainstPerson	0.10
Findings of the Arrest	Type of Seizure	NumOfDrugSeizures(3-5)	0.45
		Pounds(up1000)	0.33
		Pounds(up500)	0.29
		NumOfCashSeizures(over-1)	0.24
		NumOfCashSeizures(1)	0.24
		Pounds(over-5000)	0.21
		Pounds(up5000)	0.13
	Drugs Associated	Cocaine	0.20
		Cannabis	0.18
Tactics and Arrest Mode	Type of Tactics	NumOfArrests(2)	0.62
		GenericTactic_Search_of_Premises	0.50
		Non-Law_Enforcement_Agent	0.46
		GenericTactic_Search_of_Person	0.36
		NumOfTactics(3)	0.31
		NumOfArrests(3)	0.21
		NumOfTactics(2)	0.18
		GenericTactic_Search_of_Object	0.16
		NumOfTacticSequences(2)	0.16
		No_in_Operation	0.13
	Arrest Mode	ArrMode_Direct(2)	0.63
		ArrMode_Other(2)	0.36
		ViolentOnArrest(more-1)	0.27
		ArrMode_Result_of_Enquiries(1)	0.17
		ArrMode_Result_of_Enquiries(2)	0.15
		OnBailAtTimeOfOffence(2)	0.12
		ArrMode_Direct(3-5)	0.11
		ArrMode_Given_into_custody	0.10

During training, they develop for each connection only positive values. Therefore, the Auto-CM does not present inhibitory relations among nodes, but only different strengths of excitatory connections.

Auto-CM can also learn in hard conditions, that is, when the connections of the main diagonal of the second connections matrix are removed. When the learning process is organized in this way, Auto-CM seems to find specific relationships between each variable and any other. Consequently, from an experimental point of view, it seems that the ranking of its connections matrix is equal to the ranking of the joint probability between each variable and the others.

After the learning process, any input vector, belonging to the training set, will generate a null output vector. So, the energy minimization of the training vectors is represented by a function trough which the trained connections absorb completely the input training vectors. Auto-CM seems to learn to transform itself into a dark body.

At the end of the training phase ($\Delta w_{i,j} = 0$), all the components of the weights vector **v** reach the same value:

$$\lim_{n \to \infty} v_{i_{(n)}} = C. \tag{14.8}$$

The matrix **w**, then, represents the Auto-CM knowledge about the entire dataset.

It is possible to transform the **w** matrix also as a probabilistic joint association among the variables m:

$$p_{i,j} = \frac{w_{i,j}}{\sum_{j=1}^{N} w_{i,j}}; \tag{14.9}$$

$$P(m_j^{[s]}) = \sum_{i}^{N} p_{i,j} = 1. \tag{14.10}$$

The new matrix **p** can be read as the probability of transition from any state-variable to any other:

$$P(m_i^{[t]} \left| m_j^{[s]} \right.) = p_{i,j}. \tag{14.11}$$

At the same time the matrix **w** may be transformed into a non-Euclidean distance metric (semi-metric), when we train the Auto-CM with the main diagonal of the **w** matrix fixed at value N.

Now, if we consider N as a limit value for all the weights of the **w** matrix, we can write:

$$d_{i,j} = N - w_{i,j}. \tag{14.12}$$

The new matrix **d** is also a squared symmetric matrix where the main diagonal represents the zero distance between each variable from itself.

14.3.3 Auto-CM and Minimum Spanning Tree

Equation (14.12) transforms the squared weights matrix of Auto-CM into a squared matrix of distances among nodes. Each distance between a pair of nodes becomes, consequently, the weighted edge between that pair of nodes.

At this point, matrix **d** may be analyzed via graph theory.

The Minimum Spanning Tree (MST) problem is defined as follows: find an acyclic subset T of E that connects all of the vertices in the graph and whose total weight is minimized, where the total weight is given by:

$$d(T) = \sum_{i=0}^{N-1} \sum_{j=i+1}^{N} d_{i,j}, \forall d_{i,j}. \tag{14.13}$$

T is called the spanning tree, and MST is T with the minimum sum of its edges weighted.

$$\mathrm{MST} = \mathrm{Min}\{d(T_k)\}. \tag{14.14}$$

Given an undirected Graph G, representing a **d** matrix of distances, with V vertices, completely linked to each other, the total number of their edges (E) is:

$$E = \frac{V \cdot (V - 1)}{2}; \tag{14.15}$$

and the number of its possible tree is:

$$T = V^{V-2}. \tag{14.16}$$

In 1956 Kruskal (Kruskal 1956; Cormen et al. 2001) derived an algorithm able to determinate the MST of any undirected graph in a quadratic number of steps, in the worse case. Obviously, the Kruskal algorithm generates one possible MST. In fact in a weighted graph more than one MST is possible.

From a conceptual point of view the MST represents the *energy minimization* state of a structure. In fact, if we consider the atomic elements of a structure as vertices of a graph and the strength among them as the weight of each edge, linking a pair of vertexes, the MST represents the minimum of energy needed because all the elements of the structure continue to stay together (Karger et al. 1995; Fredman and Willard 1990; Gabow et al. 1986).

In a closed system, all the components tend to minimize the overall energy. So the MST, in specific situations, can represent the most probable state of a system.

To define the MST of an undirected graph, each edge of the graph has to be weighted. Equation (14.12) shows a way to weight each edge where the nodes are the variables of a dataset and where the weights of a trained Auto-CM provides the metrics.

Obviously, it is possible to use any kind of Auto-Associative ANN or any kind of Linear Auto-Associative algorithm to generate a weight matrix among the variables of an assigned dataset. But it is hard to train a two-layer Auto-Associative Back Propagation with the weights main diagonal fixed (to avoid auto-correlation of variables) (Buscema et al. 1994; Chauvin and Rumelhart 1995; Fahlman 1988; McClelland and Rumelhart 1988, Rumelhart and McClelland 1986). In most cases, the Root Mean Square Error stops decreasing after a few epochs. Especially when the orthogonality of the records increase. This is usually the case when it is necessary to weight the distance among the records of the assigned dataset. In this case, in fact, it is necessary to train the transposed matrix of the assigned dataset.

By the way, if a linear Auto-Associative algorithm is used, all the nonlinear associations among variables will be lost.

So, actually, Auto-CM seems to be the best choice to compute a complete and nonlinear matrix of weights among variables or among records of any assigned dataset.

14.3.4 The Graph Complexity: The H Function

This *degree of protection* in a graph defines the rank of centrality of each node within the graph, when an iterative pruning algorithm is applied to the graph.

This algorithm was found and applied for the first time as a global indicator for graph complexity by Giulia Massini at Semeion Research Center in 2006 (Buscema et al. 2008c).

Pruning Algorithm

```
Rank=0;
Do
{
Rank++;
Consider_All_Nodes_with_The_Minimum_Number_of_Links ();
Delete_These_Links();
Assign_a_Rank_To_All_Nodes_Without_Link(Rank);
Update_The_New_Graph();
Check_Number_of_Links();
} while at_least_a _link_is_present;
```

Higher the rank of a node, bigger is the centrality of its position within the graph. The latest nodes to be pruned are also the kernel nodes of the graph.

The pruning algorithm can be used also to define the *quantity of graph complexity* of any graph.

In fact, if we assume μ as the mean number of nodes without any link in each iteration, during the pruning algorithm, we can write the Hubness Index, H_0, of a graph with N nodes as:

$$H_0 = \frac{\mu \cdot \varphi - 1}{A}; \quad 0 < H_0 < 2; \tag{14.17}$$

$$\text{where:}\mu = \frac{1}{M}\sum_i^M Nd_i = \frac{A}{M}; \quad \varphi = \frac{1}{P}\sum_j^P S_{TGj};$$

A = number of links of the graph (N–1 for tree graphs); M = number of iterations of the pruning algorithm; P = number of types of pruning; Nd_i = number of nodes without link at the j-th iteration; S_{TGj} = series of pruning gradient types.

Using H_0, as a global indicator, it is possible to define how much a graph is *hub-oriented.*

14.3.5 Auto-CM and the Maximally Regular Graph

The MST represents the nervous system of any dataset. In fact, the summation of the strength of the connection among all the variables represents the total energy of that system. The MST selects only the connections *that minimize this energy.*

Consequently, all the links shown by MST are fundamental, but not every fundamental link of the dataset is shown by MST.

Such a limit is intrinsic to the nature of MST itself: every link able to generate a cycle into the graph is eliminated, whatever its strength.

To avoid this limit and to explain better the intrinsic complexity of a dataset, it is necessary to add more links to the graph according to two criteria:

1. The new links have to be *relevant* from a quantitative point of view.
2. The new links have to be able to generate new *cyclic regular microstructures*, from a qualitative point of view.

Consequently, the MST Tree-graph is transformed into an undirected graph with cycles. Because of the cycles, the new graph is a dynamic system, involving in its structure the *time* dimension.

This is the reason why this new graph should provide information not only about the structure but also about the *functions* of the variables of the dataset.

To build this new graph we need to proceed in the following way:

Assume the MST structure as a starting point of the new graph;

Consider the sorted list of the connections skipped during the MST generation;

Estimate the H function of the new graph each time we add a new connection to the MST structure, to monitor the variation of the complexity of the new graph at every step.

So, we have named *Maximally Regular Graph* (MRG) the graph whose *H function* is the highest, among all the graphs generated adding to the original MST the new connections skipped before to complete the MST itself.

Consequently, starting from Eq. (14.17), the MRG is given by the following equations:

$$\begin{array}{ll}
H_i = f\left(G\left(A_p, N\right)\right); & \text{/*Generic Function on a graph with } A_p \text{ arcs e } N \text{ Nodes*/} \\
H_i = \frac{\mu_p \cdot \varphi_{p-1}}{A_p}; & \text{/*Calculation of H Function, where } H_0 \text{ represents MST complexity*/} \\
MRG = \mathrm{Max}\{H_i\}. & /*\text{ Graph with highest H } */ \\
i \in [0,1,2,\ldots,R]; & /*\text{ Index of H Function } */ \\
p \in [N-1, N, N+1, \ldots, N-1+R]. & /*\text{ index for the number of graph arcs } */ \\
R \in \left[0,1,\ldots,\frac{(N-1)\cdot(N-2)}{2}\right]; & /*\text{ Number of the skipped arcs during the MST generation } */
\end{array} \tag{14.18}$$

The R variable is a key variable during the MRG generation. R, in fact, could also be null, when the generation of MST implies no connections to be skipped. In this case, there is no MRG for that dataset.

The R variable, further, makes sure that the last and consequently the weakest connection added to generate the MRG is always more relevant than the weakest connection of MST.

The MRG, finally, generates, starting from the MST, the graph presenting the *highest number of regular microstructures using the most important connections* of the dataset.

The higher the H function selected to generate the MRG, the more meaningful the microstructures of the MRG.

14.3.6 Application of Auto-CM to the Persons Dataset

Auto-CM provides a typology of drug use that is slightly different from SOM. The following Tables 14.5a–e show the Auto-CM prototypes of the five drugs with the same number we used for SOM analysis. The only difference is in the number close to each variable: in the SOM table this number is the value of linear correlation between the variable with variables at the head of the table, while in Auto-CM the number points out the strength of membership of the variables over the mean (zero representing the average membership). We outline with boldface the shared associations between Auto-CM and SOM.

14.4 Comparison of Data Mining Techniques

It is hard to make a comparison between two or more Auto-poietic (not supervised) ANN, because there is not in this case a set of dependent variables that we can use as a "gold standard." Only the experimental findings can say to us something about their associative power and this is not true under every condition.

In any case, to compare the capability of SOM and AutoCM on the same dataset we will use a new validation strategy, composed of different steps:

Table 14.5a Auto-CM prototype of cannabis user

Cannabis			
Places	Home borough	NA_Borough	0.193
		Lewisham	0.176
		Havering	0.171
		Hounslow	0.147
		Lambeth	0.145
	Borough of Arrest	Arr_PL_NA	0.188
		Arr_Hounslow	0.055
		Arr_Havering	-0.031
Anagraphic Data	Gender	Sex_Male	0.726
		Sex_Female	0.212
	Nation Group	UK	0.725
		NK	0.327
		VTN	0.297
		AFR	0.044
		JAM	0.033
	Ethnic Group	**(EA1)_White_European**	0.618
		(EA3)_Afro-Caribbean	0.525
		(EA4)_Asia	0.483
	Age	**Age(21-25)**	0.622
		Age(25-35)	0.475
		Age(Over45)	0.456
Past Criminal Curriculum	Convictions	ConvictionsNumber(5-10)	0.428
		ConvictionsNumber(1)	0.407
		ConvictionsNumber(4)	0.404
		ConvictionsNumber(11-20)	0.388
	Offences	**OffencesNumber(6-10)**	0.537
		OffencesNumber(3-5)	0.513
		OffencesNumber(11-20)	0.367
		OffencesNumber(0)	0.366
	Age at the first Conviction	Off_FirstConvAge(up-to-18)	0.633
		Off_FirstConvAge(19-21)	0.662
		Off_FirstConvAge(22-27)	0.478
		Off_FirstConvAge(34-39)	0.140
	Offences at the last Conviction	Off_LastConvAge(1)	0.613
		Off_LastConvAge(2)	0.551
		Off_LastConvAge(0)	0.474
	Types and Number of Offences	**Other_offences**	0.770
		Off_AgainstPerson(0)	0.727
		Off_Fraud(0)	0.727
		Off_Sexual(0)	0.726
		Off_AgainstProperty(0)	0.711
Findings of the Arrest	Type of Seizure	**NumOfDrugSeizures(3-5)**	0.791
		NumOfDrugSeizures(over-5)	0.779
		Pounds(0)	0.663
		NumOfCashSeizures(0)	0.657
		NumOfDrugSeizures(2)	0.621
	Drugs Associated	**MDMA**	-0.105
Tactics and Arrest Mode	Type of Tactics	**GenericTactic_Search_of_Premises**	1.030
		GenericTactic_Search_of_Person	0.825
		InOperation(0)	0.779
		NumOfTacticSequences(1)	0.747
		NumOfTactics(3)	0.632
	Arrest Mode	ViolentOnArrest(0)	0.727
		OnBailAtTimeOfOffence(0)	0.723
		ArrMode_Result_of_Enquiries(0)	0.715
		ArrMode_Other(0)	0.710
		ArrMode_Direct(1)	0.576

1. We analyze the dataset with three different, independent, limited but grounded techniques:

   a. Linear Correlation among all the couples of the dataset variables (LC Algorithm):

$$R_{i,j} = \frac{\sum_{k=1}^{N} (x_{i,k} - \bar{x}_i) \cdot (x_{j,k} - \bar{x}_j)}{\sqrt{\sum_{k=1}^{N} (x_{i,k} - \bar{x}_i)^2 \cdot \sum_{k=1}^{N} (x_{j,k} - \bar{x}_j)^2}}; \qquad (14.19)$$

$$-1 \leq R_{i,j} \leq 1; \; i,j \in [1,2,\ldots,M].$$

Table 14.5b Auto-CM prototype of cocaine user

Cocaine			
Places	Home borough	Sutton	0.077
		Lewisham	0.042
		Islington	-0.078
		Bromley	-0.106
	Borough of Arrest	**Arr_Bromley**	0.023
		Arr_Sutton	-0.110
		Arr_Lambeth	-0.132
Anagraphic Data	Gender	**Sex_Female**	0.127
		Sex_Male	-0.078
	Nation Group	**SAME**	0.225
		UK	-0.068
		EU	-0.164
	Ethnic Group	**(EA2)_Dark_European**	0.272
		(EA1)_White_European	0.012
	Age	**Age(25-35)**	0.079
		Age(35-45)	-0.139
Past Criminal Curriculum	Convictions	**ConvictionsNumber(0)**	-0.021
		ConvictionsNumber(1)	-0.031
	Offences	**OffencesNumber(0)**	-0.018
		OffencesNumber(1)	-0.092
	Age at the first Conviction	**Off_FirstConvAge(22-27)**	-0.002
		Off_FirstConvAge(28-33)	-0.108
	Offences at the last Conviction	Off_LastConvAge(1)	0.033
		Off_LastConvAge(0)	-0.052
	Types and Number of Offences	**Drug_trafficking_Offences(2-5)**	0.098
		Off_RelatedToPolice(0)	0.048
		Off_TheftKindred(0)	0.032
		Off_Sexual(0)	0.013
		Drug_trafficking_Offences(over-5)	0.012
Findings of the Arrest	Type of Seizure	**NumOfDrugSeizures(over-5)**	0.615
		NumOfCashSeizures(over-1)	0.003
		Pounds(0)	-0.020
		NumOfCashSeizures(0)	-0.037
		NumOfDrugSeizures(3-5)	-0.074
	Drugs Associated		
Tactics and Arrest Mode	Type of Tactics	InOperation(1)	0.352
		GenericTactic_Search_of_Premises	0.173
		GenericTactic_Other	0.070
		NumOfTactics(2)	0.015
		NumOfTactics(over-3)	0.012
	Arrest Mode	**ArrMode_Direct(over-5)**	0.079
		OnBailAtTimeOfOffence(0)	0.019
		ViolentOnArrest(0)	0.012
		ArrMode_Direct(2)	0.012
		ArrMode_Result_of_Enquiries(0)	0.006

b. Co-occurrence probability among all the couplets of the dataset variables (PP Algorithm):

$$A_{i,j} = -\ln \frac{\frac{1}{N^2} \cdot \sum_{k=1}^{N} x_{i,k} \cdot (1 - x_{j,k}) \cdot \sum_{k=1}^{N} (1 - x_{i,k}) \cdot x_{j,k}}{\frac{1}{N^2} \cdot \sum_{k=1}^{N} x_{i,k} \cdot x_{j,k} \cdot \sum_{k=1}^{N} (1 - x_{i,k}) \cdot (1 - x_{j,k})}; \tag{14.20}$$

$$-\infty \leq A_{i,j} \leq +\infty; x \in [0,1]; i,j \in [1,2,...,M].$$

Table 14.5c Auto-CM prototype of heroin

Heroin			
Places	Home borough	Enfield	0.100
		Kensington_and_Chelsea	0.087
		Haringey	0.025
		Camden	0.019
	Borough of Arrest	**Arr_Haringey**	0.013
		Arr_Kensington_and_Chelsea	0.010
		Arr_Camden	-0.022
Anagraphic Data	Gender	Sex_Male	0.122
	Nation Group	**TU-CY**	0.611
		JAM	0.073
		UK	-0.047
	Ethnic Group	**(EA2)_Dark_European**	0.257
		(EA3)_Afro-Caribbean	0.052
		(EA4)_Asia	-0.014
	Age	Age(Over45)	0.100
		Age(25-35)	0.062
		Age(35-45)	0.031
Past Criminal Curriculum	Convictions	ConvictionsNumber(1)	0.019
		ConvictionsNumber(0)	-0.004
	Offences	OffencesNumber(20-50)	0.147
		OffencesNumber(0)	-0.005
		OffencesNumber(6-10)	-0.054
		OffencesNumber(11-20)	-0.089
	Age at the first Conviction	**Off_FirstConvAge(over-51)**	0.323
		Off_FirstConvAge(40-45)	0.032
		Off_FirstConvAge(22-27)	-0.026
		Off_FirstConvAge(up-to-18)	-0.042
	Offences at the last Conviction	**Off_LastConvAge(0)**	0.044
		Off_LastConvAge(1)	0.014
	Types and Number of Offences	**Drug_trafficking_Offences(over-5)**	0.578
		Off_Drug(over-10)	0.476
		NumOfArrests(over-3)	0.450
		Off_Total(20-50)	0.122
		Off_Sexual(0)	0.115
Findings of the Arrest	Type of Seizure	**NumOfDrugSeizures(over-5)**	0.817
		Pounds(0)	0.142
		NumOfCashSeizures(0)	0.132
		NumOfDrugSeizures(3-5)	-0.008
	Drugs Associated	**Crack**	0.460
Tactics and Arrest Mode	Type of Tactics	**InOperation(over-5)**	0.591
		NumOfTacticSequences(over-5)	0.591
		GenericTactic_Covert_Purchase	0.537
		NumOfTactics(over-3)	0.354
		GenericTactic_Search_of_Premises	0.117
	Arrest Mode	**ArrMode_Direct(over-5)**	0.251
		ArrMode_Other(over-2)	0.128
		ViolentOnArrest(0)	0.113
		OnBailAtTimeOfOffence(0)	0.108
		ArrMode_Result_of_Enquiries(0)	0.097

Table 14.5d Auto-CM prototype of crack user

Crack			
Places	**Home borough**	**Haringey**	0.261
		Kensington_and_Chelsea	0.191
		Southwark	0.189
		NA_Borough	0.087
		Camden	0.032
	Borough of Arrest	**Arr_Hackney**	0.307
		Arr_Kensington_and_Chelsea	0.168
		Arr_Southwark	0.157
		Arr_Camden	0.046
		Arr_Lewisham	-0.015
Anagraphic Data	**Gender**	**Sex_Male**	0.271
		Sex_Female	0.154
	Nation Group	**JAM**	0.836
		UK	0.058
	Ethnic Group	**(EA3)_Afro-Caribbean**	0.510
		(EA4)_Asia	-0.091
	Age	**Age(25-35)**	0.297
		Age(35-45)	0.191
		Age(Over45)	0.022
Past Criminal Curriculum	**Convictions**	ConvictionsNumber(1)	0.263
		ConvictionsNumber(2)	0.162
		ConvictionsNumber(5-10)	0.033
		ConvictionsNumber(3)	0.011
	Offences	OffencesNumber(6-10)	0.241
		OffencesNumber(20-50)	0.204
		OffencesNumber(11-20)	0.164
		OffencesNumber(3-5)	0.108
	Age at the first Conviction	**Off_FirstConvAge(28-33)**	0.206
		Off_FirstConvAge(up-to-18)	0.157
		Off_FirstConvAge(34-39)	0.125
		Off_FirstConvAge(22-27)	0.115
	Offences at the last Conviction	**Off_LastConvAge(1)**	0.285
		Off_LastConvAge(2)	0.276
	Types and Number of Offences	Drug_trafficking_Offences(over-5)	0.980
		NumOfArrests(over-3)	0.956
		Off_Drug(over-10)	0.601
		Off_Drug(6-10)	0.449
		Drug_trafficking_Offences(2-5)	0.389
Findings of the Arrest	**Type of Seizure**	**NumOfDrugSeizures(over-5)**	0.927
		NumOfDrugSeizures(3-5)	0.306
		Pounds(0)	0.275
		NumOfCashSeizures(0)	0.263
		NumOfCashSeizures(1)	0.196
	Drugs Associated	**Heroin**	0.460
Tactics and Arrest Mode	**Type of Tactics**	**InOperation(over-5)**	0.979
		NumOfTacticSequences(over-5)	0.979
		GenericTactic_Covert_Purchase	0.927
		NumOfTactics(over-3)	0.835
		InOperation(2-5)	0.586
	Arrest Mode	**ArrMode_Direct(over-5)**	0.683
		ArrMode_Other(over-2)	0.504
		OnBailAtTimeOfOffence(0)	0.293
		ViolentOnArrest(0)	0.287
		ArrMode_Other(0)	0.265

Table 14.5e Auto-CM prototype of MDMA user

MDMA			
Places	Home borough	**NA_Borough**	0.293
		Southwark	0.045
		Lambeth	0.028
	Borough of Arrest	**Arr_Wandsworth**	0.050
		Arr_Westminster	-0.018
Anagraphic Data	Gender	Sex_Male	0.125
		Sex_notknown	0.075
		Sex_Female	-0.002
	Nation Group	EU	0.312
		UK	0.175
		ASIA	-0.052
	Ethnic Group	**(EA1)_White_European**	0.368
		(EA2)_Dark_European	0.180
		(EA6)_Arab	-0.074
	Age	**Age(25-35)**	0.182
		Age(21-25)	0.121
		Age(35-45)	-0.015
Past Criminal Curriculum	Convictions	**ConvictionsNumber(1)**	0.236
		ConvictionsNumber(11-20)	0.012
		ConvictionsNumber(2)	-0.007
	Offences	**OffencesNumber(1)**	0.072
		OffencesNumber(3-5)	-0.036
		OffencesNumber(11-20)	-0.051
		OffencesNumber(6-10)	-0.069
	Age at the first Conviction	**Off_FirstConvAge(22-27)**	0.193
		Off_FirstConvAge(up-to-18)	0.010
	Offences at the last Conviction	Off_LastConvAge(2)	0.192
		Off_LastConvAge(1)	0.089
	Types and Number of Offences	**Drug_Possession_Offences**	0.472
		NumOfArrests(3)	0.213
		Off_RelatedToPolice(0)	0.213
		AR_OFF_Other_Drug_Offences	0.197
		Off_Fraud(0)	0.186
Findings of the Arrest	Type of Seizure	**NumOfDrugSeizures(3-5)**	0.355
		NumOfDrugSeizures(over-5)	0.338
		NumOfCashSeizures(1)	0.299
		Pounds(up100)	0.186
	Drugs Associated	**Cannabis**	-0.105
Tactics and Arrest Mode	Type of Tactics	**Non-Law_Enforcement_Agent**	0.799
		GenericTactic_Search_of_Person	0.548
		GenericTactic_Search_of_Premises	0.326
		NumOfTactics(over-3)	0.230
		InOperation(0)	0.229
	Arrest Mode	**ArrMode_Given_into_custody**	0.281
		ViolentOnArrest(0)	0.195
		OnBailAtTimeOfOffence(0)	0.187
		ArrMode_Result_of_Enquiries(0)	0.179
		ArrMode_Other(0)	0.171

c. Euclidean Distance among all the dataset variables (ED Algorithm):

$$d_{i,j}^{[E]} = \sqrt{\sum_{k=1}^{M}(x_{i,k} - x_{j,k})^2};\ i,j \in [1,2,..N];\ x \in [0,1]. \tag{14.21}$$

All three techniques are very robust: The LC Algorithm determines the proportionality among the variables; the PP Algorithm defines their probability of co-occurrence; and the ED algorithm measures their distances in a flat space. At the same time, all these techniques are very limited: the LC and the PP algorithms consider only the first order of effects among variables and the ED algorithm assumes the Euclidean space as the only metric able to explain the closeness among the variables. So, these algorithms represent three tools to analyze three manifestations of evidence in a dataset: *the evidence of linearity, the evidence of probability, and the evidence of distance*. But there is no linear correlation among these three techniques: each technique can determine what is hidden for the others. Consequently, the LC, PP, and ED algorithms are three robust, independent, and limited techniques. When a highly nonlinear and multivariate algorithm (like SOM or AutoCM) determines some association supported by at least one of these three techniques, we can say that this complex algorithm has discovered something that is trivial, but grounded.

2. We calculate for each linear algorithm (LC, PP, and ED) and for SOM and AutoCM, the Minimum Spanning Tree (obviously, to do that some intelligent pre-processing is needed).
3. We compare the agreement of MST of each algorithm with the MST of the others; in this way we can define for each algorithm three different basic indexes and one composed index:

   a. **The Intersection Index**: to what extent the associations of any two of the algorithms agree:

$$\text{Iindex}_{i,j} = \sum_{k}^{M} \frac{(\text{link}_i = \text{true} \cap \text{link}_j = \text{true})}{(\text{link}_i = \text{true} \cup \text{link}_j = \text{true})}; \qquad (14.22)$$

   where:
   $i, j \in N$
   $K \in M$
   $N =$ Number of different MST coming from different algorithms;
   $M = (\text{Num Variables})^2$

   b. **The Evidence Index**: how much the associations of each algorithm are supported by the associations of the others:

$$\text{Eindex}_i = \frac{1}{2(N-1)(M-1)} \sum_{z=1}^{M} \sum_{k=1}^{M} \sum_{j=1;j\neq i}^{N} (\text{link}_{i,z,k} = \text{true} \cap \text{link}_{j,z,k} = \text{true}); \qquad (14.23)$$

   where:
   $i, j \in N$
   $K \in M$
   $N =$ Number of different MST coming from different algorithms;
   $M = \text{Num Variables}^2$

c. **The Singularity Index**: How many times the associations of each algorithm are only self-supported:

$$\text{Sindex}_i = \frac{1}{2(N-1)(M-1)} \sum_{z=1}^{M} \sum_{k=1}^{M} \text{link}_{i,z,k} = \text{true} \cap \left(\sum_{j=1;j \neq i}^{N} \left(\text{link}_{j,z,k} = \text{false}\right) \right) = 0; \tag{14.24}$$

where:
$i, j \in N$
$K \in M$
N = Number of different MST coming from different algorithms;
M = Num Variables^2

d. **The E-S Ratio Index**: this is for each algorithm the balance between associations supported by other algorithms and associations that are self-supported:

$$\text{Ratio}_i = -\ln\left(\frac{\text{Sindex}_i}{\text{Eindex}_i}\right); -\infty \leq \text{Ratio}_i \leq +\infty. \tag{14.25}$$

14.4.1 The Intersection Index

The Intersection Index shows the agreement and disagreement between any two algorithms, in respect to their fundamental associations among the dataset variables.

From a global point of view the behavior of the five algorithms considered is shown in Fig. 14.8 and in Tables 14.6 and 14.7:

Table 14.6 points out that more than half of the Auto-CM connections are supported by Linear Correlation (LC) and more than one-third of the SOM connections are supported by Euclidean Distance (ED). LC seems to behave as a bridge between Auto-CM and SOM, while the PP Algorithm shows a completely different logic.

Table 14.6 Intersection indexes of algorithms

Algorithms	Agreement
CM-LC	52.22%
ED-SOM	37.01%
ED-LC	34.73%
LC-SOM	30.36%
ED-CM	27.74%
CM-SOM	23.37%
LC-PP	14.10%
CM-PP	14.06%
ED-PP	11.36%
PP-SOM	8.62%

Table 14.7 Means of intersection indexes of the algorithms

Algorithms	Mean Agreement
LC	32.85%
CM	29.35%
ED	27.71%
SOM	24.84%
PP	12.03%

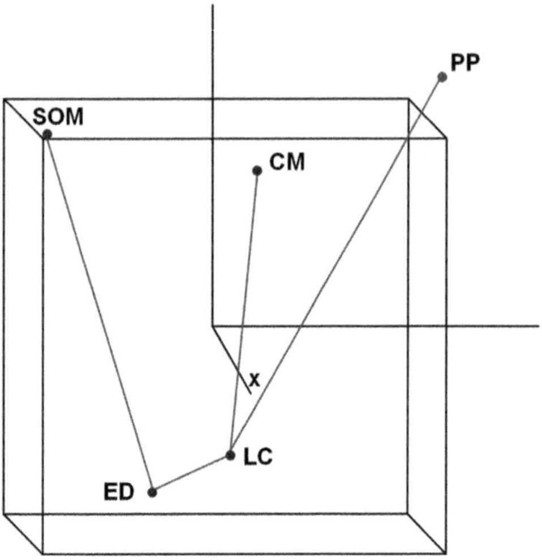

Fig. 14.8 Projection into a 3 dimensional space of the behavior of the five algorithms intersection values according to the similarity of results for the "Persons" dataset

If we translate the algorithms intersection values into a matrix distance and if we project this matrix distance into a three-dimensional space, we obtain the following map:

We can conclude the analysis of this index with this observation:

Auto-CM is supported by LC as SOM is supported by LC and ED, while PP seems to be an outlier.

14.4.2 The Evidence and the Singularity Indexes

The Evidence Index measures to what extent the associations of each algorithm are supported by the associations of the others. The Singularity Index measures the opposite: how many associations in each algorithm are not supported at all by the others.

The Evidence Index is important to establish to what extent the connections of each algorithm are supported and shared by the others. The greater the support and sharing among some connections, the more reliable those connections.

The Singularity Index, instead, is fundamental to understanding to what extent the connections of each algorithm are specific and hidden to the others. Obviously, it is not possible to know a priori if this specificity is grounded.

For this reason we have proposed a new index: the *ratio between Evidence and Singularity*. According to the *Ratio Index* we can distinguish three classes of algorithms:

1. Conservative Algorithms, where Ratio $\gg 0$.
2. Creative Algorithms, where Ratio $\ll 0$.
3. Moderate Algorithms, where Ratio $\cong 0$.

Furthermore, if, for each algorithm, we calculate the *variance* of the algorithms that support or do not support at all every connection, then we can also define the *specificity* of the research area of each algorithm.

Table 14.8 shows the behavior of the five algorithms after the analysis of the "Persons" dataset from the point of view of:

1. Evidence Index;
2. Singularity Index;
3. Ratio Index;
4. Variance of Association Support.

Table 14.8 The behavior of the five algorithms after the analysis of the "Persons" dataset

Algorithms	Support	Singulatiries	Variety	Ratio
LC	0.7469	0.2531	0.4166	1.0824
CM	0.6816	0.3184	0.4142	0.7613
ED	0.5224	0.4776	0.4188	0.0899
SOM	0.4735	0.5265	0.4139	-0.1062
PP	0.1837	0.8163	0.4281	-1.4917

Table 14.8 describes the basic profile of each algorithm:

1. The fundamental associations of the LC algorithm agree with most of the other algorithms, but its capability to discover new associations is limited.
2. The associations of the Auto-CM algorithm are also well supported, but also the number of its specific connections is high.
3. Around 1/2 of the associations of the ED algorithm are supported by the other algorithms, but most of these associations are singular (47.76%).
4. The basic associations of the SOM algorithm are partially supported by the other algorithms, while its creativity is pretty high (52.65%).
5. The associations of the PP Algorithm are very creative (81.63%), but the number of associations supported by the other algorithms is very low.

14.4.3 The Models Fusion Methodology (MFM)

When we use Auto-poietic systems, such as nonsupervised ANNs, it is not easy to establish which algorithm is more consistent than the others. The only "gold standard" in this case is to explore every algorithm hypothesis on the field. But for these algorithms we need to organize a detective strategy. So we need to define "a priori" which of the proposed links are more believable.

Because each of the presented algorithms follows different mathematics, the best way is via a fusion:

a. Each of the presented algorithms proposes a specific tree of dependencies among the variables of the same dataset (the MST);
b. We need to extract from all these trees only one graph whose links among the variables are the more robust and believable;
c. So, we overlap all the trees and we conserve only the connections selected by at least two different algorithms; in other words: if two different algorithms, using different mathematics, outline the same link between two variables, then it is more probable that between these two variables the link is "real."

Consequently, we generate a graph with interesting features:

a. The resulting graph can present cycles;
b. the resulting graph could also be a disconnected graph (see Fig. 14.9a).

Working in this way we discover a new scenario: the graph generated by the fusion is a disconnected graph divided into at least four frames as follows:

1. The variables without links: 16 of the analyzed variables belong to this group:
   Sexual Offences (typically one)
   Sexual Offences (typically two)
   Offences against Property (typically one)
   Voilence on the Arrest (typically one)
   One years from the last Conviction
   Two years from the last Conviction
   3-5 years from the last Conviction
   11-20 years from the last Conviction
   East Europe Nationality
   Sex: Female
   Fraud Offences (typically one)
   Fraud Offences (typically between 2-5)
   Residence borough not available
   Non UK Nationality
   Result of Enquiries (typically two)
   On Bail at the time of Offence (typically one)

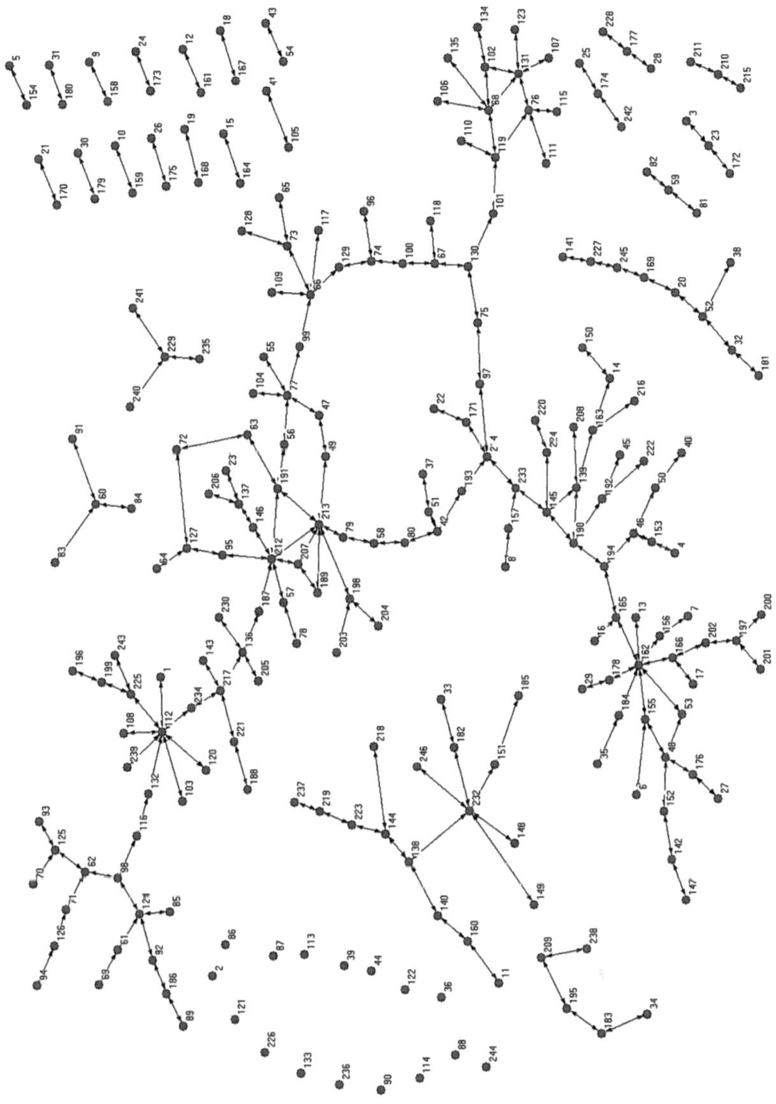

Fig. 14.9a The final graph of the associations among variables

For these variables it is not possible to make specific inferences. Maybe, in some cases the number of records is too small, or too different. In any case, for these variables there is no minimum of convergence among the algorithms.

2. The twin variables: 28 variables are clustered into 14 couples, but any couple is completely disconnected from all the other variables of the dataset: 12 of these couples represent the link between the "borough of the arrest" and "the borough where the arrested person lives":

   The other two couples show a specific relationship between nationality and behavior and nationality and ethnic group:

Arrest: Lambeth	Home: Lambeth
Arrest: Islington	Home: Islington
Arrest: Hammesmith	Home: Hammesmith
Arrest: Hillingdon	Home: Hillingdon
Arrest: Croydon	Home: Croydon
Arrest: Sutton	Home: Sutton
Arrest: Merton	Home: Merton
Arrest: Havering	Home: Havering
Arrest: Southwark	Home: Southwark
Arrest: Barnet	Home: Barnet
Arrest: Enfield	Home: Enfield
Arrest: Camden	Home: Camden

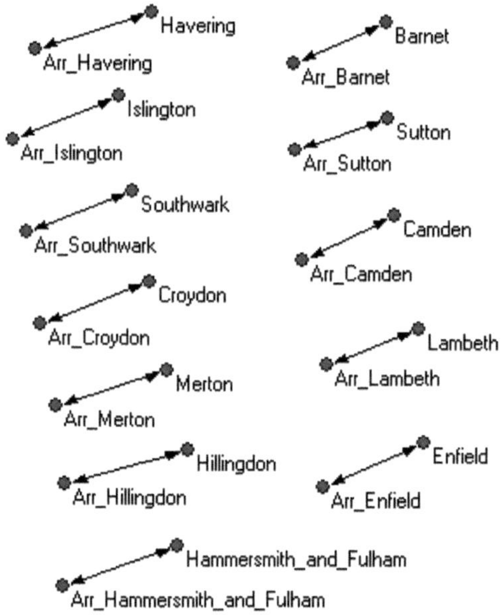

Irish	Offences against Persons (typically 2)
Middle East	Arab

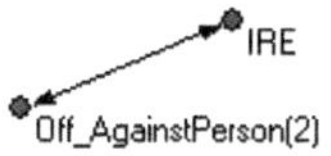

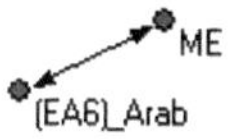

This clustering means that more than one algorithm finds a strong relationship between the two variables, but this link is the only one.

3. The next frame is formed by groups of three, four or more variables with specific links to each other, clustered into isolated small worlds (see Figs. 14.9b–f):

   a. "Other Law-Enforcement Agent" is the common point linking "Controlled Delivery" and "Search of Object."
   b. Persons whose age is between 35 and 45 have their first conviction within the same interval of age.
   c. Persons living in Kingston upon Thames are arrested in the same borough (and this seems to be typical), but with these persons the agents typically declare that they are not able to define their gender.
   d. Persons arrested in Lewisham often live in the same borough, but typically they are arrested many times in a nondirect mode.
   e. Persons arrested in Redbridge often live in the same borough, but typically their arrest mode is not declared by the police.
   f. Persons over 45 received their last conviction 20 years ago and typically they actually come back to commit offences.
   g. Persons not arrested in a direct mode are obviously arrested in other ways and often as a result of enquiries.
   h. MDMA is typically found by non Law-Enforcement Agents. They arrest the persons involved taking them into custody. This is typical for the borough of Wandsworth, the place where the arrested persons live.
   i. One graph is about the Asian world: Asian persons, with Asian nationality, are arrested fundamentally in two boroughs: Tower Hamlets and Hounslow, where typically these persons also live. But the Asian people of Hounslow have interesting features: they have already been arrested more than one time in a violent mode, because of offences against persons, and very often they were on bail at the time of the offence.
   j. The last small world is about the direct arrest of violent persons, with firearms and weapons; most of these persons are old criminals, with an impressive curriculum in drugs trafficking and other types of offences. Typical places where these persons live and where they are arrested are Waltham Forest and Ealing.

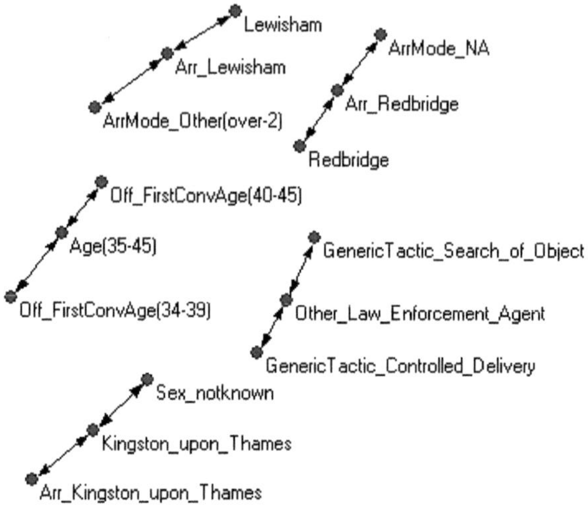

Fig. 14.9b Example of "small worlds"

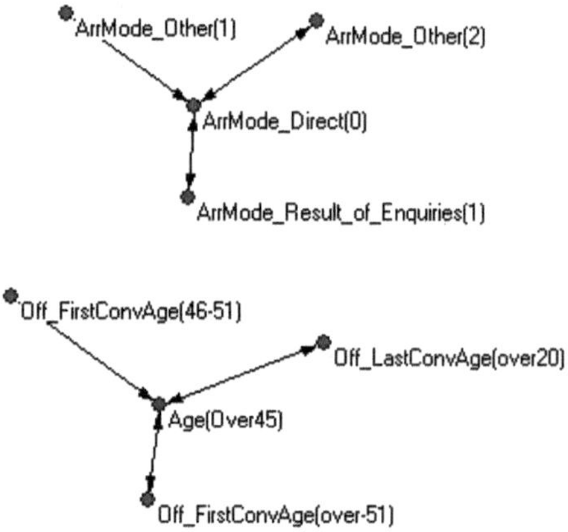

Fig. 14.9c Example of "small worlds"

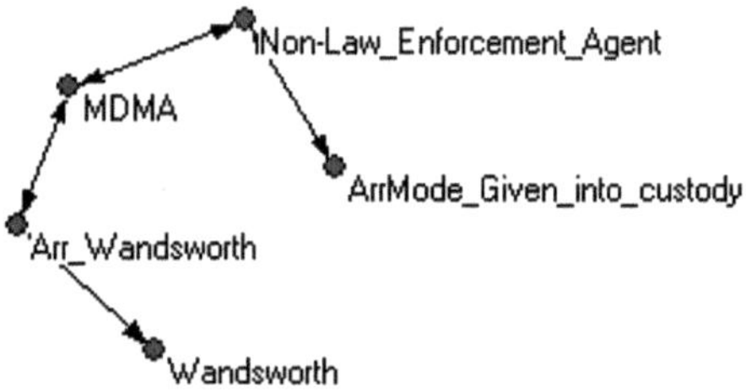

Fig. 14.9d Example of "small worlds"

Fig. 14.9e Example of "small worlds"

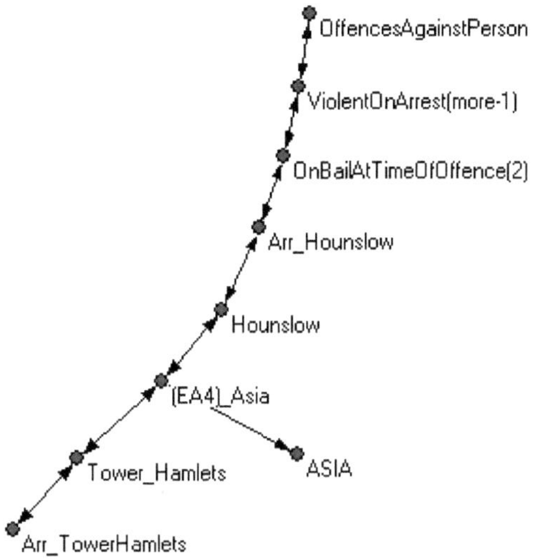

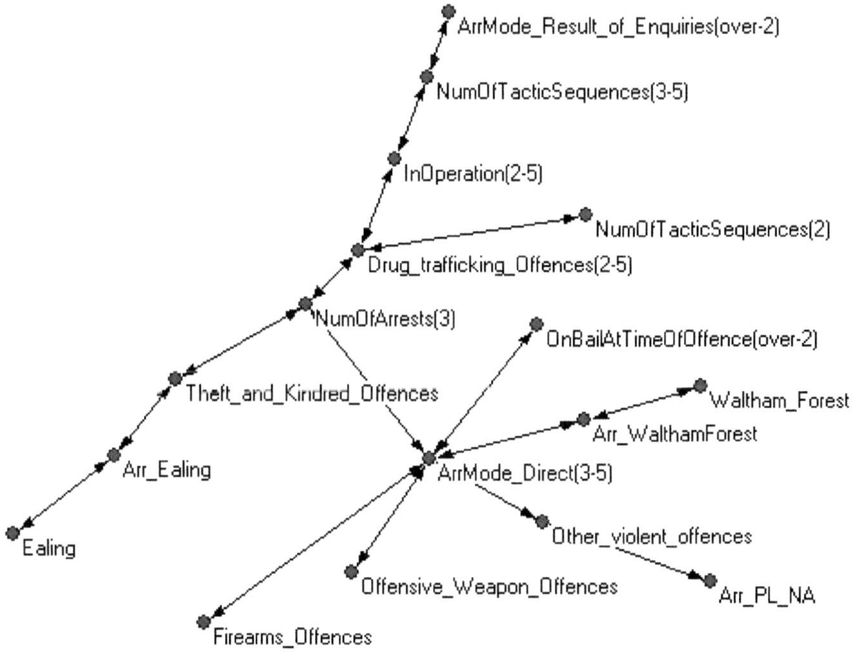

Fig. 14.9f Example of "small worlds"

Of course the other 146 variables are connected in the same big graph. Each one of these connections is proven by at least two independent algorithms, so they should be quite strong and robust.

This big graph (see Fig. 14.10a) shows many cycles and a thorough analysis of the graph would take many pages. In any case, if we look only at the positions of the four drugs and of their neighbors, we can define a robust and a synthetic prototype of each drug (see Figs. 14.10b and 14.10c).

Table 14.9 should be a road map for the anti-drug strategy in London: showing in which boroughs police should look for which type of drug, which persons, with which criminal curricula, with which tactics, etc.

Table 14.9 Prototypes for the five drugs according to the MFM

Drugs	First Order Neighbors	Second Order Neighbors
Crack	Jamaican	Afro-Caribbean
		Age of first Convictions(28-33)
	Covert Purchase	Arr_Kensignton_and_Chelsea
		Drugs Offences (over 10)
		Arrest in Direct Mode (over 5)
Heroin	Arr_Haringay	Home Haringay
		Arr_Grrenwhich
	Turkish-Cypriots	Dark-European
		Arr_Baking_and_Dagenham
	NumOfDrugSeizures(over 5)	Drug_Trafficking_Offences(over 5)
		NumOfArrests(over 3)
		Cocaine
Cocaine	InOperation(1)	
	SAME (South Americans)	
	NumOfDrugSeizures(over 5)	Drug_Trafficking_Offences(over 5)
		NumOfArrests(over 3)
		Heroin
Cannabis	Convictions Number (2)	Offences Number(3-5)
	Age(18-21)	First_Conviction_Age(up to 18)
	Tactic Search of Persons	Tactic Search of Premises
		Drug Offences (3-5)
		Drug Possesion Offences
		Num of Drug Seizures (1)
		Age(21-25)
		Num of Tactics(3)
	Tactic Search of Premises	Tactic Search of Person
		White European
		Num of Tactics(3)
		Num of Drug Seizures (3-5)
		Num of Cash Seazures (over 1)
		First_Conviction_Age(22-27)
MDMA	Non-Law Enforcement Agent	Arrest Mode : Given into Custody
	Arrest: Wandsworth	Home: Wandsworth

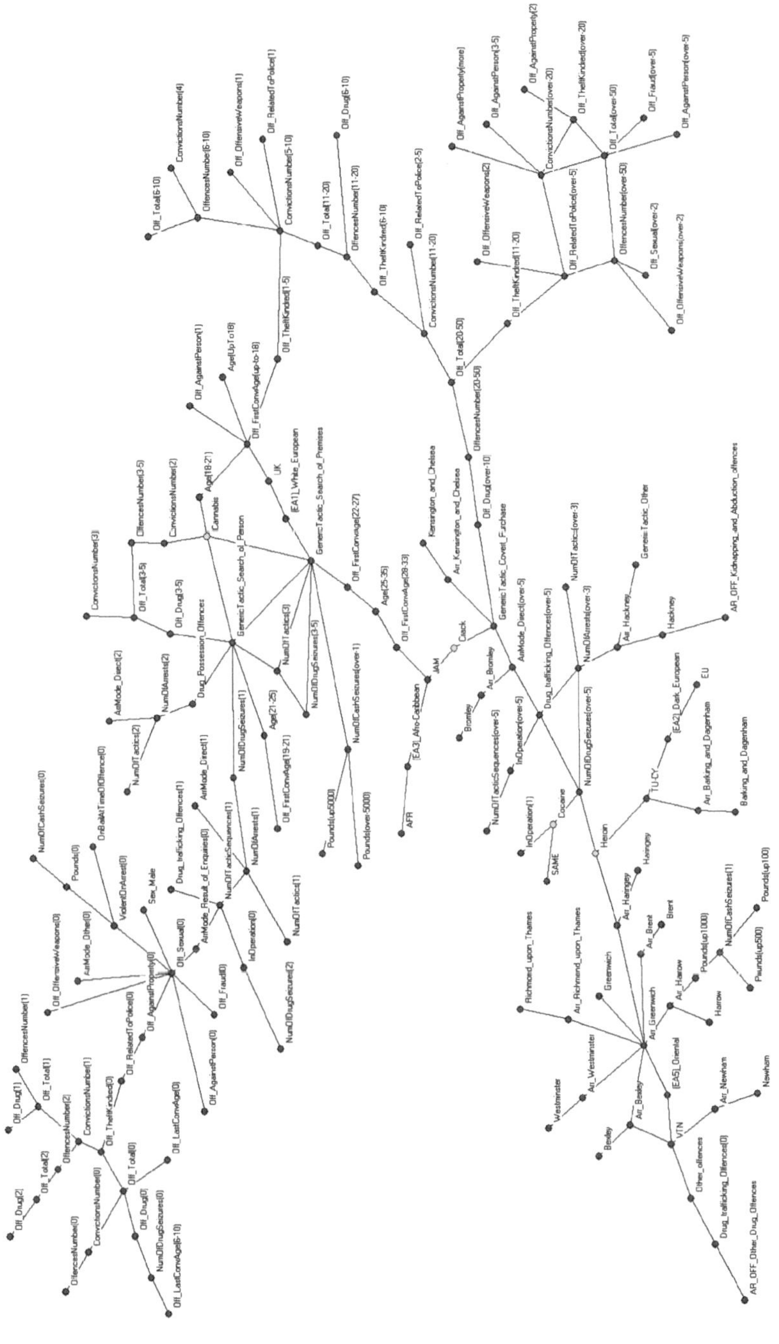

Fig. 14.10a The big graph. From the position of the four drugs and of their neighbors, we can define a robust and a synthetic prototype of each drug

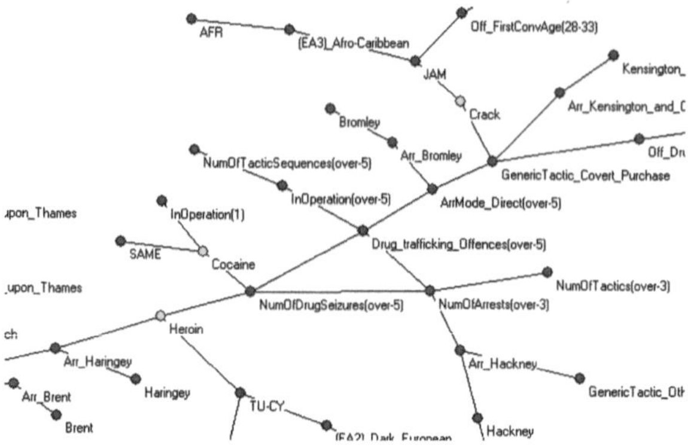

Fig. 14.10b Close-up of three drugs

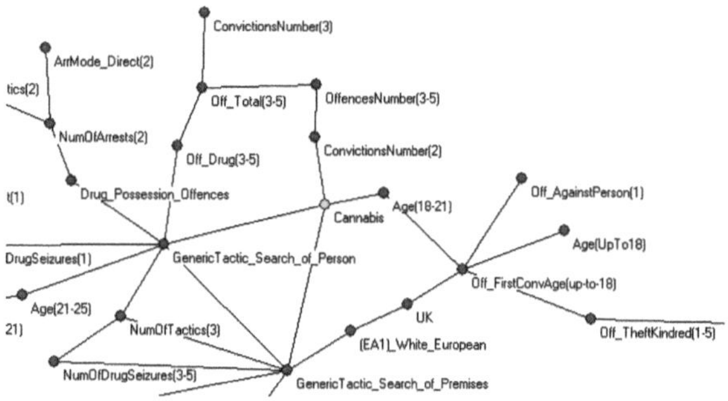

Fig. 14.10c Close-up of Cannabis

14.5 Conclusions

This paper presents an example of how to apply nonlinear auto-associative systems to data analysis. For this reason we have presented data and equations in a style that is unusual for such a paper.

Nonlinear auto-associative systems are often known by the generic name of non-supervised Artificial Neural Networks (ANNs). These systems, however, represent a powerful set of techniques for data mining and they do not deserve simply a generic name. We propose to name this set of ANNs "Auto-poietic ANNs" (that is, systems that organize their behaviors by themselves).

Auto-poietic ANNs are a complex mix of different topologies, learning rules, signal dynamics, and cost functions. So, their mathematics can be very different from one to another and their capability to discover hidden connections within the same dataset can be very different too. This represents both the strength and the weakness of these algorithms.

All the Auto-poietic ANNs, in fact, can determine within a dataset how each (independent) variable is associated with the others, also considering nonlinear associations involved in parallel many-to-many relationships. But, because of the specific mathematics of each one of these algorithms, the final findings of their application to the same dataset can be different. Consequently, when we apply different Auto-poietic ANNs to the same sample of data, we can find as the result of their learning process different frames of associations among the same set of variables. The problem, at this point, is: which of these frames is more grounded? If the dataset represents a real situation, which of the resulting frames should we follow to organize a productive strategy of manipulation in the real world?

A weak, but politically correct, answer could be: every algorithm shows us different features of the same world. But we need to know, indeed, which one of these features is more robust and fundamental than the others. In fact, strategies and actions in the real world are expensive and we should spend our energy aiming directly at the critical points of a real situation. The main target of a data analysis is exactly this.

When we use supervised ANNs or other types of supervised classifiers out target is different: because our dataset presents dependent variables, we need to believe that these dependent variables represent the "gold standard" and consequently we can size the effectiveness of our supervised algorithms following different and robust validation protocols: K-fold cross validation, 5×2 Cross Validation, Training-Testing-Prediction protocol, etc.

When using Auto-poietic ANNs we do not have dependent variables, so we do not have a gold standard.

To be honest we have to say that many validation protocols were proposed to analyze the performances of Auto-poietic systems. But all these validation protocols aim at controlling the self-consistency and flexibility (capability to react in similar ways to unseen inputs, when the last ones are similar to known inputs) of the Auto-poietic ANNs.

This is not enough.

The only effective validation protocol for these systems should consist of a field analysis able to control their association schemes in real situations. This is the best of the possible worlds, following the right methodology to execute a validation of the field; but this method has some counter-indications: it is a very expensive method (the number of possible connections among N variables is 2^N, only considering the limit case where each connection can be present or absent), and the data-mining target should be known a priori.

These are the reasons why we have proposed a new probabilistic method for validating the performances of Auto-poietic ANNs, when they are used for data mining.

We have organized our methodology into different steps:

1. We have chosen a representative dataset of a real situation: the arrests executed in London for drug trafficking over a sequence of four months.
2. We have chosen two very powerful and very different Auto-poietic ANNs: the Auto-contractive maps (AutoCM) and the Self-organizing maps (SOM). These two algorithms present completely different mathematics (topology, learning rule, signal dynamics, and cost function), but they have the same general goal:

to analyze the global similarities of the records of a dataset according to their variables, including the nonlinear associations among the variables themselves.

3. We have chosen the Minimum Spanning Tree (MST) as a filter to synthesize the main associations among variables that the two Auto-poietic ANNs have found at the end of their learning process. The MST has many suitable properties, considering its capability to put in evidence the fundamental backbone of a structure. In this case the "structure" is the matrix of associations among variables generated by each one of our Auto-poietic ANNs.
4. We have selected three simple linear algorithms, very different to each other and very robust and mathematically grounded:

   a. The Linear Correlations algorithm (LC), based on the co-variance of any couple of variables;
   b. the Prior Probability algorithm (PP), based on the probabilistic co-occurrence of any couple of variables;
   c. the Euclidean Distance (ED), based on the assumption that the distance from any variable and the others is in a flat space of N dimensions.

   These three algorithms are very orthogonal to each other, but at the same time each is able to determine very robust, but sometimes trivial relationships among variables. We have used these three algorithms as "sapiens sauvage": they are not educated to discover nonlinear relations among variables, or complex many-to-many associations, but they are expert in determining evidences among data. And what is more important is that each of these three algorithms is oriented towards looking for evidences within the data in three different areas of the whole space of the variables possible associations.
   Using these three algorithms as "basic analysts," we are able to understand when the associations found by the two complex Auto-poietic ANNs are:

   a. Evident for one or more of the "basic analysts";
   b. original and supported by the two ANNs together;
   c. original and supported by only one of the two ANNs;
   d. evident for at least one of the "basic analysts," but unseen by one or both the ANNs.

5. At this point we have generated the MST of the five algorithms (the three basic analysts and the two ANNs) and we have made a point-to-point comparison among them. The goal of this match is to create a new graph, where only the associations among variables, supported by at least two algorithms, were present. Obviously, each connection will have a different membership of plausibility according to the number of algorithms supporting it. In the same way, each connection will have also a different grade of originality, if supported only by the ANNs (if the number of ANNs in our experiment were greater than two, the cut-off of two algorithms to accept the connections, will work all the same).

Using this methodology, which we named Model Fusion Methodology, we can also produce a sparse graph (some nodes and/or groups of nodes disconnected from the others), with many and complex cycles. This is good. We are able to determine for which variables nothing can be said (nodes isolated), for which variables we can say "something" (group of nodes isolated), and which simple or complex circuits (cliques) are grounded into the dataset.

We can consider the ANN as an "individual" with its own point of view about a dataset. So a group of ANNs/individuals makes an hypothesis about the kind of relationship among the entities of a dataset, that is to say the variables. Greater is the number of these points of view, higher is the probability of convergence towards a single and stable hypothesis on the relationship among the variables which can be considered as the "soul" of a dataset.

Bibliography

Buscema, M. (2007a). A novel adapting mapping method for emergent properties discovery in data bases: experience in medical field. In *2007 IEEE International Conference on Systems, Man and Cybernetics (SMC 2007)*. Montreal, Canada, 7–10 October.

Buscema, M. (2007b). Squashing Theory and Contractive Map Network, Semeion Technical Paper #32, Rome.

Buscema, M., Didoné, G., and Pandin, M. (1994). *Reti Neurali AutoRiflessive, Teoria, Metodi, Applicazioni e Confronti*. Quaderni di Ricerca, Armando Editore, n.1, *[Self-reflexive networks: Theory, methods, applications and comparison*. Semeion Research book by Armando Publisher, n.1].

Buscema, M. and Grossi E. (2008a) The semantic connectivity map: An adapting self-organizing knowledge discovery method in data bases. Experience in Gastro-oesophageal reflux disease. *Int. J. Datamining and Bioinfo.* 2(4), 362–404.

Buscema, M., Helgason, C., and Grossi, E. (2008b). *Auto-contractive maps, H function and maximally regular graph: theory and applications*. Special session on artificial adaptive systems in medicine: applications in the real world, NAFIPS 2008 (IEEE), New York, May 19–22.

Buscema, M., Grossi, E., Snowdon, D., and Antuono, P. (2008c) Auto-contractive maps: An artificial adaptive system for data mining. An application to Alzheimer disease. *Curr. Alzheimer Res.* 5, 481–498.

Fredman, M. L. and Willard, D. E. (1990). Trans-dichotomous algorithms for minimum spanning trees and shortest paths. 31st IEEE Symp. *Foundations of Comp. Sci.* 719–725.

Chauvin, Y. and Rumelhart D. E., (Eds.). (1995). *Backpropagation: Theory, architectures, and applications*. 365 Broadway Hillsdale, New Jersey: Lawrence Erlbaum Associates, Inc. Publishers.

Cormen, T. H., Leiserson, C. E., Rivest, R. L., and Stein, C. (2001). *Introduction to Algorithms* (2nd edn, pp. 567–574). MIT Press and McGraw-Hill. ISBN 0-262-03293-7. Section 23.2: The algorithms of Kruskal and Prim.

Fahlman, S. E. (1988). An empirical study of learning speed in back-propagation networks. CMV Technical Report, CMV-CS-88-162.

Gabow, H. N., Galil, Z., Spencer, T., and Tarjan, R. E. (1986). Efficient algorithms for finding minimum spanning trees in undirected and directed graphs. *Combinatorica* 6, 109–122.

Karger, D. R., Klein, P. N., Tarjan, R. E. (1995). A randomized linear-time algorithm to find minimum spanning trees. *J. ACM* 42, 321–328.

Kohonen, T., (1990). The self-organizing map. *Proceedings IEEE* 78, 1464–1480.

Kohonen, T. (1995). Learning vector quantization. In Arbib (Ed.), *The handbook of brain theory and neural networks*. A Bradford Book, Cambridge MA, London, England: The MIT Press.

Kohonen, T. (1995b). *Self-organizing maps*. Berlin, Heidelberg: Springer Verlag.

Kruskal J. B., (1956). *On the shortest spanning subtree of a graph and the traveling salesman problem*. In Proc Amer. Math. Soc. 7(1), 48–50.

Licastro, F., Porcellini, E., Chiappelli, M., Forti, P., Buscema, M. et al. (2010). *Multivariable network associated with cognitive decline and dementia, in Neurobiology of Aging*, 31, 257–269.
McClelland, J. L., and Rumelhart, D. E., (1988). *Explorations in parallel distributed processing.* Cambridge MA: The MIT Press.
Rumelhart, D. E., McClelland J. L, (Eds.). (1986). Parallel distributed processing. Vol. 1: *Foundations, explorations in the microstructure of cognition*. Vol. 2: *Psychological and biological models*. Cambridge MA: The MIT Press.

Research Software

Buscema, M. (2002). Contractive Maps, Ver. 1.0, Semeion Software #15, Rome, 2000–2002.
Buscema, M. (2007). Constraints Satisfaction Networks, Ver 11.0, Semeion Software #14, Rome, 2001–2007.
Buscema, M. (2008). MST, Ver 5.1, Semeion Software #38, Rome, 2006–2008.
Massini, G. (2007a). Trees Visualizer, Ver 3.0, Semeion Software #40, Rome, 2007.
Massini, G. (2007b). Semantic Connection Map, Ver 1.0, Semeion Software #45, Rome, 2007.

Chapter 15
Medicine and Mathematics of Complex Systems: An Emerging Revolution

Enzo Grossi

Abstract The entrance of mathematics in medicine is relatively recent, dating back to nineteenth century. This entrance has coincided with a spectacular progress in the quality and accuracy of health care provided, till the unexpected predominance of chronic degenerative disease characterized by high complexity and nonlinearity and not affordable with the traditional mathematics of linear systems.

A new mathematics, borrowed from chaos theory, nonlinear dynamics, and complexity theory, is now slowly helping physicians in affording a second revolution by which we expect to substantially improve the application of basic research discoveries to the real world.

The coupling of computer science and these new theoretical bases coming from complex systems mathematics allows the creation of "intelligent" agents able to adapt themselves dynamically to problem of high complexity: the artificial neural networks (ANNs).

ANNs are able to reproduce the dynamical interaction of multiple factors simultaneously, allowing the study of complexity; they can also draw conclusions on individual basis and not as average trends. These tools can allow a more efficient technology transfer from the science of medicine to the real world overcoming many obstacles responsible for the present translational failure. They also contribute to a new holistic vision of the human subject contrasting the statistical reductionism which tends to squeeze or even delete the single subject sacrificing him to his group of belongingness. Some examples of the added value obtainable by the use of advanced intelligent systems in different medical fields are described.

E. Grossi (✉)
Medical Department, Bracco Spa, Milano, Italy; Centro Diagnostico Italiano, Milano, Italy; Semeion Research Centre, Rome, Italy
e-mail: enzo.grossi@bracco.com

V. Capecchi (eds.), *Applications of Mathematics in Models, Artificial Neural Networks and Arts*, DOI 10.1007/978-90-481-8581-8_15,

15.1 Introduction: Some Milestones of Mathematics in Medicine

For many centuries medicine has not considered the use of mathematics for its evolution.

Harvey waited from 1615 to 1628 to publish his results about the use of mathematics to infer the existence of blood circulation and blood volume, contradicting Galen's views dating for over 1400 years.

The result of Harvey is the most significant achievement in physiology and medicine of the seventeenth century.

In seventeenth century the strong message by Galileo about the existence of a language of universe, written in mathematical terms, is not immediately captured by medical science:

> Questo grandissimo libro che continuamente ci sta aperto innanzi a gli occhi (io dico l'universo), non si può intendere se prima non s'impara a intender la lingua, e conoscer i caratteri, ne' quali è scritto. Egli è scritto in lingua matematica, e i caratteri son triangoli, cerchi, ed altre figure geometriche, senza i quali mezi è impossibile a intenderne umanamente parola; senza questi è un aggirarsi vanamente per un oscuro labirinto.
>
> Galileo Galilei, 1623; Il Saggiatore p. 171.

We have to wait till nineteenth century for a formal entrance of mathematics in medicine, when two outstanding pioneers, one French and the other British, come into the scene.

15.1.1 Pierre Louis and the Numerical Method

In the aftermath of the French Revolution, Victor Broussais, a Parisian doctor, claimed that all fevers had the same origin: they were manifestations of the inflammation of organs. Accordingly, leeches were applied on the surface of the body corresponding to the inflamed organ and the resultant bloodletting was deemed to be an efficient treatment. For example, the chest of a patient suspected of having pneumonitis was covered with a multitude of leeches. Broussais' theories were highly regarded by contemporary French physicians. His influence can be assessed using an economic measure: In 1833 alone, France imported 42 million leeches for medical use. Before he began practising in France, Pierre-Charles-Alexandre Louis (1787–1872) had had some experience as a clinician in Russia. He doubted of the validity of Broussais' theory and published several monographs arguing against it. Louis was a meticulous clinician and this had important implications for the quality of his research. He had a large collection of case records, which he had assembled during years of intensive clinical activity and autopsy in the Parisian hospital La Charité. The 77 patients that he selected for his bloodletting analysis were a very homogeneous group with the same, well-characterized form of "pneumonia." They had all been in perfect health at the time of the first symptoms of their disease. After establishing as accurately as he could the timing of the onset of the disease in each of his 77 patients, Louis analyzed the duration of the disease and the frequency of death by the timing of the first bloodletting. He grouped patients by whether they had been bled early (days 1–4 of the illness) or late (days 5–9). This division resulted in two comparison groups of 41 and 36 patients, which were of comparable average age (41 and 38 years, respectively). He found that the duration of disease was an average of 3 days shorter in those who had been bled early compared with those who had been bled late. However, "three sevenths" (i.e., 44%) of the patients who had been bled early died compared to "only one fourth" (i.e., 25%) of those bled late, a result that Louis remarked was "startling and apparently absurd" (1836, p. 9). In the light of these findings, Louis concluded that there were useful effects of bloodletting, but only for specific indications. Louis also believed, without providing supporting quantitative evidence, that abundant bleeding worked better than local bleeding: "These observations seem to show that the use of the lancet should be preferred to that of leeches in the diseases which we have been considering."

We are indebted to Pierre Louis for the first introduction of a "numeric method" in medicine which evaluates the effectiveness of a given therapeutic measure.

> You should take as many cases as possible, of as similar description as you could find, and would count how many recovered under one mode of treatment, and how many under another; in how short a time they did so; and if the cases were in all respects alike, except in the treatment, you would have some confidence in your conclusions; and if you are fortunate enough to have a sufficient number of facts from which to deduce any general law, it would lead to your employment in practice of the method you had seen oftenest successful. Louis PCA (1835)

15.1.2 John Snow and the 1854 Golden Square Cholera Epidemic

Dr. John Snow (1813–1858) is a legendary figure in the history of public health, epidemiology, and anesthesiology. He is considered to be one of the fathers of epidemiology for his persistent efforts to determine how cholera was spread and for the statistical mapping methods he invented.

Snow was a skeptic of the then-dominant miasma theory that stated that diseases such as cholera or the Black Death were caused by pollution or a noxious form of "bad air." The germ theory had not been formulated at this time, so he was unaware of the mechanism by which the disease was transmitted, but evidence led him to believe that it was not due to breathing foul air. He first publicized his theory in an essay *On the Mode of Communication of Cholera* in 1849. In 1855 a second edition was published, with a much more elaborate investigation of the effect of the water supply in the Soho, London epidemic of 1854.

Snow talked to local residents and conducted door-to-door investigation, thus collecting the data to create a spot map to illustrate how cases of cholera were centered around the pump. He used bars to represent deaths that occurred at the specified households, and by weighting the density of these bars and relating them to the distance of neighborhood pumps, he was able to identify the Broad Street pump as the origin of the spread of the cholera outbreak (Fig. 15.1). A full visual confirmation of the communication between the cesspool near number 40 and the pump

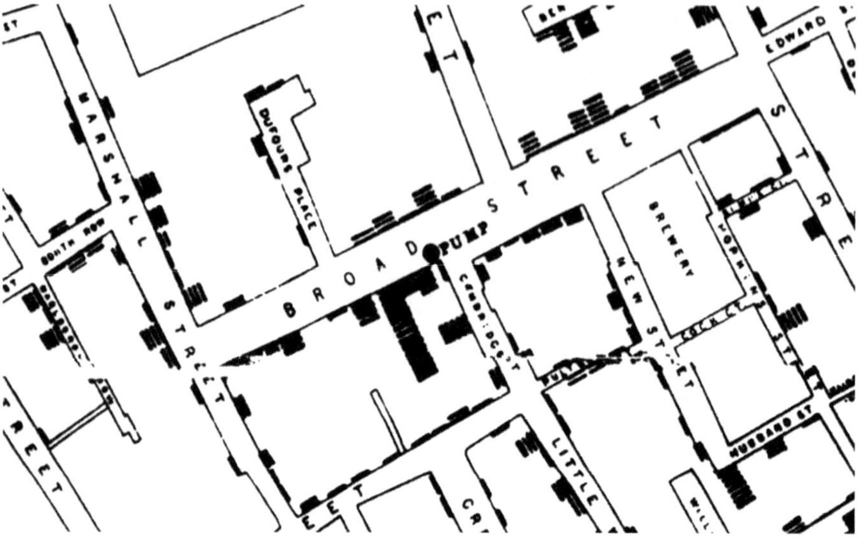

Fig. 15.1 Detail of the John Snow map with Broad Street pump

well was given 4 months after the publication of Snow's classic on the Mode of Communication of Cholera in December 1854, following a complete excavation by the parish council. It now seems likely that the index case had been living with her parents at number 40 and her mother Sarah Lewis washed the sick baby's diapers in the cesspool, allowing the vibrios to enter the water supply through communication between the cesspool and the pump well.

In Snow's own words:

> On proceeding to the spot, I found that nearly all the deaths had taken place within a short distance of the [Broad Street] pump. There were only ten deaths in houses situated decidedly nearer to another street pump. In five of these cases the families of the deceased persons informed me that they always sent to the pump in Broad Street, as they preferred the water to that of the pumps which were nearer. In three other cases, the deceased were children who went to school near the pump in Broad Street...
>
> With regard to the deaths occurring in the locality belonging to the pump, there were 61 instances in which I was informed that the deceased persons used to drink the pump water from Broad Street, either constantly or occasionally...
>
> The result of the inquiry, then, is, that there has been no particular outbreak or prevalence of cholera in this part of London except among the persons who were in the habit of drinking the water of the above-mentioned pump well.
>
> I had an interview with the Board of Guardians of St James's parish, on the evening of the 7th inst [Sept 7], and represented the above circumstances to them. In consequence of what I said, the handle of the pump was removed on the following day.
>
> —John Snow, letter to the editor of the Medical Times and Gazette

15.2 The Progress with Acute Disease and the Languish with Chronic Diseases

The introduction of mathematics in medicine has coincided, not by chance, with a spectacular improvement of the quality and accuracy of medical science, which has been translated in a substantial reduction of mortality and control of most endemic diseases.

However, the impression gained in the last two decades is that this improvement is not proportional to the basic science advancements, especially when we refer to chronic degenerative disorders like cancer or Alzheimer disease.

If we consider the body of medical literature as evidence of the amount of medical data processed all over the world, it is clear that the growth has been exponential. The number of currently published medical journals is estimated to be around 20,000 and is still increasing due also to the advent of e-publishing. This figure is at strong discrepancy with the scenario of the first decades of 1900 when the number of medical journals was in the order of a few dozens, mirroring the difficulties associated with systematic data collection and the lack of knowledge of the basic rules of clinical epidemiology, a discipline that was founded only in the 1950s. At the time, the application of statistics to the medical field was in its infancy and this is not surprising since many techniques were originally developed for different fields like agriculture and only subsequently applied to the medical setting.

In fact the most powerful and well-established statistical methods were developed in the first half of the past century when the size as well as the understanding of figures coming from clinical observations was rather limited and certainly negligible in comparison with today. These methods are still widely used today to analyze medical data and are indeed considered as standard tests by the regulatory agencies. It is noteworthy that all these methods rely on the basic assumption that medical variables are normally distributed and, more importantly, that they are linear in nature.

The reasons underlying this belief are quite easy to understand: on the one hand linear models are undoubtedly more user-friendly as compared to nonlinear ones which require stronger theoretical assumptions in the pre-analysis phase; on the other hand the limited historical exposure of physicians to medical data has led them to assume that biological phenomena share the linear laws that govern physical systems and that have their grounds in Newtonian mechanics.

The issue of nonlinearity of medical data has very rarely been raised in the literature. Clearly epidemiologists and statisticians devoted to the medical field are quite happy with linear techniques, since they have been trained from the beginning with them; physicians and other health professionals, due to their proverbial poor mathematical competence, are also happy, provided that statisticians and regulatory agencies do not think differently.

There is now the reason to ask a fundamental question: Is the mathematics used in medicine what it should be? It is perhaps useful to remind ourselves that nowadays research and practice in medicine, diagnosis, and therapy have become formidable due to the contribution of physics with all its complex mathematics behind.

15.3 The Increasing Complexity of Clinical Data

A simple way to define complexity is to differentiate a complex system from a complicated one. Complicated systems like a Boeing 747 consist of a huge number of different elementary components (approximately 200,000 in the case of Boeing 747). The assembly of this Jumbo is clearly deterministic; there is only one way to assemble these components to ensure that the Jumbo Jet will be able to fly. A screw used in the assembly remains a screw whether the Jumbo is a child's model for play or an actual jet plane taking him for a visit. The structure originated from that assembly determines the relationship between the various components, and the mathematics underlying it is often based on linear functions. For systems like this the time elapsing along their use and existence is just "noise" and does not give any special advantage. In other words, we cannot expect a better adaptation to a dynamic environment from a complicated system. With complex systems on the contrary, the rules are rather different as one might see from Table 15.1, which summarizes the principal differences between "complicated systems" and "complex systems." These systems can adapt themselves to a dynamic environment, and time for them is not "noise" but is rather a way to reduce potential errors. Complexity is an adaptive process; it is time sensitive, and over time complex processes evolve and/or degenerate. Complexity is based on small elementary units working together in small populations of synchronous processes.

Table 15.1 Complicated vs. complex systems

Complicated systems	Complex systems
Linear functions	Nonlinear functions
Adaptation to static environment	Interaction with dynamic environment
Simple casualty	Mutual casualty
Deterministic	Probabilistic
Structure determines relationships	Structure and relationships interact
Average dominate outliers irrelevant	Outliers key determinants
Components maintain their essence	Components change their essence

The experience with these relatively new concepts has helped us to understand that "acute disease," for example, behaves more as complicated systems, while degenerative chronic diseases resemble complex systems. Table 15.2 tries to summarize the principal features in this regard.

It is noteworthy the fact that in early XXth century the prevalent cause of death was attributable to acute diseases, while after one century the scenario has been dominated by chronic diseases, among which infarction, cancer and stroke are the most prevalent cause of death (See Table 15.3). Mathematical and physical techniques combined with physiological and medical studies are addressing these questions and are transforming our understanding of the rhythms of life and the processes resulting in the "failures" of life – a range of temporary and chronic disabilities, decreased quality of life, and one's ultimate final death.

Table 15.2 Complicated acute diseases and complex chronic diseases

Complicated acute disease	Complex chronic disease
Abrupt onset	Gradual onset over time
Often all causes can be identified and measured	Multivariate cause, changing over time
Diagnosis and prognosis are often accurate	Diagnosis is uncertain and prognosis obscure
Specific therapy or treatment is often available	Indecisive technologies and therapies with adversities
Technological intervention is usually effective: Cure is likely with return to normal health over time	No cure, pervasive uncertainty: management, coaching, and self-care is needed to improve health
Profession is knowledgeable while laity is inexperienced	Profession and laity must be reciprocally knowledgeable to improve health

Table 15.3 Evolution of prevalent death cause in the last 100 years

Scoring	1900	2000
1°	Pneumonia/influenza	Infarction
2°	Tuberculosis	Cancer
3°	Diarrhea	Stroke

There is therefore an emerging concept of complexity in medicine as well as an increasing awareness of and sensitivity to the network multi-dimensionality of both health and disease.

The human body is not a machine and its malfunctioning cannot be adequately analyzed by breaking the system down into its component parts and considering each in isolation.

A small change in one part of this network of interacting systems may lead to a much larger change in another part through amplification effects. For all these reasons neither illness nor human behavior is predictable and neither can safely be "modeled" in a simple cause and effect system.

As E. O. Wilson, known as the father of biodiversity, said: "The greatest challenge today, not just in cell biology and ecology but in all science, is the accurate and complete description of complex systems" (http://rainforests.mongabay.com/10complexity.htm). Scientists have broken down many kinds of systems. They think they know most of the elements and forces. The next task is to reassemble them, at least in mathematical models that capture the key properties of the entire ensembles, including their linkages, their nodes, and their hubs.

15.4 Nonlinear Dynamics in Human Physiology

Chaos theory can be considered a paradigm of the so-called nonlinear dynamics.

Mathematical analyses of physiological rhythms show that nonlinear equations are necessary to describe physiological systems (Gollub 2000).

The physiological variation of blood glucose, for example, has traditionally been considered to be linear.

Recently a chaotic component has been described both in diabetic patients and in normal subjects.

This chaotic dynamic is common in other physiological systems (Kroll 1999).

Table 15.4 summarizes some of the best examples of nonlinear dynamics in human physiology.

Table 15.4 Examples of nonlinear dynamics in human physiology

Processes with chaotic behavior	Processes with complex fractal fluctuations
Shape of EEG waves	Heart frequency
Insulin blood levels	Respiration
Cellular cycles	Systemic arterial pressure
Muscle action potential	Gait control
Esophagus motility	White blood cells number
Bowel motility	Liver regeneration patterns
Uterine pressure	

It has for instance been shown that the interbeat interval of the human heart is chaotic and that a regular heart beat is a sign of disease and a strong predictor of imminent cardiac arrest (Singer 1988).

The work of Goldberger has nicely pointed out how traditional statistics can be misleading in evaluating heart time series in health and disease. In fact there are circumstances in which two data sets belonging to two subjects can have nearly identical mean values and variances and, therefore, escape statistical distinction based on conventional comparisons. However, the raw time series can reveal dramatic differences in the temporal structure of the original data which can be explained from the fact that while one time series is from a healthy individual, the other is from a patient during episodes of severe obstructive sleep apnea.

The time series from the healthy subject reveals a complex pattern of nonstationary fluctuations. In contrast, the heart rate data set from the subjects with sleep apnea shows a much more predictable pattern with a characteristic timescale defined by prominent, low-frequency oscillations at about 0.03 Hz. Both the complex behavior in the healthy case and the sustained oscillations in the pathologic one suggest the presence of nonlinear mechanisms (Goldberger 2002).

Other researchers as McEwen and Wingfield have introduced the concept of allostasis, i.e., maintaining stability through change, as a fundamental process through which organisms actively adjust to both predictable and unpredictable events. Allostatic load refers to the cumulative cost to the body of allostasis, with allostatic overload being a state in which serious pathophysiology can occur. In this regard chaos theory seems to fit quite well with biological adaptation mechanisms (McEwen and Wingfield 2003).

The importance of chaotic dynamics and related nonlinear phenomena in medical sciences has been only recently appreciated. It is now quite clear that that chaos is not mindless disorder; it is a subtle form of order and that approximate results of treatment can be predicted (Ruelle 1994).

Chaotic dynamics are characterized most of the time by what is called a strange attractor. This roughly means that during the chaotic evolution, the variables characterizing the state of the system remain in a restricted range of values. This leads to the possibility of characterizing the system evolution in terms of probabilities (Firth 1991).

15.5 Examples of Applications of Chaos Theory to Medical Settings

One promising application of dynamic analysis involves strategies to restore complex biological variability including fractal fluctuations to cardiopulmonary systems. Initial results using artificial ventilation in experimental animals and clinical settings suggest the possibility of improving physiological function with "noisy" vs. "metronomic" parameter settings. The use of dynamic assays to uncover basic and clinical information encoded in time series also promises to provide new, readily implemented diagnostic tests for prevalent conditions such as sleep-disordered breathing. The extent to which dynamic measures and complexity-informed models and interventions will enhance diagnostic capabilities and therapeutic options in chronic obstructive lung disease is an intriguing area for future study (Goldberger 2006).

Another paradigmatic area of interest and application is represented by electroencephalography (EEG). The 19 channels in the EEG represent a dynamic system characterized by typical asynchronous parallelism. The nonlinear implicit function that defines the ensemble of electric signals series as a whole represents a meta-pattern that translates into space (hyper-surface) what the interactions among all the channels create in time.

The behavior of every channel can be considered as the synthesis of the influence of the other channels at previous but not identical times and in different quantities, and of its own activity at that moment. At the same time, the activity of every channel at a certain moment in time is going to influence the behavior of the others at different times and in different quantities. Therefore, every multivariate sequence of signals coming from the same natural source is a complex asynchronous dynamic system, highly nonlinear, in which each channel's behavior is understandable only in relation to all the others.

In a recent paper (Buscema 2007) the results obtained with the innovative use of special types of artificial neural networks (ANNs) assembled in a novel methodology named IFAST (implicit function as squashing time) capable of compressing the temporal sequence of electroencephalographic (EEG) data into spatial invariants have been presented.

The principal aim of the study was testing the hypothesis that automatic classification of MCI and AD subjects can be reasonably correct when the spatial content of the EEG voltage is properly extracted by ANNs.

Resting eyes-closed EEG data were recorded in 180 AD patients and in 115 MCI subjects. The spatial content of the EEG voltage was extracted by IFAST step-wise procedure using ANNs. The data input for the classification operated by ANNs were not the EEG data, but the connection weights of a nonlinear auto-associative ANN trained to reproduce the recorded EEG tracks.

These weights represented a good model of the peculiar spatial features of the EEG patterns at scalp surface. The classification based on these parameters was binary (MCI vs. AD) and was performed by a supervised ANN. Half of the EEG database was used for the ANN training and the remaining half was utilized for the automatic classification phase (testing).

The results confirmed the working hypothesis that a correct automatic classification of MCI and AD subjects can be obtained extracting spatial information content of the resting EEG voltage by ANNs and represent the basis for research aimed at integrating spatial and temporal information content of the EEG. By the way the best results in distinguishing between AD and MCI reached 92.33%. The comparative results obtained with the best method so far described in the literature, based on blind source separation and Wavelet pre-processing, were 80.43% ($p < 0.001$).

15.6 Artificial Adaptive Systems and Medical Decision Support

The aim of the vast majority of clinical studies is to acquire enough knowledge of the phenomena underlying the medical problem under study to be able to make some sort of prediction. Traditional statistics has addressed this goal with the use of techniques based on regression. For studies with binary endpoints (event–no event; disease A, disease B, etc.) logistic regression is considered the method of choice, while for multinomial endpoints discriminant analysis is frequently used. The regression models are the standard techniques used to address the problem of prediction (logistic regression for binomial problems and linear discriminant analysis for the multifactorial ones). These techniques have become standards due to their relative simplicity and widespread availability of adequate and validated computer software.

The best justification for the ANNs use is the additional functionality they provide to traditional statistical methods when the representation of a problem and the kind of data observed are difficult to treat with linear models (Lisboa 2000). The signal-to-noise ratio of medical data is typically very low; the high level of noise is due to the combined effects of random error in measurements, variation in clinical protocols, and geo-demographical differences between patient populations (Kennedy 1997). Data configuration coming from clinical observation often shows complex interaction between medical variables and the function connecting the data is difficult or expensive to compute (typically a nonlinear function). The current clinical application of neural networks in nonlinear inference has followed two principal aims:

- prediction of outcome and diagnosis in individual patients;
- data mining of complex data set.

From a theoretical point of view, we can say that the advantage of using ANNs as data mining tools is the following: the function connecting the data is approximated by a mathematical model; different kinds of ANNs may provide different mathematical models for the same database, in other words, different ANNs respond to different questions on the same problem. Despite the widespread use of artificial neural networks (ANNs) in several medical intervention domains, their success has been rather limited so far and from a technological point of view they remain a nonlinear modeling and inference tool that could be accessible to skilled statisticians (Cross 1995).

On the base of this observation, in recent years we have developed the hypothesis that different ANN models may cooperate, when applied on the same database in sequential or parallel order, and the outcome of such cooperation is a more articulate model of the problem in study. The organization of different kinds of ANNs in order to simulate the behavior of complex systems leads to the conception of the artificial organisms (AO). These organisms are able both to optimize training and testing splitting and the selection of the variables which contain the real information. The association of ANN with evolutionary algorithms like T&T (Training&Testing) and IS (Input Selection) which we will describe later on creates the conditions for a substantial improvement of the prediction capability. If we compare the performances of such artificial organism with the traditional statistical tools, then the differences in efficacy and accuracy in some of the data sets considered become impressive (Buscema 2004, 2005).

Our group in the last 6 years has systematically employed AO vis-à-vis "standard" and advanced (recurrent) ANNs in a variety of medical fields. Most of these analyses have been published in journals or book chapters.

Some of them have just been presented in national or international congresses. Since in all these analyses a standard protocol has been adopted we felt interesting and appropriate to perform a sort of meta-analysis of these results in order to achieve a quantitative evaluation of the real contribution yielded by the AO previously mentioned (T&T and IS) on the performance of standard ANN models processing medical database. The framework we adopt to discuss the potential value of AAS approach, both at diagnostic and prognostic level, takes into account specific medical intervention domain such as gastroenterology, Alzheimer disease, and cardiovascular medicine. Table 15.1 summarizes the overall experience with the use of AO.

We have employed AO in 19 analyses pertaining to 13 different applications concerning five major clinical areas: gastroenterology, Alzheimer disease, cardiology, pediatrics, and medical imaging. For this review of each analysis we have considered the following features: the size of the samples, the number of input variables, the number of variables selected by IS, and the obtained results in terms of sensitivity, specificity, and overall accuracy.

The sample size distribution ranged between 117 and 1001 cases (454 subjects on average), while the number of variables ranged between 14 and 105 (50.5 variables on average). A simple comparison between the performances obtained by the ANNs coupled with the AO and those of standard ANNs and traditional statistical methods (linear discriminant analysis and logistic regression) is proposed in Table 15.5.

Table 15.5 Performances obtained by the ANNs + AO, Standard ANNs and traditional statistical methods (Linear Discriminant Analysis, LDA, and Logistic Regression, LR)

		Overall accuracy %		
Medical area	Ref. Bibl.	LDA/LR	Standard ANN	ANN + AO
Gastroenterology	Andriulli 2003	64.82	68.89	79.6
	Andriulli 2003	55.05	69	88.6
	Pagano 2004	61.27	76.23	89.32
	Lanher 2005	94.6	96.6	98.8
	Pace 2005	78.31	73.43	100
	Grossi 2005	82.75	89.11	93.43
	Caspani 2005	69.74	71.59	80.52
	Dominici 2005	72.59	79.39	96.87
Alzheimer	Buscema 2004	72.36	79.86	89.92
	Buscema 2004	73.8	84.16	90.36
	Buscema 2004	75.52	83.95	87.68
	Buscema 2004	69.77	83.68	89.92
	Buscema 2004	65.1	76.6	82.21
	Buscema 2004	77.02	80.65	90.65
	Grossi 2003	73.33	76.44	83.82
Cardiology	Baldassarre 2004	69.4	71.7	85
	Penco 2005	68.37	69.81	80.8
Imaging	Vomweg 2003	79.7	81.55	92.75
Pediatrics	Buscema 2005	54.15	61.53	73.13
Mean		71.46	77.59	88.07

where the percentage of overall accuracy reached in classification/prediction tasks using ANNs + AO, standard ANNs, and LDA or LR is compared. As one can see, the performances obtained by the standard ANNs are significantly increased, in terms of the overall accuracy percent, compared with those of traditional statistical methods, even if, as stated previously, the absolute difference is not high. This trend is confirmed in all the experiments we considered with only one exception in which the standard ANNs obtained a lower performance level in comparison to traditional statistics.

The mean gain of the global accuracy in percent scores is 6.74 (see chart in Fig. 15.1). On the other hand it can be observed that the ANNs' performance obtains a large increase when these are used in combination with the AO. In fact, thanks to the combined use of T&T and IS systems, an overall accuracy of over 88% is reached (Table 15.5).

The increase exceed, on average, 10% scores. Consequentially, also the comparison between the performances of traditional statistics and ANNs coupled with AO shows a dramatic increase in the overall accuracy, equal to 16.3% scores.

In most experiments considered (89.5%) the AO performance reached an overall accuracy clearly superior to 80%; only the 36.84% of the standard ANNs and the 10.4% of traditional statistics were able to obtain the same performances. On the 36.7% of experiments with AO the overall accuracy we have obtained was higher to 90% and in one experiment the AO performance reached 100% of accuracy, with a real increase of 26% scores compared to traditional statistics and 21.7% scores compared to standard ANNs. An overall accuracy higher to 90% was obtained only in one of our experiments both by standard ANNs and by traditional statistics. Finally, we have compared the mean overall accuracy gain obtained by the standard ANNs and the AO, considering only the ten experiments where the LDA/LR techniques reached an overall accuracy ≥70%. Even when the performance of the traditional statistics is quite good, the gain obtained in the overall accuracy by both standard ANNs and AO is significantly high (5.59 and 13.63% scores, respectively). It is interesting to note that the artificial organism IS selects, on average, the 50% of the total number of observed variables.

Despite the widespread use of artificial neural networks (ANNs) in several medical intervention domains, the general appreciation of these tools remains low from the large audience and also from expert statisticians. As stated before, ANNs remain an exotic nonlinear modeling and inference tool that is accessible only to very expert statisticians. The appropriateness of the generalization performance of such nonlinear models on medical data is yet under discussion. ANNs are perceived as complex and essentially poorly available and not adequately validated techniques even if the inherently parallel architecture of neural networks enhances their noise tolerance and potential for analysis of medical data in which the signal-to-noise ratio of medical data is typically very low. One of the reasons about this skeptical attitude vs. ANNs is probably based on the discrepancy between the huge potency of these tools and the modest advantage in terms of predictive capacity in comparison with cheap and simple statistical approaches. Discriminant analysis and logistic regression typically employ a limited number of variables in building up their model (those with a prominent linear correlation with the dependent variable); ANNs on the other hand being a sort of universal approximators use all information available, independently from an eventual poor linear correlation index. This would be clearly an advantage but only in the lucky situations in which all the variables considered would be pertinent to the problem under study. Unfortunately this happens almost never and if some of the considered would be pertinent to the problem under study. Unfortunately this happens almost never and if some of the variables are actually reflecting white noise rather than true information, then the ANN lose a major part of their potential in the generalization during the testing phase. In other words, by definition ANNs can learn almost everything during the training phase, but if they learn white noise, their comprehension of the problem is rather poor, like a child who is able to repeat a foreign poetry by memory but does not understand its meaning. There are two main messages coming out from this article. The first immediate evidence is that ANNs have obtained better results than discriminant analysis or logistic regression in 18 out of 19 analyses. The advantage of ANN resulted to be striking in specific situations like diagnosis of subclinical hypothyroidism, outcome of dyspeptic symptoms, and diagnosis of GERD, with an increase in overall accuracy in the range of 20% or more. In other contexts, like the atrophic gastritis model and the Alzheimer study, the difference resulted less marked.

The variability in the outperformance of ANN reflects necessarily different degrees on nonlinearity in clinical data related to the specific nature of the medical problem in study. From the table it is also evident that standard supervised multilayer network outperforms linear discriminant, but in many cases without big differences in accuracy.

On average, in absence of AO, the results we obtained with standard ANNs would have been exactly in the range of the literature. Otherwise, if we compare the performances of such artificial organism with the traditional statistical tools, then the differences in efficacy and accuracy in some of the data sets considered become impressive. The second emerging message is that a big part of the variables considered in our analyses (50% on average) resulted to be important for the problem under evaluation for ANNs. Most of these variables would not have been considered in classical statistics modeling either for collinearity problems or for being too low linearly correlated with dependent variable. As complement of this, a big part of variables collected are redundant for the problem of study being discarded by the intelligent selection systems. This fact underlies a crucial theme in current medical practice, from economic point of view: the collection of indifferent information both for classical statistics (about 90%) and for artificial intelligence (about 50%).

Considered in this perspective AO pose themselves in the middle of a strategic behavior temperating the massive use of information typical of standard ANNs, not followed by dramatic accuracy improvement on one hand and the miserly use of information typical of classical statistical models, which stresses the paradox of the cost-utility of data collection in medical practice.

15.7 Conclusions

On the basis of previous considerations and findings we should start to systematically address the analyses of our nonlinear and complex diseases setting with a different kind of approach. In my view the use of artificial neural networks, evolutionary algorithms, and other systems of "knowledge discovery in databases" should be supported and encouraged by scientific community. The cooperation with "bio" mathematicians keen on complex adaptive systems should be strongly advocated in the interest of the community and of the quality of health care delivery.

Bibliography

Andriulli, A., Grossi, E., Buscema, M., Festa, V., Intraligi, N. M., Dominici, P., Cerutti, R., and Perri, F. (2003). NUD LOOK study group: Contribution of artificial neural networks to the classification and treatment of patients with uninvestigated dyspepsia. *Dig. Liver Dis.* 35(4), 222–231.

Baldassarre, D., Grossi, E., Buscema, M., Intraligi, M., Amato, M., Tremoli, E., Pustina, L., Castelnuovo, S., Sanvito, S., Gerosa, L., and Sirtori, C. R. (2004). Recognition of patients with cardiovascular disease by artificial neural networks. *Ann. Med.* 36(8), 630–640.

Buscema, M. (2004). Genetic doping algorithm (GenD): Theory and applications. *Expert Syst.* 21(2), 63–79.

Buscema, M., Grossi, E., Snowdon, D., Antuono, P., Intraligi, M., Maurelli, G, and Savare, R. (2004). Artificial neural networks and artificial organisms can predict Alzheimer pathology in individual patients only on the basis of cognitive and functional status. *Neuroinformatics* 2(4), 399–416.

Buscema, M., Grossi, E., Intraligi, M., Garbagna, N., Andriulli, A., and Breda, M. (2005). An optimized experimental protocol based on neuro-evolutionary algorithms application to the classification of dyspeptic patients and to the prediction of the effectiveness of their treatment. *Artif Intell Med.* 34(3), 279–305.

Buscema, M., Pingitore, G., Tripodi, S., Calvani, M., Caramia, G., Grossi, E. Intraligi, M., and Mancini, A. (2005). Allergie nei bambini: la statistica e le reti neurali artificiali nell'analisi dei fattori di rischio in gravidanza. In *Proceedings of convegno progetto bambino salute* (pp. 18–20). Portonovo-Italy.

Buscema, M., Rossini, P., Babiloni, C., and Grossi, E. (2007). The IFAST model, a novel parallel nonlinear EEG analysis technique, distinguishes mild cognitive impairment and Alzheimer's disease patients with high degree of accuracy. *Artif. Intell. Med.* 40(2), 127–141.

Caspani, G., Intraligi, M., Massini, G., Capriotti, M., Carlei, V., Maurelli, G., Mancini, A., and Buscema, M. (2005). Progetto Esonet – Applicazione delle Reti Neurali Artificiali nella diagnosi della MRGE. *Sistemi Artificiali Adattivi in Biomedicina*, 2, 118–157.

Cross, S. S., Harrison, R. F., and Kennedy, L. R. (1995). Introduction to neural networks. *Lancet* 346, 1075–1079.

Dominici, P., Grossi, E., Buscema, M., and Intraligi, M. (2005). Reti Neurali Artificiali e Screening nella MRGE Sistemi Artificiali Adattivi in Biomedicina. *Sistemi Artificiali Adattivi in Biomedicina* 2, 104–117.

Firth, W. J. (1991). Chaos, predicting the unpredictable. *Br.Med.J.*, 303, 1565–1568

Goldberger, A. L. (2006). Giles F. Filley lecture. Complex systems. *Proc. Am. Thorac. Soc.* 3(6), 467–471.

Goldberger, A. L., Amaral, L. A. N., Hausdorff, J. M., Ivanov, P. C. H., Peng, C. K., and Stanley, H. E. (2002). Fractal dynamics in physiology: alterations with disease and aging. *Proc. Natl. Acad. Sci. USA.* 99, 2466–2472

Gollub, J. P. and Cross, M. C. (2000). Nonlinear dynamics: Chaos in space and time. *Nature* 404, 710–711.

Grossi, E., Astegiano, M., Demarchi, B., Bresso, F., Sapone, N., Mancini, A., Intraligi, M., Dominici, P., and Buscema, M. (2005). Dolore addominale e alterazione dell'alvo: è possibile semplificare l'iter diagnostico attraverso l'uso di Sistemi di Intelligenza Artificiale? *Sistemi Artificiali Adattivi in Biomedicina* 1, 66–102.

Grossi, E., Buscema, M., Intraligi, M., et al. (2003). Artificial Neural Networks can recognize individual patients affected by dementia only on the basis of previous history. In *Proceedings of VII annual meeting Italian interdisciplinary network on Alzheimer disease* (pp. 22–24, 92–93). Sorrento .

Kennedy, R. L., Harrison, R. F., Burton, A.M., Fraser, H.S., Hamer, W. G., McArthur, D., Mc Allum, R., and Steedman, D. J. (1997). An artificial neural network system for diagnosis of acute myocardial infarction (AMI) in the accident & emergency department: evaluation and comparison with serum myoglobin measurements. *Comput. Meth. Prog. Bio.* 52, 93–103.

Kroll, M. H. (1999). Biological variation of glucose and insulin includes a deterministic chaotic component. *Biosystems* 50, 189–201.

Lahner, E., Grossi, E., Intraligi, M., Buscema, M., Delle Fave, G., and Annibale, B. (2005). Possible contribution of advanced statistical methods (artifical neural networks and linear discriminant analysis) in the recognition of patients with suspected atrophic body gastritis. *World J. Gastroenterol.* 11, 37, 5867–5873.

Lisboa, P. J. G., Ifeachor, E. C., and Szczepaniak, P. S. (eds.). (2000). *Artificial neural networks in biomedicine*. London: Springer.

Louis, P. C. A. (1835). *Recherches sur les effets de la saignée dans quelques maladies inflammatoires, et sur l'action de l'émétique et des vésicatoires dans la pneumonie*. Paris: J-B Ballière.

Snow, J. (1855). *On the mode of communication of cholera*. 2nd edn. London: John Churchill.

McEwen, B. S. and Wingfield, J. C. (2003). The concept of allostasis in biology and biomedicine. *Horm. Behav*. 43(1), 2–15.

Pace, F., Buscema, M., Dominici, P., Intraligi, M., Grossi, E., Baldi, F. et al. (2005). Artificial neural networks are able to recognise GERD patients on the basis of clinical data solely. *Eur. J. Gastroenterol. Hepatol.* 17, 605–610.

Pagano, N., Buscema, M., Grossi, E., Intraligi, M., Massini, G., Salacone, P. et al. (2004). Artificial neural networks for the prediction of diabetes mellitus occurrence in patients affected by chronic pancreatitis. *J. Pancreas*. Suppl. 5, 405–453.

Penco, S., Grossi, E., Cheng, S., Intraligi, M., Maurelli, G., Patrosso, M.C., Marocchi, A., and Buscema, M (2005). Assessment of the role of genetic polymorphism in venous thrombosis through artificial neural networks. *Ann. Hum. Genet*. 69(6), 693–706.

Ruelle, D. (1994). Where can one hope to profitably apply the ideas of chaos? *Phys. Today*, 47, 24–30.

Singer, D. H., Martin, G. J., Magid, N. et al. (1988). Low heart rate variability and sudden cardiac death. *J. Electrocardiol.* Suppl 21, S46–S55.

Vomweg, T. W., Buscema, M., Kauczor, H. U., Teifke, A., Intraligi, M., Terzi, S., Heussel, C. P., Achenbach, T., Rieker, O., Mayer, D., and Thelen, M. (2003). Improved artificial neural networks in prediction of malignancy of lesions in contrast-enhanced MR-mammography. *Med. Phys*. 30(9), 2350–2359.

Chapter 16
J-Net System: A New Paradigm for Artificial Neural Networks Applied to Diagnostic Imaging

Massimo Buscema and Enzo Grossi

Abstract In this chapter we present a new unsupervised artificial adaptive system, able to extract features of interest in digital imaging, to reduce image noise maintaining the spatial resolution of high-contrast structures and the expression of hidden morphological features. The new system, named J-Net, belongs to the family of ACM systems developed by Semeion Research Institute. J-Net is able to isolate in an almost geological way different brightness layers in the same image. These layers seem to be invisible to the human eye and for the other mathematical imaging system. This ability of the J-Net can have important medical applications.

Keywords Image processing · Artificial neural networks · Active connections matrixes

16.1 Introduction

Significant progress in the development of machine vision and image processing technology has been made in the past few years in the medical field in conjunction with improvements in computer technology (Davies 1990, Gonzalez and Woods 1992, Haralick and Shapiro 1992, Horn 1986, Marr 1982, Vernon 1991, CANDY 2003, Jahne 2003).

With the introduction of multislice spiral CT scanners, the number of images of body organs, like the lung for example, is steadily increasing and it is critical to develop fast, accurate algorithms that require minimal to no human interaction to identify emergent features of interest.

Artificial neural networks (ANNs) can overcome some of these difficulties by interpreting images quickly and effectively. ANNs are composed of numerous processing elements (PEs) arranged in various layers, with interconnections between pairs of PEs (Haykin 1994, Kartalopoulos 1996, Kasabov 1996).

M. Buscema (✉)
Semeion Research Center, Via Sersale, Rome, Italy
e-mail: m.buscema@semeion.it

V. Capecchi (eds.), *Applications of Mathematics in Models, Artificial Neural Networks and Arts*, DOI 10.1007/978-90-481-8581-8_16,

They are designed to emulate the structure of natural neural networks such as those of a human brain. For most ANNs, PEs in each layer are fully connected with PEs in the adjacent layer or layers, but are not connected to other PEs in the same layer. The PEs simulate the function of the neurons in natural neural networks, while the interconnections between them mimic the functions of dendrites and axons.

There have been many applications of ANNs reported for the interpretation of images in medicine.

The main problems in many image processing applications still are the abundance of features and the difficulty of coping with concomitant variations in position, orientation and scale. This clearly indicates the need for more intelligent, *invariant feature extraction* and *feature selection mechanisms* (Egmont-Petersen 2002). In a recent review about the role of ANNs in medical decision support with digital imaging, the authors concluded that ANNs can play a role in image processing, although it might be a role as a supporting tool rather than a major one (Chua and Roska 2002, Harrer and Nossek 1992, 1992b, Schamschula et al. 2000).

The Active Connection Matrix (ACM) is a new unsupervised artificial adaptive system developed by Semeion Research Institute (Buscema 2006). The system is able to automatically extract features of interest (e.g. edges, tissue differentiation) from digital images when activated by original non-linear equations. ACM systems copy with the feature selection problems in digital imaging: ACM activation allows the reduction of image noise while maintaining the spatial resolution of high-contrast structures and the expression of hidden morphological features.

16.2 General Overview on ACM Families: Basic Notions

The relationship that develops, in space and time, between the entity (the *thing-in-itself*) and the context in which it interacts and which enables one to define the *phenomenon* is expressed through strains and stresses, the existing forces between the minimal elements of the phenomenon.

These forces are called

- *finite* when they acquire true finite values in any space and time neighbourhood of a considered initial point.
- *continue* when there is no point of a space and time neighbourhood where the value of the force depends on the direction reached in the considered point, and
- *local* when the propagation of the effects of these forces continues through every single space and time point subsequent to the initial one being considered.

The ability of a *phenomenon* to keep the forces *finite*, *local* and *continue* among its minimal elements is the space–time *cohesion* the *phenomenon* itself.

The *relevant topology* of a *phenomenon* is its intrinsic geometry which expresses the form which can be taken from the frequency spectra where the phenomenon is analysed and from the respective variations of energy. These variations of energy become *relevant information* because they are an expression of the *relevant topology* of the phenomenon, that is to say of its form or intrinsic geometry. In this case the *phenomenon* is called a *visual phenomenon*.

Every relevant topological phenomenon manifests an identity and unity of the phenomenon itself which is determined by its space–time cohesion. This means that each minimal element of the phenomenon is directly or indirectly contiguous and connected by specific forces to the others. Therefore the quantitative value of each minimal element of the analysed phenomenon results from the action of these forces. It can be demonstrated that in a relevant topological phenomenon the forces which connect each of the minimal elements to each other in its local neighbourhood are enough to explain the space–time cohesion of the whole phenomenon.

This allows one to say that each visual phenomenon can be expressed as a *matrix of values*, locally connected each other, by other values (weights), representing the local *cohesion forces* of the minimal units of that phenomenon.

As already noted elsewhere (Buscema 2006), the *phenomenon* we refer to, in general, in our research concerns the image which is perceived by our senses when a light-shrouded subject appears to us precisely as a *phenomenon*. The image of the subject caught and made available as a *phenomenon* can be represented for its analytic treatment by a matrix of points corresponding to the pixels of the assumed initial image. Trying to extract from this image – from this *phenomenon* – other information about the subject producing it, which is not visible in the initial image which is being considered, allows us to consider the initial image's matrix of pixels as a dynamic system which develops in its phase space until it creates a final configuration matrix of the pixels. It is important not to mistake this space phase with the two-dimensional or three-dimensional space of the initial image. In fact, it is the other dimension which is derived by the intensity of the connection forces of the pixels to each other which is added to the latter space's dimension. This occurs when the point matrix is considered and when its *active* meaning is considered that the initial matrix will result in a final matrix precisely because of a dynamic evolution of these connections.

The functioning of ACM systems is based on *local*, *deterministic* and iterative operations:

- *Local*, because in each elaboration cycle the operations involve a central pixel and its relations with the very contiguous pixels (neighbourhood of the central pixel).
- *Deterministic*, because the static state towards which the dynamic system tends is represented by the matrix of pixels with the new image, is based on deterministic equations; therefore the elaboration can be repeated always resulting in the same outcome.
- *Iterative*, because the operations of the dynamic system repeat themselves, iteratively, until the evolution in the space of phases reaches its attractor.

Figure 16.1 schematically presents the previously published ACM system (Buscema 2006).

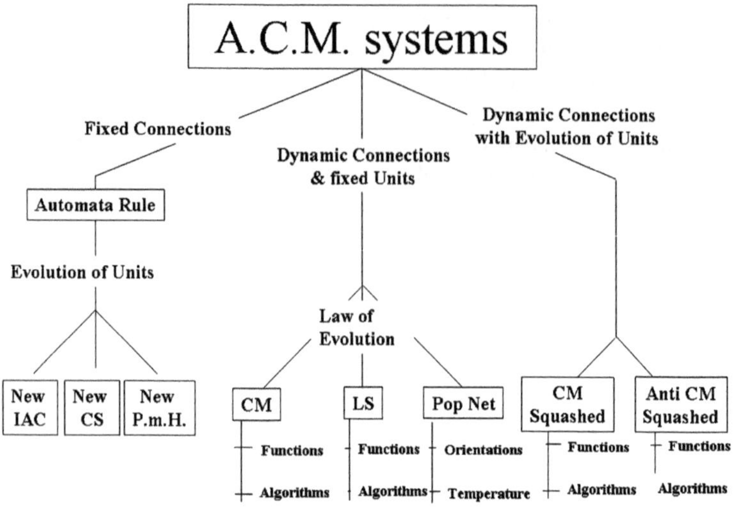

Fig. 16.1 A general schematic representation of the ACM system

ACM families, as previously noted, differ according to how they let units and connections evolve. They are divided, more specifically, into three families, shown in Fig. 16.1, according to the following evolution rules:

a. *Fixed Connections*: Units u_x are allowed to evolve until they reach a static state showing the presence of an attractor. The static state, and therefore the attractor, changes according to the evolution rule which is used. A connection matrix is initially determined by an equation called *Automata Rule* which uses the pixel's matrix of the assigned image.
b. *Fixed Units*: Connections $w_{x,xs}$ are allowed to evolve until they reach a static state showing the presence of an attractor. The static state, and therefore the attractor, changes according to the evolution rule that is used. It uses the pixel's matrix of the assigned image, which remains constant in every elaboration cycle.
c. *Dynamic Connections and Units*: Connections $w_{x,xs}$ reaches their attractor according to the matrix of the units u_x updating in every elaboration cycle. In this case, the brightness of the matrix pixel of the units u_x is updated during the evolution of the system, participating in the correction of the matrix of the *connections*.

16.3 J-NET: A New ACM System

The ACM research, as noted earlier, was carried out assuming that the new morphological and dynamic regularities visible in the images resulted from any of the three ACM families noted above. These were the product of *local, deterministic* and *iterative* operations carried out on the pixel's matrix of the initial image and on the connection matrix of each single pixel with its local neighbourhood.

It would obviously be useful to discover the way in which to widen the relationships between the central pixel and its neighbourhood pixel. This would also include the relationships among these latter pixels when each one of them is also a neighbourhood pixel of every pixel which is contiguous to it. Considering the totality of these contributes, at every elaboration cycle, for the construction of the new image. It would also mean widening the range of the operations which would no longer be strictly *local*. This occurs by virtue of the fact that each pixel would give an immediate feedback contribution to determine all the other pixels. It is the same as if every solicitations coming from each point of the territory participated simultaneously in the creation of a mountain landscape.

This current research presents a new ACM family that has already occurred, in a stronger way than in the previous case (c). This includes the participation of every single neighbourhood pixel in the evolution of the connections matrix, which will be finally used in order to create the pixel matrix with the new image.

This happens because the new equation not only considers the value of the neighbourhood pixels and the one of their connections with the central pixel but also the subsequent relationships which emerge when each one of them is considered as a neighbourhood pixel of each of their contiguous pixel and when this latter one is considered to be the central pixel. It is possible, in each elaboration cycle, for each pixel to give its contribution to each iterating pixel, even those which are far from it due to neighbourhood pixels spreading this contribution as waves.

We called this new ACM family J-NET ACM[1] (Buscema et al. 2007).

The equations defining the J-Net system are divided in two sets: the set of the equations expressing the evolution of the connection's value of each pixel of the assigned image and the set of the equations expressing the evolution of the value of the internal state of each pixel of the assigned image.

Neighbourhoods having a radius of the central pixel equal to 1, that is local neighbourhoods, will be considered later. We will use the synthetic notation applied to the case of two-dimensional images, in which the indexes *i,j* represent the two dimensions of a plane image, where *i* indicates the position of the central pixel of the neighbourhood and *j* represents one of any other remaining *N* positions of the neighbourhood pixels. If the neighbourhood radius is equal to 1, $N = 8$.

A legend of the symbols we are going to use, their initial values and their meaning are as follows:

$W_{i,j}^{[0]} = 0.0$: Initial connection value between two pixels;
$u_i \in [-1+\alpha, 1+\alpha]$: Initial scaling down of the values of all of the pixels of the assigned image;
$\alpha =$: Scaling down threshold of the pixel's values;

[1] ACM J-Net is a European patent pending owner: Semeion Research Center of Sciences of Communication, Via Sersale, 117, Rome 00128, Italy. Inventor: Massimo Buscema.

$x^{[n]} = x$ at step n; any variable (connections, pixels, etc.) at a certain elaboration cycle;
$P_i^{[n]} = i$th pixel at step n;
$Out_i^{[n]} = i$th exit at step n;
$S_i^{[n]} = i$th state at step n;
$N =$ Neighbourhood nodes.

The set of the equations ruling the connection's value of each pixel can be partitioned into four steps:

$$D_i = \sum_j^N (u_j^{[n]} - W_{i,j}^{[n]}) \tag{16.1}$$

The D_i factor is not, as it appears to be, a distance. It is a simple addition of the differences between the value of each pixel and the weight of the central pixel with which it is connected. D_i can be considered to be a representative term of the *resemblance* between the pixel of the local neighbourhood of the central pixel and the connection of this latter pixel with each one of them.

$$J_i = \frac{e^{D_i} - e^{-D_i}}{e^{D_i} + e^{-D_i}} \tag{16.2}$$

The variable J_i is the result of the application of the tangent's hyperbolic function on the factor.

This operation has a three-fold aim:

a. closes the possible values of D_i in a finite spread;
b. provides a sigmoid form to the possible values of D_i;
c. operates with a differentiable function on each point.

$$\begin{aligned}\Delta W_{i,j}^{[n]} &= -(u_i^{[n]} \cdot J_i) \cdot (-2 \cdot J_i) \cdot \\ &(1 - J_i^2) \cdot (u_j^{[n]} - W_{i,j}^{[n]})\end{aligned} \tag{16.3}$$

This equation can be divided into three components:

1. The first component, $-(u_i^{[n]} \cdot J_i)$, weights the value of the central pixel with the variable J_i depending on its neighbourhood (weight and pixel). However, it inverts the classic mathematic relationships among the signs: the concordance generates a negative value, while the discordance generates a positive value in this case. In other words:

   a. if the central pixel tends towards black (negative value) and the weights connecting it to its neighbourhood are, on average, *larger* than this neighbourhood's pixel then the value of this part of the equation will be negative;

b. if the central pixel tends towards black (negative value) and the weights connecting it to its neighbourhood are, on average, *smaller* than this neighbourhood's pixel then the value of this part of the equation will be positive;
c. if the central pixel tends towards white (positive value) and the weights connecting it to its neighbourhood are, on average, *larger* than this neighbourhood's pixel, then the value of this part of the equation will be positive;
d. if the central pixel tends towards white (positive value) and the weights connecting it to its neighbourhood are, on average, *smaller* than the pixel of this neighbourhood, then the value of this part of the equation will be negative.

2. the second component of the equation (16.2), $(-2 \cdot J_i) \cdot (1 - J_i^2)$, is the second derivative of J_i in respect to D_i. It contributes to correct the weights with a term which considers how the variation of compression of the resemblance changes in respect to the resemblance itself;
3. the third component (16.3) weights the first two components of the whole equation, with the difference between each neighbourhood pixel and the weight of the central pixel to which it is connected.

$$W_{i,j}^{[n+1]} = W_{i,j}^{[n]} + \Delta W_{i,j}^{[n]} \tag{16.4}$$

This is the equation representing the update of the weights connecting the central pixel to each pixel of its neighbourhood occurs.

The first four equations point out the following:

a. every central connections between the central pixel and its neighbourhood depends on the value of *each* pixel of the same neighbourhood;
b. each connection between the central pixel and each pixel of its neighbourhood depends on *all* pixels of the same neighbourhood.

Therefore, the evolution of the weights represents a *first-order* transformation of each pixel of the assigned image (each pixel in relation with its neighbourhood).

These first J-Net equations are capable of determining interesting transformations of *any* image.

It is, in fact, sufficient to calculate at each evolutionary J-Net cycle the average of the weight values that are derived from each central pixel and to scale down this value in the most suitable way between 0 and 255 (if it is the range of values that the pixels can have the image). This is necessary in order to obtain some transformations which segment the image into two sets: picture and background.

$$\begin{aligned} P_i^{[n]} &= \text{Scale}_{\text{Pixel}} \cdot \frac{\sum_j^N W_{i,j}^{[n]}}{N} + \text{Offset}_{\text{Pixel}} \\ P_i^{[n]} &\in [0, \text{MaxPixelOut}]; \end{aligned} \tag{16.5}$$

$$
\begin{aligned}
\text{Scale}_{\text{Pixel}} &= \frac{\text{MaxPixelOut}}{(\text{MaxW} - \text{MinW})} \\
\text{Offset}_{\text{Pixel}} &= -\frac{\text{MinW} \cdot \text{MaxPixelOut}}{\text{MaxW} - \text{MinW}}
\end{aligned}
\tag{16.6}
$$

Obviously, different values of the value α in the initial scale down phase (16.2) are designed to change the outlines of the picture with respect to the background.

The set of equations designed to change the activation of the units u can also be segmented in different steps.

$$
\begin{aligned}
\text{Out}_i^{[n]} &= \text{Scale}_{\text{Out}} \cdot \frac{\sum_j^N W_{i,j}^{[n]}}{N} + \text{Offset}_{\text{Out}} \\
\text{Out}_i^{[n]} &\in [-1, +1]
\end{aligned}
\tag{16.7}
$$

$$
\begin{aligned}
\text{Scale}_{\text{Out}} &= \frac{2}{\text{MaxW} - \text{MinW}} \\
\text{Offset}_{\text{Out}} &= -\frac{\text{MaxW} + \text{MinW}}{\text{MaxW} - \text{MinW}}
\end{aligned}
\tag{16.8}
$$

The purpose of these equations is to scale down the average of the connection's value of each central pixel with its neighbourhood in a numerical set included in the spread $\{-1,+1\}$.

The outcome of this scale-down, considered in its absolute value, will define the *internal activation* state of each central pixel:

$$
S_i^{[n]} = |\text{Out}_i^{[n]}| \tag{16.9}
$$

Therefore, in terms of a pixel's value it is possible to assert that the greater the weight average connecting each central pixel to its neighbourhood is distant from a neutral value ("zero" if the values are scaled down between -1 and +1 or "grey 127" if the values are scaled down between 0 and 255), the more active the internal state of that central pixel will be.

The equations dealt with so far concern only transformations of *first-order* between pixels. In other words, each pixel is transformed on the basis of the pixels of its neighbourhood, using nonlinear transformations of the connection's weights.

Actually we believe that it is useful to also consider that each central pixel, in turn, is also a neighbourhood pixel of the pixels which are contiguous to it. That is to say that in the two-dimensional case with radius equal to 1, the central pixel u_i belongs to eight different neighbourhoods, each one centred in the u_j pixel of its initial neighbourhood. To consider the central pixel as being a neighbourhood pixel of each of the near pixels means expecting *second-order* transformations.

A "delta factor", $\Delta S_{i,j}^{[n]}$, is given to each pixel through the following equation considering its activation value, $S_i^{[n]}$, and the activation value of each pixel $u_j^{[n]}$ having this factor as a neighbourhood:

$$\Delta S_{i,j}^{[n]} = -\mathrm{Tan}H(S_i^{[n]} + u_j^{[n]}) = -\frac{e^{(S_i^{[n]}+u_j^{[n]})} - e^{-(S_i^{[n]}+u_j^{[n]})}}{e^{(S_i^{[n]}+u_j^{[n]})} + e^{-(S_i^{[n]}+u_j^{[n]})}} \quad (16.10)$$

Equation (16.10) is fundamental for different reasons.

Each pixel of a two-dimensional image, if its radius is equal to 1, has a neighbourhood formed by eight other pixels. This means that in equation (16.30), the more the internal state of the central pixel tends towards 1 and the more the activation of the neighbourhood pixel is greater than zero, the more the $\Delta S_{i,j}^{[n]}$ will have a sign which is opposite to the neighbourhood pixel's value. The more the internal state of the central pixel tends towards 1 and the more the activation of the neighbourhood pixel tends towards -1, the more the $\Delta S_{i,j}^{[n]}$ will tend towards zero.

Equation (16.10) considers the effects and counter-effects of each pixel on the contiguous ones. These effects, in this case, are *second-order effects*.

The addition of the complements to one of the squares of the $\Delta S_{i,j}^{[n]}$ of each neighbourhood belonging to each neighbourhood pixel, weighted in the most suitable way, will define $\varphi_i^{[n]}$ of the *second-order* of each of the image's pixels.

$$\varphi_i^{[n]} = \mathrm{LCoef} \cdot u_i^{[n]} \cdot \sum_j^N (1 - \Delta S_{j,i}^{[n]^2}) \quad (16.11)$$

At this point, if we transform the mutual terms of a second-order $\varphi_j^{[n]}$ with a hyperbolic tangent in order to contain them in the spread {– 1,+1}, and then we add all terms referring to the same neighbourhood of u_i , as each neighbourhood pixel become central pixel, we also consider the propagation of the mutual effects, that is the variations of *third-order* of each pixel:

$$\psi_i^{[n]} = \sum_j^N \tanh(\varphi_j^{[n]}) = \sum_j^N \frac{e^{\varphi_j^{[n]}} - e^{-\varphi_j^{[n]}}}{e^{\varphi_j^{[n]}} + e^{-\varphi_j^{[n]}}} \quad (16.12)$$

While the vector $\varphi_i^{[n]}$ defines the close outline of the assigned image, the vector $\psi_i^{[n]}$ is responsible for the progressive creation of outline waves moving from the initial outline to the brightest part of the image. Through its constructive and destructive interferences, these waves define a sort of "skeleton" of the image itself, taking shape slowly inside it.

The following equation unifies in a single term both second- and third-order contributions that define the final variation which each unit of the image has to receive. Actually we have discovered two forms for this equation: we have named the first one "*Union of n-order effects*":

$$\delta u_i^{[n]} = \varphi_i^{[n]} + \psi_i^{[n]} \tag{16.13}$$

The second one has as target the "*Intersection of n-order effects*":

$$\delta u_i^{[n]} = \varphi_i^{[n]} \cdot \psi_i^{[n]} \tag{16.13b}$$

Consequently, the final equation, which at the next cycle will modify the activation of each unit of the assigned image, will have the following form:

$$u_i^{[n+1]} = u_i^{[n]} + \delta u_i^{[n]} \tag{16.14}$$

The stop criterion of the J-Net system is connected to the stabilization of the connection's value (see equation (16.3)).

More precisely, the energy of the J-Net system, $E^{[n]}$, will result from the addition of the changes of the connection's values relating to the whole image to each processing cycle, according to the following equation:

$$E^{[n]} = \sum_{x=1}^{X} \sum_{s=1}^{N} \left(\Delta w_{x,x_s}^{[n]}\right)^2 \tag{16.15}$$

$X =$ Number of pixels of the source image;
$N =$ Number of pixels into
the central pixel neighborhood (ray $= 1$);
$x,x_s = x$ th pixel and its neighborhood.

The evolution of the J-Net system determines a reduction of the system energy when the processing cycles increase:

$$\lim_{n \to \infty} E^{[n]} = 0 \tag{16.16}$$

It means that the energy E^* of the J-Net system will be minimal at the end of the evolution:

$$E^* = \min\{E^{[n]}\} \tag{16.17}$$

The J-Net system of the ACM family can be represented by the following flow chart in a more abstract way:

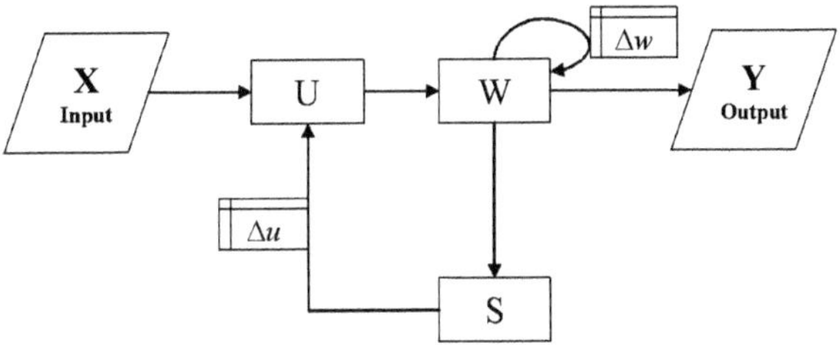

Fig. 16.2 Flow chart of the J-Net system

16.4 J-Net: Medical Applications

Before deciding to apply J-Net system to medical images we have assessed its ability to extract the outline of an image in few cycles in different toy models with noisy images, comparing with standard software available. The results have been surprisingly remarkable (Buscema 2003–2006, 2007).

The J-Net system has demonstrated its ability to detect internal stenosis which appeared to be invisible to the surgeon even in the case of particularly sophisticated images, such as the digital subtraction angiography:

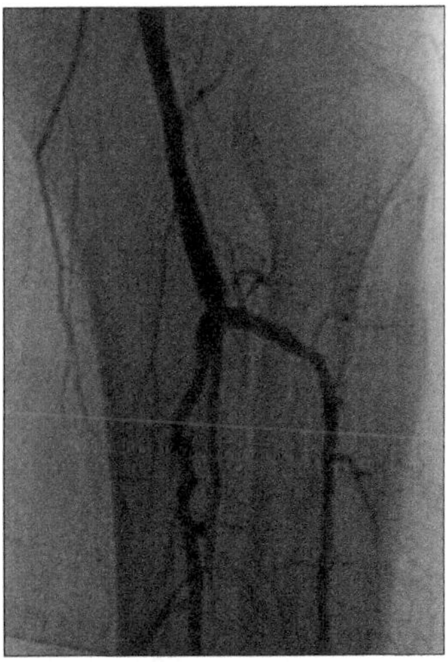

Fig. 16.3a Digital subtraction angiography: popliteal artery (Galeazzi Hospital, Milan)

In the previous J-Net elaborations the values of the initial image were scaled down between -1 and $+1$; so, the scaling factor alpha was implicitly equal to zero. This factor determines the sensitivity threshold of the system to the brightness of the image. Table 16.1 summarizes what has been noted up to this point:

The same image can be elaborated by J-Net with a different threshold α independently. The pictures which were developed with the different threshold α will

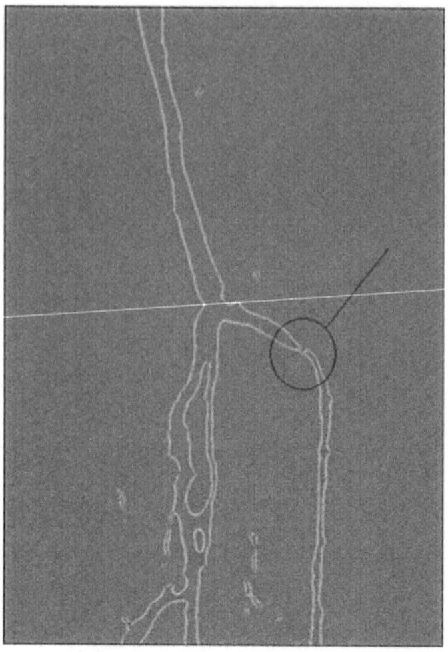

Fig. 16.3b J-Net "Intersection mode"

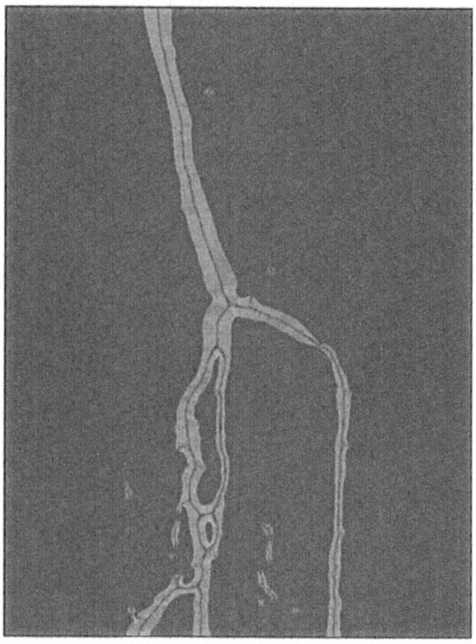

Fig. 16.3c J_Net "Union mode"

highlight the final images with *different pictures*. The lower factors α will highlight *only* the picture with a more intense brightness, while the higher factors α will highlight *only* the picture having a decreasing intensity of brightness.

Therefore, different values of α operate on the assigned image through a *scanning* of the different bright intensities.

In cases in which the intensity of brightness in a medical picture is quite proportional to the activity of the pathology in question, it is possible to use different J-Net scanning in order to detect a temporal order of development of the pathology itself.

In lung cancers, for example, it can be supposed that the different bright intensity in the computerized tomography (CT) reflects the areas where the cancer is more active. In the case of malignant cancer the most peripheral parts can appear to be

Table 16.1 Ratio between the threshold and the scale-down of the units

Threshold	Scale-down
$\alpha = -1.0$	$u \in [-2.0, 0.0]$
$\alpha = -0.9$	$u \in [-1.9, +0.1]$
$\alpha = -0.8$	$u \in [-1.8, +0.2]$
$\alpha = -0.7$	$u \in [-1.7, +0.3]$
$\alpha = -0.6$	$u \in [-1.6, +0.4]$
$\alpha = -0.5$	$u \in [-1.5, +0.5]$
$\alpha = -0.4$	$u \in [-1.4, +0.6]$
$\alpha = -0.3$	$u \in [-1.3, +0.7]$
$\alpha = -0.2$	$u \in [-1.2, +0.8]$
$\alpha = -0.1$	$u \in [-1.1,+0.9]$
$\alpha = 0.0$	$u \in [-1.0, +1.0]$
$\alpha = +0.1$	$u \in [-0.9, +1.1]$
$\alpha = +0.2$	$u \in [-0.8, +1.2]$
$\alpha = +0.3$	$u \in [-0.7, +1.3]$
$\alpha = +0.4$	$u \in [-0.6, +1.4]$
$\alpha = +0.5$	$u \in [-0.5, +1.5]$
$\alpha = +0.6$	$u \in [-0.4, +1.6]$
$\alpha = +0.7$	$u \in [-0.3, +1.7]$
$\alpha = +0.8$	$u \in [-0.2, +1.8]$
$\alpha = +0.9$	$u \in [-0.1, +1.9]$
$\alpha = +1.0$	$u \in [-0.0, +2.0]$

dark like the background of the human eye, while actually they should present "light shadows" of brightness, indicating the explorative and diffusive strategies of the cancer itself. These micro variations of brightness can be so thin that other analysis algorithms could easily classify them as "noise" and erase them. The J-Net system, on the contrary, seems to be able to distinguish between those cases in which the bright oscillations of the background represent simple noise and those in which oscillations represent a just-traced model of a picture.

The scanning of the picture operated by J-Net through the variation of the threshold α has been demonstrated to be able to point out some kinds of development of lung's cancer 1 or 2 years earlier.

In order to verify this assumption we have used research and the picture published by a group of researchers in 2000 in the well-known scientific journal (Aoki et al. 2000).[2]

[2] In order to give a complete overview, the entire abstract is included as published by PubMed: Aoki et al. (2000). Objective: This study was performed to evaluate the evolution of peripheral lung adenocarcinomas using CT findings and histologic classification related to tumour doubling time. Materials and Methods: The subjects were 34 patients, each with an adenocarcinoma smaller than 3 cm. All patients underwent chest radiography and 10 of them had previously undergone CT more than 6 months before surgery. Tumour doubling time was estimated by examining sequential radiographs using the method originally described by Schwartz. Tumour growth was also observed by studying the changes on CT in the 10 patients who had previously undergone CT. The histologic classification (types A–F) was evaluated according to the criteria of Noguchi et al. Results: Five (83%) of the six adenocarcinomas with tumour types A or B showed localized ground-glass

We took two pairs of lungs cancer images from this research. Each pair shows the cancer as it was when the first CT was done (time 0) and one or three years later (time 1). The researchers report that in the time 0 the picture did not allow for an accurate and differential cancer diagnosis.

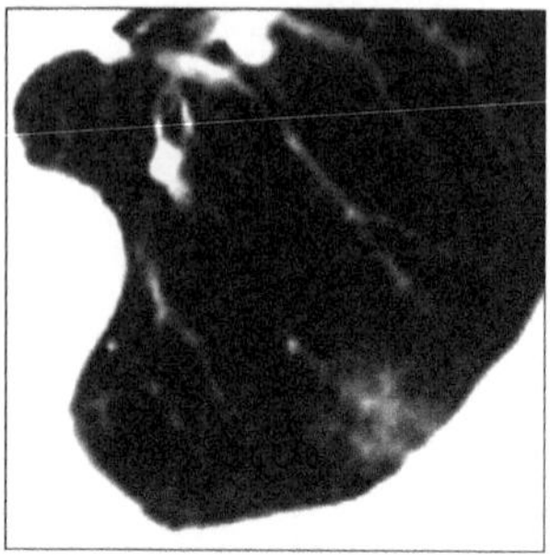

Fig. 16.4a Type B adenocarcinoma in 74-year-old man. Initial CT scan shows localized 22 × 22-mm ground-glass opacity in left lower lobe of lung

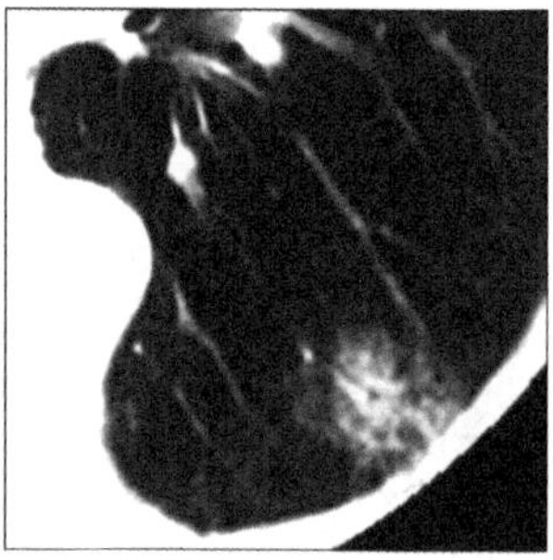

Fig. 16.4b Type B adenocarcinoma in 74-year-old man. CT scan obtained 349 days after initial CT scan shows an increase in size (to 23 × 26 mm) and the development of vascular convergence. Attenuation at the centre of the tumour is slightly increased

Two experiments were carried out with this pair of images: The first experiment elaborated the first image (Fig. 16.3a) with different positive values of α. This was designed to increase the sensitivity of J-Net at each elaboration and to discover hidden background patterns.

---

opacity on high-resolution CT. All six tumours had a tumour doubling time of more than 1 year. Fifteen (71%) of the 21 tumours with type C showed partial ground-glass opacity mixed with localized solid attenuation on high-resolution CT. Ten (48%) of these 21 type C tumours had a tumour doubling time of more than 1 year. In types B and C, the solid component or the development of pleural indentation and vascular convergence increased during observation before surgery. All seven tumours with types D, E and F showed mostly solid attenuation, and the tumour doubling time was less than 1 year in six (87%) of the seven tumours. Conclusion: Two main types of peripheral lung adenocarcinoma exist. The first type appears on CT as localized ground-glass opacity with slow growth, and the other appears as a solid attenuation with rapid growth. PMID: 10701622 [PubMed – indexed for MEDLINE].

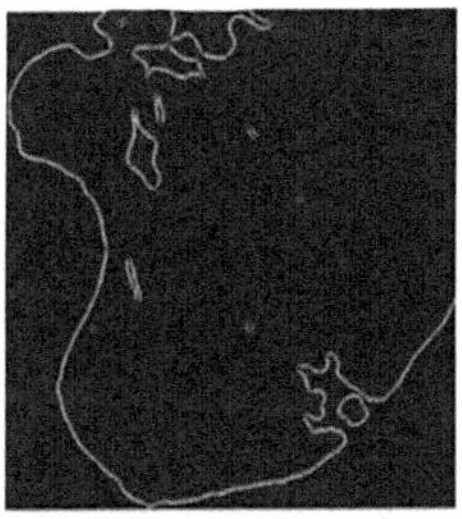

Fig. 16.4a1. (α = 0.0)

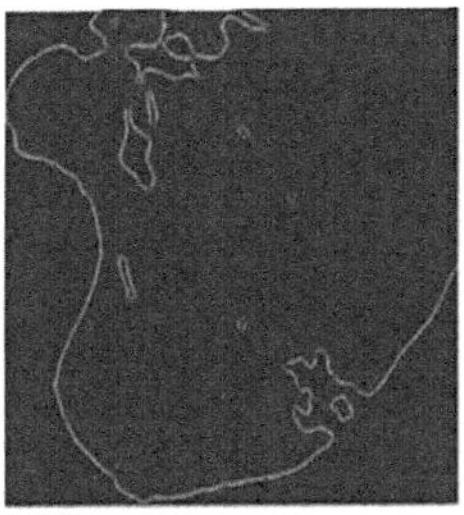

Fig. 16.4a2. (α = 0.1)

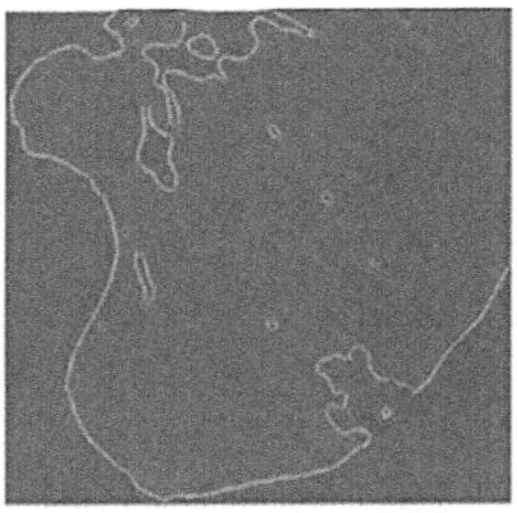

Fig. 16.4a3. (α = 0.2)

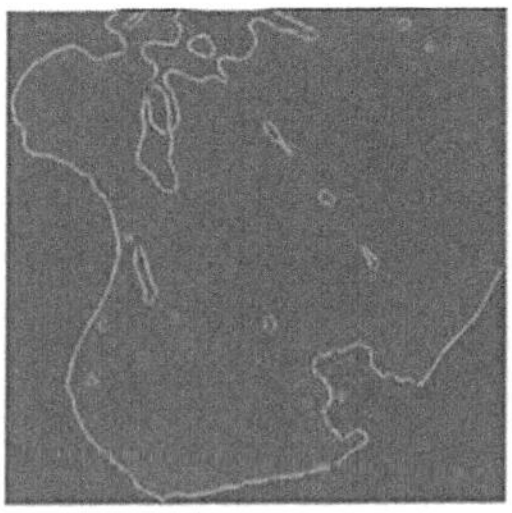

Fig. 16.4a4. (α = 0.3)

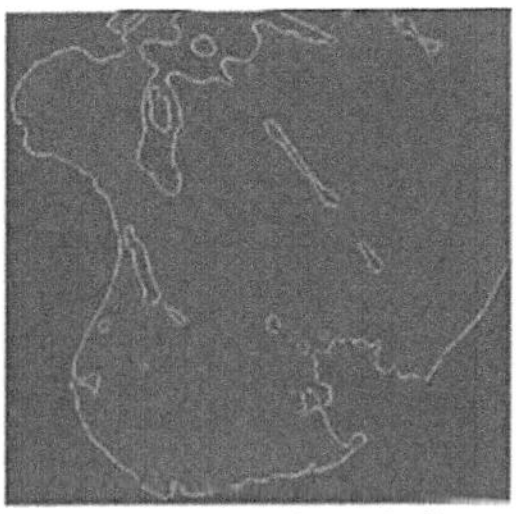

Fig. 16.4a5. (α = 0.4)

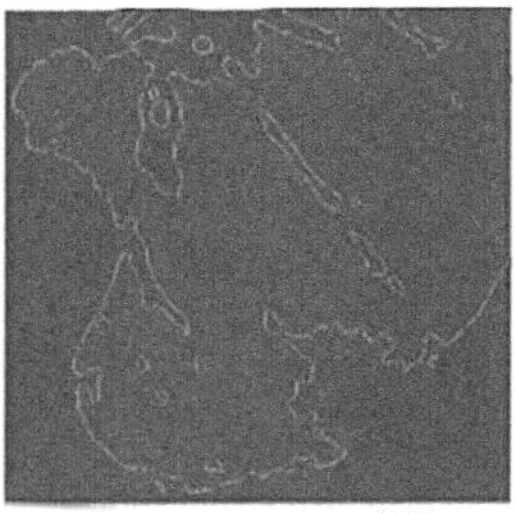

Fig. 16.4a6. (α = 0.5)

Figure 16.4a1 documents a very clear photograph of the outline of the cancer which is contained in the source Figure (Fig. 16.4a). The outline of the cancer is increasingly modified from Fig.16.4a2 to Fig.16.4a5 apparently without a known reason with respect to the original figure (Fig 16.4a).

It is, however, to be noted that the outline of the Figs. 16.4a5 and 16.15a6 are very similar to the shape that the cancer will have in the same patient 1 year later (see Fig. 16.4b).

In the second experiment, 1 year later, only the image of the cancer was developed (Fig. 16.4b). This time, the different J-Net developments were carried out decrementing the values of α. This was designed to make J-Net less sensitive to certain brightness intensities at every elaboration, as if we wanted to go back in time.

It can be noted that the outline of the cancer in Fig. 16.4b2 is similar to the outline of the cancer in Fig. 16.4a5. The outline of the cancer in Fig. 16.4a1 can be practically superimposed upon the outline of the cancer in Fig. 16.4b6 in the same way.

The transformation of the cancer shape at time 0 during the J-Net elaboration having $\alpha = 0.0$(present time) and having $\alpha = 0.4$(possible future) is clearly visible:

The photographed superimposition of Fig. 16.4a5 (prognosis of cancer development) upon Fig. 16.4b1 (the real situation 1 year later) documents the extent to which the J-Net system could discover and diagnoses the hidden development model of the cancer:

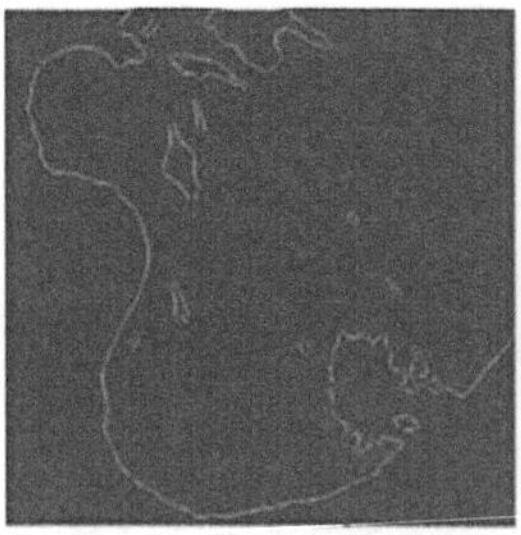

Fig. 16.4b1. (α = 0.0)

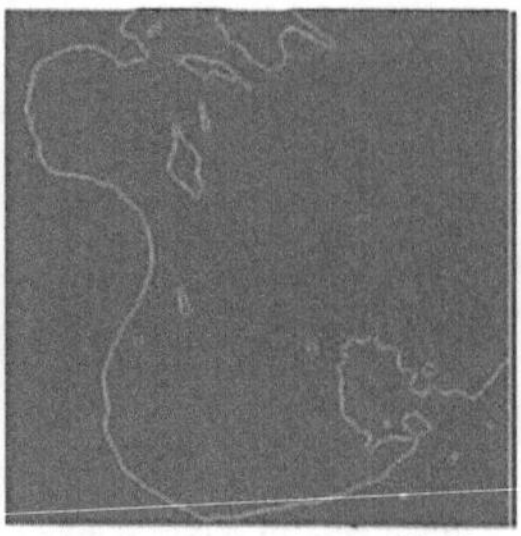

Fig. 16.4b2. (α = -0.1)

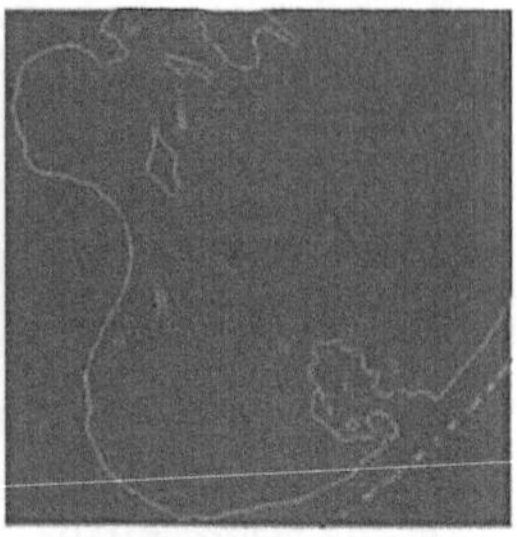

Fig. 16.4b3. (α= -0.2)

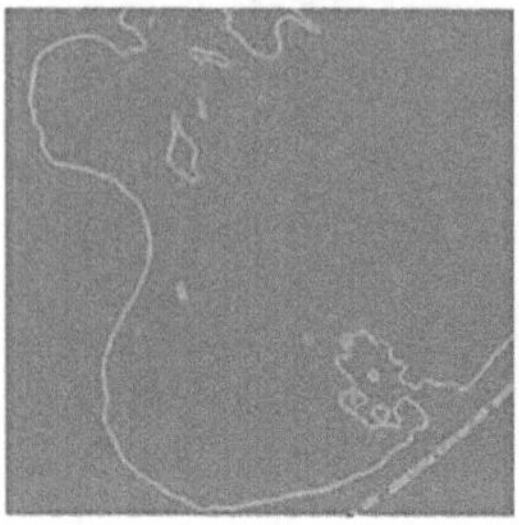

Fig. 16.4b4. (α = -0.3)

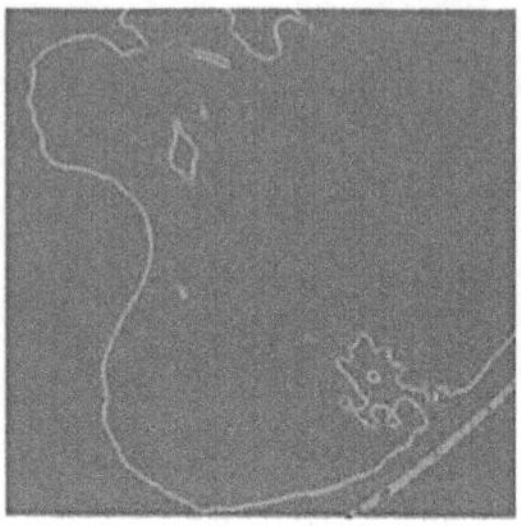

Fig. 16.4b5. (α= -0.4)

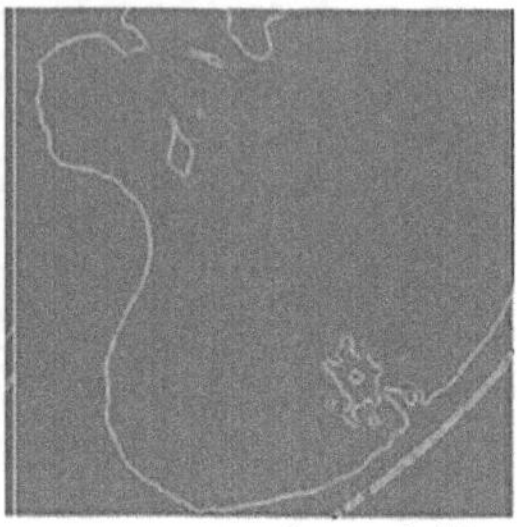

Fig. 16.4b6. (α = -0.5)

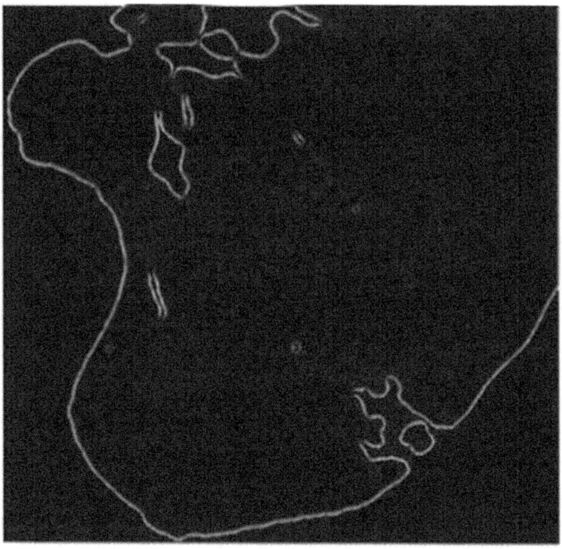

Fig 16.4a1 Time 0 – present – $\alpha = 0.0$

The transformation of the cancer shape at time 1, during the J-Net elaboration with $\alpha = 0.0$(present time) and $\alpha = -0.4$ (possible past), is more clearly visible in the same way:

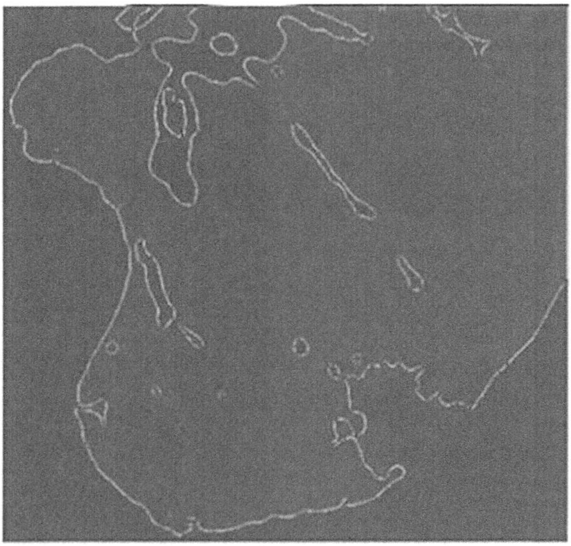

Fig 16.4a5 Time 0 – possible future – $\alpha = 0.4$

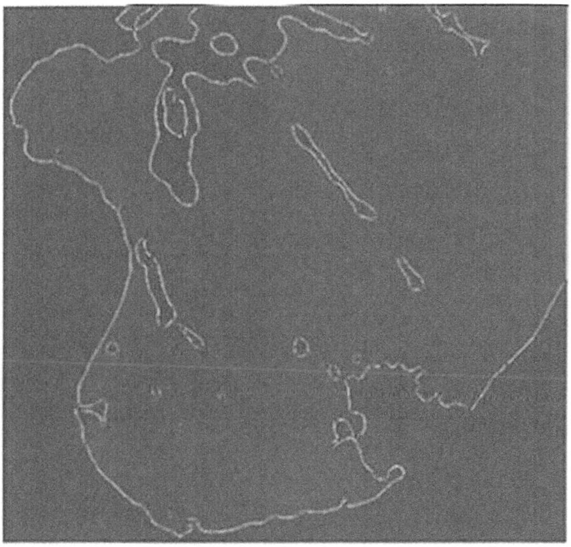

Fig. 16.4c Fig.16.4b1 (*Black*: Real cancer 1 year later) and **Fig**. 16.4a5 (*White*: Prognosticated cancer 1 year before). [The images were manually superimposed without trying to register or stretch them. A imperfect registration results because of the different sizes of the images, taken at two different times]

The photographic superimposition of Fig. 16.4b5 (prognosis of cancer origin) upon Fig.16.4a1 (the real situation 1 year earlier) documents the extent to which the J-Net system could diagnose the hidden degenerative model of the cancer:

The same experimental procedure was used with a second pair of images from the same patient approximately 3 years later with a different type of cancer:

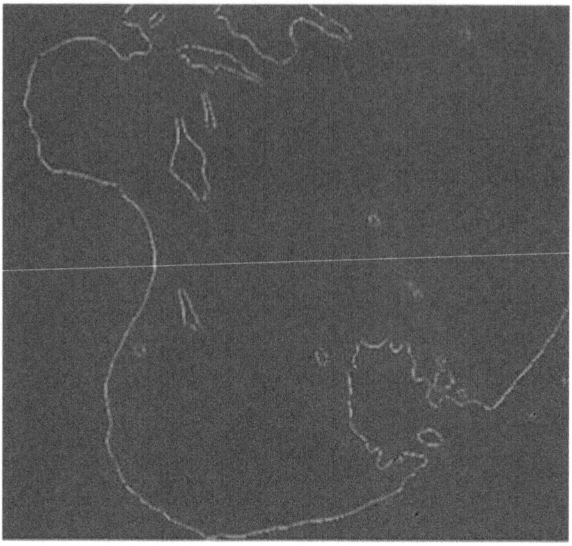

Fig. 16.4b1 Time 1 – present – $\alpha = 0.0$

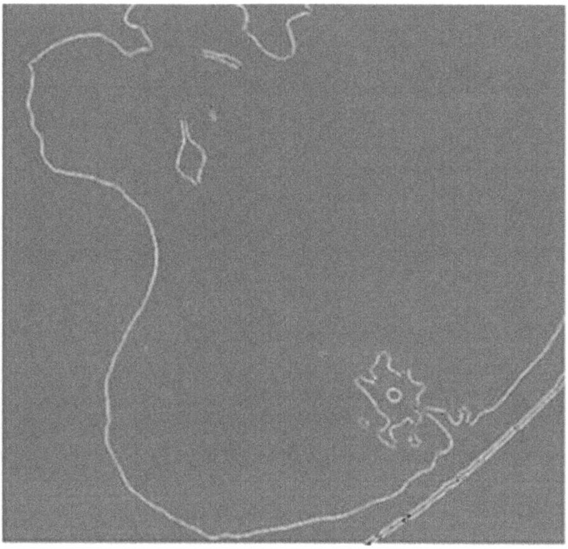

Fig. 16.4b.6 Time 1 –possible past – $\alpha = -0.5$

The J-Net system developed the image at time 0 (Fig 16.4a) with different kind of positive values of α:

The elaboration of the cancer shape in Fig. 16.5a5 and 16.5a6 appears to be an accurate prognosis of the spread of the same cancer 3 years later.

The superimposition of the real cancer shape at time 1 (3 years later) upon the two prognoses of the J-Net system, having two independent parameters of α on

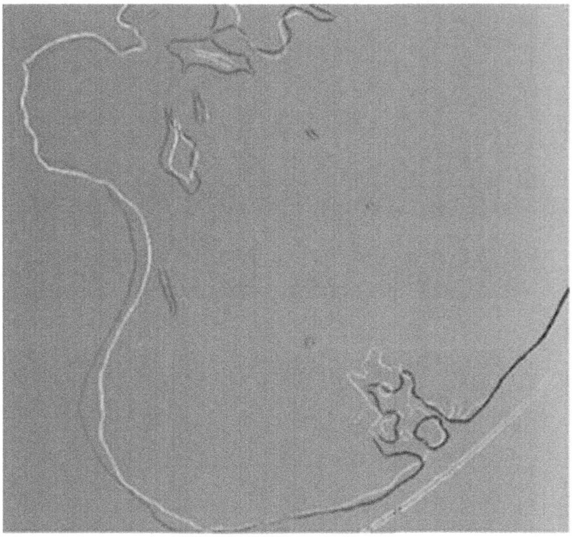

Fig. 16.4d Fig16.4a1 (Black: Cancer 1 year earlier) and **Fig**. 16.4b6 (White: Possible past of the cancer reconstructed 1 year later). [The images were manually superimposed without trying to register or to stretch them. Therefore we have a non-perfect registration because of the different size of the images, taken in two different moments].

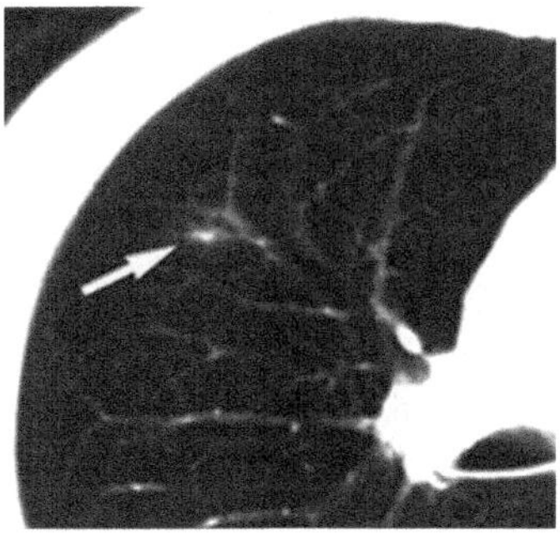

Fig. 16.5a Type C adenocarcinoma in a 64-year-old man. The initial CT scan shows a tiny solid nodule (*arrow*) with minimal adjacent ground-glass opacity (15 × 10 mm) in the right middle lobe

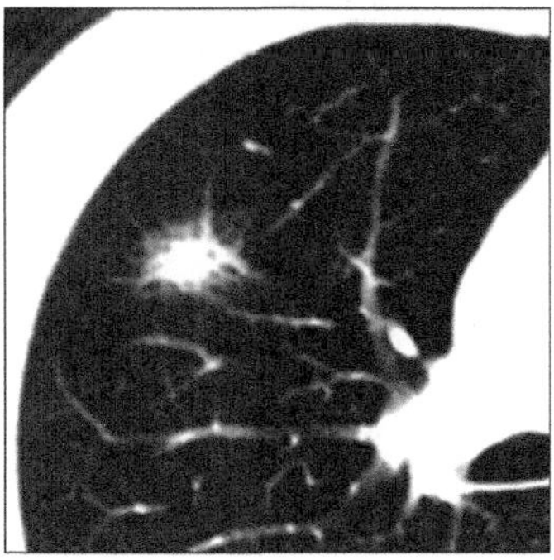

Fig. 16.5b Type C adenocarcinoma in a 64-year-old man. This CT scan, obtained 1137 days after the initial CT scan, shows an increase in size (25 × 20 mm) and vascular convergence. The area of solid attenuation is also increased

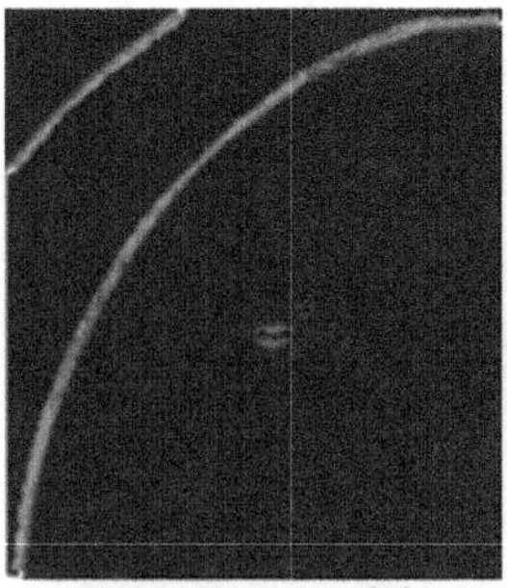
Fig. 16.5a1. $\alpha = 0.0$

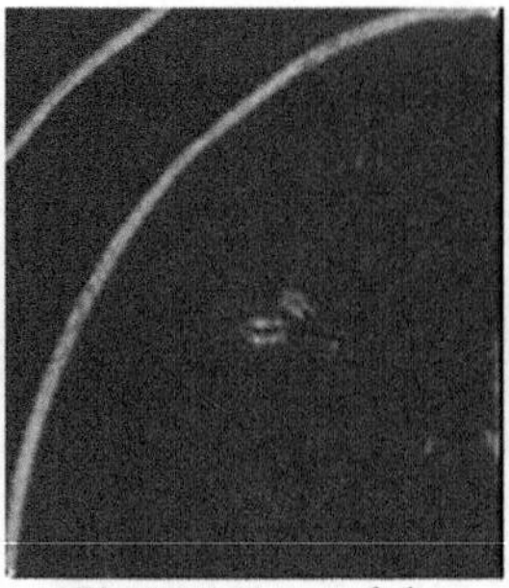
Fig. 16.5a2. $\alpha = 0.1$

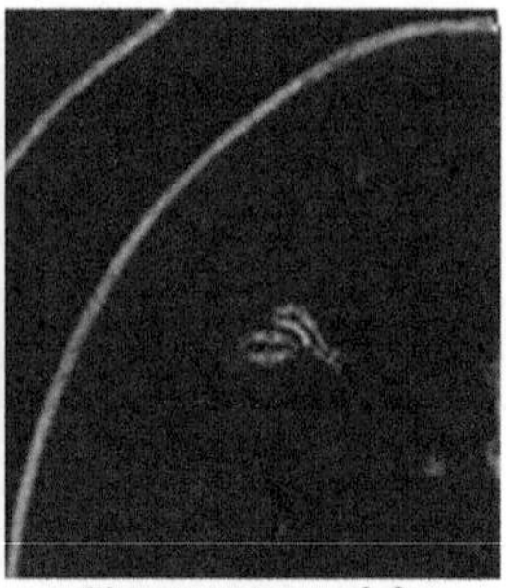
Fig. 16.5a3. $\alpha = 0.2$

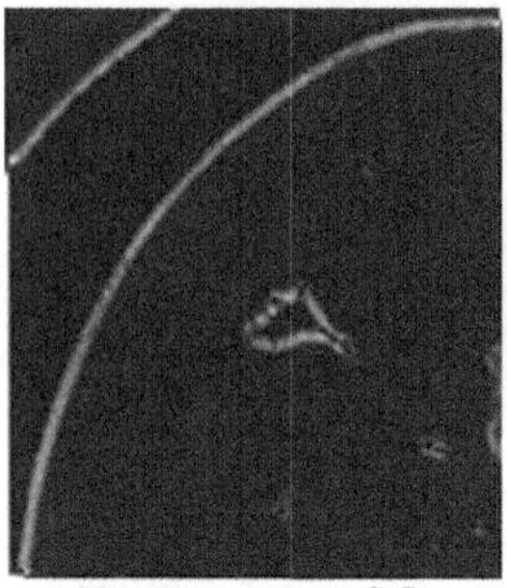
Fig. 16.5a4. $\alpha = 0.3$

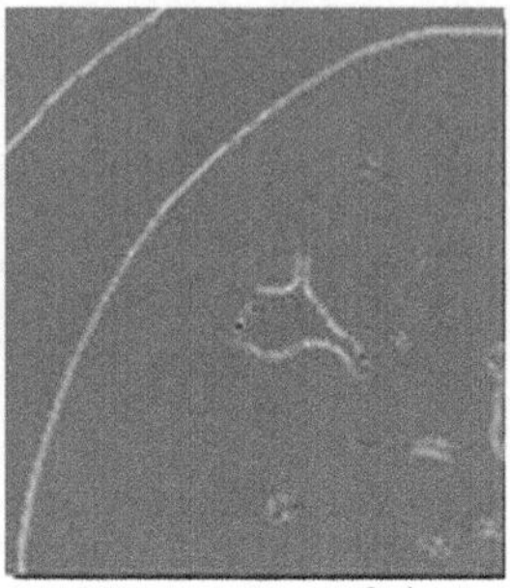
Fig. 16.5a5. $\alpha = 0.4$

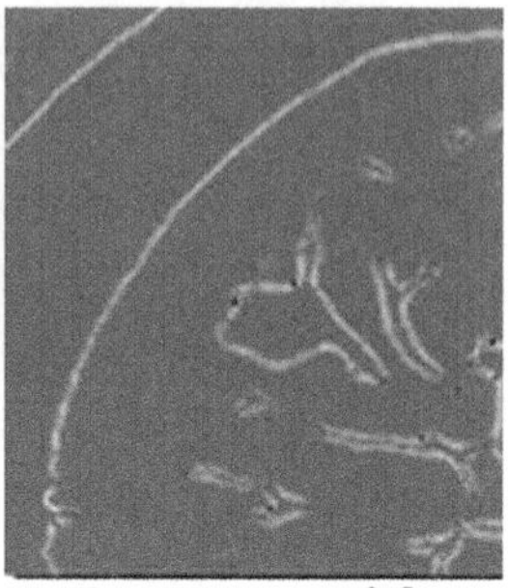
Fig. 16.5a6. $\alpha = 0.5$

the image, scanned 3 years earlier (see further) confirms a specific ability of the system. The J-Net system can isolate and highlight informative models existing on the initial image with such thin and specific levels of brightness that they appear as noisy oscillations to other algorithms and are invisible to the human eye.

These experiments clearly and visibly document that the J-Net system is able to read some brightness variations into the image at time 0, which are very difficult to see. These thin brightness variations appear to delineate the cancer's pattern of spread that will occur at time 1.

16.5 Discussion

16.5.1 A Medical Perspective

In principle, cancer cells can spread within the body by different mechanisms, such as direct invasion of surrounding tissues spread via the blood vascular system (hematogenous metastasis) and spread via the lymphatic system (lymphatic metastasis).

The metastatic spread of tumour cells is responsible for the majority of cancer deaths, and with few exceptions, all cancers can metastasize. Clinical findings have

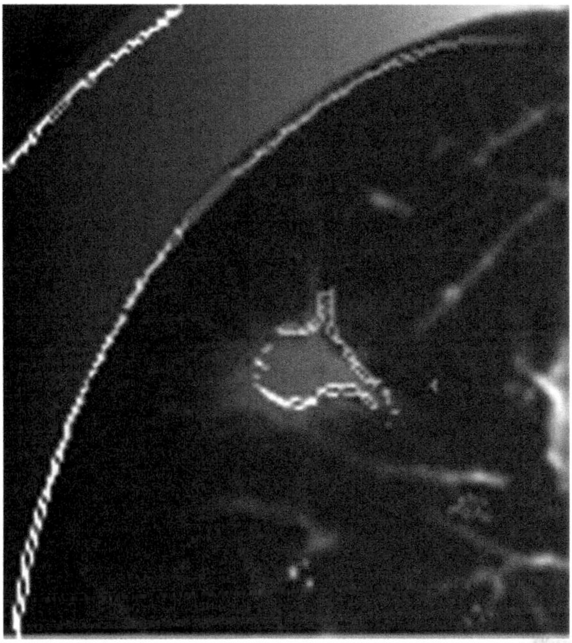

Fig. 16.5c = Fig 16.5b + 16.5a5 Prognosis of the cancer shape made by J-Net with $\alpha = 0.4$

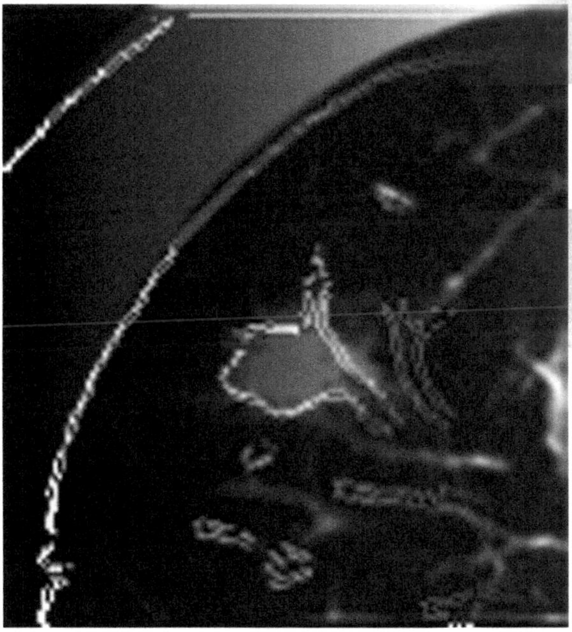

Fig. 16.5d = Fig 16.5b + 16.5a6 Prognosis of the cancer shape made by J-Net with $\alpha = 0.5$. [The images were manually superimposed without trying to register or to stretch them. An imperfect registration results because of the images' different sizes of the, taken at two different times]

long suggested that by providing a pathway for tumour cell dissemination, tumour-associated lymphatics are a key component of metastatic spread.

Despite its clinical relevance, surprisingly little is known about the mechanisms leading to the spread via the lymphatics. It is not known, however, whether pre-existing vessels are sufficient to serve this function, or whether tumour cell dissemination requires de novo lymphatic formation (lymphangiogenesis) or an increase in lymphatic size. Lymphangiogenesis has traditionally been overshadowed by the greater emphasis placed on the blood vascular system (angiogenesis).

In recent years four separate research groups provide direct evidence that two recently cloned members of the vascular endothelial growth factor (VEGF) family, VEGF-C and VEGF-D are not only important regulators of lymph vessel growth (lymphangiogenesis) in vivo but also enhance lymphatic metastasis (Plate 2001, Boardman and Swartz 2003).

The lymphatic system is important for tissue fluid balance regulation, immune cell trafficking, oedema and cancer metastasis, yet very little is known about the sequence of events that initiate and coordinate lymphangiogenesis.

We know very well that angiogenesis occurs in embryonic development, wound healing and tumour growth through a polypeptide growth factor-related sprouting process (e.g. VEGF-A and angiopoietin-2). The primary physiological driving force for blood angiogenesis is oxygen concentration, which is directly correlated with the primary function of the blood vasculature. Indeed, a number of growth factors including VEGF-A and erythropoietin are expressed under the influence of the hypoxia inducing factor-I, an oxygen-sensitive transcription factor 12. The primary function of the lymphatic system, in contrast to the blood circulation, is to maintain interstitial fluid balance and provide lymphatic clearance of interstitial fluid and macromolecules, thereby sustaining osmotic and hydrostatic gradients from blood capillaries through the interstitium and stimulating convection for interstitial protein transport.

In a recent paper a group of authors employing a new model of skin regeneration using a collagen implant in a mouse tail has shown that (1) interstitial fluid channels form *before* lymphatic endothelial cell organization and (2) lymphatic cell migration, vascular endothelial growth factor-C expression, and lymphatic capillary network organization are initiated primarily in the direction of the lymphatic flow. These data suggest that interstitial fluid channelling precedes and may even direct lymphangiogenesis (in contrast to blood angiogenesis, in which fluid flow proceeds only after the vessel develops). A novel and robust model is introduced for correlating molecular events with functionality in lymphangiogenesis.

In exploring one possible mechanism for these events, the authors observed that in the upstream region of interstitial flow, MMP activity is increased, which could lead to preferential cell migration in the direction of the flow. They also documented that increased expression of the LEC mitogen VEGF-C occurs primarily in upstream regions of the CDE, which (with subsequent unidirectional transport) could then enhance cell migration and proliferation even further in the direction of the flow. Thus, interstitial flow may represent an important transport mechanism to help guide growth and organization of a developing lymphatic capillary network.

The J-Net system's ability to document the neo-formed network of interstitial flow channels preceding the lymphangiogenesis surrounding the malignant tumour makes it possible to anticipate very reliably what the tumour mass, which will grow alongside these direction lines, will be in the future.

16.5.2 A Mathematical Perspective

The J-Net system belongs to the ACM system's family (Marr 1982).

It is a new ACM system, which can change in space and time with dynamic evolution both of the local connection's values and of the state value of each single unit.

In this complex evolutionary dynamics, the modified image, at each cycle, is a suitable scaling down of the average of all local connections values around each pixel unit.

The most important features of the J-Net system are the following:

a. The J-Net isolates a closed picture and background in each image on the basis of a specific bright intensity (factorα) in few cycles.
b. When factor α changes, J-Net selects different figures and background, "as if" it could read the bright intensity as "different kinds of frequencies".
c. At the end of its evolution J-Net has filled up the inside of the figures or the background (according to which part is the brightest) with waves, which have started to propagate from the isolated figures. The shape of each wave will be homologated with the shape of the figure working as its source. The destructive and constructive differences between these waves create the skeleton of the figures.
d. The J-Net evolves with different values of the parameter α scans different parts of the same image, having different brightness. In the case of lung cancers detected by a CT it seems that J-Net is able to read both the past and the future history of the cancer itself, due to the different bright tracks left by the cancer and to those revealing its diffusion patterns. This is possible because J-Net is able to isolate in an almost geological way different brightness layers in the same image. These layers seem to be invisible to the human eye and for the other mathematical imaging system.

These features of the J-Net system, which still have to be examined more closely, are being presented in an early research stage. J-Net's operation seems to result from some of their mathematical characteristics:

- The architecture of the J-Net system, providing for the independent evolution in space and time of its both local connections and units (Marr 1982).
- The algorithm is designed for the projection of each image from the pixels to the local connections net among the pixels themselves. In fact, during the evolution

of the system the user does not see the evolution of the pixel units of the image, but just the value of the weights locally connecting each pixel to its immediate neighbours (Marr 1982).

- The equations are designed to create attractions between different pixels, and repulsions between similar pixels (from equations (16.1), (16.2), (16.3) and (16.4)) implement the development of closed figures inside the image.
- The equation modifying the internal state of each unit considers the third delta order between each pixel and the neighbourhoods of the neighbourhood of its neighbourhood (from equations (16.5), (16.6), (16.7), (16.8), (16.9), (16.10), (16.11), (16.12), (16.13) and (16.14)). This cascade propagation helps the system to spontaneously close the figures detected and to generate homothetic waves to the source figure.
- The initial scaling-down parameter α of the image allows for the isolation of different "bright intensity frequencies" which are so thin that they appear to be invisible or as simple noises. Starting from a parameter α, which is suitably defined, its equations permit J-Net to be able to only isolate those bright signals, even if they are weak, tending to create a closed form, and it anchor them. Those signals which are "foreign" to any closed figure, specifically at that brightness level, are automatically removed.

Acknowledgments A special thanks to the Gruppo Bracco for the financial support given for this basic research.

Bibliography

Amendolia, S. R., Bisogni, M. G., Bottigli, U., Ceccopieri, A., Delogu, P., Fantacci, M. E., Marchi, A., Marzulli, V. M., Palmiero, M., and Stumbo, S. (2001). The calma project: A CAD tool in breast radiography. *Nucl. Instr. Meth. Phys. Res.* A460, 107–112.

Aoki, T., Nakata, H., Watanabe, H., Nakamura, K., Kasai, T., Hashimoto, H., Yasumoto, K., and Kido, M. (2000). Evolution of peripheral lung adenocarcinomas : CT findings correlated with histology and tumor doubling time. *Am. j. roentgenol.* 174(3), 763–768.

Boardman K. C. and Swartz M. A. (2003). Interstitial flow as a guide for lymphangiogenesis. *Circ. Res.* 92(7), 801–808.

Boyle, R., and Thomas, R. (1988). *Computer vision: A first course.* Cambridge: Blackwell Scientific Publications.

Buscema, P. M. (2006). *Sistemi ACM e imaging diagnostico. Le immagini mediche come matrici attive di connessioni* [ACM systems and diagnostic imaging. Medical images as active connections matrices, in Italian]. Italy: Springer-Verlag.

Buscema, M. (2003–2006). ACM: Active connection matrix, v. 10.0, SemeionSoftware #30, Roma.

Buscema, M. (2007), ACM batch, v. 2.0, Semeion Software #33, Roma.

Buscema, M., Catzola, L., and Grossi, E., (2007). Images as active connection matrixes: The J-net system. *IC-MED (Int. J. Intelligent Computing in Med. Sci.* 2(1), 27–53.

CANDY – Multilayer CNN Simulator© (2003). *Analogical and neural computing laboratory.* Budapest, Hungary: MTA-SzTAKI.

Chua, L. O. and Roska, T. (2002). *Cellular neural networks and visual computing. Foundations and applications.* Cambridge: Cambridge University Press.

Davies, E. (1990). *Machine vision: Theory, algorithms and practicalities.* London: Academic Press.

Delogu, P., Fantacci, M. E., Masala, G. L., Oliva, P., and Retico, A. (2004–2005) Documents D8.2: Evaluation of new developments for CADe and report; D8.4: Preliminary tests on MammoGrid/CADe and report. www.mammogrid.vitamib.com

Egmont-Petersen, M., De Ridder, D., Handels, and H. (2002). Image processing using neural networks – a review, *Pattern Recogn.* 35(10), 2279–2301.

Gonzalez, R. C. and Woods, R. E. (2008). *Digital image processing*, 3rd. edn. Upper Saddle River, NJ: Prentice-Hall.

Fantacci, M. E., Bottigli, U., Delogu, P., Golosio, B., Lauria, A., Palmiero, R., Raso, G., Stumbo, S., and Tangaro, S., Search for microcalcification clusters with the Calma CAD station. *SPIE* 4684, 1301–1310.

Hansen, T. and Neumann, H. (2004) A simple cell model with dominating opponent inhibition for a robust image processing. *Neural Networks* 17, 647–662.

Haralick, R. and Shapiro, L. (1992). *Computer and robot vision* (Vol. 1). Reading: Addison-Wesley.

Harrer, H. and Nossek, J. A. (1992a). Discrete-time cellular neural networks. *Int. J. Circuit TheoryAppl.*, 20(5), 453–467.

Harrer, H. and Nossek, J. A. (1992b). Skeletonisation: A new application for discrete-time cellular neural networks using time-variant templates. Proceedings IEEE International, 10-13 May, San Diego. *Circuits and Systems*, 6, 2897–2900.

Haykin, S. (1994). *Neural networks. A comprehensive foundation*. New York: Macmillan College Publishing Company, Inc.

Horn, B. (1986). *Robot vision*. Cambridge: MIT Press.

Jahne, B. (2003). *Digital image processing*, (5th revised and extended edition). Heidelberg: Springer-Verlag.

Kartalopoulos, S. V. (1996). *Understanding neural networks and fuzzy logic. Basic concepts and applications*. New York, NY: The Institute of Electrical and Electronics Engineers, Inc.

Kasabov, N. K. (1996). *Foundations of neural networks, fuzzy systems, and knowledge Engineering*. Cambridge MA: The MIT Press.

Marr, D., (1982) *Vision*. San Francisco: Freeman.

MATLAB (1984–2005). The language of technical computing, ver. 7.1, MathWorks Inc.

Plate, K. H. (2001). From angiogenesis to lymphangiogenesis. *Nat. Med.,*, 7, 151–152.

Vernon, D. (1991). *Machine vision*. London: Prentice-Hall.

Schamschula, M. P., Johnson, J. L., Inguva, R. (2000). *Image processing with pulse coupled neural networks*. The second international forum on multimedia and image processing, world automation congress, Maui, 2000.

Chapter 17
Digital Image Processing in Medical Applications, April 22, 2008

Sabina Tangaro, Roberto Bellotti, Francesco De Carlo, and Gianfranco Gargano

Abstract A number of methods for medical image analysis will be presented and their application to real cases will be discussed. In particular, attention will be focused on computer-aided detection (CAD) systems for lung nodule diagnosis in thorax-computed tomography (CT) and breast cancer detection in mammographic images. In the first case both a region growing (RG) algorithm for lung parenchymal tissue extraction and an active contour model (ACM) for anatomic lung contour detection will be described. In the second case, we will focus on a Haralik's textural feature extraction scheme for the characterization of the regions of interest (ROIs) of the mammogram and a supervised neural network for the classification of the ROIs.

Keywords Medical images · Textural features · Neural network

17.1 Introduction

The use of digital technologies in the medical field is becoming more and more diffuse. They aim at making the medical aid more efficient, economic, and safe by reducing the risk of human errors. The main tools of the digital technology are electronic clinical sheets containing all the data of the patient, anywhere they are recorded, and computer-aided diagnosis (CAD) systems for an automatic detection of pathologies. In the USA 18% of the hospitals make use of electronic clinical sheets and 42% have installed hardware and software resources. In 54% of the hospitals, the staff is equipped with notebooks with wireless connections to record the data and share remote information.[1] In Europe, 82% of the physicians make use of

S. Tangaro (✉)
National Institute of Nuclear Physics, Bari Section, Bari, Italy
e-mail: sonia.tangaro@ba.infn.it

[1] Study of the Healthcare Information and Management System Society, 2004.

V. Capecchi (eds.), *Applications of Mathematics in Models, Artificial Neural Networks and Arts*, DOI 10.1007/978-90-481-8581-8_17,

the PC for their work, 80% have access to the Internet. On the other side only 27% make use of the Internet to transmit or receive results of the examinations, to share with other physicians data related to their patients, and to remotely interact with the patients themselves.[2] To exploit the full power of the digital technologies it is necessary to realize large band information networks able to connect all hospitals. This is one of the main national goals in the USA to realize before 2010 and is one of the objectives of e-Health in Europe (approved by UE, 30 April 2004). It has been proved that the use of automatic systems for the image analysis is very useful to the radiologists, above all in the frame of the screening programs. In fact, during a screening program, the radiologists must diagnose on the basis of noisy images only, most of them corresponding to healthy subjects, where the pathological structures resemble the anatomical ones. For this reason the independent double reading is strongly recommended, and the CAD systems can be used as a second reader. The attention is focused on the pulmonary and mammographic CAD, as lung and breast tumors have the highest degree of mortality among the tumor pathologies affecting the western population. It is worth remembering that the performance of a CAD system can be provided in terms of (1) sensitivity, that is the percentage of pathological patients correctly diagnosed; (2) specificity, that is the percentage of healthy subjects correctly detected; and (3) the ROC curve subtending an area *AZ* that is a good index of the effectiveness of the method: the closer to 1 the value *AZ*, the best the classification system.

In Italy cancer of the breast represents a quarter of the total women's tumors and it affects about 3000 women every year. The living women struck down with this disease are about 300,000 while only 10% of people in jeopardy is currently subjected to a breast screening. Also, it is generally known that women regularly subjected to screening have a statistically significant reduction of mortality for cancer of the breast compared to women not subjected to screening (Tabar et al. 1985). Besides, the double, independent of mammogram, reading executed by two radiologists improves the sensibility of mammogram screening (Thrflell et al. 1994, Beam et al. 1996, Burhenne Warren et al. 2000) of the 4–15% of the number of revealed cancers. The most diffused method of diagnosis is the mammography. The reliability of this method is not optimal; in fact about 15% of the pathologies are not diagnosed for various reasons: mammogram with non-optimal exposure, errors of reading, fatigue from the radiologists, etc. In the mammography a tumoral lesion is often visible as a clear zone, distinguishable from the surrounding tissue, but sometimes it can be confused with the parenchymal structure, especially in the case of dense tissue. In the mammography a tumoral lesion is often visible as a clear zone, distinguishable from the surrounding tissue, but sometimes it can be confused with the parenchymal structure, especially in the case of dense tissue.

The early detection of lung neoplasia is the best way to achieve a reduction of the lung cancer mortality rates. Screening programs, dedicated to the control of

[2]Study of Eurobarometro, 2003.

asymptomatic population, chosen according to epidemiologic and statistical criteria, are more and more encouraged. In these screening programs it has been demonstrated that the use of automatic systems to analyze images is very useful for the radiologists. In fact the diagnosis is made only by means of images, the larger part of healthy patients, images usually rather noisy where potential pathological structures may be confused with anatomical details. The routine of double independent lecture is therefore strongly recommended and CAD (computer-aided detection) system can play the role of the second lecturer (Gurcan et al. 2002). In the case of lung neoplasia it has been proved that early detection followed by surgical treatment can significantly improve the prognosis: the 14% 5 years' overall survival rate rises to 49% if the lesion is localized, to 67% for tumor at stage 1, while drops to 2% if the tumor has produced metastases. The main problem is that treatable early stage lung tumors usually do not give any illness signal. So far the results of experimental screening programs based on thorax radiography and cytological sputum examination have failed to reduce the mortality (Itoh et al. 2000, Armato et al. 2002) possibly because of the low sensitivity of thorax radiography to detect micro nodules. Recently, attempts have been made in Japan to apply helical CT to lung cancer screening (Itoh et al. 2000). The preliminary results, in populations at high risk to develop lung cancer, have shown that helical CT is a potentially more useful screening method for the detection of early peripheral lung cancer with respect to chest radiography (Diederich 2002). However, since the radiation dose associated with this method is about 10 times higher than that associated with conventional chest radiography, a further reduction in radiation dose is required before this method can be applied to the general population. Many studies (Diederich et al. 2002) have suggested that dose reduction in CT does not decrease its sensitivity for small pulmonary nodules. The efficacy of low-dose helical CT protocols (Armato et al. 2002) has renewed the interest in (and also the demand for) lung cancer screening because it is able to detect small tumors, even if the effect of any lung cancer screening program, including screening with low-dose helical CT, remains a topic of debate in the medical community (Swensen et al. 2005). At present several experimental screening trials for high-risk population based on low-dose high-resolution CT to investigate if there is an effective reduction of mortality are being performed around the world and mainly in the USA and Japan. Many observational arm study have been activated in Italy, in the last years/months and randomized controlled trial studies. The number of images that need to be interpreted in CT screening is high (Gurcan et al. 2002), particularly when multi-detector helical CT and thin collimation are used, and most of them correspond to non-pathological patients. Because missed cancers are not uncommon in CT interpretation (Gurcan et al. 2002), double reading is being used in a Japanese CT screening program to reduce missed diagnosis, but it doubles the demand of radiologist's time. So researchers have recently begun to explore CAD methods in this area (Gurcan et al. 2002, Li et al. nd).

17.2 Methods

17.2.1 Region Growing

The region growing (RG) is an image analysis technique that consists in searching for connected regions of pixels satisfying a given inclusion rule. The algorithm works as follows:

1. a *seed* point is chosen and its neighbors are considered;
2. if the neighbors satisfy the inclusion rule, they are included into the growing region, otherwise they are ruled out;
3. all points included at a certain step become seed points for the following step;
4. the routine is iterated until no more points satisfy the inclusion rule.

The main problem of an RG algorithm relies in the selection of a proper seed point, which is usually done by hand. As our aim is the implementation of an automated CAD system, the seed point could be automatically selected as follows: a scan of the 3D matrix is carried out and the first voxel satisfying the inclusion rule is chosen to start the growth. When the growth is finished, the segmented region is removed from the image and the matrix scan restarts to search for a new seed point. This routine is iterated until no more seeds are found. In this way, a number of not connected regions satisfying the same inclusion rule are obtained.

Different inclusion rules may be adopted. Some examples are the following ones:

1. *Simple Bottom Threshold/Simple Top Threshold (SBT/STT)*: if the intensity I is greater/lower than a certain threshold θ, the voxel is included into the growing region:

$$I \geq \theta(\text{SBT})$$
$$I \leq \theta(\text{STT})$$

2. *Mean Bottom Threshold/Mean Top Threshold (MBT/MTT)*: the intensities of the voxel and its 26 neighbors are averaged; if the average $\langle I \rangle$ is greater/lower than the threshold θ, the voxel is included into the growing region:

$$\langle I \rangle \geq \theta(\text{MBT})$$
$$\langle I \rangle \leq \theta(\text{MTT})$$

17.2.2 Active Contour Model

The active contour model (ACM), first introduced in (Kass et al. 1988), is an image analysis technique used to define the contours of complex objects. Kass developed a novel technique for image segmentation, which was able to solve a large class of segmentation problems that had eluded more conventional techniques. He was interested in developing a model-based technique that could recognize familiar objects in the presence of noise and other ambiguities. Kass proposed the concept of active contour model that use "an energy minimizing spline guided by external constraint forces and influenced by image forces that pull it toward features such as lines and edges." The focus of this technique consists in positioning a closed curve, a *spline*, joining a number of nodes, in a certain position of the image, and leaving it to evolve until an equilibrium position is reached. The evolution of the spline is driven by both internal forces (generally elastic forces) attracting (or repelling) the nodes one another and external forces based on the image suitably transformed into a potential or a force field. Different results can be obtained depending on the initial position of the spline and on the kind of transformation of the image. ACMs are used in many fields as tracking of moving objects for traffic monitoring (Tai 2004), facial feature extraction (Wan 2005), or, as in our case, in medical image analysis for anatomical contour selection (Dong 1999).

17.2.3 Features Extraction: Gray-Level Co-occurrence Matrix

Transforming the input data into the set of features is called features extraction. If the features extracted are carefully chosen it is expected that the features set will extract the relevant information from the input data in order to perform the desired task using this reduced representation instead of the full size input. Texture analysis offers interesting possibilities to characterize the structural heterogeneity of classes. The texture of an image is related to the spatial distribution of the intensity values in the image and as such contains information regarding contrast, uniformity, rugosity, regularity, etc. A considerable number of quantitative texture features can be extracted from images using different methodologies in order to characterize these properties and then can be used to classify pixels following analogous processes as with spectral classifications. To provide useful information about the texture of an image it is possible to use the gray-level co-occurrence matrix (GLCM) (Haralik et al. 1973), also known as spatial gray-level dependence (SGLD) (Conners and Harlow 1980). As the name suggests, the GLCM is constructed from the image by estimating the pairwise statistics of pixel intensity, thus relying on the assumption that the texture content information of an image is contained in overall or average spatial relationship between pairs of pixel intensities (Haralik et al. 1973). A co-occurrence matrix M is a $G \times G$ matrix, whose rows and columns are indexed by the image gray levels $i = 1,...,G$, where $G = 2^n$ for a n-bit image. Each element p_{ij} represents an estimate of the probability that two pixels with a specified polar separation (d, θ) have gray levels i and j. Coordinates d and θ are, respectively, the distance and the angle between the two pixels i and j. In their seminal paper, Haralik et al. (1973) considered only displacements $d = 1$ at quantized angles $\theta = k\pi/4$, with $k = 0, 1, 2, 3$, thus having $M_{d,\theta}(j,i) = M_{d,\theta+\pi}(i,j)$. Symmetry is achieved by averaging the GLCM with its transpose, thus leading to invariance under π-rotations too. Textural features can be derived from the GLCM and used in texture classification in place of the single GLCM elements. A number of 14 features are introduced, related to a textural property of the image such as homogeneity, contrast, presence of organized structure, complexity, and nature of gray tone transitions. The values of these features are sensitive to the choice of the direction θ, given that the parameter d is fixed to 1. Invariance under rotation should be restored in order to avoid describing two images, one obtained by rotating the other, with different feature sets. This is achieved by considering average and range of each feature values over the θ angles, thus obtaining a number of 28 textural variables, even if only few of them are used as inputs to the classifier (Conners and Harlow 1980, Conners et al. 1984, Weszka 1976). As the texture is gray tone independent, either the image must be normalized or one should choose features which are invariant under monotonic gray-level transformation. If no kind of normalization is applied it is possible to use, among all the GLCM features, the ones that are invariant under monotonic gray tone transformation:

1. energy:

$$f_1 = \sum_{ij} p_{ij}^2 \tag{17.1}$$

2. entropy:

$$f_2 = -\sum_{ij} p_{ij} \ln(p_{ij}) \tag{17.2}$$

3. information measures of correlation:

$$f_3 = \frac{f_2 - H_1}{\max\{H_x, H_y\}} \tag{17.3}$$

$$f_4 = (1 - \exp\{-2(H_2 - f_2)\})^{1/2} \tag{17.4}$$

where

$$P_x(i) = \sum_j p_{ij} \tag{17.5}$$

$$P_y(j) = \sum_i p_{ij} \tag{17.6}$$

$$H_1 = -\sum_{ij} p_{ij} \ln\{P_x(i) P_y(j)\} \tag{17.7}$$

$$H_2 = -\sum_{ij} P_x(i)P_y(j) \ln \{P_x(i)P_y(j)\} \tag{17.8}$$

$$H_x = -\sum_{i} P_x(i) \ln \{P_x(i)\} \tag{17.9}$$

$$H_y = -\sum_{j} P_y(j) \ln \{P_y(j)\} \tag{17.10}$$

For each of the above-mentioned features $\{f_i\}_{i=1,\ldots,4}$,{ average and range are computed for the angles $\theta = k\pi/4$, with $k = 0, 1, 2, 3$, and $d = 1$, thus obtaining eight textural features.

17.2.4 Feed-Forward Neural Network

A feed-forward neural network is an artificial neural network where connections between the units do not form a directed cycle. The feed-forward neural network was the first and arguably simplest type of artificial neural network devised. In this network, the information moves in only one direction, forward, from the input nodes, through the hidden nodes (if any), and to the output nodes. There are no cycles or loops in the network. This class of networks consists of multiple layers of computational units, usually interconnected in a feed-forward way. Each neuron in one layer has directed connections to the neurons of the subsequent layer. In many applications the units of these networks apply a sigmoid function as an activation function. The universal approximation theorem for neural networks states that every continuous function that maps intervals of real numbers to some output interval of real numbers can be approximated arbitrarily closely by a multi-layer perception with just one hidden layer. This result holds only for restricted classes of activation functions, e.g., for the sigmoidal functions. Multi-layer networks use a variety of learning techniques, the most popular being back-propagation. Here the output values are compared with the correct answer to compute the value of some predefined error function. By various techniques the error is then fed back through the network. Using this information, the algorithm adjusts the weights of each connection in order to reduce the value of the error function by some small amount. After repeating this process for a sufficiently large number of training cycles the network will usually converge to some state where the error of the calculations is small. In this case one says that the network has learned a certain target function. To adjust weights properly one applies a general method for non-linear optimization that is called gradient descent. For this, the derivative of the error function with respect to the network weights is calculated and the weights are then changed such that the error decreases (thus going downhill on the surface of the error function). For this reason back-propagation can only be applied on networks with differentiable activation functions.

17.3 Application

The analysis of medical images is gathering, in the last years, a growing interest from the scientific community working at the crossover point among physics, engineering, and medicine. The development of computer-aided detection (CAD) systems for the automated search for pathologies could be very useful for the improvement of physicians' diagnosis. In the next section will be presented some procedure used in the case of a CAD for breast neoplasia detection in mammographic images and of a CAD for lung nodule detection in thorax computed tomography (CT) images.

17.3.1 RG Application: Internal Lung Volume Segmentation

In a previous study, our group proposed a CAD for lung nodule detection in thorax computed tomography (CT) images (Bellotti et al. 2007). The first step of the CAD scheme consists in the segmentation of the internal lung volume. In thorax CT images the internal lung volume, which consists of air and bronchial tree, typically appears as low-intensity voxels surrounded by high-intensity voxels corresponding to the pleura (see Fig. 17.1). This suggests to segment the internal lung volume by means of a 3D RG algorithm. The choice of the inclusion rule with the optimal

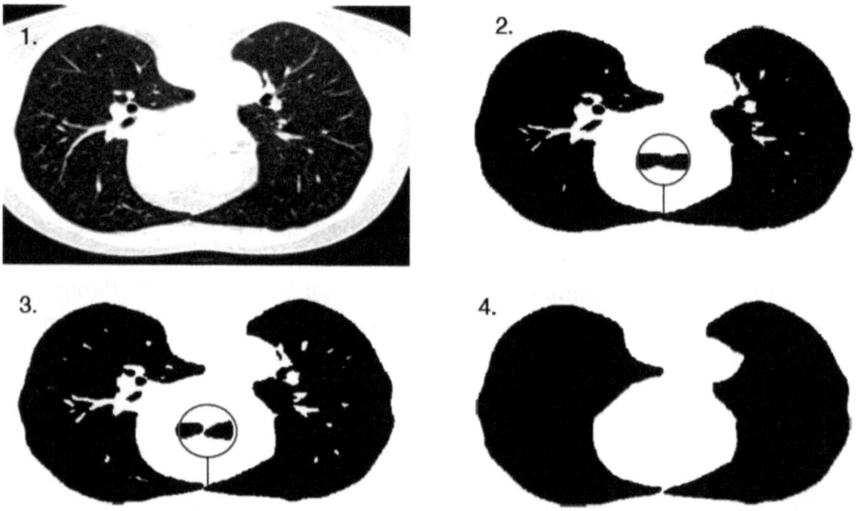

Fig. 17.1 (1) Original section of a CT scan: low-intensity (black) voxels correspond to air and bronchial tree; high-intensity voxels correspond to pleura, fat, muscles, vascular tree, bones, and, eventually, nodules. (2) Section of the volume segmented by the MTT RG; an enlargement of the two lungs joined together is displayed in the circle. (3) The same slice as in (2) with separated lung sections, as displayed by the enlargement in the circle. (4) A section of the *working volume*, obtained after the ACM contour detection (see Section 17.3.2)

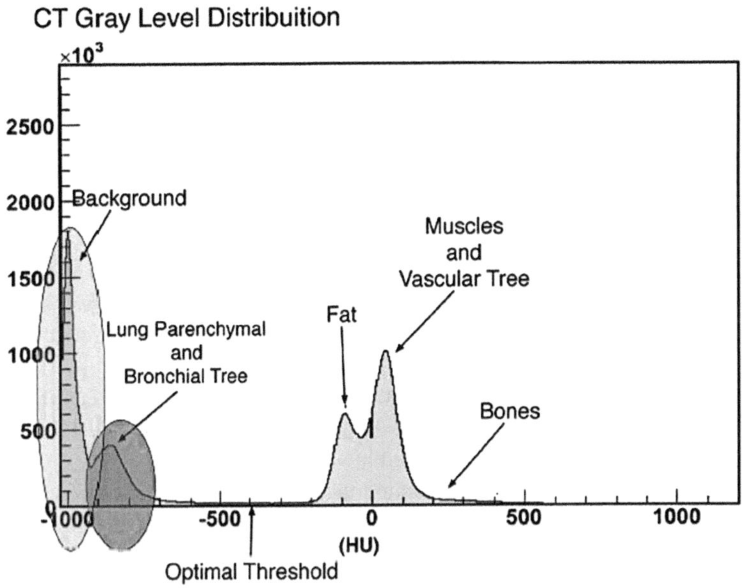

Fig. 17.2 Gray-level distribution of the voxels of one of the analyzed CT. Similar distributions can be obtained from the other CTs. The region segmented by the RG algorithm refers to the lung parenchymal and the bronchial tree. The voxels corresponding to the background, though having an intensity lower than the threshold $\bar{\theta}$, are not included in the grown region because they are not geometrically connected with the seed point

threshold and the selection of a proper seed point are of great relevance for the best performance of the algorithm. Our choice is the MTT rule that allows to reduce the "noise" of the low-dose CT, thus obtaining a volume with quite regular contours. The threshold value $\bar{\theta}$ is automatically selected with the method adopted in (Ridler and Calvard 1978); it is based on the gray tone distribution of the CT voxels that typically shows two well distinct parts (see Fig. 17.2 obtained from one of the analyzed CTs): one containing air, lung parenchyma, trachea, and bronchial tree and the other one containing vascular tree, bones, muscles, and fat. The optimal threshold, set at the *plateau* between these two regions, is selected as follows:

- the CT gray tone histogram is divided in two regions with equal number of bins and the mean values of the bins in the two regions are computed;
- the previously computed mean values are averaged and the bin having the intensity nearest to the new mean is selected as the threshold to divide the histogram;
- the routine is iterated until the threshold bin does not change any more.

The seed point of the RG is automatically selected as the first voxel that satisfies the inclusion rule in a cubic region located as follows: the CT is divided lengthwise, thus obtaining two parts of equal sizes; the center of the cube is positioned at the cross-point of the diagonals of, say, the left part (the choice of the right part would be equivalent). In this way, we are quite sure that the cubic region where the seed point is searched is inside the lung, for less than abnormal anatomical deformities. Once this voxel is found the growth of the internal lung volume is started, otherwise the search is repeated in a greater cubic region until a voxel satisfying the inclusion rule is found.

The volume thus segmented shows some slices with joined lungs (see the magnified circle in Fig. 17.2). To draw the correct lung volume contour (see Section 17.3.2) it is necessary that the two lung sections are separated in all slices. To this purpose, a lower number of voxels should be included in the growing region, along the contour of the sections where the lungs are joined. This is achieved as follows:

1. starting from the top, the slices where the lung sections are joined are found, and a 2D RG is carried out in each slice with MTT inclusion rule and 1% decreased threshold with respect to the initial value $\bar{\theta}$;
2. the threshold is decreased at the same rate in order to include a lower number of voxels into the 2D growing region, until the lung sections are disjoined.

The previously described routine is repeated for all slices where the lung sections are joined. As an example Fig. 17.3 shows the result (see the magnified circle) of the above-described routine when applied to the image displayed in Fig. 17.2.

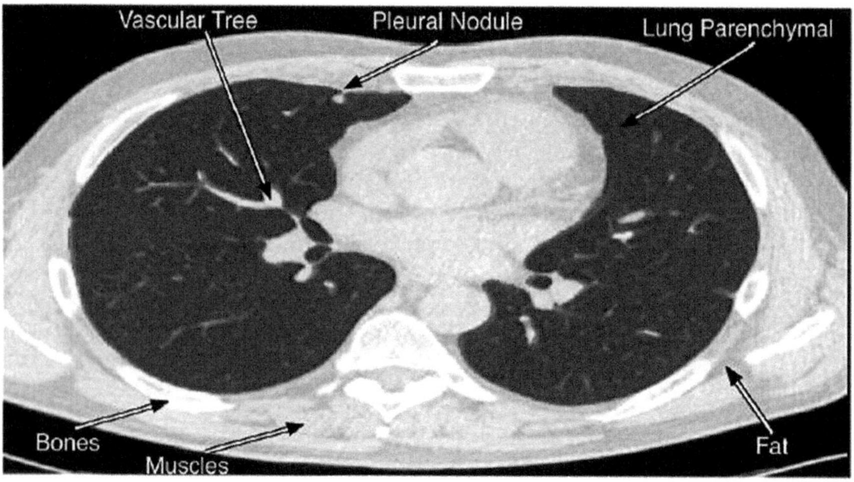

Fig. 17.3 An example of one slice of the internal lung volume obtained after the first step of our CAD. It should be stressed the presence of a pleural nodule which has not been included into the segmented region

Figure 17.3 shows another typical example of one slice of the segmented region. It should be stressed that the volume thus obtained includes the lung parenchyma, the bronchial tree, and the trachea, while structures outside the lung, as bones, fat, and vascular tree are ruled out. Also internal and pleural nodules are not included at

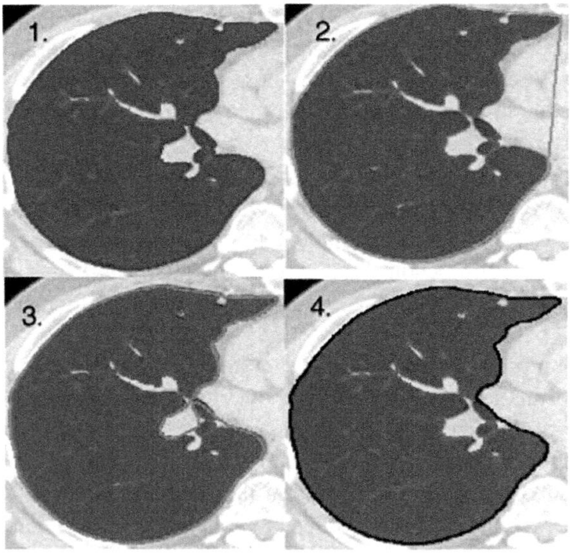

Fig. 17.4 (1) the 2D lung contour obtained after the segmentation with the RG: the pleural nodule, marked by a *circle*, is ruled out; this contour is the initial position of the spline in the GEB dynamics and corresponds to the case $q = +\infty$; (2) the 2D lung contour obtained with a CH: the pleural nodule is included into the contour but the right part of the lung is roughly approximated by a *straight line*; this contour is also obtained by the GEB dynamics for $q = 0$; (3) the 2D lung contour obtained by the GEB with a suboptimal value of the parameter q; (4) the 2D lung contour obtained by the GEB with the best value of q

this stage because they do not satisfy the MTT inclusion rule. On the other side, not only the nodules but also the vascular tree inside the lung must be included into the parenchymal volume, because there may be some nodules attached to its external walls. To this purpose, the contour of the lung must be outlined and all voxels inside this contour must be considered (see Section 17.3.2).

17.3.2 ACM Application: Anatomic Lung Contour Selection

The anatomic lung contour selection is implemented slicewise; after that, all pixels inside the 2D contours will be combined together to obtain the 3D-segmented volume. Fig. 17.4(1) shows an example of segmented lung slice, as obtained with the RG, together with the contour of the lung section. As one can see, the lung slice includes a pleural nodule, marked by the black circle, that is ruled out by the contour. To avoid this drawback one can think to apply a convex hull (CH) algorithm, that is the intersection of all convex regions containing a given object. The result of such application is shown in Fig.17.4(2): the pleural nodule is correctly included into the contour but other concave structures, as the section of the vascular tree near the lung hilum, are roughly approximated by a straight line.

Other approaches can be followed for the detection of the pleural nodules, as comparing the curvatures at points on the lung border (Ko and Betke 2001): a rapid change in curvature indicated a nodule, large vessel, or bronchus that formed an acute or obtuse angle with the lung border, and the lung border was then corrected by means of insertion of a border segment.

We have developed a new kind of ACM algorithm, named *Glued Elastic Band (GEB)* (Gargano 2007) that simulates the dynamics of a spline *glued* to the nodes along the contour. The algorithm implements a sort of *local* CH, able to include concave parts with little bending radius, such as pleural nodules, and to rule out concave parts with great bending radius, such as the section of the vascular tree near the lung hilum.

The algorithm relies on one parameter q that can be considered as the quantity of glue. The results are shown in Fig. 17.4(3) and (4): in particular, Fig. 17.4(3) shows the results obtained with a non-optimal value of q, while Fig. 17.4(4) shows the lung contour obtained with the optimal quantity of glue. As one can see, the spline has reached an equilibrium position that includes concave parts with little bending radius as pleural nodules, while concave parts with great bending radius, as the section of the vascular tree near the lung hilum, are ruled out.

The dynamics of the spline is driven by the following forces:

1. constant internal forces that the nodes exchange one another with the nearest neighbors (the previous and the following along the spline);
2. constant adhesive forces acting toward the inside of the object when the nodes are in contact with the section contour of the object, as if there was some glue on the spline;
3. the constraint reactions acting when the nodes are pushed inside the contour.

In detail, let us consider the constant internal forces $\vec{F}_{i+1}$ and $\vec{F}_{i-1}$ acting on node i due to the neighboring nodes $i+1$, $i-1$; if a Cartesian system is considered with origin on the node i and axis versus $\vec{u}_x$ and $\vec{u}_y$, we have

$$\begin{cases} \vec{F}_{i-1} = \cos\vartheta_{i-1}\vec{u}_x + \sin\vartheta_{i-1}\vec{u}_y \\ \vec{F}_{i+1} = \cos\vartheta_{i+1}\vec{u}_x + \sin\vartheta_{i+1}\vec{u}_y \end{cases} \tag{17.11}$$

where the angles ϑ_{i-1} and ϑ_{i+1} define the directions of the neighboring nodes with respect to node i. The resultant internal force on node i has the following intensity and orientation:

$$|R_i| = \sqrt{(\cos\vartheta_{i-1} + \cos\vartheta_{i+1})^2 + (\sin\vartheta_{i-1} + \sin\vartheta_{i+1})^2} \tag{17.12}$$

$$\tan\vartheta_{R_i} = \frac{\sin\vartheta_{i-1} + \sin\vartheta_{i+1}}{\cos\vartheta_{i-1} + \cos\vartheta_{i+1}} \tag{17.13}$$

The adhesive force $\vec{F}_a$ due to the glue is assumed to have the same direction as $\vec{R}_i$, versus pointing always toward the inside of the contour, and constant strength

$|F_a|$. If the sum $\vec{F}_{TOT_i} = \vec{R}_i + \vec{F}_a$ points toward the outside ($\vec{R}_i$ and $\vec{F}_a$ have opposite versus, with $|\vec{R}_i| > |\vec{F}_a|$), node I detaches from the contour. If $\vec{F}_{TOT_i}$ points toward the inside ($\vec{R}_i$ and $\vec{F}_a$ have the same versus), then a constraint reaction $\vec{N}_i$ (equal strength and direction of $\vec{F}_{TOT_i}$, opposite versus) forbids node i to move inside the contour: as a result the node remains glued to the contour. Figure 17.5 provides a pictorial explanation of this dynamics: for nodes on concave parts of the contour with great bending radius, as node number 1, the sum of the internal forces, due to nearest neighbors, is smaller than the adhesive force due to the glue; hence, such nodes remain glued to the contour: this is the typical case of nodes near the lung hilum. On the other side, for nodes on concave parts of the contour with little bending radius, as node number 2, the sum of the internal forces is strong enough to exceed the adhesive forces of the glue; the effect is that the spline is pulled out and the concave part is included inside the spline: this is the typical case of the pleural nodules. Finally, for node number 3 the sum of the internal forces points toward the inside of the region: such node feels a constant reaction as for an object on a plane; the effect is that this node does not move. This dynamics is applied to all nodes of the spline.

The only parameter of the GEB is quantity of glue that is given by the ratio between adhesive and internal forces:

$$q = \frac{F_a}{F} \tag{17.14}$$

It is interesting to note that in the limit $q = +\infty$, the internal forces are irrelevant with respect to the adhesive forces and the spline remains perfectly glued to the 2D contour: this case corresponds to the initial position of the spline (Fig. 17.4(1)).

On the other side, for $q = 0$, the adhesive force is zero and the result is the same of a CH (Fig. 17.4(2)). Between these two cases, one can have intermediate values implementing a *local* CH with different results: the highest the q, the greater the bending radius of the concave parts that are ruled out. The parameter q is set slicewise by varying its value until the following condition holds:

$$\frac{A_i}{A_f} = a \tag{17.15}$$

where A_i and A_f are, respectively, the initial and the final area inside the 2D contours. The parameter a should be optimized in order to maximize the number of the nodules included into the contour and minimize the segmented volume. However changes of a in the neighborhood of the best value do not affect in a substantial way both the number of detected nodules and the volume of the segmented region, thus suggesting that the method is stable. All voxels inside the final position of the spline are considered (see Fig. 17.1(4)) and combining together the regions inside the 2D contours of each slice, we obtain the 3D-segmented volume which contains bronchial and vascular trees inside the lung, trachea, internal, and pleural nodules. Fig. 17.6 shows two 3D images obtained as a result of this procedure.

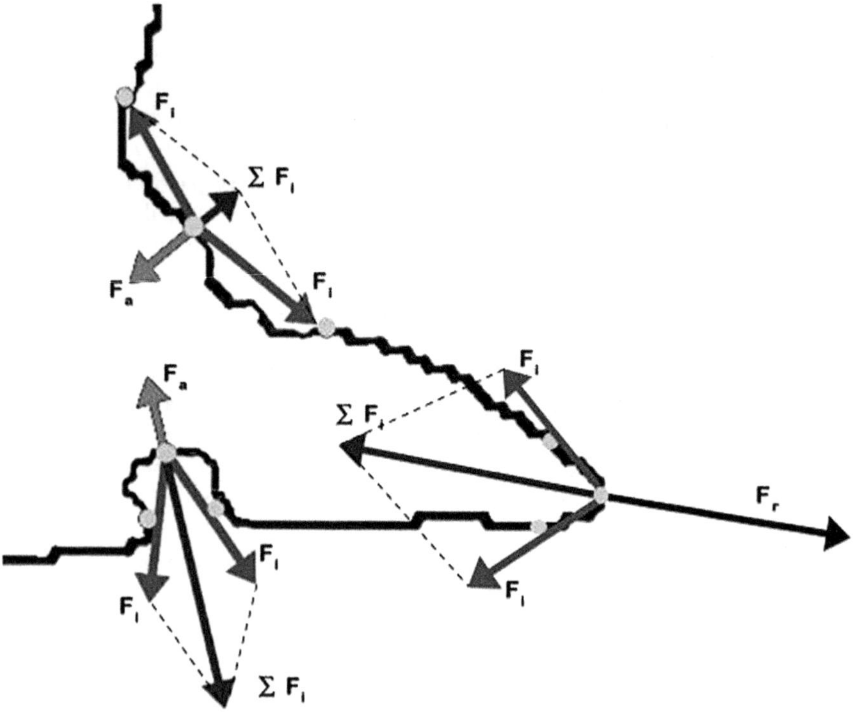

Fig. 17.5 A pictorial explanation of the GEB dynamics: node number 1 is on a concave part of the contour with great bending radius where the sum of the internal forces, due to nearest neighbors, is smaller than the adhesive force due to the glue; hence, such node remains glued to the contour: this is the typical case of the nodes near the lung hilum. Node number 2 is on a concave part of the contour with little bending radius where the sum of the internal forces is strong enough to exceed the adhesive forces; the effect is that the spline is pulled out and the concave part is included inside the spline: this is the typical case of the pleural nodules. For node number 3 the sum of the internal forces points toward the inside of the region: such node feels a constant reaction as for an object on a plane; the effect is that this node does not move. This dynamics is applied to all nodes of the spline

17.3.3 Feed-Forward Neural Network Application: Classification of Massive Lesions in Breast Mammographic Images

In a previous study, our group proposed a CAD scheme based on ROI localization, textural feature extraction, and neural network classification (Bellotti 2006). Suspect regions were detected by edge-based segmentation algorithm where regions of interest (ROIs) are defined by iso-intensity contours. The ROIs thus obtained were characterized using the Haralik's features set (see Section 17.2.3) and then classified using a feed-forward neural network (see Section 17.2.4). We used a supervised two-layered feed-forward neural network, trained with gradient descent learning rule (Hertz et al. 1991) for the ROI pattern classification:

$$\Delta w_{ij}(\tau) = -\eta \frac{\vartheta E(\tau)}{\vartheta w_{ij}} + \alpha \Delta w_{ij}(\tau - 1) \tag{17.16}$$

$$E(\tau) = \frac{1}{2} \sum_{\mu} \left[t^{\mu} - y^{\mu} \right]^2 \tag{17.17}$$

where the $E(\tau)$ function measures the error of the network outputs y^{μ} in reproducing the targets $t^{\mu} = 1{,}0$, at iteration τ, and w_{ij} are the network weights. The second term in (17.16), known as *momentum*[22], represents a sort of inertia which is added to quickly move along the direction of decreasing gradient, thus reducing the computational time to the solution. Different values of the momentum parameter α were tested and the best trade-off between performance and computational time was reached for $\alpha = 0.1 \div 0.2$. The learning rate was $\eta = 0.01$. A sigmoid transfer function is used:

$$g(x) = \frac{1}{1 + e^{-\beta x}} \tag{17.18}$$

with gain factor$\beta = 1$.

The network architecture consisted of $N_i = 8$ input neurons and one output neuron. The size of the hidden layer was tuned in the range $[N_i - 1{,}2N_i + 1]$ optimizing the classification performance. All the true positive (including e pre diagnosed lesion) ROIs at our disposal ($N_{TP} = 1207$) and as many negative ones were used to train the neural network. To make sure that the negative training patterns were representative, they were selected with a probability given by the distribution of the whole negative ROI set at our disposal, in the eight-dimensional feature space. With a random procedure we build up two sets (A and B), each one made of 1207

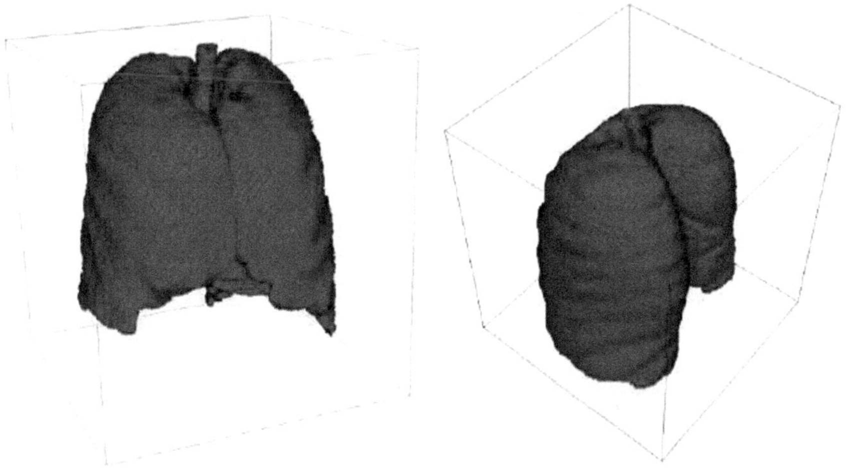

Fig. 17.6 3D images obtained as a result of this procedure

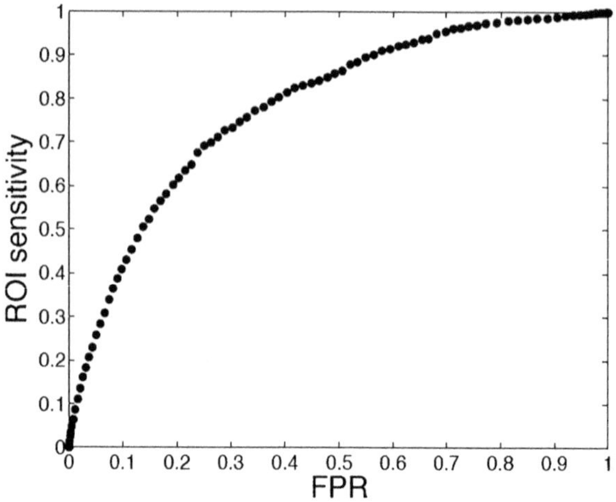

Fig. 17.7 ROC curve for ROI-based classification. The area under the curve (AUC) is $A_z = 0.783 \pm 0.008$

patterns, which are used, in turn, for both training and test, according to the cross validation technique (Stone 1974): first, the network is trained with set A and tested with set B, then the two sets are reversed. In addition, we take care that the occurrence for each kind of mass and tissue present in the database is balanced in set A and set B, in order to train and test the network in the most complete and correct way. All the other patterns (negative ROIs not selected for the training stage and FP) are used for validation only. The results are presented in the form of receiver operating characteristic (ROC) curves in Fig. 17.7. The ROC curve is particularly suitable when testing a binary hypothesis (Swets 1988): it is obtained by plotting the ROI sensitivity against the ROI false-positive rate (FPR), at different values of the decision threshold on the neural network output.

Bibliography

Armato, S. G., Li, F., Giger, M. L., MacMahon, H., Sone, S., and Doi, K. (2002). Lung cancer: Performance of automated lung nodule detection applied to cancers missed in a CT screening program. *Radiology* 225, 685–692.

Beam, V. et al. (1996) *Acad. Radiol.* 3, 891-897.

Bellotti, R., De Carlo, F., Gargano, G., Maggipinto, G., Tangaro, S., Castellano, M., et al. (2006). A completely automated CAD system for mass detection in a large mammographic database. *Med. Phy.* 33(8), 3066–3075.

Bellotti, R., De Carlo, F., Gargano, G., Tangaro, S., Cascio, D., Catanzariti, E., et al. (2007). ACAD system for nodule detection in low-dose lung CTs based on Region Growing and a new Active Contour Model. *Med. Phy.* 34(12), 4901–4910.

Burhenne Warren L. J., et al. (2000). *Radiology* 215, 554–562.

Conners, R. W. and Harlow, C. A., (1980). A theoretical comparison of texture algorithm. *IEEE Trans. Patt. Anal. Machine Intell.* 2, 204–222.

Conners, R.W., Trivedi, M. M., and Harlow, C. A., (1984). Segmentation of a high-resolution urban scene using texture operators. *Comp. Vision, Grap. Image Process.* 25, 273–310.

Diederich, S., Lentschig, M. G., Overbeck, T. R., Wonnanns, D., and Hemdel, W. (2002). Detection of pulmonary nodules at spiral CT: comparison of maximum intensity projection sliding slabs and single-image reporting. *Eur. Radiol.* 11, 1345–1350.

Diederich, S., Wormannas, D., Semik, M., Thomas, M., Lenzen, H., Roos, N., Heindel, W. (2002). Screening for early lung cancer with low-dose spiral CT: Prevalence in 817 asymptomatic smokers. *Radiology* 222, 773–781.

Gurcan, M. N, Sahiner, B., Petrick, N., Chan, H.-P., Kazerooni, E.A., Cascade, P.N., and Hadjiiski, L. (2002). Lung nodule detection on thoracic computed tomog-raphy images: Preliminary evaluation of a computer-aided diagnosis system. *Med. Phy.* 29(11), 2552–2558.

Gargano, G., Bellotti, R., De Carlo, F., Tangaro, S., Tommasi, E., Castellano, M., et al. (2007). *A novel active contour model algorithm for contour detection in complex objects*. Proceedings of the 2007 IEEE inter-national conference on computational intelligence for measurement systems and applications, Ostuni, Italy, 27–29 June.

Hanley, J. A. and McNeil, B. J. (1982). The meaning and use of the area under a receiver operating characteristic (ROC) curve. *Radiology* 143, 29–36.

Haralik, R. M., Shanmugam, K., and Dinstein, I., (1973). Textural features for image classification. *IEEE Trans. Sys., Man and Cybernet.* SMC-3, 610–621.

Hertz, J., Krogh, A., Palmer, and R. G. (1991). *Introduction to the theory of neural computation.* Addison-Wesley.

Itoh, S. Ikeda, M., Arahata, S., Kodaira, T., Isomura, T., Kato, T., and Yamakawa, K., Maruyama, V., Ishigaki, T. (2000). Lung cancer screening: Minimum tube current required for helical C. *Radiology* 215, 175–183.

Joong K. D., (1999). A fast and stable snake algorithm for medical images. *Patt. Recog. Lett.* 20(5), 507–512.

Kass, M., Witkin, A., and Terzopoulos, D. (1988). Snakes: Active contourmodels. *Int. J. Comp. Vision* 1(4), 321–331.

Ridler, T. W. and Calvard, S. (1978). Picture thresholding using an iterative selec-tion method. *IEEE Trans. Sys., Man and Cybernet.* 8, 630–632.

Ko, J. P. and Betke, M. (2001). Chest CT: Automated nodule detection and assessment of change over Time preliminary experience. *Radiology* 218, 267–273.

Li, Q. Some, S., and Doi, K., (nd). Selective enhancement filters for nodules, vessels, and airway walls in two-an three-dimensional CT scans.

Rumelhart, D. E. and McClelland, J. L. (1986). *Parallel Distribuited rocessing* (Vol.I). Cambridge MA: MIT Press.

Stone, M. (1974). Cross-validatory choice and assessment of statistical predictions. *J. Royal Stat. Soc.* B, 36(1), 111–147.

Swensen, J. S., Jett, J. R., Hartman, T. E., Midthun, D. E., Mandrekar, S. J., Hillman, S. L., et al. (2005). CT screen-ing for lung cancer: Five-year prospective experience. *Radiology* 235, 259–265.

Swets, J. A. (1988). Measuring the accuracy of diagnostic systems. *Science* 240, 1285–1293.

Tabar, L., et al. (1985). *Lancet* 1, 829–83.

Tai, J. -C., Tseng S. -T., Lin, C. -P., Song., K. -T, (2004). Real-time image tracking for automatic traffic monitoring and enforcement applica-tions. *Image Vision Comp.* 22(6), 485–501.

Thrflell, E. L., et al. (1994). *Radiology* 191, 241–244.

Wan, K.-W., Lam, K.-M., Ng, K.-C., (1999). An accurate active shape model for facial feature extraction. *Patt. Recog. Lett.* 26(15), 2409–2423.

Weszka, J. S., Dyer, C. R., and Rosenfeld, A. (1976). A comparative Study of texture measures for terrain classification. *IEEE Trans. Sys. Man and Cybernet.* 6, 269–285.

Part III
Mathematics and Art

Chapter 18
Mathematics, Art, and Interpretation: A Hermeneutic Perspective

Giorgio T. Bagni

Abstract Since the beginning of the 19th century, Schleiermacher pointed out the presence of a circle (*hermeneutic circle*) in the comprehension: A particular element can be considered only taking into account the universe to which it belongs, and vice versa. Heidegger reconsidered the mentioned issue, so the comprehension is not understood according to the model of textual interpretation; it is based on the relationship between human beings and the world. When we consider a "historical" piece of knowledge (both an artistic masterpiece and an ancient mathematical idea) we can try to frame it in its historical period; nevertheless we can read it from our present, actual viewpoint. As regards mathematical knowledge, for instance, it is not really meaningful to look for "general rules" of mathematical evolution. Every culture clearly influenced the development of its own mathematics, for instance, by using artefacts and semiotic representations (Peirce). Both historico-cultural approaches (Radford) and anthropological approaches (D'Amore and Godino) ask us to investigate how cultural contexts determined mathematical experiences. Therefore art and mathematics can be linked by a hermeneutic approach: they are human enterprises and they are not to be considered as paths towards a form of truth "out there" (in Richard Rorty's words).

Sommario A partire dall'inizio del XIX secolo, Schleiermacher segnalò la presenza di un circolo (*circolo ermeneutico*) per il quale il particolare può comprendersi soltanto partendo dall'universale di cui esso stesso è parte e viceversa. Il problema fu ripreso da Heidegger: dunque la comprensione non viene più ad essere orientata sul solo modello della spiegazione teoretica dei testi, bensì sullo stesso rapporto che gli esseri umani hanno con il mondo. Quando ci accostiamo ad un'opera "storica" (un capolavoro dell'arte di alcuni secoli fa ma anche un contenuto matematico antico) possiamo osservarla cercando di collocarla rigorosamente nel proprio periodo storico, ma anche leggerla con i nostri occhi. Per quanto riguarda la matematica, non ha ad esempio molto senso tentare di individuare le "regole generali" che

G.T. Bagni (✉)
Department of Mathematics and Computer Science, University of Udine, Udine, Italy
e-mail: giorgio.bagni@dimi.uniud.it

V. Capecchi (eds.), *Applications of Mathematics in Models, Artificial Neural Networks and Arts*, DOI 10.1007/978-90-481-8581-8_18,

avrebbero determinato l'evoluzione della matematica. Ogni cultura ha chiaramente influenzato lo sviluppo della propria matematica, ad esempio mediante l'uso di artefatti e di rappresentazioni semiotiche (Peirce). Sia gli approcci storico-culturali (Radford) che quelli antropologici (D'Amore e Godino) ci chiedono di stabilire come i contesti culturali abbiano determinato le esperienze matematiche. L'arte e la matematica possono dunque legarsi ad un approccio ermeneutico: sono costruzioni umane, non momenti di accesso ad una qualche Verità "là fuori" (nelle parole di Richard Rorty).

Keywords Artefact · Pistemology · Hermeneutics · History of mathematics · Language

18.1 Introduction

Since the beginning of the 19th century, Schleiermacher pointed out the presence of a circle (the so-called *hermeneutic circle*) in the human comprehension: as a matter of fact, frequently a particular element can be considered only taking into account the universe to which it belongs, and vice versa (Bagni 2007). In the 20th century, Heidegger reconsidered the mentioned issue, so now the comprehension is not understood according to the model of textual interpretation; it is based on the relationship between human beings and the world.

When we consider a "historical" piece of knowledge (both an artistic masterpiece and an ancient mathematical idea) we can try to frame it into its historical period; nevertheless we can read it from our present, actual point of view. Concerning mathematical knowledge, for instance, is it really meaningful to look for "general rules" of mathematical evolution? Every culture influenced the development of its own mathematics, for instance, by using artefacts and semiotic representations (D'Amore 2005). Both historico-cultural approaches (see, for instance, Radford 2000, 2003) and anthropological approaches (D'Amore and Godino, 2006, 2007; Font et al. 2007; D'Amore et al. 2006) ask us to investigate how cultural contexts determined mathematical experiences (Grugnetti and Rogers 2000).

18.2 Artefacts and Tools

Mathematical practice, from the educational viewpoint too, is influenced by the use of artefacts and tools (it is possible to make reference to a theoretical framework discussed in Arzarello 2000, Bartolini Bussi and Boni 2003, Bartolini et al. 2005; it is based on basic works by Vygotskij 1978, 1997, Wartofsky 1979, and Engestroem 1990; as regards semiotic aspects, we shall consider some Peircean ideas).

According to Vygotskij, the function of semiotic mediation can be connected to tools. A first distinction is to be performed between technical and psychological tools (signs, or tools of semiotic mediation). It is worth highlighting that Wartofsky identifies technical gadgets as *primary artefacts*; *secondary artefacts* are used in order to transmit the acquired “skills or modes of action” (Wartofsky 1979: 200; Engestroem 1990). A mathematical theory is a *tertiary artefact* which organizes the secondary artefacts and hence the models constructed in order to represent the modes of action by which primary artefacts are used.

With regard to the processes by which a gadget becomes a real tool for the students, we must consider the distinction between artefact and tool (Rabardel 1995), i.e. the artefact associated with a personal or social *schema* of action (Artigue 1998, Radford 2005). For instance, if we make reference to a symbolic object as artefact, in order to be able to consider it as a tool, we need a constructive mediated activity on the part of the subject (Radford 2002, 2003) and it must be framed into a wider social and cultural context. So approaching the meaning of a piece of knowledge, with reference to both mathematics and art, must be considered within a cultural context, which involves the shared symbols of a community, its traditions, its artefacts, and its gadgets.

18.3 A Semiotic Reflection, Following Peirce

The theoretical framework previously described can be linked with some considerations about semiotic issues, based on a Peircean approach. We are going to consider some features of mathematical expressions leading us to make reference to mathematics as a human enterprise to be constructed, and not just to be contemplated.

According to Hoffmann (2007), cognitive systems are first of all semiotic systems since they are dependent on signs and representations as mediators. According to Peirce we cannot “think without signs” and signs consist of three inter-related parts: a sign, an object, and an interpretant (Peirce 1998: 478). The interpretant can be considered as the understanding that sign users have of the relation between sign and object, so according to Peirce the meaning of a sign is manifest in the interpretation generated in sign users (see, for instance, Atkin 2006, Liszka 1996, Savan 1988, 41). The sign determines an interpretant by using some features of the way the sign signifies its object to generate and shape our understanding (Bagni 2006a, 2006b).

Peirce thought that representations generate interpretants in three possible ways, with reference to the division of a sign into icon, index, and symbol (although Peirce’s ideas about this division changed at various steps in the development of his theory). If we interpret a sign as standing for its object because of some shared quality, then it is an icon. If our interpretation comes because of a causal connection, then the sign is an index. Finally, if we generate an interpretant in virtue of some conventional connection between sign and object, then the sign is a symbol. In a letter to Lady Welby (1904), Peirce wrote (1931–1958, § 8.328)

> Firstness is the mode of being of that which is such as it is, positively and without reference to anything else. Secondness is the mode of being of that which is such as it is, with respect to a second but regardless of any third. Thirdness is the mode of being of that which is such as it is, in bringing a second and third into relation to each other.

In 1903, Peirce wrote that "an *icon* is a representamen whose representative quality is a firstness of it as a first" (Peirce 1998, § 2.273; "representamen" is employed by the Author for the term "sign"); and «an *index* [...] is a representamen whose representative character consists in its being and individual second» (Peirce 1998, § 2.274). Finally, the concept of habit (Zeman 1986) induced Peirce to relate symbols with his category named thirdness (Atkin 2006).

If we want to frame systems of mathematical signs into the original Peircean theoretical account, we are induced to ask ourselves what is "the object" in play, and a similar position can be discussed with reference to art. Nevertheless this question can be misleading (D'Amore and Fandiño Pinilla 2001, Dörfler 2006): as a matter of fact, our reflection does not deal with the problem of the existence of "mathematical objects" (Radford, forthcoming). A Platonic view of mathematics cannot be stated uncritically, so we shall not force our readers to make reference to a particular object.

Nevertheless, it is important to underline that Peircean approach associates signs with cognition, and this can be taken into account both with reference to mathematics and with reference to Art. All objects (whatever we intend by that) "determine" their signs, so the cognitive nature of the considered object influences the nature of the sign in terms of what successful signification requires. As previously noticed, Peirce thought the nature of these constraints fell into three classes: qualitative, physical, and conventional; if the constraints of successful signification require that the sign reflects qualitative features of the object, then the sign is an icon; if they require that the sign utilizes some existential or physical connection between it and its object, then the sign is an index; if they require that the sign utilizes some convention or law that connects it with its object, then the sign is a symbol (Atkin 2006).

If, for instance, we make reference to our modern algebraic expression, we must take into account that, according to Peirce, the very formulas of algebra are icons, i.e. signs which represent by resemblance, which are mappings of that which they represent (Zeman 1986). Let us quote Peirce himself (1931–1958, § 2.279, *MS* 787):

> Particularly deserving of notice are icons in which the likeness is aided by conventional rules. Thus, an algebraic formula is an icon, rendered such by the rules of commutation, association, and distribution of the symbols; that it might as well, or better, be regarded as a compound conventional sign. It may seem at first glance that it is an arbitrary classification to call an algebraic expression an icon; that it might as well, or better, be regarded as a compound of conventional sign. But it is not so. For a great distinguishing property of the icon is that by direct observation of it other truths concerning its object can de discovered than those which suffice to determine its construction.

In his *On the Algebra of Logic: A Contribution to the Philosophy of Notation* (Peirce 1885), Peirce underlined the importance of iconicity and noticed (1931–1958, § 3.363) that "reasoning consists in the observation that where certain relations subsist certain others are found, and it accordingly requires the exhibition of the relations reasoned within an icon" and "deduction consists in constructing an icon or diagram the relations of whose parts shall present a complete analogy with those of the parts of the object of reasoning, of experimenting upon this image in the imagination, and of observing the result so as to discover unnoticed and hidden relations among the parts" (more generally, see, for instance, Stjernfelt 2000).

An inscription can be considered a diagram when it is manipulable according to some operation rules; according to Peirce, algebraic expressions and sequences of formulas are diagrams. L. Radford (forthcoming) writes

> Diagrammatic thinking is a central piece in Peirce's endeavour to rescue the epistemological import of perception. It is strongly linked to a heuristic process that exhibits, via intuition (i.e. in a sensual manner), some aspects of the object under scrutiny, thereby making these aspects available for observation, in order to help us discover new conceptual relations. The epistemological potential of diagrammatic thinking rests then in making apparent some relations that have thus far remained hidden from perception or beyond the realm of our attention. This is why, etymologically speaking, diagrammatic thinking relates to actions of objectification and a diagram, considered as a semiotic artifact, is a semiotic means of objectification.

A point to be considered is that pure icons, according to Peirce (1931–1958, 1.157), only appear in thinking, if ever. Pure icons, pure indexes, and pure symbols are not actual signs (Sonesson 1989, III, 1). In fact, every sign "contains" all the components of Peircean classification, although frequently one of them is predominant, so, for instance, we call "symbol" a sign whose components of iconicity and indicality are minor (Marietti 2001, 36). Different cultures can give very different roles to these components and expressions of a piece of knowledge can be remarkably different in different cultural contexts, so they need a particular interpretation, both with reference to artistic language and with reference to mathematical language.

18.4 Rorty and the "Conversation"

According to Richard Rorty, it is possible to perform a distinction between "normal" and "abnormal" discourse, so a distinction which generalizes Kuhn's distinction between "normal" and "revolutionary" science (Kuhn 1962): as a matter of fact, in Rorty's own words, "normal discourse is that which is conducted within an agreed-upon set of conventions about what counts as a relevant contribution, what counts as answering a question, what counts as having a good argument for that answer or a good criticism of it. Abnormal discourse is what happens when someone joins in the discourse who is ignorant of these conventions or who sets them aside. [...] Hermeneutics is the study of an abnormal discourse from the point of view of some normal discourse" (Rorty 1979, 640). "For epistemology, to be rational is to find a proper set of terms into which all the contributions should be translates if agreement is to become possible. For epistemology, conversation is implicit inquiry. For hermeneutics, inquiry is routine conversation" (Rorty 1979, 636). Of course, "the two [epistemology and hermeneutics] do not compete, but rather help each other out. Nothing is so valuable for the hermeneutical inquirer into an exotic culture as the discovery of an epistemology written within that culture" (Rorty 1979, 692).

So Rorty conceived knowledge as a matter of "conversation" (see, in particular, Rorty 1979) and, in particular, as a social practice, rather than as the ancient attempt to mirror nature "out there". His philosophical approach was explicitly against the supposed presence of general underlying structures: in fact, Rorty refused the traditional western conception of philosophy as a discipline trying to obtain absolute truths about the world, according to a misguided reliance on Platonic metaphysics (Bagni 2008). More precisely, according to Rorty (1989, 11)

> we need to make a distinction between the claim that the world is out there, and the claim that the truth is out there. To say that the world is out there, that it is not our creation, is to say, with common sense, that most things in space and time are the effects of causes which do not include human mental states. To say that truth is not out there is simply to say that where there are no sentences, there is no truth, that sentences are elements of human languages, and that human languages are human creations. Truth cannot be out there – cannot exist independently of the human mind – because sentences cannot so exist, or be out there. The world is out there, but descriptions of the world are not. Only descriptions of the world can be true or false. The world on its own – unaided by the describing activities of human beings – cannot.

As a consequence, "philosophy makes progress not by becoming more rigorous but by becoming more imaginative", once again in Rorty's own words (Rorty 1998), and this statement can be very interesting for mathematics educators. As a matter of fact, a Platonic approach cannot be stated uncritically, for instance, in educational practice: didactics of mathematics must take into account that a major point is related to the frequent attempt to model knowledge on perception and to treat "knowledge of" by grounding "knowledge that" (see Rorty 1979, 316).

Rorty strongly underlined the crucial importance of the community as a source of epistemic authority (Rorty 1979, 380) and stated, "We need to turn outward rather then inward, toward the social context of justification rather than to the relations between inner representations" (Rorty 1979, 424). His approach leads us to consider both mathematics and art as products of human activity, whose comprehension can be framed into a hermeneutic perspective.

18.5 Final Reflections

To conclude, we can say that both mathematics and art are not merely "dumb things" (Bachtin 2000, 377) to be contemplated: as previously noticed, for instance, some mathematical contents can be reconstructed practically by using the primary artefacts and with reference to the secondary artefacts that have characterized their historical development (Bussi et al. 2005), and this makes reference to an important hermeneutic activity. An artistic masterpiece, of course, needs an essential comprehension connected to its interpretation.

Therefore, in general, mathematics and art can be really and effectively framed into (and linked by) a hermeneutic approach: both of them are important human enterprises, so they are not to be considered as paths towards a form of Truth "out there" (Rorty 1989).

Acknowledgments The author would like to thank Bruno D'Amore (University of Bologna) and Willibald Dörfler (University of Klagenfurt, Austria) for their very valuable suggestions.

Bibliography

Artigue, M. (1998). L'évolution des problématiques en didactique de l'analyse. *Recherches en Didactique des Mathématiques*, 18(2), 231–262.

Arzarello, F. (2000). Inside and outside: spaces, times and language in proof production. *Proc. PME-24*, 1, 22–38.

Atkin, A. (2006). *Peirce's theory of signs*. http://plato.stanford.edu/entries/peirce-semiotics

Bachtin, M. (2000). *L'autore e l'eroe*. Torino: Einaudi (*Estetica slovesnogo tvorčestva*. Moskva: Izdatel'stvo Iskusstvo, 1979).

Bagni, G. T. (2006a). Some cognitive difficulties related to the representations of two major concepts of Set theory. *Educa. Stud. Math.*, 62(3), 259–280.

Bagni, G. T. (2006b). Linguaggio, storia e didattica della matematica. Bologna: Pitagora.

Bagni, G. T. (2007). *Rappresentare la matematica*. Roma: Aracne.

Bagni, G. T. (2008). Richard Rorty (1931–2007) and his legacy for mathematics educators. *Educ.Stud. Math.*, 67(1), 1–2.

Bartolini Bussi, M. G. and Boni, F. (2003). Instruments for semiotic mediation in primary school classrooms. *For the Learn. Math.*, 23(2), 12–19.

Bartolini Bussi, M. G., Mariotti, M. A., and Ferri, F. (2005). Semiotic mediation in primary school: Dürer's glass. In M. H. G. Hoffmann, J. Lenhard, and F. Seeger (Eds.), *Activity and sign. Grounding mathematics education. Festschrift for Michael Otte* (pp. 77–90). New York: Springer.

D'Amore, B. (2005). Secondary school students' mathematical argumentation and Indian logic (Nyaya). *For the Learn. Math.*, 25(2), 26–32.

D'Amore, B. and Fandiño Pinilla, M. I. (2001). Concepts et objets mathématiques. In Gagatsis, A. (Ed.), *Learning in mathematics and sciences and educational technology* I (pp. 111–130). Nicosia: Intercollege Press.

D'Amore, B. and Godino, D. J. (2006). Punti di vista antropologico ed ontosemiotico in Didattica della Matematica. *La matematica e la sua didattica*, 1, 9–38.

D'Amore, B. and Godino, J. D. (2007). El enfoque ontosemiótico como un desarrollo de la teoría antropológica en Didáctica de la Matemática. *Revista Latinoamericana de Investigación en Matemática Educativa*, 10(2), 191–218.

D'Amore, B., Radford, L. and Bagni, G. T. (2006). Ostacoli epistemologici e prospettive socioculturali. *L'insegnamento della matematica e delle scienze integrate* 29B, 1, 11–40.

Dörfler, W. (2006). Inscriptions as objects of mathematical activities. In J. Maasz, and W. Schloeglmann (Eds.), *New mathematics education research and practice* (pp. 97–111). Rotterdam-Taipei: Sense.

Engestroem, Y. (1990). When is a tool? Multiple meanings of artifacts in human activity. In *Learning, working and imagining: twelve studies in activity theory* (pp. 171–195). Helsinki: Orienta-Konsultit Oy.

Font, V., Godino, J. D., and D'Amore, B. (2007). An ontosemiotic approach to representations in mathematics education. *For the Learn. Math.*, 27(2), 9–15.

Grugnetti, L. and Rogers, L. (2000). Philosophical, multicultural and interdisciplinary issues. In J. Fauvel and J. van Maanen (Eds.), *History in mathematics education* (pp. 39–62). Dordrecht: Kluwer.

Hoffmann, M. H. G. (2007). Learning from people, things, and signs. *Stud. Philos. Educ.*, 26(3), 185–204.

Kuhn, T. S. (1962). *Die Struktur wissenschaftlicher Revolutionen*. Frankfurt a.M.: Suhrkamp.

Liszka, J. (1996). *A general introduction to the semeiotic of Charles S. Peirce*. Bloomington: Indiana University Press.

Marietti, S. (2001). Icona e diagramma. Il segno matematico in Charles Sanders Peirce. Milano: LED.

Peirce, C. S. (1885). On the algebra of logic: A contribution to the philosophy of notation. *Am.J. Math.*, 7(2), 180–196.

Peirce, C. S. (1931–1958). *Collected papers*, I–VIII. Cambridge: Harvard University Press.

Peirce, C. S. (1998). *The essential peirce*. Peirce Edition Project. Bloomington: Indiana University Press.

Rabardel, P. (1995). *Les hommes et les technologies: Approche cognitive des instruments contemporains*. Paris: Colin.

Radford, L. (2000). Signs and meanings in the students' emergent algebraic thinking: a semiotic analysis. *Educ. Stud. Math.*, 42 (3), 237–268.

Radford, L. (2002). The seen, the spoken and the written. A semiotic approach to the problem of objectification of mathematical knowledge. *For the Learn. Math.*, 22(2), 14–23.

Radford, L. (2003). Gestures, speech and the sprouting of signs. *Math. Think. Learn.*, 5(1), 37–70.

Radford, L. (2005). The semiotics of the schema. Kant, Piaget, and the calculator. In M. H. G. Hoffmann, J. Lenhard, and F. Seeger (Eds.), *Activity and sign. Grounding mathematics education* (pp. 137–152). New York: Springer.

Radford, L. (forthcoming). Rescuing Perception: Diagrams in Peirce's theory of cognitive activity. In de Moraes, L. and Queiroz, J. (Eds.), *C.S. Peirce's Diagrammatic Logic*. Catholic Univ. of Sao Paulo, Brazil.

Rorty, R. (1979). *Philosophy and the mirror of nature*. Princeton: Princeton University Press.

Rorty, R. (1989). *Contingency, irony, and solidarity*. Cambridge: Cambridge University Press.

Rorty, R. (1998). *Truth and progress. Philosophical papers III*. Cambridge: Cambridge University Press.

Savan, D. (1988). *An introduction to C.S. Peirce's full system of semeiotic*. Toronto: Toronto Semiotic Circle.

Sonesson, G. (1989). *Pictorial concepts. Inquiries into the semiotic heritage and its relevance for the analysis of the visual world*. Lund: Lund University Press.

Stjernfelt, F. (2000). *Diagrams as centerpiece of a peircean epistemology. Trans. Charles S. Peirce Soc.*, 36, 357–384.

Vygotsky, L. S. (1978). Interaction between learning and development. In M. Cole, V. John-Steiner, S. Scribner, and E. Souberman (Eds.), *Mind in society: The development of higher psychological processes* (pp. 79–91). Cambridge: Harvard University Press.

Vygotskij, L. S. (1997). *Collected works*. R. Rieber (Ed.). New York: Plenum.

Wartofsky, M. (1979). Perception, representation and the forms of action: towards an historical epistemology. In *Models. Representation and the scientific understanding* (pp. 188–209). Dordrecht: Reidel.

Zeman, J. J. (1986). Peirce's philosophy of logic. *Trans. Charles S. Peirce Soc.*, 22, 1–22.

Chapter 19
Point, Line and Surface, Following Hilbert and Kandinsky

Giorgio Bolondi

Abstract Kandinsky's attempt of developing a systematic theory of fundamental elements of painting has a key step in the publication of *Punkt und Linie zu Fläche*. This book is indirectely influenced by, and in some sense related to, the general beginning of the century debate on fundamental elements of geometry. We examine some existing *liaison* between Kandinsky and geometry, pointing out that his way of looking to the generation of lines has surprising "vector field" connotations.

Kandinsky spent the year 1923 in Weimar. After the break caused by the First World War and the time spent in Revolutionary Russia, once he came back to Germany he met again some old friends of his like Paul Klee and Alexej von Jawlensky. He took up again a project that he had carried on during summer 1914 in Goldach, on the Bodensee: the writing of the *organic development* of his previous book *Über das Geistige in der Kunst*, published in 1912. The aim of Kandinsky is the foundation of a systematic theory of fundamental elements of painting, and after the treatment of *colours* he considers *shapes* (the third component being, in his project, the *subjects*). Therefore he devoted 3 years to writing *Punkt und Linie zu Fläche- Beitrag zur Analyse der malerischen Elemente*, a book that since the dryness of his title presented itself as a "strict" treatment of the fundamental elements of the shape.

This book, even if published in 1926, was born in the atmosphere of the beginning of the twentieth century, when the osmosis of ideas, keywords and metaphors between distinct (as we see them today) cultural circles was intense.

To a mathematician, words like *point, line* and *surface*, in that context, immediately recall the systematization of the foundations of geometry. In 1899 David Hilbert had published the *Grundlagen der Geometrie*, a book which was at the same time the final step of a long work of organization and axiomatization of elementary geometry going back to Pasch, Pieri, Padoa, Peano and many others, and the starting point of a new epoch, the era of formalization. Arguing with Frege, Hilbert wrote

G. Bolondi (✉)
Department of Mathematics, University of Bologna, Bologna, Italy
e-mail: giorgio.bolondi@unibo.it

V. Capecchi (eds.), *Applications of Mathematics in Models, Artificial Neural Networks and Arts*, DOI 10.1007/978-90-481-8581-8_19,

that for a mathematician the words *Punkte, Geraden und Ebenen* had no other meaning than the (logical) one imposed by the axioms and could be replaced by *Tische, Stühle und Bierseidel*. The ideas of *rigour* and *objective theory* (using Kandinsky's words) are different in mathematics and in arts, and Kandinsky would not have ever written a book like *Tische und Stühle zur Bierseidel*.

The main point is another one, in fact. Hilbert' setting is a crucial step which changed (due to its intrinsic value and to the prestige of the author) our way of thinking and looking to the way of expounding mathematics. There is no doubt, on the other hand, that during those years the discussions about this topic were intense and open. We can read the review that Poincaré wrote about Hilbert's *Grundlagen* (he repeated some years later almost *verbatim* the same ideas in *Science et méthode*):

> Le poin de vue logique, parait seul l'interesser. Etant donnée une suite de propositions, il constate que toutes se déduisent logiquement de la première. Quel est le fondement de cette première proposition, quelle en est l'origine psychologique? Il ne s'en occupe pas... Son œuvre est donc incomplète, mais ce n'est pas une critiques que je lui adresse. Incomplet, il faut bien se résigner à l'etre. Il suffit qui il ait fait faire à la philosophie des mathématiques un progrès considérable comparable à ceux que l'on devait à Lobatchebsky, à Riemann, à Helmoltz et à Lie.
>
> *English Translation*
>
> Only the logical point of view seems to interest him. Given a sequence of proposition, he verifies that all of them are deduced from the first one. Which is the foundation of this first proposition, which is its psychological origin? He does not take care of it... Its work is therefore incomplete, but this is not a crtiticism that I direct to him. Everyone must resign himself to be incomplete. It is sufficient to say that his work is for the philosophy of mathematics a progress comparable to the progresses due to Lobatchevsky, Riemann, Helmoltz and Lie.

We underline, in this little *querelle* between two giants of mathematics, that Poincaré says *progress to the philosophy of mathematics* (and not *progress to mathematics*). An attempt to study the *psychological origin* of the postulates of geometry was performed by Federigo Enriques in 1901 with his essay *Sulla spiegazione psicologica dei postulati della geometria*, which was taken over by Gonseth and (later on) Jean Piaget; hence a completely different history.

Poincaré's worries were also of didactical nature:

> Or, pour comprendre une théorie, il ne suffit pas de constater que le chemin que l'on a suivi n'est pas coupé par un obstacle, il faut se rendre compte des raisons qui l'ont fait choisir. Pourra-t-on donc jamais dire qu'on comprend une théorie si on veut lui donner d'emblée sa forme définitive, celle que la logique impeccable lui impose, sans qu'il ne reste aucune trace des tâtonnements qui y ont conduit ? Non, on ne la comprendra pas réellement, on ne pourra même la retenir, ou on ne la retiendra qu'à force de l'apprendre par cœur.
>
> *English Translation*
>
> Well, in order to understand a theory, it is not sufficient to verify that the path that one has followed is not interrupted by an obstacle. It is necessary to realize the reasons of the choice of that path. Is it possible to say that a theory is understood if we want to give it from the

beginning its final form, the form imposed by an impeccable logic, without any trace of the attenpts which led to that organization? No, we will not really understand it, and we will not be able to remember it, or we will only remember it by learning by mind.

Anyway, even if today it is easy for us, fed during our studies with Hilbert'formalism and Bourbaki's didactics, to consider the *meaning* of entity like point, line and plane a non-problem, from the mathematical point of view, the situation was different when Kandinsky was writing his book. If we succeed in seeing things out the hilbertian paradigm, it is easier to understand Kandinsky's effort in the correct context.

First of all, the *point*. Mario Pieri, who was the author of a systematization of elementary geometry before Hilbert, at the epoch considered even more elegant and complete, used just two primitive notions: *point* and *rigid motion*, the *straight line* being defined as a derivate notion (he notes by the way that it would be possible to use, as primitive notions, *point* and *omography*, but that this would be a rash choice from the didactical point of view). In Pieri's opinion, one cannot do without using the notion of *point*, since it is the *substratum* of every geometrical construction. According to Kandinsky, the point is the absolute conciseness, which creates lines through drawing. It is worth noting that Hilbert himself, in 1894, wrote that geometry is based upon the simplest experiment we can do, that is to say upon *drawing*. Points and lines are abstractions coming principally from the experience of drawing, not from vision or tactile experience. These ideas were developed in another foundational book, *Les étapes de la philosophie mathématique*, by Léon Brunschvicg, written in 1912, exactly the year of *Über das Geistige in der Kunst*. Brunschvicg identifies in the practice of drawing the *origin of geometrical truth*.

Enriques, in the above-quoted *Sulla spiegazione psicologica dei postulati della geometria*, considers the point as the starting element of the representation of spatial concepts (his cognitive approach is point-based, not at all *gestaltic*) – without points it is impossible to give *meaning* to geometrical entities.

These topics were *à la mode*. Frans Brentano, who was a *maitre à penser* very influential, in a letter to Vailati discusses Euclid's axioms, implicitly trying to enucleate the essential being of concepts assumed as primitive, like point and straight line. Vailati answers that

> alla domanda: quali sono i veri assiomi della geometria? Non si può dare, secondo me, una risposta precisa senza rispondere prima a quest'altra domanda: qual è il miglior modo di ordinare le nostre conoscenze sulle proprietà dello spazio, in modo che esse compaiano come conseguenze d'un numero limitato di ipotesi fondamentali? E, dei vari modi in cui questo scopo può essere raggiunto, alcuni possono essere preferibili per certi caratteri altri per altri (per esempio, alcuni per la grande evidenza delle ipotesi, altri invece per il loro piccolo numero).

English Translation

> to the question: which are the ture axioms of geometry? It is impossible to give a precise answer, in my opinion, without answering in a preliminary way to this other question: which is the best way of ordering our knowledges on the properties of the space, in such a way that they will appear as consequences of a limited numebr of fundamental hypothesis? And,

among the many ways this puropose can be achieved, some of them may be preferable for some of thier fueatures other for other features (for instance, some for the great evidence of the hypothesis, other for ther limited number).

During those years, the *milieu* who was elaborating abstract art was interested, sometimes fascinated, by the "discovering" of mathematicians. The members of the Puteaux group (Kupka, Leger, Gleizes, Metzinger, Dillon, Duchamp, Le Fauçonnier – or at least someone among them) read Poincaré and some Einstein, and even tried to incorporate some hints of these works into their productions. For instance, the fourth dimension was a recurring theme – we must remember that it was a *geometrical* fourth dimension, the medley with space–time being a modern fact. At the same time, the attempts to represent pictorially the motion led to results that are related to Kandinsky's approach. For instance, we may look to Kupka, who paints with lines which are trajectories of object in motion – getting curves as a result of motion of points.

Surely, these artistic circles read at the same time Poincaré and Madame Blavatsky, but in some sense even this is typical of the period. Kandinsky himself, following Peter Ouspensky, thought to the spiritual world as a multidimensional structure – there were people trying to explain supernatural or paranormal facts with the new discoverings in geometry. Someone showed how Jesus entered into the refectory where all doors were closed simply by passing through the fourth dimension.

Vladimir Lenin (!) in *Materialism and Empiriocriticism* attacked Poincaré since his theories about multidimensional spaces gave arguments to idealists and spiritualists.

Anyway, even if the theoretical explanations of artists like Duchamp, nowadays, may appear *naives* (for instance, when he tries to explain how every tridimensional object in a painting is the projection of a fourth-dimensional one) the artistic result, as in the case of *La mariée mise à nu par ses célibataires, même*, is extraordinary.

Kandinsky examines, in his book, the problem of motion of a point in the plane and his analysis is essentially *local*. A point is subjected to two *tensions*, the first horizontal and the second vertical – the composition of these two forces is the resulting direction of the motion. At every moment this composition changes, following the changement of intensity of the basic forces. This is an idea very "vectorial" of the generation of curves, recalling us vector fields and integral curves.

Lines are *not*, for Kandinsky, simple unions of single points. Their *continuous* nature is strong and inalienable. At a given moment, he arrives to speak about the *mark of the moving point*. This is exactly the psychological origin of curves, in Enriques' approach, who will go on by considering surfaces as generated by systems of curves. On the contrary, for the physicist Poincaré the immediate reality is tridimensional, and we get surfaces and points via hyperplane sections. Note, however, that Kandinsky too said that a characteristic feature of lines is of generating surfaces.

These tensions on points are generated by an *inner perception*. It must be remarked here that this theory of shapes developed by Kandinski is the theoretical instrument which allows him to leave the figurative art, without losing the prophetic value which is a structural constitutive element of art in general. How to maintain the prophetical function of arts, if we abandon the representation of objects? Kandinsky's solution is to pass to the representation of *inner perceptions*, which results in tensions over the points. Kandinsky spoke, in relation with points and lines, of a *soul experience*. Hence, a line is generated by a point coming out of itself in a non-isotropic plane, where two privileged directions (horizontal = warm, vertical = cold) have different meanings. Hence, Kandinsky seeked for an inner generation of fundamental elements of drawing and Enriques for a psychological founding of the same elements.

In more modern words, Kandinsky says that in abstract thinking, in our "ideas" (whatever is the meaning of this expression), a point is ideally small, ideally round, like an infinitely small circle and that it materializes when we *draw* it: he is dealing with what is today called the dialectic between the figural aspects and the conceptual ones. The different shapes of points reproduced in Kandinsky's book are called *relative colouring variations of the fundamental character, which is unalterable*.

Some words about a last point. Kandinsky's ideas are surprisingly explanatory when we compare them with what our pupils do and say in our classrooms, when dealing with the first constructions of geometry. For instance, there is the horizontal direction and the vertical one, of course; but often there is *the* diagonal direction that one forming a 45° angle with the horizontal and the vertical. The other lines are just *deviations* more or less important from *the* diagonal. Why children differentiate horizontal and vertical? This is quite natural; but why this intuitive non-isotropy is still influencing them when they deal with euclidean geometry or formal reasoning? Why do they speak about "standing up rectangles" or they are not able to recognize trapezoids in non-canonical positions? These are well-known problems in didactics of mathematics.

There are three basic angles, for Kandinsky: right, acute (= 45°!) and obtuse (= 135°!), the other angles simply being just variations of these, bearing different personalities. The frame of a painting is a very strong framing, which is continuously evocated in the composition of the work and his analysis helps us to understand why it is so difficult, for many pupils, to do geometry without being influenced by the positions of the objects or of the sheet.

Kandinsky recalls us, with the power of his art, that the geometrical elements, when are graphically represented, are full of meanings and understatements, and psychologically non-neutral.

Chapter 20
Figurative Arts and Mathematics: Pipes, Horses, Triangles and Meanings

A Contribution to a Problematic Theory of Conceptual Meaning, from Frege and Magritte up to the Present Time

Bruno D'Amore

Abstract In this chapter we describe a proposal for a problematic interpretation of the concept of signification, taken from conceptual signification theory, not only in the field of mathematics but also presenting examples of analogous behaviour from another field of study, that of figurative art. The aim is to show how a totally satisfactory signification theory has still not been constructed, while other fields of study continue to rediscover the basic stages of the epistemological domain.

20.1 Meaning and Its Representation: The Case of Mathematics

When we speak of "theory of meaning" thought runs fast to psychology, semiotics, linguistic or mathematics. But we must not think that this kind of problems regards only these fields of research and analysis. Every self-respecting discipline that wants to put into the field a reflection about objects of its knowing and of its specific representing is sooner or later obliged to go deeply into this matter. This is even more true in mathematics (Duval 1993, D'Amore 2000, 2001a, b, c, 2003a), since it is obliged to use "representations of meaning" (for the moment an expression we use in a naïve sense).

B. D'Amore (✉)
NRD Department of Mathematics, University of Bologna, Bologna, Italy; ASP High Pedagogical School, Locarno, Switzerland; MESCUD Districtal University "Fr. José de Caldas", Bogotá, Colombia
e-mail: damore@dm.unibo.it

This chapter was published in Italian: (2005) on *L'insegnamento della matematica e delle scienze integrate*. [Paderno del Grappa, Italia]. 28B, 5, 415–433; in Spanish: D'Amore B. (2005). Pipas, caballos, triánguloy significados. Contribución a una teoría problemática del significado conceptual, de Frege y Magritte, hasta nuestros días. *Números*. [Tenerife, Spagna], 61, 3–18.

V. Capecchi (eds.), *Applications of Mathematics in Models, Artificial Neural Networks and Arts*, DOI 10.1007/978-90-481-8581-8_20,

Indeed in mathematics, because evoked "objects" do not have a real nature (in a naïve realism with a concrete character),[1,2] we can do nothing else but turn to their *representations* within an appropriate semiotics, so that the mathematician, while he mentions and speaks about objects that belong to the domain of mathematics, in fact, he chooses, handles and transforms their representations within semiotic registers.[3, 4]

20.2 The Case of Figurative Art: Pipes and Horses

A case analogous to mathematics, unexpected by most of the people, is definitely constituted by figurative art. Even if we do not complicate this issue and we assume, in a decidedly uncritical and historically outdated manner, that art studies the interpretation of objects' and natural phenomena's problematic figural representations, it is rather evident that every representation in the figural world alludes to an object or a phenomenon but it is distinct from them. Every artistic product in end is itself an object or a phenomenon of nature.

---

[1]Here "object" is intended as "real object" or "thing", in the meaning well expressed by Aristotle in *metaphysics* when he declares that the "thing", as part of reality, is that which presents the following characteristics: (1) three dimensionality, (2) multiple sensory accessibility (that is more senses at a time) independent from semiotic representations and (3) possibility of material separation and from other parts, i.e. from other "things". This acceptation is enclosed in the Greek word πράγμα that expresses it. But we must wait for Descartes for a distinction between "corporal things" and "things that think" (*Méd*., II), until Locke to have the term "substances" (*An Essay Concerning Human Understanding*, 1690, II, 12, 6), taken up and made his own by Berkeley with the acceptation of "real things" to distinguish them from the ones "excited by imagination" that owe the name *ideas* "or images of Things that they copy or represent" (*Principles*, I, 33).

[2]With "naïve realism" (*Naiven Realismus*) I intend that so defined by G. Schuppe (*Grundriss der Erkenntnistheorie und Logik*, 1910), i.e. that in which one recognizes the independence of the known object from the act (psychic) with which it is known. But it draws its origin from a famous article of G.E. Moore of 1903 (published on *Mind*, entitled: *The Refutation of Idealism*), inspired by W. Hamilton's positions (*Natural Realism*) who ascribes this way of thinking to Scottish philosophy. But I believe that all these positions are born from Kant's *empiric realism*.

[3]Here I am explicitly referring to the three "fundamental operations of semiotics" (Duval 1993, D'Amore 2003):

4

- choice of the distinctive features of the object that we want to represent;
- *treatment* transformation, that allows to transform a semiotic representation into another but in the same register;
- *conversion* transformation, that allows to transform a semiotic representation into another but in a different register.

So, the reflections of the Belgian surrealist painter René Magritte (1898–1967) on the nature of art's language and on the sense of the relationship between meaning and representation appeared immediately necessary and revealing.

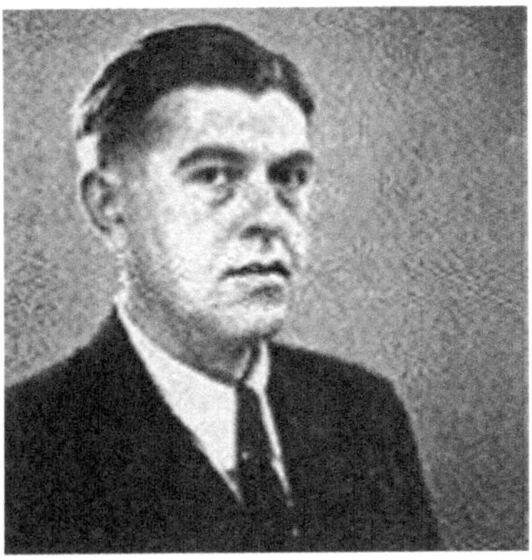

His reflections often constituted on their part true artistic works, like the renowned *Ceci n'est pas une pipe* that Magritte made in several versions between 1929 and 1946.

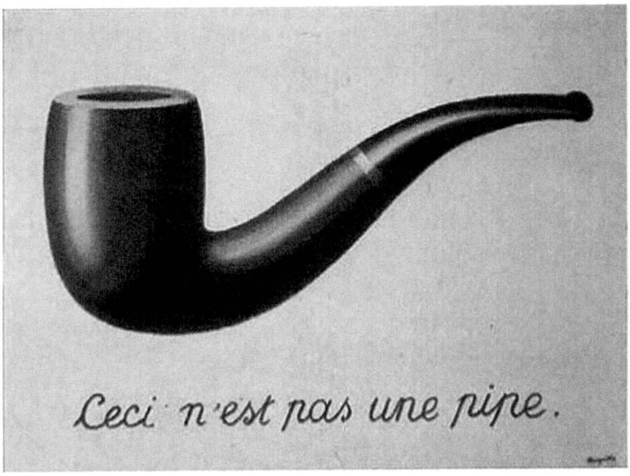

Beyond the embarrassment it provoked when it was exhibited, seen with today's critical and sharp eyes, the sense of this work, intentionally popular, is completely clear: what the observer indeed sees is *not* a pipe but one of its representations which alludes to a pipe; in other words what we see is a representation, an allusion, an evocation, not the object itself.

Sometimes, instead, Magritte loves to work out real theoretical studies, as the same famous *Les mots et les images* (1929) that although, as I said, is a theoretical study, it was also exhibited as a work.

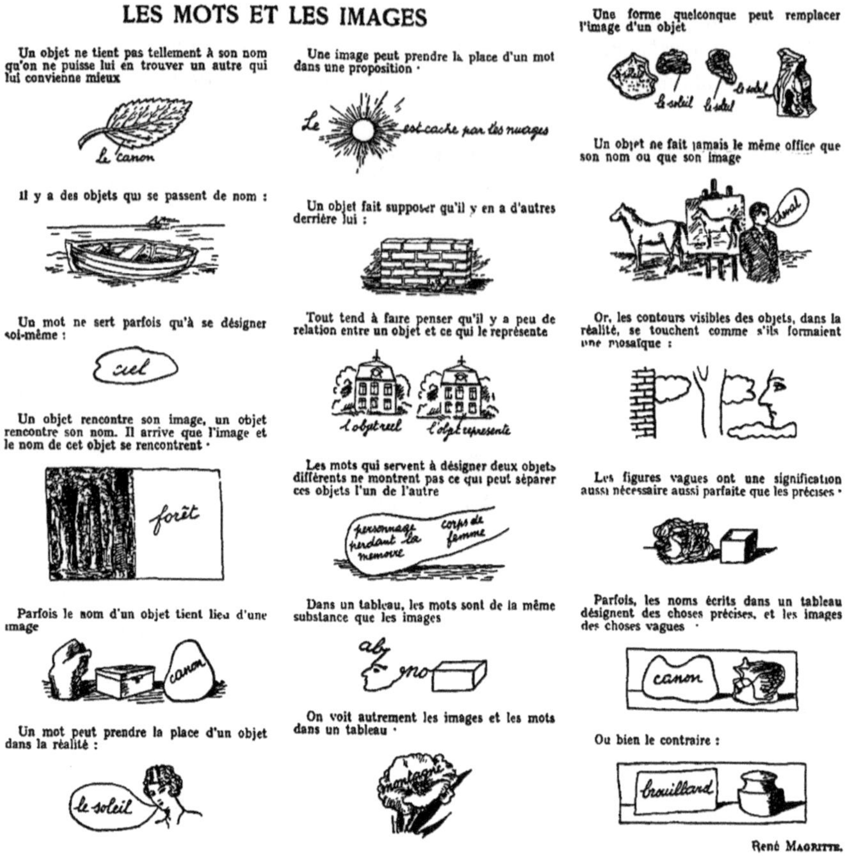

LES MOTS ET LES IMAGES

Un objet ne tient pas tellement à son nom qu'on ne puisse lui en trouver un autre qui lui convienne mieux

le canon

Il y a des objets qui se passent de nom :

Un mot ne sert parfois qu'à se désigner soi-même :

ciel

Un objet rencontre son image, un objet rencontre son nom. Il arrive que l'image et le nom de cet objet se rencontrent :

forêt

Parfois le nom d'un objet tient lieu d'une image

canon

Un mot peut prendre la place d'un objet dans la réalité :

le soleil

Une image peut prendre la place d'un mot dans une proposition :

Le … est caché par les nuages

Un objet fait supposer qu'il y en a d'autres derrière lui :

Tout tend à faire penser qu'il y a peu de relation entre un objet et ce qui le représente

l'objet réel l'objet représenté

Les mots qui servent à désigner deux objets différents ne montrent pas ce qui peut séparer ces objets l'un de l'autre

personnage perdant la mémoire corps de femme

Dans un tableau, les mots sont de la même substance que les images

On voit autrement les images et les mots dans un tableau :

montagne

Une forme quelconque peut remplacer l'image d'un objet

le soleil le soleil le soleil

Un objet ne fait jamais le même office que son nom ou que son image

cheval

Or, les contours visibles des objets, dans la réalité, se touchent comme s'ils formaient une mosaïque :

Les figures vagues ont une signification aussi nécessaire aussi parfaite que les précises :

Parfois, les noms écrits dans un tableau désignent des choses précises, et les images des choses vagues :

canon

Ou bien le contraire :

brouillard

René Magritte.

Maybe, in this study, the most famous and discussed detail is that relative to the horse's image which is completely evident.

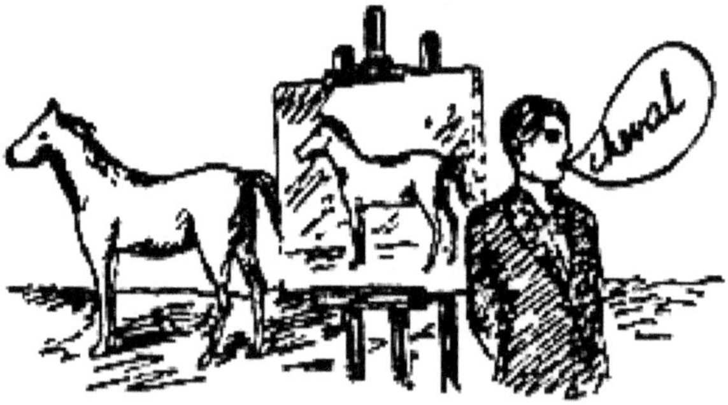

You can see a horse, a pictorial representation of the horse, a verbal enunciation of the horse (in the "oral language" semiotic register). But you must not forget that the horse that appears on the left of this figure is, on his turn, a drawing.

20.3 Gottlob Frege and Meaning in Mathematics

This analysis of the pictorial language cannot recall the work of the German mathematical logician Gottlob Frege (1848–1925).

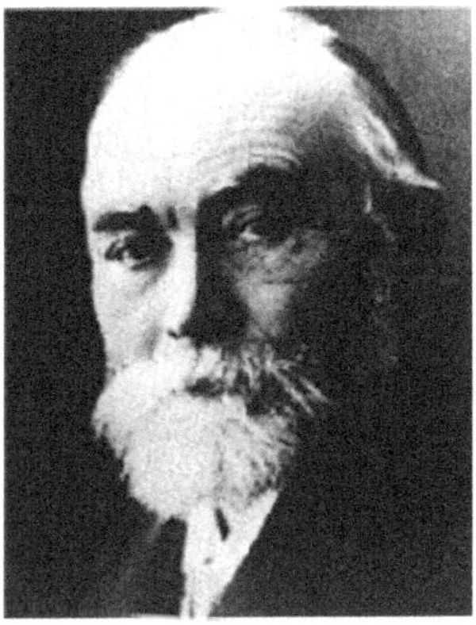

Along with other everlasting works, Frege wrote an article regarding the nature and the sense of mathematics and its language: *Über Sinn und Bedeutung* (*On sense and denotation*, published in 1891); it was a real bombshell in the world of mathematical reflection and contributed to opening the way to that period of critical thought named *Foundational Crisis* that lead to the present way of conceiving mathematics (D'Amore and Matteuzzi 1975). In that article, that was at that time an occasion for a hoary controversy with G. Peano (1858–1932) (D'Amore and Matteuzzi 1975), Frege sharply proposed a distinction between "concept" and "object". According to Frege, a concept is an expression (it will be so also for Wittgenstein); however, such an expression is not able to denote in a specific way (that which it would/ should denote), if it only uses its functional characteristics, i.e. those typical of expressions; actually, the expression as such does not succeed in denoting specifically concepts but it needs something else. Instead, the object works as an argument to which several connotations give sense. For example, a number is identified with the object denoted by a concept, i.e. with the extension of that concept.[5]

In the other renowned work, *Die Grundlagen der Arithmetik – Eine logisch-matematische Untersuchung über den Begriff der Zahl*, published in Wroclaw in 1884, at p. 59 Frege affirms "The attribution of a number always contains a statement about a concept. The thing is particularly clear for the number 0. When we say 'The planet Venus has 0 satellites', there really isn't any satellite or aggregate of

[5]The distinction and then the conceptual organization that regards the dialectics between "intensional" and "extensional" was launched in a modern sense by G.W. Leibniz (1646–1716); Leibniz always preferred the first picture that, however, did not have success in mathematics (D'Amore and Matteuzzi 1975). You can also see D'Amore (2001c).

satellites on which we can state something. Instead on the concept 'Venus's satellite' the aforementioned statement ascribes a property (i.e. that of not including any object under its influence)".[6]

This position, that I do not hesitate to count among the today so-called realistic ones, had a great success until the 1970s of the twentieth century, but at the present time is in crisis in favour of "pragmatists positions" (D'Amore 2001a, c, D'Amore and Fandiño Pinilla 2001).

20.4 Horses and Meanings Before and After Frege

Since 1883, that is *before* Frege, the American mathematician, physicist and philosopher Charles Sanders Peirce (1839–1914) already started using triangular schemes to study the relationships between objects and their representations, using the term interpretant–representamen–object; it seems interesting to find a description of Magritte's reflection according to Peirce's scheme:

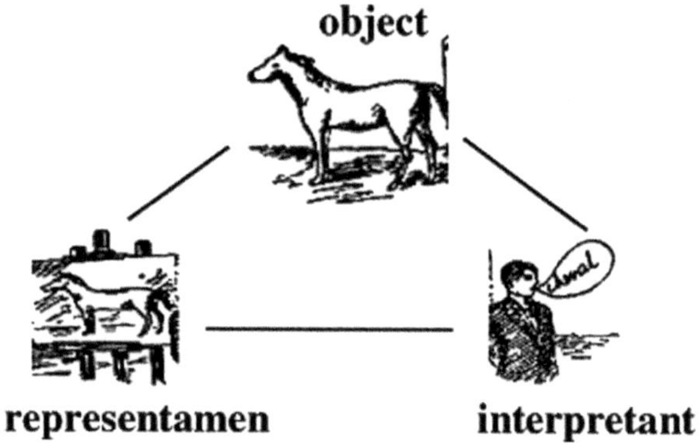

but who is willing to do so can create its own ternary interpretation of Magritte's "horse", using the triangle of

- Gottlob Frege: Sinn (sense)–Zeichen (symbol)–Bedeutung (denotation), published in 1892, as we already said,

or the more recent one of

- C.K. Ogden, I.A. Richards: reference–symbol–referent (published in 1923).

[6]The specific history about the meaning of number according to mathematicians and philosophers is of great interest but I avoid it here because it is not specific of this chapter; it involves, just to quote some of the personalities who had a leading role, H. Poincaré (1854–1912), Giuseppe Peano (1858–1932), Richard Dedekind (1831–1916) and Bertrand Russell (1872–1970). In a certain sense, the dispute regarding sense and meaning of the concept of number has never appeased.

20.5 Art and Meaning After Magritte

Dwelling again upon the world of figurative arts, I acknowledge the thesis supported by the outstanding art critic Filiberto Menna (1975) who maintains that the "analytical line of modern art" had in Magritte's studies and reflections a great artificer "(...) Magritte proposes a coming a part between image and word, between visual definition (the image of the pipe) and verbal definition (the legend "Ceci n'est pas une pipe"), disavowing the traditional assertive role traditionally ascribed to the painting because of the (implicit or explicit) presence of a caption (...). As regards art, and paintings in particular, he says that it is not possible to predicate about true or false clauses and, to prove this assumption, he faces the issue from gnoseological foundations established by the laws of the theory of identity (...)" (Menna 1975, 58–59).

The idea of Magritte had a long continuation (not yet extinguished) among artists the world over, especially among those artists who in the 1960–1980s have been artificers of the so-called conceptual scientific[7] current, among whom I recall here only the American Joseph Kosuth, quoting two of his most famous works.

Neon electrical light English glass letters white eight (1965)

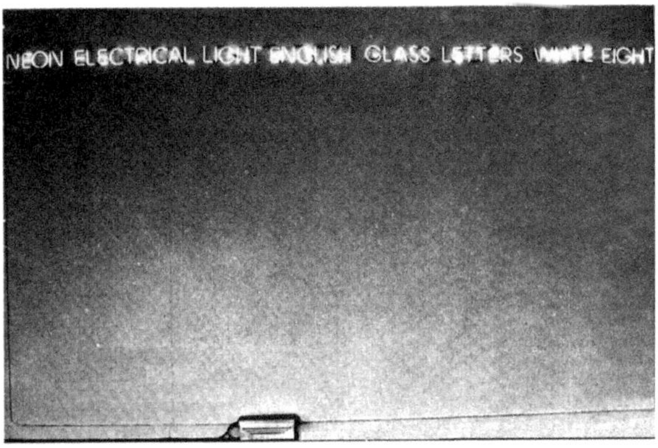

"The content of this work is that which is described in the title", in the *exact* sense of this sentence. Therefore it is an autonimus reference whose "sense" is the reference to itself, as it happens to the majority of mathematical signs.

This work consists of an object (the chair), the photograph of that chair and the definition of "chair" taken from a dictionary; it cannot recall, at the same time, a synthesis of Magritte's and Frege's works. Is it (a representation of) "one" or "three" chairs?

---

[7]In the 1970s and in the 1980s I have dedicated great attention to this artistic current that draws much inspiration from the world of science in general and of mathematics in particular, promoting several exhibition initiatives and carrying out many critical analyses on both the artistic movement and the single artists.

One and three chairs (1965)

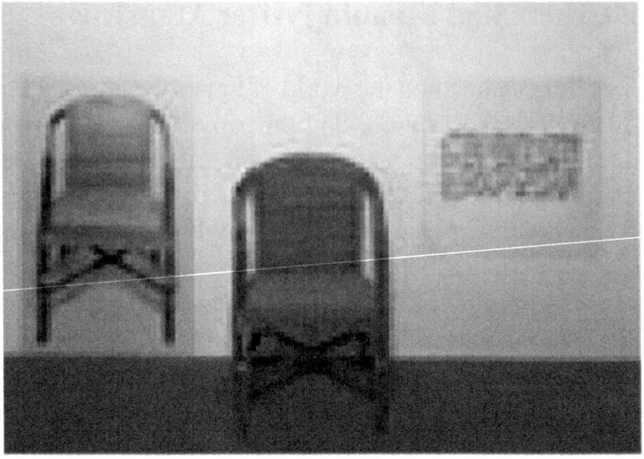

To have further critical references on figurative art of the time you can see the catalogue of a famous international art exhibition on this theme (D'Amore and Menna 1974), the proceedings of a study meeting that gathered together mathematicians and art critics (D'Amore and Speranza 1977) and the history of that period (1970–1990) written by Giorgio Di Genova (1993), one of the most outstanding scholars in art history.

20.6 Ternary Schemes of Meaning

Let us turn back to interpretations of conceptual meaning.

The "triangle" schemes would like to grasp "the semiotic study of content" (Eco 1975, 89), but they fail as soon as we try to define in a univocal way (for all languages and codes) what we should intend for the "signified" of a "signifier" (which is of great relevance if we want to understand mathematics or art).

The most naïve and immediate position is that the signified of a signifier is the object itself, to which the signifier refers. This position leads to a fallacy ("extensional fallacy") (Eco 1975, 93ff) that, if it is true that it puts into crisis every code theory having the need of objectual extensions regarding reality, it does not disturb mathematics whose objects can be defined in an extensive form but without the need of referring to the empiric objective reality (I think that the same identical discourse, changing references that have to be changed, fits figurative art).

It is not by chance that the mathematical logician Frege can allow himself to consider *Bedeutung* in a strictly extensional sense since he thought only about mathematics and not natural language.[8]

[8]Interesting didactical considerations are obtained applying Frege's ideas to the semantic of algebra; you can see a presentation in Arzarello et al. (1994), p. 36 ff.

One of the most recent and remarkable three-term schematization is certainly that of Gérard Vergnaud (1990),[9] at least in the field of didactics and of epistemological reflections, above all as regards mathematics. According to this renowned French author, [10] the decisive point of conceptualization of reality (and in mathematics education) is the passage from *concepts-as-instruments* to *concepts-as-objects*, and an essential linguistic operation in this transformation is nominalization.

It is therefore fundamental to give a pertinent and effective definition of a *concept*; according to Vergnaud:

a concept C is a tern of sets $C = (\mathbf{S}, \mathbf{I}, S)$, such that

- **S** is the set of situations that give sense to the concept (the *referent*) **I** is the set of invariants (defined and exemplified in other of his works) on which the operativity of the schemes is based (idem) (the *signified*)
- S is the set of linguistic and non-linguistic forms that allow to symbolically represent the concept, its procedures, the situations and treatment procedures (the *significant*)

According to Vergnaud, studying how a concept develops and works means considering, from time to time, these three planes separately and in mutual relationship.

20.7 Binary Schemes of Meaning

In more recent times, Raymond Duval (1993) has replaced the ternary scheme with a binary scheme, that which is expressed through the pair "signified–object" or the pair "sign–object"; the fact is that in Duval the term "signified" groups the different signifiers of the same object; therefore the terms "signified" and "sign" are in a certain sense interchangeable. It is obvious that if we stress the pair (*sign*, *object*), all the triadic representations (of C. S. Peirce, of G. Frege, of C. K. Ogden and I. A. Richards, of G. Vergnaud, etc.) fall in defect.

Therefore conceptualization passes through the sign that expresses its same object.

The case of mathematics is in this field peculiar at least for three reasons:

- Every mathematical concept, as we have already said, refers to "non-objects"; therefore conceptualization is not and it cannot be based on meanings that lie on concrete reality; in other words in mathematics ostensive references are impossible

[9] A broad discussion of Vergnaud's theses is in D'Amore (1999).

[10] See my entry on G. Vergnaud in the *Enciclopedia Pedagogica* (D'Amore 2002).

- Every mathematical concept is obliged to make use of representations since there are not any "objects" to exhibit in their place or for their evocation[11]; therefore conceptualization must necessarily pass through representative registers that, for several reasons, especially if they have a linguistic character, cannot be univocal.
- In mathematics we more often speak of "mathematical objects" rather than "mathematical concepts" because in mathematics we preferably study objects rather than concepts; "the notion of object is a notion that we cannot avoid using when we question knowledge's nature, conditions of validity and value" (Duval 1998).

It is absolutely necessary to underline that the term "concept" in Duval does not lead to the same circumstances and use of Piaget, Kant, Vergnaud, Vygotsky, Chevallard, etc.

In the path traced by Duval the notion of concept, preliminary and anyway priority in almost all the Authors, becomes secondary while that which assumes a character of priority is the pair (*sign, object*).

Duval (1996) often quotes a passage of Vygotsky who basically declares that there is not a concept without a sign:

> All higher psychological functions have the common higher characteristic of being mediated processes, i.e. to include in their structure, as central and essential part of the process as a whole, the use of sign as a fundamental means of orientation and domain of psychological processes... The core [of the concepts' formation process] is the functional use of signs, or words, as a means that allows the adolescent to submit to his power his own psychological operations, to dominate the course of his own psychological processes... (Vygotsky 1962; in the French edition, 1985, 150, 151, 157).

[As regards this quotation of Vygotsky, or better profiting by it, it is appropriate to make a quick remark on the word "sign" suggested by personal conversations and exchanges of ideas with Raymond Duval because he declares that, among some scholars in didactics, we notice a reduction of *sign* to *conventional symbols* that connote objects directly and separately. This is restrictive.]

Referring to De Saussure (1915) (that Vygotsky knew well because of his formation as a linguist) there is not a sign outside a "system of signs". For example, words do not have a meaning but within the system of the language (the well-known translating problems come from here). When in Duval (and therefore here) we speak of "semiotic representation register" we refer to a system of signs that allow to fulfil the functions of communication, treatment and objectification, and instead we do not refer to conventional notations that do not form a system. For example, the binary numeration system or the decimal one forms a system but it is not so for the letters or symbols that we use to indicate algebraic operations.

Maybe it would be more appropriate to translate Vygotsky replacing the word "sign" with the expression "system of signs".

---

[11] I recall here the definition of "thing" given a few pages before quoting Aristotle.

Notice also that from this point of view and in opposition to the widespread opinion, a semiotic system is not an instrument: It is constitutive of the same functioning of thought and knowledge. Only a code that is used to re-encode an already-expressed message can be an instrument.

20.8 The Complex and Problematic Nature of Conceptual Meaning and of Its Representations

Like Magritte used to do, we can ironically escape from the issue of conceptual meaning or try to capture the essence of the relationship between conceptual meaning and its representations like Frege and other scholars tried to do, searching for schemes suitable to grasp that essence in general, independently from codes; or assimilate the conceptual meaning with the set of representative signs that evoke the represented but in specific semiotics; etc.

I believe that the result does not change; what it stands out with strength is that the nature of conceptual meaning is *complex* and *problematic*.

Complex means that it is not definable in a univocal manner, since it involves different human activities and in each of them it assumes different specific identities, depending on the context; it can also happen that there actually are interpretative analogies (and in this study I tried to put in relation the field of mathematics and of figurative art), but it is not possible to highlight more than analogies. A general univocal theory of conceptual meaning does not exist.

Problematic means that the nature of conceptual meaning cannot undergo to reductionisms that refer to pre-existent models (Speranza 1997). Every attempt to categorize opens new interpretations and therefore the need for new, deeper and deeper, models. In other words the answers to questions on the nature of conceptual meaning are never definite, and if they are not self-referent, they open the way to new questions.

We have seen that conceptual meaning representations cannot even be ostensive, at least as regards the two creative human activities I have reflected on, mathematics and figurative art. At most the representation can turn to signs with different semiotic natures and expect coincidence with them (there are Duval's famous examples in mathematics and of several artists in the field of figurative art like Kosuth and others that for the sake of brevity I did not recall here). Therefore, also the representation of conceptual meaning has complex problematic characteristics.

Taking as a starting point the distinction that we make in epistemology of mathematics between realistic and pragmatist positions (D'Amore and Fandiño Pinilla 2001, D'Amore 2001a, 2003b), we should be ready to recognize a double analogy between absolutism and realism and between problematicism and pragmatism: according to this analogy, the complex and problematic nature of the conceptual meaning theory becomes relative to the context; this makes it difficult to "capture" with classical systems that are successful in realistic positions: logic, for example, or an a priori semantic.

We must forcely turn to "human practices" (Godino and Batanero 1994) recognizing that, as Luis Radford underlines, knowledge is indissolubly linked with activities which individuals are engaged in (Radford 1997, 2003a, 2003b) and this must be considered in close relationship with the cultural institutions of the social context time by time considered (Crombie 1995, p. 232).

Radford underlines the specificity of the environments which, in the historical development, the scientific research evolved in: "In fact, a simple inspection of different cultures through the history shows that each culture had its own scientific interests. Moreover, each culture had its own ways of defining and delimiting the form and the content of the objects of their inquiry" (Radford 1997, p. 30); I believe that we can say exactly the same for figurative art without even forcing someone's hand. This clearly illustrates the sense I wanted to give to the adjectives *complex* and *problematic* that I used in this text. The results of mathematics and figurative art are human artefact products, indissoluble from the cultural society that produced them and strictly determined by the human practice through which they have been carried out.

So, rather than a theory of meaning of something general that includes these products, there is instead the specific meaning of that something in that given context in which they have emerged. Complexity and problematic nature are reduced to a local fact relative and specific to that product of human creativity in that given also specific context.

Acknowledgments The authors wish to thank George Santi for the translation.

Bibliography

Arzarello, F., Bazzini, L., and Chiappini, G. (1994). L'algebra come strumento di pensiero. Analisi teorica e considerazioni didattiche. *Quaderno 6, Progetto Strategico del CNR "Innovazioni didattiche per la matematica"*. Pavia. [Account of the IX national seminar of research in Mathematics education. Pisa. November 5–7, 1992].

Crombie, A. C. (1995). Commitments and Styles of European Scientific Thinking. *Hist. Sci.* 33, 225–238.

D'Amore, V. (1999). *Elementi di didattica della matematica*. Bologna: Pitagora.

D'Amore, B. (2000). "Concetti" e "oggetti" in Matematica. *Rivista di Matematica dell'Università di Parma*. 3(6), 143–151.

D'Amore, B. (2001a). Un contributo al dibattito su concetti e oggetti matematici: la posizione "ingenua" in una teoria "realista" vs il modello "antropologico" in una teoria "pragmatica". *La matematica e la sua didattica*, 1, 4–30.

D'Amore, B. (2001b). Concettualizzazione, registri di rappresentazioni semiotiche e noetica. *La matematica e la sua didattica*, 2, 150–173.

D'Amore, B. (2001c). *Scritti di Epistemologia Matematica 1980–2001*. Bologna: Pitagora.

D'Amore, B. (2002). Gérard Vergnaud. Entry in *Enciclopedia Pedagogica* (pp. 1508–1509). Appendix A–Z. .Brescia: La Scuola Ed.

D'Amore, B. (2003a). La complexité de la noétique en mathématiques ou les raisons de la dévolution manquée. *For the Learn. Math.*, 23(1), 47–51.

D'Amore, B. (2003b). *Le basi filosofiche, pedagogiche, epistemologiche e concettuali della Didattica della Matematica*. Bologna: Pitagora.

D'Amore, B., and Fandiño Pinilla, M. I. (2001). Concepts et objects mathématiques. In: Gagatsis A. (Ed.), *Learning in mathematics and science and educational technology*. Nicosia (Cyprus): Intercollege Press Ed. [Proceedings of the Third intensive programme socrates-erasmus, Nicosia, University of Cyprus, June 22–July 6, 2001. 111–130].

D'Amore, B., and Matteuzzi, M. (1975). *Dal numero alla struttura*. Bologna: Zanichelli.

D'Amore, B., and Menna, F. (1974). *De Mathematica*. Roma: L'Obelisco. [Book catalogue of an international exhibition]

D'Amore, B., Speranza, F., et al. (1977). *Alcuni aspetti della critica analitica. Rapporti tra critica analitica e ricerca nelle arti visive*. Bologna: Modern Art Gallery. [Proceedings of a conference, birth certificate of the school of exact art that stemmed into an infinite quantity of exhibitions].

De Saussure, F. (1915). *Cours de linguistique générale*. Paris et Lausanne: Payot. [5th edn., 1960]. [Italian translation: 1968, Bari: Laterza].

Di Genova, G. (1993). *Storia dell'arte italiana del 900*. Bologna: Bora.

Duval, R. (1993). Registres de représentations sémiotiques et fonctionnement cognitif de la pensée. *Annales de Didactique et de Science Cognitives, ULP, IREM Strasbourg*. 5, 37–65.

Duval, R. (1996). Il punto decisivo nell'apprendimento della matematica. La conversione e l'articolazione delle rappresentazioni. In B. D'Amore (Ed.), *Convegno del decennale*. 11–26. Bologna: Pitagora.

Duval, R. (1998). Signe et objet (I). Trois grandes étapes dans la problématique des rapports entre répresentations et objet. *Annales de Didactique et de Sciences Cognitives*, 6, 139–163.

Eco, U. (1975). *Trattato di semiotica generale*. Milano: Bompiani.

Godino, J. D., and Batanero, C. (1994). Significado institucional y personal de los objetos matemáticos. *Recherches en didactiques des mathématiques*. 14(3), 325–355.

Menna, F. (1975). *La linea analitica dell'arte moderna*. Milano: Einaudi.

Radford, L. (1997). On psychology, historical epistemology and the teaching of mathematics: Towards a socio-cultural history of mathematics. *For the Learn. Math.*, 17(1), 26–33.

Radford, L. (2003a). On the epistemological limits of language. Mathematical knowledge and social practice in the Renaissance. *Educa. Stud. Math.*, 52(2), 123–150.

Radford, L. (2003b). On culture and mind. A post-vygotskian semiotic perspective, with an example from Greek mathematical thought. In M. Anderson, et al. (Eds.), *Educational perspectives on mathematics as semiosis: From thinking to interpreting to knowing* (pp. 49–79). Ottawa: Legas.

Speranza, F. (1997). *Scritti di epistemologia della matematica*. Bologna: Pitagora.

Vergnaud, G. (1990). La théorie des champs conceptuels. *Recherches en didactique des mathématiques*. 10, 133–169.

Vygotsky, L. S. (1962). *Thought and language*. Cambridge, MIT Press. [It is a summary taken from the original Russian edition written in Russian language, a collection of articles published in Moscow in 1956. French edition: 1985, Paris: Èd. Sociale. Italian Edition: 1990, Bari: Laterza].

Chapter 21
The Idea of Space in Art, Technology, and Mathematics

Michele Emmer

Abstract Both art and architecture have always been influenced by scientific and mathematical ideas of space. In the 20th century, artists and architects profoundly changed their view of the structure of the external world in the light of the new geometrical ideas of space. New technologies further contributed to change the idea of space.

Keywords Art · Architecture · Technology · Computer graphics · Mathematics

21.1 Introduction: Visual Mathematics

Over the past several years, there has been a notable increase in the use of computer graphics in mathematics; this had led not only to the development of a new branch of mathematics that can be called *Visual Mathematics* (Emmer 1992, 1999) but also to a renewed interest in mathematics and the mathematical images on the part of artists and architects and, on the part of mathematicians, a new attention to the aesthetic aspects of some of the new scientific images that have been generated. The major tool in this new way of doing mathematics is computer graphics, which is by no means ousting what we may call the traditional method. What is involved here is not simply visualizing well-known phenomena by means of graphic tools but using visual tools in order to form an idea of still unsolved problems in mathematical research. That is, the computer is a genuine tool for experimentations. This very large diffusion has strongly raised intuition and creativity in that part of mathematical research connected to the possibility of visualizing not only

M. Emmer (✉)
Department of Mathematics, University of Rome 1, Rome, Italy
e-mail: emmer@mat.uniroma1.it

V. Capecchi (eds.), *Applications of Mathematics in Models, Artificial Neural Networks and Arts*, DOI 10.1007/978-90-481-8581-8_21,

known phenomena but to *make visible the invisible*. What may most interest people concerned with the relationships among art, architecture, and mathematics is the fact that the mathematician's use of graphics has greatly expanded their creative capacity.

Roger Penrose in his essay *The Emperor's New Mind* wrote (Penrose 1989)

> It is a feeling not uncommon amongst artists, that in their greatest works they are revealing eternal truths which have some kind of prior ethereal existence...but the case for believing in some kind of ethereal, eternal existence, at least for the more profound mathematical concepts, is a good deal stronger than in those other cases. There is a compelling uniqueness and universality in such mathematical ideas which seems to be of quite a different order from that which one could expect in the arts.

Mathematical ideas are not subjects to fashions, they do not vary in centuries; a theorem proved by Euclid is valid today and it will be valid for centuries; it will never be over. "Of course the creative process must produce a work that has design, harmony and beauty. These qualities too are present in mathematical creations" wrote Morris Kline in his essay *Mathematics in Western Culture* (Kline 1953).

It is possible to discuss the new possibilities opened for the relationships among art, architecture, and mathematics by the new technologies. It is possible to focus on the main directions along which to obtain results of interest for each fields. The mathematicians have obtained in the visual investigation of scientific problems images that have arose the interest not only of the scientific community but of a large audience, artists, and architects in particular. The great possibility that has been opened with the use of computer graphics of seeing mathematical objects of which it was not even possible to imagine the enormous graphic complexity has opened wide spaces to artistic creativity.

Mathematicians very soon became aware of this not secondary aspect of their researches. For example, talking of *Fractal Geometry* Mandelbrot wrote

> I believe I can safely say that fractal geometry' contribution to science and art is absolutely original.

Mandelbrot has repeatedly stressed the importance of fractals in art (Mandelbrot 1989)

> We can say that fractal geometry has given rise to a new category of art, close to the idea of art for art's sake: art for science's (and mathematics') sake. The origin of fractal art lies in the recognition that very simple mathematical formulas, seemingly dry and dust, can actually be very rich, so to speak, in huge graphic capacity. The artist's taste can intervene only in the choice of formulas, their arrangement and visual rendering. By bringing the eye and the hand into mathematics, we not only rediscovered the ancient beauty, which remains intact, but also discovered a hidden, extraordinary new beauty.

The example of fractals is not at all the only case of intrusion by mathematicians in the arts' field. To give an idea of the growing importance of the visual aspects and to point out the possible connections between some of the most recent mathematical research and the work of artists using visual techniques influenced by mathematical ideas, see the volumes *The Visual Mind: Art and Mathematics* (Emmer 1993, 2005, 2006).

Talent and creativity of mathematicians, assisted by graphic tools unimaginable until a few years ago, have opened new fields to mathematical research and gave the chance to catch the great graphic complexity in very simple problems and formulas.

Impossible to imagine, until a few years ago, a book like *Symmetry in Chaos: A Search for Pattern in Mathematics, Art and Nature*. The authors, the mathematicians Michael Field and Martin Golubitsky, wrote in the introduction (Field and Golubitsky 1992):

> In our mathematics research, we study how symmetry and dynamics coexist. This study has led to the pictures of symmetric chaos that we present throughout this book. Indeed, we have two purposes in writing this book: to present these pictures and to present the ideas of symmetry and chaos – as they are used by mathematicians – that are needed to understand how these pictures are formed.... One of our goals for this book is to present the pictures of symmetric chaos because we find them beautiful, but we also want to present the ideas that are needed to produce these computer-generated pictures.

The authors recall the volume of Peitgen and Richter *The Beauty of Fractals* (Peitgen and Richter 1986) and add:

> It is worth noting that the images we present have a different character from those found in fractal art. While fractal pictures have the sense of avant-garde abstract modernism or surrealism, ours typically have the feel of classical design.

Who could have imagined a few years ago that such declarations could have been found in the introduction of a volume written by two mathematicians?

Probably the creativity and capability of mathematicians have put to artists the problem of an active confrontation with the ideas of mathematicians.

"And since mathematics possesses these fundamental elements and puts them into meaningful relationships, it follows that such facts can be represented or transformed into images....which have an unquestionably aesthetic effect." wrote in 1949 the famous artist Max Bill, who died in 1994 (Emmer 2006).

Several elements have created a new possibility of cooperation and exchange of both visual and virtual ideas between artists, architects, and mathematicians. We need to go back to several years ago.

21.2 Space Is Mathematics

> I seem to detect a firm belief that, in philosophising, it is necessary to depend on the opinions of some famous author, as if our minds should remain completely sterile and barren, when not wedded to the reasoning of someone else. Perhaps he thinks that philosophy is a book of fiction written by some man, like the *Iliad*, or *Orlando Furioso* – books in which the least important thing is whether what is written there is true. This is not how the matter stands. Philosophy is written in this vast book, which continuously lies upon before our eyes (I mean the universe). But it cannot be understood unless you have first learned to understand the language and recognise the characters in which it is written. It is written in the language of mathematics, and the characters are triangles, circles, and other geometrical figures. Without such means, it is impossible for us humans to understand a word of it, and to be without them is to wander around in vain through a dark labyrinth. Galileo Galilei in *The Assayer* (*Il Saggiatore*), published in Rome in 1623.

Only a few years ago the Catholic Church recognized its errors regarding Galileo. It is interesting to note Pope Benedetto XVI's recent words:

> A fundamental characteristic of the modern sciences and of its related new technologies consists in the systematic use of mathematical tools to interface with nature and put at our service its immense energies. Mathematics in its own is a creation of our mind: the correspondence between its structures and the real structures of the universe – which is the basis of all modern developments, both scientific and technological, already explicitly formulated by Galileo Galilei with his famous statement that the book of nature is written in mathematical language – generates our admiration and poses a very important question. In fact it implies that even the universe has been structured in an intelligent way, in such a manner that there is a profound correspondence between our subjective mind and the objective mind of nature...The tendency to give the foremost place to the irrational, to chance and need, and to relate to these our intelligence and our freedom is reversed. On this basis it is possible again to widen the space of our rationality, to reopen it to the great questions of truth and goodness, to link theology, philosophy and the sciences, fully respecting their own methods and their autonomy, with the understanding of the intrinsic unity that binds them together. [1]

Thus, without mathematical structures we cannot understand nature. Mathematics is the language of nature. Now let's jump forward a few centuries. In 1904 a famous painter wrote to Emile Bernard:

> To treat nature by the cylinder, the sphere, the cone, the whole in perspective, such that is each side of an object, a plane, goes to a central point. The parallel lines on the horizon give the extension, or a section of nature. The lines perpendicular to the horizon give the depth. But nature for us humans is more depth than surface hence the necessity to introduce into our light vibrations, represented by red and yellow a suficient amount of blue, to feel the air. (Venturi 1970)

The art historian Lionello Venturi commented that in Cezanne's (the artist in question) paintings there are no cylinders, spheres, and cones, so the artist's quote represents nothing but an ideal aspiration to an organization of shapes transcending nature.

During the period when Cezanne was painting, and even a few years earlier, the panorama of geometry had changed since Galileo's time. In the second half of the nineteenth century geometry had mutated significantly. Between 1830 and 1850 Lobacevskij and Bolyai built the first examples of non-Euclidean geometry, in which the famous fifth postulate by Euclid was not valid. Not without doubt and conflicts, Lobacevskij would later call his geometry (which today is called non-Euclidean hyperbolic geometry) imaginary geometry, because it was in such strong contrast with common sense. For some years non-Euclidean geometry remained marginal to the field, a sort of unusual and curious form, until it was incorporated into and became an integral part of mathematics through the general ideas of G. F. B. Riemann (1826–1866). In 1854 Riemann held his famous dissertation entitled Ueber die Hypothesen welche der Geometrie zur Grunde liegen (On the hypotheses which lie at the foundation of geometry) before the faculty of the University of Göttingen (it was not published until 1867). In his presentation Riemann held a

[1] Papa Benedetto VXI (2006). Verona, 19/10/2006.

global vision of geometry as the study of varieties of any dimension in any kind of space. According to Riemann, geometry did not necessarily need to deal with points or space in the traditional sense, but with sets of ordered n-tuples.

In 1872 in his inauguration speech after becoming professor at Erlangen (known as the *Erlangen Program*), Felix Klein (1849–1925) described geometry as the study of the properties of figures with invariant character in respect to a particular group of transformations. Consequently each classification of the groups of transformations became a codification of the different types of geometry. For example, Euclidean plane geometry is the study of the properties of the figures that remain invariant in respect to the group of rigid transformations of the plane, which is formed by translations and rotations.

Jules Henri Poincaré (1968) held that

> the geometrical axioms are neither synthetic a priori intuitions nor experimental facts. They are conventions. Our choice among all possible conventions is guided by experimental facts; but it remains free, and is only limited by the necessity of avoiding every contradiction, and thus it is that postulates may remain rigorously true even when the experimental laws which have determined their adoption are only approximate.
>
> In other words the axioms of geometry are only definitions in disguise. What then are we to think of the question: Is Euclidean geometry true? It has no meaning. We might as well ask if the metric system is true and if the old weights and measures are false; if Cartesian coordinates are true and polar coordinates are false. One geometry cannot be more true than another; it can only be more convenient. Euclidean geometry is and will remain the most convenient.

Poincaré, in *Analysis Situs* (Latin translation of the Greek), published in 1895, is also responsible for the official birth of the sector of mathematics which today is called *Topology*:

> As far as I am concerned, all of the various research that I have performed has brought me to *Analysis Situs* (literally analysis of place).

Poincaré defined topology as the science that introduces us to the qualitative properties of geometric figures not only in ordinary space but also in more than 3-D space. Adding the geometry of complex systems, fractal geometry, chaos theory, and all of the "mathematical" images discovered (or invented) by mathematicians in the last 30 years using computer graphics, it is easy to see how mathematics has contributed to changing our concept of space – the space in which we live and the idea of space itself. Because mathematics is not merely a means of measurement in recipes but has contributed, if not determined, the way in which we understand space on earth and in the universe, specifically in regard to topology, the science of transformations, and the science of invariants. An example is Frank O. Gehry's project for the new Guggenheim Museum in Manhattan, an even more stimulating and more topological project than that of the Guggenheim in Bilbao.

There is certainly a remarkable cultural leap: construction using techniques and materials that allow for the realization of an almost continuous transformation, a sort of contradiction between the finished product and its distortion.

It is interesting to note that the study of contemporary architecture begins with the instruments that mathematics and science make possible, more than technical instruments, cultural instruments. It is important to mention that the discovery (or invention) of non-Euclidean geometry and of the higher dimensions (from the fourth on), the new idea of space to summarize, is one of the most interesting examples of the profound repercussions that mathematical ideas will have on humanistic culture and on art.

Here are the elements necessary to give sense to the word *Space*.

21.3 Fundamental Elements

Without a doubt the first element is the space that Euclid outlined, with definitions, axioms, the properties of objects that must find room in this space: Perfect space and Platonic space. Man as the blueprint and measure of the universe, an idea which spans centuries. Mathematics and geometry that explain everything, even the form of human beings: *The Curves of Life*, title of the famous twentieth century book by Cook, who could not have fathomed how true it could be to find mathematical curves in forms in nature, including those which make up the beginnings of life: from the famous 1914 book by D'Arcy Thompson *On Growth and Form*, to Rene Thom's catastrophe theory, to complexity and the Lorentz effect, to non-linear dynamic systems.

The second element is freedom; mathematics and geometry seem to create an arid realm. For those who are not interested in mathematics, and never studied it with interest in school, it is difficult to understand the intense emotion that mathematics can provoke and to realize that mathematics is an extremely creative field. It is not only a realm of great freedom where inventions (or discoveries) of new subjects, theories, and fields of research are made, but also where problems are invented. And because mathematicians generally do not need considerable financial resources, it is not only a realm of freedom but of imagination. And of course rigour. Rigorous reasoning.

The third element to consider is how all of these ideas are transmitted and assimilated, perhaps not completely understood, or only heard in passing by various sectors of society. In her book *Nuove bidimensionalità* (Imperiale 2001) in the chapter "Tecnologie digitali e nuove supefici" the architect Alicia Imperiale writes "Architects freely appropriate specific methodologies from other disciplines. This can be attributed to the fact that ample cultural changes take place more quickly in contexts other than architecture".

She adds

> Architecture reflects the changes that take place in culture, and according to many people, at a painfully slow speed. Architects, constantly trying to be on the forefront, believe that the information borrowed from other disciplines can be rapidly assimilated into architectural design. Nevertheless the translatability, the transfer from one language to another, is a problem. Architects look more and more frequently to other disciplines and other industrial

processes for inspiration, and use an increasing amount of computer design and software for industrial production that was originally developed for other sectors.

Later she reminds us that "It's interesting to note that in the information era disciplines that were once separate are bound to each other through an international language: the digital binary code." Do computers solve all of our problems?

The fourth element is computer, the graphic computer, the ultimate logical and geometrical machine, the fulfilment of an idea of an intelligent machine that is able to resolve various, diverse problems if we are able to make it understand the language we use. The genius idea of a mathematician, Alan Turing, brought to completion thanks to the stimulus of war. A machine built by man, using a logic built by man, created by man. A sophisticated instrument, irreplaceable not only in architecture. An instrument.

The fifth element is progress, the word progress. Can we speak of progress considering non-Euclidean geometry, new dimensions, topology, the explosion of geometry, and mathematics in the twentieth century? We can speak of knowledge, but not in the sense that new results take the place of previous ones.

Mathematicians often say (referring to an Italian saying) "Mathematics is like a pig, nothing is wasted, eventually even the most abstract and senseless things become useful." Imperiale writes that topology is an integral part of Euclidean geometry. That what escaped the author of this article is what the word space means in geometry. Words. That changing geometry is necessary in order to confront problems that are different because of the difference in the structure of space. Space is the properties, not the objects contained. Words.

The sixth element is words. One of the great gifts of humans is the ability to name things. Often in naming, we use words that are already in use. This habit is problematic because hearing these words we have the impression that we understand, or at least can guess, the meaning. In mathematics this has happened frequently in recent years with words like fractal, catastrophe, complex, hyperspace. Symbolic words, metaphors. Even topology, dimensionality, and seriality have become part of a common lexicon, at least among architects.

One word will have great importance for the idea of space: topology. For more details see *Mathland: from Flatland to Hypersurfaces* (Emmer 2004).

21.4 Topology

In the middle of the nineteenth century there began a completely new development in geometry that was soon to become one of the great forces of modern mathematics.

Courant and Robbins write in the famous book *What is Mathematics?* (1940)

The new subject, called analysis situs or topology, has as its object the study of the properties of geometrical figures that persist even when the figures are subjected to deformations so drastic that all their metric and projective properties are lost.

Poincaré defined topology as the science that introduces us to the qualitative properties of the geometric figures not only in ordinary space but in more than 3-D space.

Thus topology is the study of the properties of geometric figures that, undergoing intense distortions which cause them to lose all of their metric and projective qualities, for example, shape and size, are still invariant. In other words, the geometrical figures maintain their qualitative properties. We can consider figures that are made of materials that can be arbitrarily deformed, that cannot be lacerated or welded: there are properties that these figures conserve even when they are deformed.

In 1858 the German mathematician and astronomer August Ferdinand Moebius (1790–1868) described for the first time in a work presented to the Academy of Sciences in Paris a new surface of 3-D space, a surface which is known today as the *Moebius Strip*. In his work Moebius described how to build (quite simply) the surface which bears his name. Among other things, the Moebius Strip is the first example of a non-orientable surface – it is impossible to distinguish between two faces.

Courant and Robbins write "At first, the novelty of the methods in the new field left mathematicians no time to present their results in the traditional postulational form of elementary geometry. Instead, the pioneers, such as Poincaré, were forced to rely largely upon geometrical intuition. Even today [Courant and Robbins' book is from 1941] a student of topology will find that by too much insistence on a rigorous form of presentation he may easily lose sight of the essential geometrical content in a mass of formal detail."

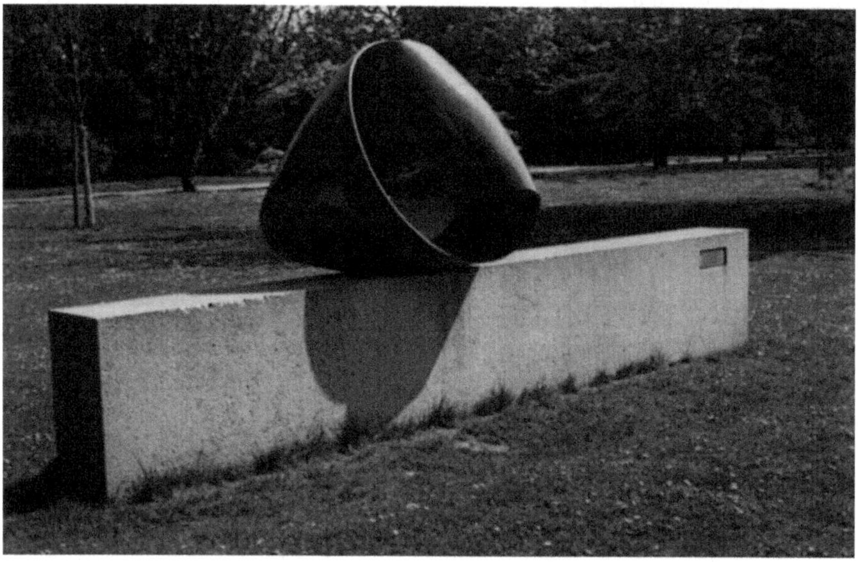

Max Bill, *Endless Ribbon*, Marble, 1936

The key word is geometrical intuition. Obviously over the years mathematicians have tried to bring topology into the realm of more rigorous mathematics, but there is still a strong sense of intuition involved. These two aspects, the distortions which maintain some of the geometrical properties of the figure, and intuition play an important role in the idea of space and shape from the 19th century to today. Some of the topological ideas were *sensed* by artists and architects in the past decades, first by artists, then much later by architects.

These shapes that so interested Max Bill in the 1930s (Bill 1970) could not go unnoticed in architecture, although it took some time: until the diffusion of computer graphics, which allows the visualization of the mathematical objects discussed, thus giving concrete support to the intuition which otherwise, for the non-mathematician, is hard to grasp.

21.5 International Architecture Exhibition 2004

In 2004 I attended the International Architecture Exhibition in Venice. The theme of the exhibition was *Metamorph*.

> Many of the great creative acts in art and science can be seen as fundamentally metamorphic, in the sense that they involve the conceptual re-shaping of ordering principles from one realm of human activity to another visual analogy. Seeing something as essentially similar to something else has served as a key tool in the fluid transformation of mental frameworks in every field of human endeavour. I used the expression "structural intuitions" to try to capture what I felt about the way in which such conceptual metamorphoses operate in the visual arts and the sciences. Is there anything that creators of artefacts and scientists share in their impulses, in their curiosity, in their desire to make communicative and functional images of what they see and strive to understand?
>
> The expression "structural intuitions" attempts to capture what I tried to say in one phrase, namely that sculptors, architects, engineers, designers and scientists often share a deep involvement with the profound sense of involvement with the beguiling structures apparent in the configurations and processes of nature – both complex and simple. I think we gain a deep satisfaction from the perception of order within apparent chaos, a satisfaction that depends on the way that our brains have evolved mechanisms for the intuitive extraction of the underlying patterns, static and dynamic.

These are the words of Martin Kemp, an art historian specialized in the relationship between art and science in the article – *Intuizioni strutturali e pensiero metamorfico nell'arte, architettura e scienze*, in *Focus* (Kemp 2004), one of the volumes that make up the catalogue of the 2004 Venice International Architecture Exhibition.

In his article Kemp writes mainly about architecture. The image accompanying Kemp's article is a project by Frank O. Gehry, an architect who obviously cannot be overlooked when discussing modern architecture, continuous transformation, unfinished architecture, and infinite architecture.

Kurt W. Forster, curator of the exhibit, discusses the great complexity, the enormous number of variations developed through essential technological innovations, the continuous surfaces in transformation. He cites the mathematician Ian Stewart's article entitled *Nature's numbers: discovering order and pattern in the universe* (1995). Some key words: pattern, structure, motif, order, metamorphosis, variations, transformations, mathematics (Forster 2004).

Forster writes

> Recent buildings predicated upon continuous surfaces make clear that they depend in conception and realization on the use of computer technology. The single hinge upon which they turn is the computer. Any number of hybrid transformations and exchanges between traditional methods and rapidly developed software have multiplied and modified the process of elaboration and realization of projects. Hardly a method that cannot be integrated within the 'loop' of numeric calculations, but more consequential than the flexibility of elaboration and the constant back-and-forth between image and object, is the fact of architecture's migration to the realm of the virtual and simulated.

Forster continues regarding Gehry:

> What really interests Gehry is the process, in the sense of dynamic process used to achieve a structural and aesthetic result.

These words, projects, and ideas at the 2004 Exhibition were visually closely connected to the ties between mathematics, architecture, topology, and transformation that I am writing about. The layout of the pavilion of the Venice Exhibition, which caused quite a stir, was assigned to two famous architects: Hani Rashid and Lise Anne Couture. In an article for the catalogue entitled *Asymptote, the Architecture of Metamorph*, they summarized their project as follows:

> Asymptote's transformation of the Corderie emerged from computer-generated morphing animation sequences derived from utilizing rules of perspective geometry with the actions and dynamics of torquing and "stringing" the space of the Corderie. The experience of Metamorph is spatial in that it is itself an architectural terrain of movement and flow. The exhibition architecture – from installation and exhibition design to graphic identity and catalogue design – provides for a seamless experience that fuses the Arsenale, Giardini and Venice, making explicit a contemporary reading of architecture where affinities and disparities co-mingle to produce the effects of flux and metamorphoses of form and thinking. (Rashid 2004)

One of the studies of the layout was described quite significantly as follows:

> Study of the topological surface that develops in the space of the Corderie and determines the movements and the curvatures used in designing levels.

Let's backtrack a bit, to the early 1990s. In 1992 the architect Eisenmann (who won the *Leone d'Oro* for his architectures at the 2004 exhibition) and his collaborators projected a skyscraper in Berlin, the *Max Reinhardt Haus*. The structure of the enormous building is based on the topological surface, the Moebius strip. In 1993 Ben van Berkel planned and built the *Moebius House*. So these two projects held the place of honor in the large hall of the *Corderie*, as if a reminder of an important step in contemporary architecture, in the idea of transformation, of metamorphosis. An explicit reference to topology.

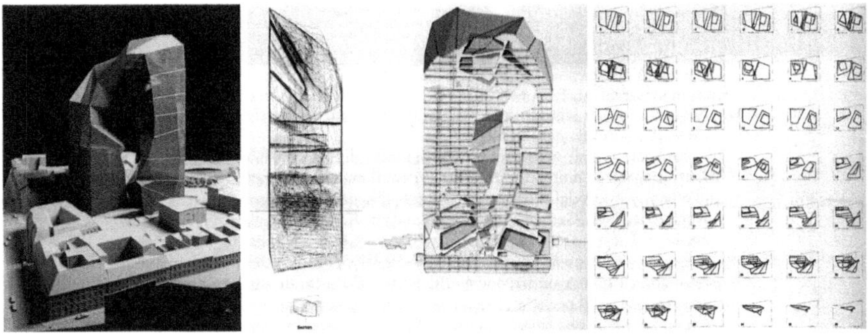

P. Eiseman, *Max Reinhardt House*, project, Berlin, 1992.

Until a few years ago these were utopic projects – and many still are; architects enjoyed creating projects that were never carried out.

21.6 Toward a Virtual Architecture

In the chapter *Topological Surfaces* Alicia Imperiale writes (Imperiale 2001)

> The architects Ben van Berkel and Caroline Bos of UN Studio discuss the impact of new scientific discoveries on architecture. The scientific discoveries have radically changed the definition of the word "Space", attributing a topological shape to it. Rather than a static model of constitutive elements, space is perceived as something malleable, mutating, and its organization, its division, its appropriation become elastic.

And the role of topology, from the architect's perspective:

> Topology is the study of the behaviour of a structure of surfaces which undergo deformations. The surface registers the changes in the differential space time leaps in a continuous deformation. This entails further potential for architectural deformation. Continuous deformation of a surface can lead to the intersection of external and internal planes in a continuous morphological mutation, exactly like in the Moebius Strip. Architects use this topological form to design houses, inserting differential fields of space and time into an otherwise static structure.

Naturally some words and ideas are changed in switching from a strictly scientific field to an artistic and architectonic one. But this is not a problem, nor a criticism. Ideas move freely and each person has the right to interpret and attempt, as with topology, to capture the essence. The role of computer graphics in all of this is essential, it allows the insertion of that deformation-time variable that would otherwise be unthinkable, not to mention unattainable.

Imperiale continues regarding the Moebius Strip:

> Van Berkel's house, inspired by the Moebius Strip (Moebius House), was designed as a programmatically continuous structure, that combines the continuous mutation of the dialectic sliding couples that flow into each other, from the interior to the exterior, from the activity of work to that of free time, from the fundamental to the non-fundamental structure.

During the same period Peiter Eisenman was designing the *Max Reinhardt Haus* in Berlin (Eisenman Architects 2004):

> The building, composed of arches, made up of intersecting and overlapping forms, presents a unified structure that separates, that compresses, transforms and finally comes back together on the horizontal plane at the height of the attic. The origin of the form is represented in the Moebius Strip, a three-dimensional geometric form characterized by a unique, unending surface that undergoes three iterative operations. In the first, the planes are generated from the extension of the vectors and triangulations of the surfaces... The second iteration overturns the strip, causing an operation similar to that in the first phase, and then appends these surfaces on top of the original form, thus creating a ghost form. The third phase applies an element of Berlinese history to the form itself, wrapping up vast public spaces between the grilled and the base of the ground floor of an already folded surface. Just as the Moebius Strip folds two sides into one surface by folding on itself, the Max Reinhardt Haus denies the dialectic tradition between internal and external and confuses the distinction between public and private.

Both van Berkel's house and Eisenman's project were at the Venice 2004 Biennial to represent the archetypes of topological architecture.

Van Berkel writes that another famous topological object, the Klein bottle, "can be translated into a canal system that incorporates all of the elements that it encounters and causes them to precipitate into a new type of internally connected integral organization." Note that the words integral and internally connected have precise meanings in mathematics.

But this is not a problem because "the diagrams of these topological surfaces are not used in architecture in a rigorously mathematically way, but constitute abstract diagrams, three-dimensional models that consent the architects to incorporate differential ideas of space and time into architecture."

As I mentioned before, architects became aware (albeit rather late) of the new scientific discoveries in the field of topology. And not only did they begin to design and build but also to reflect.

In her 1999 doctoral thesis Architettura e Topologia: per una teoria spaziale della architettura, Giuseppa Di Cristina writes

> Architecture's final conquest is space: this is generated through a sort of positional logic of the elements, that is through the arrangement that spatial relationships generate; the formal value is thus substituted by the spatial value of the configuration: the external aspect of the form is not as important as the spatial quality. And thus topological geometry, without "measure" and characteristic of non-rigid figures, is not something purely abstract that comes before architecture, but a trace left by that modality of action in the spatial concretization of architecture.

In 2001 Di Cristina edited a book on *Architecture and Science* (Di Cristina 2001). In her introduction *The Topological Tendency in Architecture* Di Cristina clarifies that

> The articles that are included here bear witness to the interweaving of this architectural neo-avant-garde with scientific mathematical thought, in particular topological thought: although no proper theory of topological architecture has yet been formulated, one could nevertheless speak of a topological tendency in architects at both the theoretical and operative levels. In particular, developments in modern geometry or mathematics, perceptual

> psychology and computer graphics have an influence on the present formal renewal of architecture and on the evolution of architectural thought. What mainly interests architects theorizing the logic of curvability and pliability is the significance of the "event", of "evolution", of "process", or the innate dynamism in the fluid and flexible configurations of what is now called topological architecture.
>
> Topological architecture means that dynamic variation of form, facilitated by information technology, by computer-assisted design, by animation software. The topologification of architectonic forms according to dynamic and complex configurations leads architectural design to a new and often spectacular plasticity, in the footsteps of the Baroque or organic Expressionism.

Stephen Perrella, one of the most interesting *virtual* architects describes *Architectural Topology* as follows (Di Cristina 2001):

> Architectural topology is the mutation of form, structure, context and programme into interwoven patterns and complex dynamics. Over the past several years, a design sensibility has unfolded whereby architectural surfaces and the topologising of form are being systematically explored and unfolded into various architectural programmes. Influenced by the inherent temporalities of animation software, augmented reality, computer-aided manufactured and informatics in general, topological "space" differs from Cartesian space in that it imbricates temporal events-within form. Space then, is no longer a vacuum within which subjects and objects are contained, space is instead transformed into an interconnected, dense web of particularities and singularities better understood as substance or filled space. This nexus also entails more specifically the pervasive deployment of teletechnology within praxis, leading to an usurping of the real (material) and an unintentional dependency on simulation.

Observations in which ideas about geometry, topology, computer graphics, and space time merge. Over the years the cultural nexus has been successful: new words, new meanings, and new connections.

21.7 Final Observations

In this article I have tried to discuss some important moments that brought about a mutation in our perception of space. I have attempted to help grasp not only the technical and formal aspects that are essential to mathematics but also the cultural aspect – using the idea of space in relation to some important aspects of contemporary architecture. I have tried to analyze the way in which the idea of space together with the development of new computer technologies have modified the way not only of working but also of thinking of modern architects. Shapes that were unthinkable can now even be realized. Without the cultural change of the idea of space, without the appearance of the new ideas in geometry, it would have been impossible not only to develop the new computer tools (just think of the essential role of Boolean Algebra in the development of computer logic) but also, most importantly, to perceive in a different way the space around us, to imagine a world full of shapes, shapes that Humanity never thought of before. Mathematics can generate great dreams.

Bibliography

Bill, M. (1949). *A mathematical approach to art*, reprinted with the author's corrections in M. Emmer (Ed.), (pp. 5–9) 1992.

Bill, M. (1970). *Come cominciai a fare le superfici a faccia unica*. In A. Quintavalle (Ed.), *Max Bill* (pp. 23–25). catalogue of the exhibition, Parma.

Courant, R. and Robbins, H. (1940). *What is mathematics? An elementary approach to ideas and methods*. Oxford University Press, New York.

Di Cristina, G., (Ed.). (2001). *Architecture and science*. Chichester: Wiley-Academy.

Eisenman Architects (2004). Max Reinhardt Haus. In Marsilio (Ed.), *Metamorph: Trajectories* (p. 252), catalogue, La Biennale di Venezia.

Emmer, M., (Ed.). (1992). *Visual mathematics*. special issue, Leonardo, Pergamon Press, vol. 25, n. 3/4.

Emmer, M., (Ed.). (1993). *The visual mind: Art and mathematics*. Boston: The MIT Press.

Emmer, M., (Ed.). (1999). Special issue on visual mathematics. *Int. J. Shape Model.* 5(1). Singapore: World Publishing.

Emmer, M. (2004). *Mathland: From flatland to hypersurfaces*. Boston: Birkhauser.

Emmer, M. (Ed.) (2005). *The visual mind 2: Art and mathematics*. Boston: The MIT Press.

Emmer, M. (2006). *Visibili armonie: arte cinema teatro matematica*. Torino: Bollati Boringhieri.

Field, M. and Golubitsky, M. (1992). *Symmetry in Chaos: A search for pattern in mathematics, art and nature*. Oxford: Oxford University Press.

Forster, K. W., (Ed.). (2004). *Metamorph: Focus* (pp. 9–10). catalog, La Biennale di Venezia, Marsilio ed.

Kemp, M. (2004). *Intuizioni strutturali e pensiero metamorfico nell'arte, architettura e scienze*. In K. W. Forster (Ed.), *Metamorph: Focus* (pp. 31–43). catalogue, La Biennale di Venezia, Marsilio (Ed.).

Kline, M. (1953). *Mathematics in Western culture*. Oxford: Oxford University Press.

Imperiale, A. (2001). *New bidimensionality*. Basel: Birkhauser.

Mandelbrot, B. (1989). Fractals and an art for the sake of Science. *ACM Siggraph 89*, Leonardo, special issue, 21–24.

Peitgen, H.-O. and Richter, P. H. (1986). *The beauty of fractals*. Berlin: Springer Verlag.

Penrose, R. (1989). *The emperor's new mind*. Oxford: Oxford University Press.

Poincaré, H. (1968). *La Science et l'Hypothèse* (pp. 75–76). Paris: Flammarion.

Rashid, H. and Couture, L. A. (2004). *Asymptote, the architecture of metamorph*. In K.W. Forster (Ed.), *Metamorph: Trajectories* (pp. 9–13), catalogue, La Biennale di Venezia, Marsilio (Ed.).

Venturi, L. (1970). *La via dell'impressionismo: da Manet a Cezanne* (pp. 268–269). Torino: Einaudi.

Chapter 22
Mathematical Structures and Sense of Beauty

Raffaele Mascella, Franco Eugeni, and Ezio Sciarra

Abstract The recognition of beauty arises from various mental operations, spontaneous or induced, passively accepted or pressingly imposed. The perception of beauty under the subjective aesthetical sensibility can be analyzed, and at least partially justified, with different approaches: neuro-psychological or evolutionary, socio-cultural and mathematical formalizing. These approaches individualize many factors in the determinations of the concept of beautiful, consequential to ancestral needs and social conventions, but also to specific mathematical characteristics.

22.1 Introduction

Beauty is an abstract concept. Each of us has his own idea about what is beautiful and what is not, but if we try to carefully define what makes them such, the assignment becomes very arduous. Identification and perception of beauty always arises by performing some mental operational processes, spontaneous or induced, passively accepted or pressingly imposed. Things, individuals, animals, plants, landscapes, dresses, images, sounds, poems, behaviours, natural or artificial operas, objects of any knowledge field, due to their chromatic and geometric structure or to the perception they induce, generate some feelings as comfort, sharing, acceptance, satisfaction, sense of positivity, astonishment, surprise, fascination. In John Keats' "Endymion" words, "A thing of beauty is a joy for ever: / its loveliness increases; it will never / pass into nothingness; but still will keep / a bower quiet for us, and a sleep / full of sweet dreams, and health, and quiet breathing."

Since antiquity, beauty has been considered an important ingredient of our lives and has got a great impact, possibly more than that we are used to conceive in our scientific and technological society. Thus, it is not surprising that philosophers have

R. Mascella (✉)
Department of Communication, University of Teramo, Teramo, Italy
e-mail: mascella@unite.it

V. Capecchi (eds.), *Applications of Mathematics in Models, Artificial Neural Networks and Arts*, DOI 10.1007/978-90-481-8581-8_22,

been interested and tried to understand the nature of experiences and judgments lying at the basis of the notion. For instance, according to the classic tradition, who saw a strong connection between mathematics and beauty, the experience of beauty is stimulated by certain perceived relations between an object and his parts, proportioned on the basis of a ratio seemed more attractive.

At first glance, mental operations connected to the beautiful look all alike, as whether the same basic stimulus would predispose such sensations, and thus with the activation of the same neuronal circuits. Probably, this would be the case, but far from discovering this functionality in human brain, we will consider the question from a series of complementary, not necessarily alternative, points of view. In this sense, some divergences seem unavoidable.

A major question concerns the possibility of existence of an anthropological canon of beauty. Many authors have claimed that a unique conception or definition of the beauty does not exist. A fixed canon is missing to allow the coding of our perception of beauty. As pointed out by Umberto Eco (2004) and Georges Vigarello (2004), we can observe that the concept of the beautiful depends upon various civilizations and upon historical moments. Eco, in particular, presented an amazing collection of different beauty ideals, theorized by philosophers and practiced by artists. Following his ideas, it is easy to show that things appreciated as beautiful, in the long history from the classic Greek world until contemporary mass media, have been many and have been changed time after time: God, nature, flowers, precious stones, human body, stars, but also the devil and fashionable clothing. Thus the concept has to be expressed with a series of stratifications and interpretations with the tendency to connect numerous principal variations meaning the various responses given by mankind.

From the beginning of western culture, the feeling of beauty has come to a close connection with the concepts of truth and goodness, thus connecting the perceiver with a consciousness or a state of being existing beyond the material world. For Plato the contemplation of beauty was the way for contemplating the truth; thus was objectively existent and an absolute principle, a transcendent entity. As in Plato's Phaedrus, the beautiful is apparently perceived through a series of properties of a particular object, but it is properly a recognition of some truths about the nature of things, known a priori by the perceiver.

The link between beauty and truth is still present in philosophical tradition, and nevertheless difficult to confirm. If we intend the truth as a correspondence between mind and reality apprehended by reason, and the beauty as a perceptually pleasing quality of objects, ordered into a harmonic and unified shape, exhibiting somehow repetition and contrast in their parts, it is complicated to make them share the same, equivalent meaning. Our perception, attitude and remembrance of things can be influenced by style and form of their expression, but whether they are true seems a matter of logical value independent of aesthetic, ethical, rhetorical or other values. But if beauty is intended in loose way, a certain relation can eventually arise. If we believe, as Aristotle, in the self-evidence, we may think on a natural inclination towards what is really true, especially if we are given two bare propositions to choose from. In other words, bad arguments may be put in a beautiful form, but they cannot be made beautiful in the way that a true argument may be. In this sense we can still appreciate Keats' final words in "Ode on a Graecian Urn":

> Beauty is Truth, Truth Beauty, – that is all
>
> Ye know on earth, and all ye need to know.

This is probably true also in scientific discovery and knowledge, and most probably true in mathematics, where the rhetorical equivalent of beauty is elegance, and an invalid theorem can badly have an elegant proof.

Ideals of physical beauty, also originated in Greece, were consequences of the classical devotion to numerical proportion and harmony. When Greeks, like Pythagoras and Euclid, discovered such mathematical relations, it seemed to their followers to have pointed towards a deep understanding. There is something in this myth sometimes discussed, probably because Euclid, in his famous textbook "*Elements*", in showing how to calculate the value of the ratios, seemed more interested in the mathematics than in architecture, for he gave them an unromantic label: *extreme* and *mean* ratio.

A canon that others have tried to develop in successive centuries, as Vitruvius, bringing in a more profound geometrical idea. The Greek sculptures, however, also if not forced by Vitruvian geometry and limiting themselves to the euclidean ratios, still at present day remain the vision of harmony and beauty, lasted and unsurpassed through the ages.

But what makes people apply the word beautiful to certain things and ugly to others? An interesting definition of the beautiful is the one given in the "Poetics" by Aristotle:

> to be beautiful a living creature, and every whole made up of parts, must not only present a certain order in its arrangements of parts, but also be of a certain definite magnitude. Beauty is a matter of size and order and therefore impossible in a very minute creature, since our perception becomes indistinct as it approaches instantaneity; or, secondly, in a creature of vast size, – one say a thousand stadia long – as in that case, the object cannot be seen all at once and the unity and wholeness of it are lost on the beholder.

In the medieval era, the perception of beauty was intended as a way to self-transcendence, a feeling of being in harmony with others, connecting the individual to the divine. Anyway, from ancient times up until after Kant, it seems philosophers have recognized two kinds of beauty: the first, universal and unchanging, who realizes itself in its objective nature; the second, a relative, dynamic one, realized through the subjective response.

The idea of an aesthetical canon based on a numerical ratio, a proportion, a measure, and thus with characteristics of computability and objectivity, grew up definitely in the first Renaissance with Luca Pacioli (1509) in a book with illustrations drawn by Leonardo da Vinci. This example was followed by the whole neoplatonic and neoplotinian Florentine school and probably influenced painters as Botticelli, Raffaello and Michelangelo. In the late Renaissance and the Baroque, the conception was enlarged, as the artistic world realized that beauty does not coincide uniquely with order and regularity. It was dependent upon the existence of something more, an added *quid* contributing to establish what the beautiful is, something neither calculable or measurable, something that one may note or, in artistic context, introduced by artist's genius. Thus, all the previous canons somehow jumped away, in the absence of a condivisibile criterion to which men may appeal. The beauty needed what will be called *taste* or a subjective dominant element.

More recent societies have modified the classical approach, losing the ancient characters and moving to a sensitive exhibition of ideas. The beauty has become contextual to a wider universe of values and a discipline is born to specifically investigate such feeling in depth. The *aesthetic* movement, whose term derives from "aesthesis", or sensation, identifies and bases its analysis on sense dimensions. The beauty is conceived as an independent pursuit, a unitary and self-sufficient type of human experience. Just view, hearing, tact, taste and sense of smell are considered, which are at the top of our perception. In this way, instead of moving away to the intelligible, the beauty ranges inside the sensible and a series of new meanings drove to considering each natural object or artificial opera as a single bearer of beauty properties.

In this way, also artistic objects became individualized under the slogan "art for art's sake". Art is not more introducing in the truth world; it does not have to be useful and convey moral or sentimental messages. It can simply show us the charm and ambiguity of the phenomena happening in this world, without any didactic purpose. Art has to be only beautiful, and thus the cult of beauty arises as a basic factor in art. But if we look at the whole modern art and the same aesthetics, as discipline, we can definitely find the necessity and the final aim to educate the taste. A simple way to explain this sight is with the actual role of museums, painting galleries, artistic schools, literature's and music classics and so on, often learned at ordinary school.

Anyway, by the eighteenth century, the nature of beauty, the way in which we experience it and the research of fundamental necessary conditions for the judgment of taste have been a central philosophical question (MacMahon 1999). According to David Hume, beauty is perceived conditionally to having a sense of beauty and involves a certain response of the perceiver. In his words (Hume 1740)

> Beauty is such an order and constitution of parts as either by the primary constitution of our nature, by custom, or by caprice is fitted to give a pleasure and satisfaction to the soul.

Kant, directing his attention to the perceptual/cognitive conditions in the perceiver, isolated two fundamental necessary conditions for a judgment to be a judgment of taste: subjectivity and universality (MacMahon 1999). Beauty and judgment of taste have to be basically subjective, i.e. based on an inner response, a feeling of disinterested pleasure or displeasure. Thus, a not-cognitive judgment and not-logical. Indeed, beauty claims a universal validity that he described in this way (Kant 1790):

> [...] when [a person] puts a thing on a pedestal and calls it beautiful, he demands the same delight from others. He judges not merely for himself, but for all men, and then speaks of beauty as if it were a property of things. Thus he says that the thing is beautiful; and it is not as if he counts on others agreeing with him in his judgment of liking owing to his having found them in such agreement on a number of occasions, but he demands this agreement

> of them. He blames them if they judge differently, and denies them taste, which he still requires of them as something they ought to have; and to this extent it is not open to men to say: Every one has his own taste. This would be equivalent to saying that there is no such thing as taste, i.e. no aesthetic judgment capable of making a rightful claim upon the assent of all men.

An antinomy arose with Kant. From one side the beauty is subjective and does not allow us an extrapolation of the object's properties that make it beautiful; thus it is very different from empirical judgment. From the opposite side, beauty is universally valid, in that we think that others "ought to have" the same judgment and should allow us to extrapolate the object's properties in such vision, because we speak "of beauty as if it were a property of things". Thus, it is like the empirical judgment. How such a subjectively universal judgment is possible?

On this question has long been debated. An interesting answer could be the one given by Jennifer MacMahon, which reincludes universality and subjectivity as complementary features of the beautiful. We may consider the principles of beauty as properties of the perceptual processes in our brain, instead of properties of the object. In this way (MacMahon 1999)

> A judgment of beauty could be understood to be both universal and subjective based on the fact that the experience of beauty is an awareness of species-specific perceptual processes or principles. If an awareness of these principles were pleasurable in themselves, it would be a disinterested pleasure, quite distinct from pleasure of the sensuous or pleasure experienced in the good.

In the following, the notion of beautiful by the subjective aesthetical sense is analysed moving through different, complementary approaches. The first, a neuro-psychological approach, ascribes to the sense of beauty some particular perceived forms, as they appear to state a deep correspondence with gratifying functions, above all reproduction and selective spreading. The second, a socio-cultural approach, ascribes the beauty to gratifying perceived forms in relation to a social convention or fashion and to beliefs connected with an equilibrium of cultural models of social communication and related to the evolving historic time. Finally, the mathematical-formalizing approach retains that human aesthetic sensibility and objective perception of the beauty has a groundwork in objective numerical structures (ratio and forms) existing in nature, which the observer may recognize in natural formalized models, in bearing the same production and acknowledgement code of the perceived beauty.

22.2 Evolutionary Beauty

The biological argument was initiated by Charles Darwin. Before him, the common view shared by the naturalists were that many plant and animal structures were created just for beauty in the eyes of man or for a mere variety. In the Darwin's view the species evolve by natural selection, where (Darwin 1859) "successive males display their gorgeous plumage and perform strange antics before the females, which standing by as spectators, at last choose the most attractive partner", and female representants at the end choose "the most melodious or beautiful males, according to their standard of beauty". Thus, the evolution of the brilliant and marvellous plumage of peacocks find explanation in sexual selection, providing reproductive advantages in terms of being chosen by females. His grandfather, Erasmus Darwin, had first the same idea (Darwin E. 1802; cited in Smith 2005):

> Our perception of beauty consists in our recognition by the sense of vision of those objects, first, which have inspired our love by the pleasure they have afforded to many of our senses; as to our sense of warmth, of touch, of smell, of taste, of hunger and thirst; and secondly which bear any analogy of form to such objects.

Taking Darwin's ideas, and the famous example of peacocks as a starting point, evolutionary biology sees the origin of our sense of beauty in the depths of our past and tries to explain how aesthetic preferences have naturally evolved as an adaptive strategy in the sexual choice mechanisms of virtually every species. Throughout history, mate selection, reproduction and survival of the species have been relied on phenotypic expressions. From the evolutionists' point of view, the perception of beauty may be governed by circuits shaped by natural selection in the human brain. This involves an inquiry on specifically features to comprehend how animals and humans appreciate physical attractiveness.

Many traits, humans and animals actually select when choosing a mate, are not just arbitrary. Instead, they seem powerful indicators of fundamental aspects in reproduction and survival: (a) physical beauty is at least in part a real indicator of health and fertility and (b) psychological traits, like kindness, creativity and intelligence, are indicators of the ability to best adaptation in the world, fidelity and parenting ability. From a certain point of view could be a fuzzyfication of what we use to regard as "inner" and "outer" beauty but it seems hard to imagine physical markers for the psychological qualities. Thus, in the biologists' evolutionary argument, physiological factors are considered components of beauty; therefore deserving an investigation, while cognitive are not.

A gender difference has been evidenced by scientific research in the process of understanding beauty and attractiveness. Among a series of determinants, in men prevail fertility and healthy status of females, while in women prevail abilities of men to obtain and defend resources also for the female. Therefore women with full lips, smooth clear skin, clear eyes, lustrous hair, good muscle tone, animated facial expression, high energy level (Buss 1994) and men with brawny and athletic body are at the top of every culture's beauty list – even if today humans muscle power has been partially replaced by financial and political possibilities.

The idea that perception of beauty may be guided by biological traits – shared universally in the species – is supported widely by researchers. Some neuro-anatomical arrangements, for their having a biological relevance, revealing certain capabilities, result in being fundamental parts in the standards of beauty. Despite aesthetic judgments have some cultural variability, scientific evidence shows that very similar patterns can be identified across diverse cultures.

First of all, some *facial features* such as symmetry, averageness and youthfulness seem to play a consistent role in revealing reproductive health and capabilities of potential sexual partners. These features suggest that such a potential mate may be pathogen free, and by the sexual selection model, only animals which are resistant to pathogens are able to develop and maintain their secondary sex characteristics. And seem predictable, however confirmed by research (Gangestad 1993), that physical attractiveness is more important in the selection of long-term mates in cultures where the pathogen prevalence is higher.

The evolutionary argument of attractiveness arising from symmetry may be explained in his recurrent association with strong and robust genes. Thus, mating with an individual which is symmetrical in appearance may improve the likelihood of survival for any offspring. In this view, a face does not seem to be beautiful because of its proportions, as suggested by people who supported the golden ratio, it is "just" due to the similarity between left and right sides. Also averageness, which generally is regarded as a signal of ordinary and normality, and thus far from the beautiful, appears as an indicator of health and resistance to parasites in genetic composition. Some studies on facial appearance (Langlois 1994) have showed that composite face, obtained by mixing adequately different parts of different faces, are judged more attractive than individual faces. An explanation could be found in the fact that averageness, above all, means similarity to the mean of the species, and then more confidence on allowing heritable resistance to disease and not carrying potentially harmful genes or mutations. Also youthfulness, mainly for women faces, has been associated with fertility.

Although one may think that the ability to well choose on the basis of such factor may be acquired as social consequence, through the exposure to cultural standards, some studies on infant have suggested that the ability is at least partly innate or acquired at the very first life months (Langlois 1987). Thus, as before cultural standards of beauty are probably assimilated.

Second, some *bodily features* as bilateral symmetry and waist–hip ratio appears a signal of attractiveness and influence sexual selection. Animal studies show symmetry to be an advantage in the partner choice competition: female peahens prefer males with long tails and large numbers of symmetrical eye spots, female barn swallows select more frequently sexual partners with more symmetrical tails, female zebra prefer males who have symmetrically coloured leg bands (Sarwer 2003). As in the facial case, bodily symmetry is closely correlated with attractiveness and seems to be a qualitative indicator for reproductive success.

Instead, the waist–hip ratio, obtained by two features who take form particularly during puberty due to increased levels of oestrogen, and which synthesize the distribution of fat between upper and lower body, appears as an indicator that a potential mate is sexually mature or biologically capable of being reproductively active. Physiologists have shown that it points out accurately most women's fertility and there is a difference coming up between women and males. Fertile and healthy women have typically a waist–hip ratio from 0.6 to 0.8 (while in menopausal is bigger), while the ratio of healthy men ranges between 0.85 and 0.95 (Sarwer 2003). As we can easily admit, a measure of hip very close to the measure of waist in females or even bigger in males is generally judged less attractive or less healthy. Such a signal is really a good indicator for healthy status, or by converse for obesity, thus carrying the possibility of a series of diseases which varies with different distributions of fat.

On the basis of this neuro-psychological approach, the factors just described, and others already found or to come, are aesthetically pleasing. In other words, they are useful in providing some information about healthy and reproductive status of the subject. We likely include all such information in a decision structure, thus having a series of information or a knowledge of the subject confirming that beauty is hardly explained by a single unique principle. A consequence of this conception of beauty, inspired by evolutionary theory, is that people who at first sight are attracting are likely to be a good representant for our mate choosing. Aesthetic judgments are not arbitrary but, instead, reflect evolutionary functional assessments and valuations of potential mates. Briefly, as suggested by Buss (1994), "Beauty may be in the eyes of the beholder, but those eyes and the minds behind the eyes have been shaped by millions of years of human evolution" and by Etcoff (1999): "Beauty is a universal part of human experience, it provokes pleasure, rivets attention, and impels actions that help ensure survival of our genes."

22.3 Socio-cultural Beauty

While the neuro-psychological approach provided by the evolutionary theory can successfully explain the standards of beauty which are stable through history and across different cultures, nevertheless it does not succeed in explaining other standards. In such cases, a socio-cultural approach is unavoidable and useful. What emerges is that many popular beauty icons, from movie stars to Leonardo's paintings, either if they provide naturally some pleasure, receive a cultural acknowledgement which is subsequently socially spreaded and, after that, are considered more beautiful than others. We may consider these beauty standards as arising, in their greatness, by induced pleasure rather than properly ancestral pleasure. To be more clear, this sort of aesthetic response is subject to societal pressure and influences.

There are many examples of different human beauty brought up by cultural and social factors. In China, for instance, extremely small feet were once considered beautiful, and physically forced (or deformed) to become such; African and South American tribes, still now, continue to wear lip plates or labrets as ornaments. But there are also tattoos and piercings in western societies. Wittgenstein (1966), among others, remarked that the sense of beauty is culturally determined. What is regarded as "aesthetically satisfying" in a social stratum, educational background or cultural and historical epoch, is often very different from what is regarded as "beautiful" in other situations. To understand an aesthetic judgment, then, we should understand life, society and culture in which the judgment is embedded.

A historical synthesis of social influences is the one provided by Georges Vigarello (2004) who has shown how human preferences for different parts of the human body have changed during historical ages. Aesthetical canons have uninterruptedly changed, at least from Renaissance until today, according to where the look has progressively been interested of.

Until Renaissance, people with higher social status were considered beauty ideals, independently by their faces or bodies. King and queens, princes and princesses, popes and bankers were glorified in paintings and poems, even if they were graceless. But, time after time, a spreading of a canon of "revealed" beauty, instead of that put aside from power, begins. This ideal was mainly feminine, ethereal, given by the oval of face and the light of the eyes, from the whiteness of hands and the littleness of mouth, without any consideration for the inferior part of the body, as a sort of statuary base transcended by the upper part. In the seventeenth century a different beauty was introduced, a canon looking at expressiveness, not characterized by physiognomic lines of an unchangeable nature, but rather opened to practices of makeup and cosmetics – a cosmetic that aims to improve natural face features, in order to express inside beauty. Faces were regarded as mirrors of souls, and eyes become streets introducing to inside spirituality. Moreover, the aesthetical appreciation has had the tendency to go progressively downwards until it concerned the whole human body, a no more ideal but relative beauty, different from person to person. And the beauty of the women was reappraised in relation to its great social function, the maternity. Again, wide hip were a signal of possibly being a good mother.

The emergence of the mass in the social environment of more and more big towns has brought to a new aesthetical logic, whose aim is the single individual: everyone is beautiful for what he/she is or able to become, thus valorizing one's good-looking feature and hiding or eliminating the ones considered ugly. Beauty is now rendered erotic, as novelists and painters of modern life express: no more a spiritual ideal, on the contrary the beautiful must satisfy human senses. And thus, we are back to present days, in which diet and exercise, then cosmetic and institutes of beauty, finally surgery and operating rooms are a supreme hymn to a new standardization of aesthetical canon, maybe partly hidden from the search of the self more in depth, partly ought to the strong assumption that a person's worth is measured by his appearance. Beauty is shaped by a set of cultural considerations and, as Eagleton (1984; cited in Zangwill 2002) notice

> The category of the aesthetic assumes the importance it does in modern Europe because in speaking of art it speaks of these other matters too [freedom and legality, spontaneity and necessity, self-determination, autonomy, particularity and universality,], which are at the heart of the middle class's struggle for political hegemony.

There is a certain evidence, indeed, that not only we think positively about beautiful people but also that we tend to treat them more favourably in interpersonal situations.

In the last century, a great variability of human beauty, especially woman's, has been progressively shaped: from an idealization of fragile and delicate features to voluptuous and rounded figures, from accentuation of breast and hip curves and musculature to thinner bodies. It appears also that, in a more recent partial change of western concept of beauty from voluptuous and round features, like the 90–60–90 breast–waist–hip ratio, to linear and thin bodies, often these beauty myths project a potentially physically unhealthy ideal to society, raising worry about mental health due to eating disorders and body mage problems (Sarwer 2003).

In the communication era, in which our perception is also a product of media influence, reasons for social success or failure of different beauty ideas and also of certain products of the culture like music, painting, architecture and so on are difficult to understand. Among two products of the same kind, with equivalent quality, one succeed while the other is destined to premature disappearance. It is often the first one to be judged beautiful while the second is not. To understand fashion processes, chaos and complexity theories are useful to understand this "inequity", which is not an effect of specific human mind and rationality, but properly the effect of what mathematicians call nonlinear chaotic phenomenon.

Georg Simmel (1905) in his essay on fashion general theory and analysis of beauty claimed that fashion is an unstable process, depending on two conflicting and interactive forces. The first is the impulse of every human being to imitate somebody else, usually someone who is felt superior or, however, worthy of imitation. Second, the impulse of each to be distinguished from the really similar one, above all from the people felt as inferior for some reason. The relationship among these tendencies, imitation and distinction varies in every human being, but both practice a noticeable strength. Let us consider, for instance, the short shirts brought by girls that show the bellybutton. After being accepted by some influential women, living on highest social classes or in the most influential cultures, first of all in the great western metropolises, gradually the exhibition of this trait has been imitated by other women, living in different social conditions or in different areas. But as the dress get propagated, becoming more and more a status symbol, it becomes also less and less distinguishing. Then, those trendies women who first proposed it will have the tendency to leaving it, passing to something else. A perennial instability, given that a mass triumph is equivalent, after a certain time, to a "forced" fashion, therefore on the sunset avenue.

But this is only the sense of fashion, which should be different from the sense of beauty. As Etcoff (1999) argues quoting Charles Baudelaire, "fashion is the «amusing, enticing, appetizing icing on the divine cake», not the cake itself."

Anyway, among other philosophical thoughts, there is an aesthetic historicism, arguing that there is not any innate and cultural universal concept of beauty. As Bourdieu writes (1984; cited in Zangwill 2002) about Kantian positions,

> Kant's analysis of the judgment of taste finds its real basis in a set of aesthetic principles which are the universalization of the dispositions associated with a particular social and economic condition.

22.4 Mathematical Formalized Beauty

During seventeenth century, Galileo, first among scientists, declared that the book of nature was written in the language of mathematics. This idea, at least for what concerns beauty, is decidedly older. In the previous paragraphs some ratios regarding human body have emerged, but not yet the king of mathematical proportions, the *golden* one. It has been often claimed, from the ancient times, that the golden section allows the division of a segment in the most aesthetically pleasant way. For this reason, it has been often incorporated in many studies, sculptures and paintings, designs and constructions of artwork and talent operas.

A segment is divided in its golden section if the ratio between the shorter and the bigger part is the same as the ratio between the bigger part and the whole segment. In mathematical terms, through the proportion $(1-x):x = x:1$, it is given by the positive solution of $x^2 + x - 1 = 0$. Its exact value is $\left(\sqrt{5}-1\right)/2$, conventionally named φ or, approximating, we may consider the value 0.618. The number $\Phi = 1 + \varphi \cong 1.618$, obtainable considering the extension instead of division, i.e. the extension of the segment in such a way that the parts and the new length are in the same ratio, together with π and e, is one of the most important irrational numbers in mathematics, due to its being solution, as the others, of a basic mathematical problem.

These numbers hold appealing infinite numerical expressions, for example, the ones represented by a continuous fraction and a continuous radix that use just the number "1":

$$\Phi = 1 + \frac{1}{1+\frac{1}{1+\frac{1}{\cdots}}}, \Phi = \sqrt{1+\sqrt{1+\sqrt{1+\sqrt{\cdots}}}}$$

The ratio, anyway, seems rooted with a millenary history, with Egyptians often credited of having this knowledge, but for sure possessed by ancient Greeks, whose painters, sculptors and architects already used it in the creation of their operas, for dividing their artwork in well-proportioned parts. Then, transmitted through the history, from Romans (as confirmed by Vitruvius) to the Medieval and Renaissance periods, artists and architects made large use of it, for legendary reasons and for its easy construction. In the sixteenth century, interest was so widespread as to convince Luca Pacioli to write the treatise *De Divina Proportione*, describing in detail its geometrical properties. Pacioli found five attributes in this proportion, making it "divine". The first four were related to the basic elements of earth, air, fire and water: it is unique, it is expressed with three terms – like trinity, it cannot be reduced to integer or rational numbers – as God is ineffable, it has self-similarity – as God is unchanging and omnipresent. The fifth attribute was instead related to the formal being of heaven, from one side expressed by Plato's dodecahedron, from the other side expressed by Aristotelian's quintessence. The section, specifically, had to be used in the construction of the 12 pentagons constituting the dodecahedron.

Just a century after, the astronomous Kepler explicited his personal and historical thought: "Geometry has got two treasures: one is the theorem of Pythagoras; the other, the division of a line into extreme and mean ratio. The first we may compare to a measure of gold; the second we may name a precious jewel" (cited in Huntley 1970).

On the origins of the name "golden section" has been long debated. For example, Fowler (1982) claims that the first English use of the term is in the 1875 edition of the *Encyclopedia Britannica*, in James Sully's article on aesthetics. The symbol Φ, indeed, comes from the first letter of the Greek sculptor and architect Phidias that, according to legend, was one of the main proponents of the aesthetic qualities of the ratio. He used it in the construction of his artistic works, such as the Parthenon. Also the usage of the symbol Φ, however, seems enough recent.

This ratio is present in many mathematical constructions: in the regular pentagon it is the relation between its sides and diagonals; in the regular pentagram (stars with five ends constructed on the regular pentagon) it is the relation between the lengths of the legs and the bases of such ends and so on. Some occurrences are also in arithmetic, for instance, the logarithmic spiral is easily constructable from a golden rectangle (whose sides respect such ratio). It seems also connected to many forms in nature, where some geometrical properties of the golden ratio are present through fillotaxis and flower and plant forms (pineapples, pine cons, sunflowers), through sea creatures (as shells, tritons, abalons) and so on.

One of the most important occurrences relies in being the limit of the ratio between two sequential numbers in Fibonacci series. Just to remind the reader, the Fibonacci series begins with 0, 1, 1, 2, 3, 5, 8, 13, ... and created through the recurrence relation $f_n = f_{n-1} + f_{n-2}$. Beyond elegance and simplicity inherent in the equation, the amount of cultural and historical tradition, the ratio f_n / f_{n-1} approaches Φ at infinity and the Binet formula $f_n = 1 \big/ \sqrt{5}\,(\Phi^n + (-1)^n \varphi^n)$ holds.

Some years ago we showed (Eugeni-Mascella 2001) that this formula could be simply generalized by taking the relation $F_n = aF_{n-1} + bF_{n-2}$ with a and b, and the initial conditions p and q, chosen as pleasant between reals. This generalized Fibonacci series includes many other series (Bell, Lucas, Bell–Lucas and their generalized versions) as particular cases. What is interesting is that considering the limit at infinity $\Phi_{a,b}$ of the ratio F_n / F_{n-1}, then nice properties arises like

$$\Phi_{a,b} = a + \cfrac{b}{a + \cfrac{b}{a + \frac{b}{\cdots}}}, \Phi_{a,b} = \sqrt{b + a\sqrt{b + a\sqrt{b + a\sqrt{b + \cdots}}}} \text{ if } a > -\sqrt{b}$$

leaving us to imagine that $\Phi_{a,b}$ could be a natural generalization of the golden section.

But does the golden section represent simply a mathematical abstraction or is really a universal aesthetic ideal? It is interesting to note that some research have been developed on the aesthetic questions arisen from this mathematical concept, for instance, whether the aesthetic questions at the base of the complex feeling of beauty find answers in a structuralist approach, being primarily psychophysical or in the combination of physical elements (Green 1995).

Fechner, considered the beginner of this experimental research on this matter, used three methods (subsequently used by others), i.e. (a) choice of figures from a certain number of alternatives, (b) production of drawings on objects with self-decided proportions and (c) use/examination of preexisting objects created by painters, architects and so on. The figures at the core of aesthetic investigation have often been the golden rectangle, and rarely other figures as golden triangle.

There seemed to be a general but ambivalent support for the idea that the golden rectangle and the ones in his closest neighbourhood are more preferred by people on average.

Remarkable works are due to Witmer, Pierce, Wundt, Titchener, Angier, Lalo, Weber, Thompson, Arhheim, Stone and Collins, Schiffman, Berlyne, Godkewitsch, Piehl, Svensson, Benjafield, McManus and others. These studies generally offer a broad vision outcoming from the general psychology theory in which the researcher used to work. Wundt, for example, tried to provide a general theory of aesthetic pleasure and, considering this a composite feeling, he observed that the aesthetic preference is connected with the associations with familiar objects and movements:

> The optical feeling of form shows itself first of all in the preference of regular to irregular forms and the in the preference among different regular forms of those which have certain simple proportions in their various parts. [...] The fact that symmetry is generally preferred for the horizontal dimensions of figures and the golden section for the vertical, is probably due to associations especially with organic forms, such as that of human body. This preference for regularity and certain simple proportions can have no other interpretations than that of measurement of every single dimension is connected with a sensation of movement and an accompanying sense-feeling which enters as a partial feeling into the total optical feeling of form (cited in Green 1995).

For Angier the symmetry is preferred because it gives rise to "a corresponding equivalence of bilaterally disposed organic energies, bought into equilibrium because acting in opposite directions [... and producing] a feeling of balance, which is, in symmetry, our aesthetic satisfaction" (Angier 1903).

After Pierce concluded that, rather than Φ, it is the equality to be the most important aesthetic division Titchener (1899) claimed that the preference for golden section could be a product at higher level of maturational process:

> The most pleasing division for a simple visual form was, originally, the symmetrical division. Symmetry is repetition with reversal: the two hands, two eyes, two halves of a circle, etc., are symmetrical. The proportion of parts, in a symmetrical figure, is accordingly that of equality. 1:1. At a higher level of aesthetic development, the symmetrical division is replaced by what is known as the golden section.

Also Piaget (1961) suggested that the individuals carry in their minds, for the purpose of comparison, some representation of parts of the visual displays. In such a way, the comparison may put in evidence the relations holding between the parts and drive to an aesthetic preference of a form.

For Thompson, the ratio is a matter of cultural transmission, not necessarily verbally. The Gestalstist Rudolf Arnheim (1974) instead wrote

> When a square is divided into two halves, the whole pattern prevails over its parts because di 1:1 symmetry of the square is simpler than the shapes of the two 1:2 rectangles. [...] If we now divide a 1:2 rectangle in the same manner, the figure breaks apart quite readily because the simplicity of the two squares imposes itself against the less compact shape of the whole. If, on the other hand, we wish to obtain a particularly coherent rectangle, we may apply our subdivision to the rectangle of the golden section [...] Traditionally and psychologically, this proportion of 1:0.618 has been considered particularly satisfying because of its combination of unity and dynamic variety. Whole and parts are nicely adjusted in strength so that the

> whole prevails without being threatened by a split, but at the same time the parts retain some self-sufficiency.

A lasting strategy of the opponents of the golden section has been to put it in contrast with the equality, but this has not put in trouble that part of psychologists, called "pythagorean", who believe that several rectangles having interesting ratios, also simple ones, show an aesthetic advantage over others. Benjafield (1980) observed:

> People tend to use two proportions more frequently than any others. When circumstances require a division into two equal parts, it seems obvious that people should be able to do so fairly accurately. However, when equal division is not required, we believe people tend to use the G[olden] S[ection].

Instead, the dominant trend of the last decades research has been to show that the golden section has not got any effect connected to beauty or pleasantness, and that the golden section is, at least psychologically, nothing more than a metaphysical speculation. So it should fade away, but the concept still remains in our interest because the phenomenon and the tradition carried by Φ seem to be mystical and difficult to let go away.

Green (1995) claimed that the traditional aesthetic effects of the golden section may be real, but are fragile and, in such a case, it is difficult to discern if they come from innate or learned structure. The history shows a continuous series of efforts to prove such effects to be illusory, followed by others who, in contrast, have restored them. In many research, apart from problem arising from the method of acquiring raw statistical data, subject scores have also been affected by various errors due to extraneous factors. In his words (Green 1995) "In the final analysis, it may simply be that the psychological instruments we are forced to use in studying the effects of the golden section are just too crude to ever satisfy the skeptic (or the advocate, for that matter) that there really is something there."

A more recent interesting subject concerns fractal geometry. Either the golden ratio rule holds or not, it seems unlikely to find a unique proportion for a mathematical formalization of the beauty and complex natural forms we constantly watch around us, whose boundaries are often characterized by irregularity and roughness. Moreover, it could be the euclidean geometry, with its perfect forms, that pertains mainly to artificial realities, whose abstract perfection is almost non-existent in nature and thus inadequate to formalize beauty.

As Mandelbrot (1977) wrote, "Clouds are not spheres, mountains are not cones, coastlines are not circles, and bark is not smooth, nor does lightning travel in a straight line." The complexity of the world we live in necessitates the use of radically different descriptive elements from those of traditional Euclidean geometry (Spehar 2003) to understand and possibly represent the irregular shapes of the real world. Fractals, that generally have a rough and fragmented geometric shape, can succeed in offering a topological representation very close to the real things. In other words, fractal principles can be used to give a mathematical description of a variety of natural phenomena, like coastlines, trees, clouds, mountain ranges, rivers and star clusters, and to create realistic and beautiful images or models of these phenomena.

Some examples are Cantor sets, Sierpinski triangle and carpet, Koch snowflake. The most famous, the Mandelbrot set, is obtained through the very simple recurrence relation $x_n = x_{n-1}^2 + c$. When these iterations are applied only to non-complex numbers (c real, rational, etc.), results are always known and predictable. But when c is a complex number, the behaviour changes completely. Depending on the values of c the iterative process will (a) immediately increase to infinity or (b) remain stable for a certain number of iterations, and later fall into infinity or (c) remain always stable, never falling into infinity. The magic of fractal images at this point arises by using colouring algorithm in order to differentiate such behaviours, also the various numbers of iterations to perform in the cases (b) before been attracted to infinity.

The constant c may initially seem non-influential, instead reveals a big sensitivity of the squaring process on complex numbers, like weather and stock markets, where negligible changes can produce unexpected chaotic effects. Thus, chaotic dynamical systems are often associated with fractals. The order behind the chaotic production of numbers by the Mandelbrot formula can only be seen through computer computation and graphic portrayal. After millions of mathematical computation and plotting, the seemingly randomness and meaninglessness vanish and the hidden geometric order is revealed, often presenting (depending on the fractal type) self-similarity over different scales, eventually at an infinite scale. For instance it happens also in real objects. If we look at the irregular shape of a coastline, then look closer at a small part of it, we will probably find the same basic shape of the whole coastline repeated on a smaller scale. But the beauty of these mathematical objects seems independent from their conformity to some existing natural object. Many representations of fractals appear aesthetically appealing and rich in structure, representatives of a new artistic dimension, strictly connected also to the choice of colours (Yaz 2004).

However, the ubiquity of fractals in nature has inspired several studies to investigate the relationship between fractals' patterns and perceived beauty. Some pioneering empirical studies (Aks 1996, Spehar 2003) pointed out, in particular, that fractals with dimensions between 1.3 and 1.5 were considered the most aesthetically appealing, with a positive correlation between preferred fractal dimension and a self-determined measure of creativity.

It might also be that, given their simplicity, elegance and beauty of their graphical representation, scientists are more confident in declaring fractals close to reality. This is what somehow happens with scientific theories, where aesthetical features – now represented by various aspects beyond physical forms – seem to the researcher a way to truth. As Paul Dirac observed "It is more important to have beauty in one's equations than to have them fit experiment."

22.5 Conclusion

Beauty is at once subjective and objective. It really exists; cultures and individuals cannot live without the ability for beauty and, nevertheless, it cannot be described by any statement, any finite algorithm or set of rules. The fact that all cultures have a sense of beauty, whatever are its roots, shows that the aesthetic response should have at least partly biological roots. From the other hand, our aesthetic judgments seem to be explained also by social factors. Not completely, but certainly our judgments are affected by social circumstances.

Some mathematical models have been found along ancient and recent history, as golden ratio and fractals. Whether mathematical structures were able to adequately represent natural or artificial beauty, may also be influenced by their mystic symbolic formulation and its semantic meaning. As Bertrand Russel affirmed "Mathematics possesses not only truth but supreme beauty, a beauty cold and austere, like that a sculpture, sublimely pure and capable of a stern perfection, such as only the greatest art can show".

As Socrates concludes in Plato's Hippias Major, beauty is possibly the pleasure that comes from seeing and hearing, but his only certainty, with an agreeable sense of humour, is that he understands in depth the Greek proverb "beautiful things are difficult".

Bibliography

Aks, D. and Sprott, J. C. (1996). Quantifying aesthetic preference for chaotic patterns. *Emp. Stud. Arts* 14, 1–16.

Angier, R. P. (1903). The aesthetic of unequal division. *Psycholo. Rev.*, 4, 541–561.

Arnheim, R. (1974). *Art and visual perception: A psychology of the creative eye*. Los Angeles: University of California Press.

Benjafeld, J., Pomeroy, E., and Saunders, M. (1980). The golden section and the accuracy with which proportions are drawn. *Canad. J. Psychol.* 34, 253–256.

Bourdieu, P. (1984). *Distinction*. London: Routledge & Kegan.

Buss, D. M. (1994). The evolution of desire: strategies of human mating. New York: Basic Books.

Darwin, C. (1859). On the origin of species by means of natural selection, or the preservation of favoured races in the struggle for life; it. Trans. L. Fratini, Boringhieri, Torino: 1980.

Darwin, E. (1802). *Zoonomia* (3rd edn). London: Johnson.

Eagleton, T. (1984). *The ideology of the aesthetic*. Oxford: Blackwell.

Eco, U. (2004). *Storia della bellezza* (3rd edn) Milano: Bompiani .

Etcoff, N. (1999). *Survival of the prettiest. The science of beauty*. New York: Random House.

Eugeni, F. and Mascella, R. (2001). A note on generalized fibonacci numbers. *J. Discr. Math. Sci. Cryp.* 4(1), 33–45.

Fechner, G. T. (1876). *Vorschule der Aesthetik*. Leipzig: Breitkopf & Härtel.

Fowler, H. D. (1982). A generalization of the golden section. *Fibonacci Quart.*, . 20, 146–158.

Gangestad, S. W. and Buss, D. M. (1993). Pathogen prevalence and human mate preferences. *Ethol. Sociobiol.*, 14, 89–96.

Green, C. D. (1995). All that glitters: a review of psychological research on the aesthetic of the golden section. *Perception*, 24, 937–968.

Hume, D. (1740). *A treatise of human nature*. E. C. Mossner (Ed.), London: Penguin Books, 1969.

Huntley, H. E. (1970). *The divine proportion: A study in mathematical beauty*. New York: Dover.

Jacobsen, T., Schubotz, R. I., Höfel, L., et al. (2006). Brain correlates of aesthetic judgment of beauty. *NeuroImage*, 29, 276–285.

Kanazawa, S. and Kovar, J. L. (2004). Why beautiful people are more intelligent. *Intelligence*, 32, 227–43.

Kant, I. (1790). *Critique of Judgment*, En. trans. J. C. Meredith. Oxford: Oxford University Press, 1997.

Langlois, J. H., Roggman, L. A., Casey, R. J., et al. (1987). Infant preferences for attractive faces: rudiments of a stereotype? *Develop. Psychol.*, 23, 363–369.

Langlois, J. H., Roggman, L. A., and Mussleman, L. (1994). What is average and what is not average about attractive faces? *Psycholo. Sci.* 5, 214–220.

Mandelbrot, B. (1977). *The fractal geometry of nature*. New York: Freeman.

McMahon, J. A. (1999). Towards a unified theory of beauty. *Literat. Aesthe.*, 9, 7–27.

McManus, I. C. (1980). The aesthetics of simple figures. *Br. J. Psychol.* 71, 505–524.

Mothersill, M. (1984). *Beauty restored*. Oxford: Clarendon Press.

Pacioli, L. (1509). *De Divina Proportione*. Turin: Aragno, 1999.

Perlovsky, L. I. (2006). Toward physics of the mind: concepts, emotions, consciousness, and symbols. *Phy. Life Rev.* 3, 23–55.

Piaget, J. (1961). *Les méchanismes perceptifs*. Paris: Presses Universitaires de France.

Rhodes, G. (2006). The evolutionary psychology of facial beauty. *Ann. Rev. Psychol.* 57, 199–226.

Sarwer, D. B., Grossbart, T. A., and Didie, E. R. (2003). Beauty and society. *Semin. Cutaneous Med. Surg.* 22(2), 79–92.

Short, L. (1991). The aesthetic value of fractal images. *Br. J. Aesthet.* 31(4), 342–355.

Simmel, G. (1905). *Die mode*. It. trans. D. Formaggio & L. Perucchi, *La moda*, Editori Riuniti, Roma, 1985.

Smith, C. U. M. (2005). Evolutionary neurobiology and aesthetics. *Perspect. Biol. Med.* 48, (1), 17–30.

Spehar, B., Clifford, C. W. G., Newell, B. R., and Taylor, R. P. (2003). Universal aesthetic of fractals. *Comput. Graph.* 27, 813–820.

Titchener, E. B. (1899). *An outline of psychology*. New York: MacMillan.

Vigarello, G. (2004). *Histoire de la beauté. Le corps et l'art d'embellir de la Renaissance à nos jours*, Seuil, Paris; it. trans., L'Erario, M. *Storia della bellezza: il corpo e l'arte di abbellirsi dal Rinascimento a oggi*, Donzelli, Roma, 2007.

Wittgenstein, L. (1966). *Lectures and conversations on aesthetics, psychology and religious belief.* C. Barrett (Ed.). Oxford: Blackwell.

Yaz, N. and Hacısalihoglu, H. H. (2004). On fractal colouring algorithms. *Dynam. Sys. Appl.. Proceed.* 706–711.

Zangwill, N. (2002). Against the sociology of the aesthetic. *Cultur. Valu.* 6(4), 443–452.

Chapter 23
Visual Impact and Mathematical Learning

Monica Idà and Cécile Ellia

Abstract In the years 2005–2007 quite a big project took place in more than 1700 Italian schools, with the aim of stimulating interest in young people toward sciences like chemistry, physics, and mathematics. This chapter is a report on one of the laboratories of the project, namely "M.C. Escher: mathematics in art." The object of the laboratory dealt with a very well-known aspect of the work of the artist, that is, tiling of the plane. The students involved in the laboratory were invited to first carefully observe some of Escher's works, and then to find the geometry lying behind them. Successively, they were asked to produce new patterns on their own. One point of interest was to observe the reaction of young people to a visual presentation, carrying a strong aesthetic component, of a mathematical problem.

In the years 2005/2006 and 2006/2007 quite a big project took place in more than 1700 Italian schools, with the aim of stimulating interest in young people toward sciences like chemistry, physics, and mathematics. The name of the project was "Progetto Lauree Scientifiche." School and university teachers joined their efforts to organize workshops where high school students could have a live approach to these sciences, different from the usual one of the teacher at the blackboard talking with the students listening.

I was the one responsible for the laboratory "M.C. Escher: mathematics in art" held in Bologna. The object of the laboratory dealt with a very well-known aspect of the work of Mauritius Cornelius Escher, that is, tiling of the plane. The artist produced wonderful work in this field, and there is a lot of mathematics hidden there, so this seemed a promising topic to work on. One point of interest from my point of view was to observe the reaction of young people to a visual presentation, carrying a strong aesthetic component, of a mathematical problem.

M. Idà (✉)
Department of Mathematics, University of Bologna, 40126 Bologna, Italy
e-mail: ida@dm.unibo.it

Illustrations by Cécile Ellia (e-mail: cecile.ellia@mail.polimi.it). The animations from which the pictures are taken are visible on http://www.dm.unibo.it/~ida/simmetrie.htm

V. Capecchi (eds.), *Applications of Mathematics in Models, Artificial Neural Networks and Arts*, DOI 10.1007/978-90-481-8581-8_23,

A regular tiling is a covering of the plane using infinitely many identical tiles, where there are no empty spaces and no overlaps, but we allow rotating the tiles or turning them upside down. Here is an example:

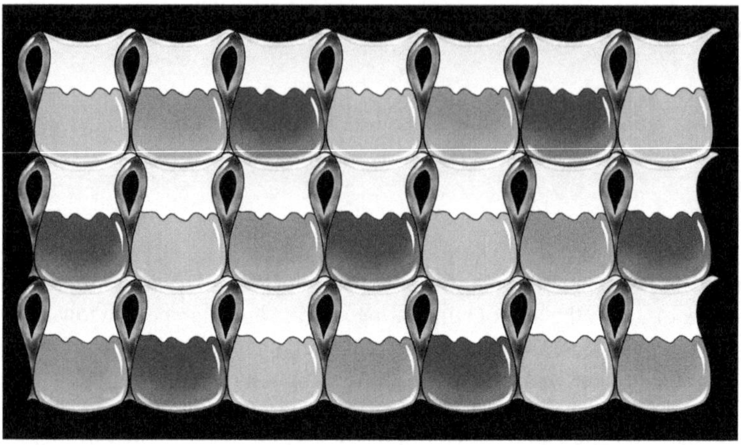

In his tilings, Escher made use of animals, devils, angels, and monsters which fitted together perfectly; he used to say that he was obsessed by this problem, and since he was an artist and not a scientist, he approached it using his imagination and manual ability, in addition to studying famous tilings and friezes, for example the ones in the Alhambra. The problem he was dealing with is in fact a mathematical problem: in how many ways can we cover the plane with a regular tiling? If we ask that there be two independent directions along which the drawing repeats, the choices are not a lot: exactly 17. In order to try to get at the heart of the question, we will not, for example, distinguish between these two tilings:

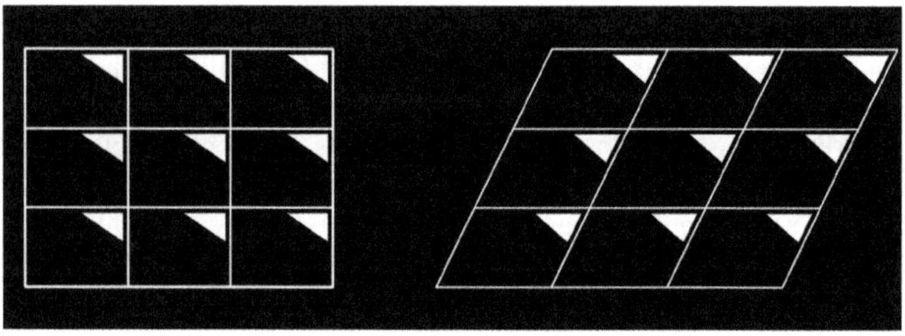

because the rigid motions occurring in these two cases are the same: merely translations. You can start with one tile and move it using translations, and if you do it an infinite number of times you cover the entire plane; or, what is the same, if you consider the entire tiling as an infinite drawing and you move it with one of these translations, you get the same drawing, that is, the tiling goes onto itself when you translate it.

If we want to get nicer compositions, we can start with a rectangular tile, cut out pieces of the tile from the lower border and add them on the upper border, and then do the same with the left and right borders, as the next figure shows.

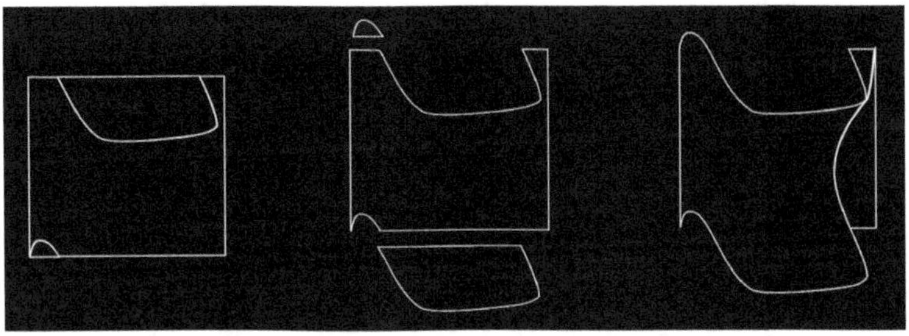

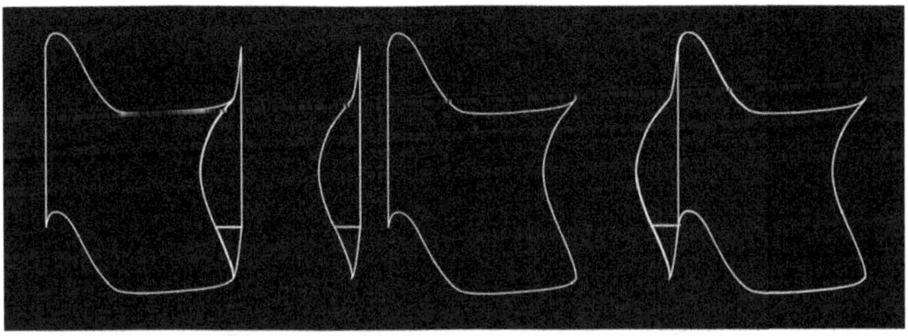

If we get a non-symmetric figure, nothing is changed from a mathematical point of view, since we get the tiling just moving the tile along two independent directions:

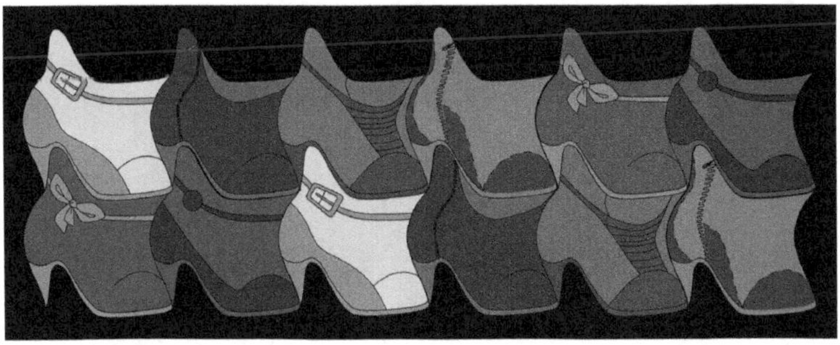

Now start with a rectangle, and cut out symmetric pieces; we get a symmetric figure:

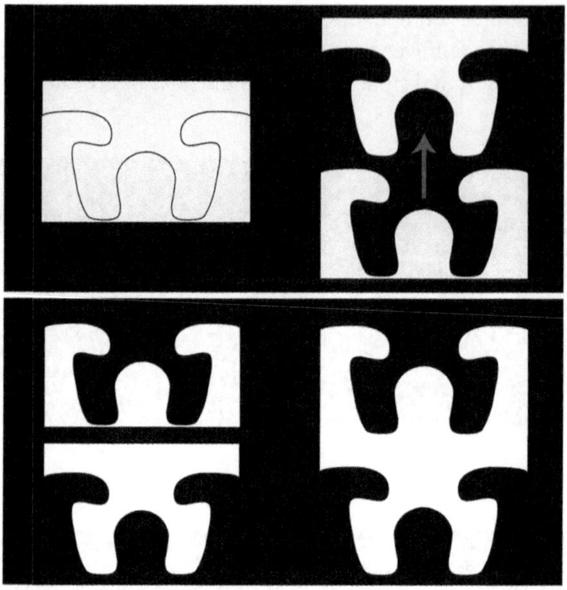

Again, we get a tiling just moving the monkey along two independent directions:

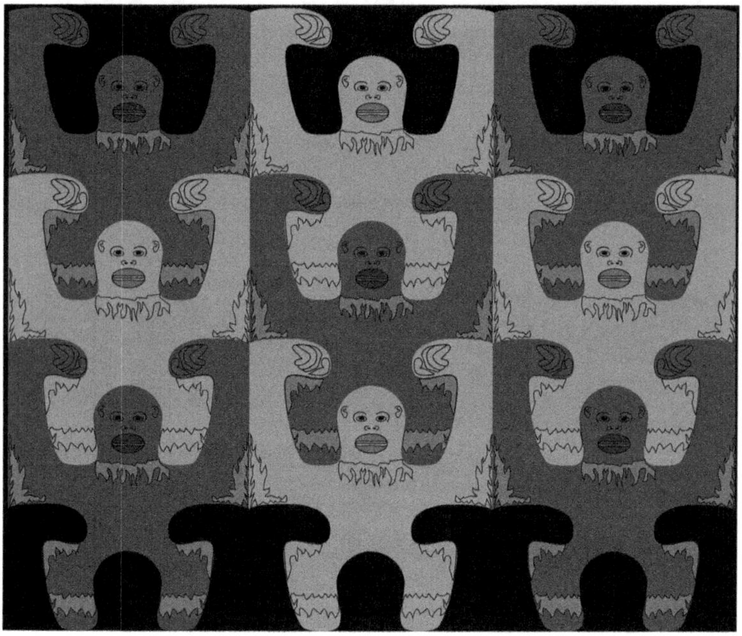

but the tiling obtained in this case is different from the previous ones, since there are more rigid motions which carry the tiling onto itself. Each monkey is symmetric with respect to its vertical axis, hence the reflection with respect to one of these axes carries the tiling onto itself; for the same reason, it is enough to use half a monkey as a tile:

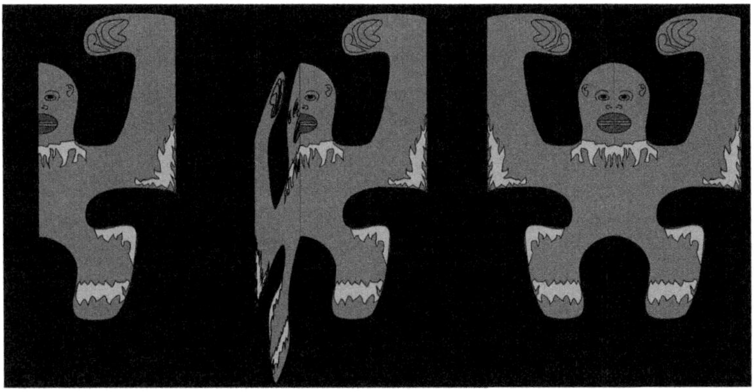

The rigid motions which carry the tiling onto itself, which is to say, which act on one tile moving it until it fills the whole plane without overlaps or empty spaces, form a group with the operation of composition, called the symmetry group of the tiling. The groups corresponding to the existing tilings are called crystallographic groups. As we saw above, the classification theorem for the plane crystallographic groups says that there are 17 such groups. These 17 types of tilings were found for the first time by a Russian chemist, E.S. Fedorov, and immediately after by A.M. Schönflies, in 1891; this is not strange if we think that the analogous problem in three dimensions consists of understanding in how many ways we can fill space with an infinitely repeated solid tile, which in this case will be a polyhedron; that is, what are the structures of the crystals.

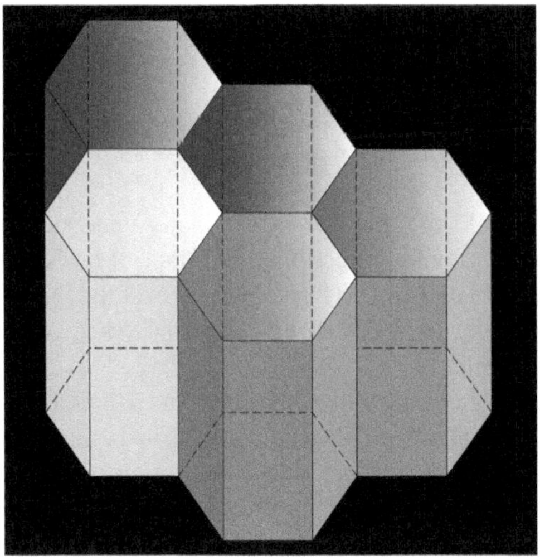

The answer is that there are 219 spatial crystallographic groups (or 230 if we classify with respect to orientation-preserving affine transformations). The n-dimensional problem appears in Hilbert's 18th Problem. If $n = 4$, there are 4783 crystallographic groups.

As one might expect, the proof of the classification theorem for the plane crystallographic groups uses tools from Euclidean geometry and group theory. One of the numerous lemmas which are used says that, if in the symmetry group of a tiling there are rotations of 90°, then in the group there are also rotations of 180°, whose centers lie in the middle points of two centers of rotations of 90°. Look, for example, at this tiling, where the dots denote the centers of rotations of 180°, while the squares denote the centers of rotations of 90°:

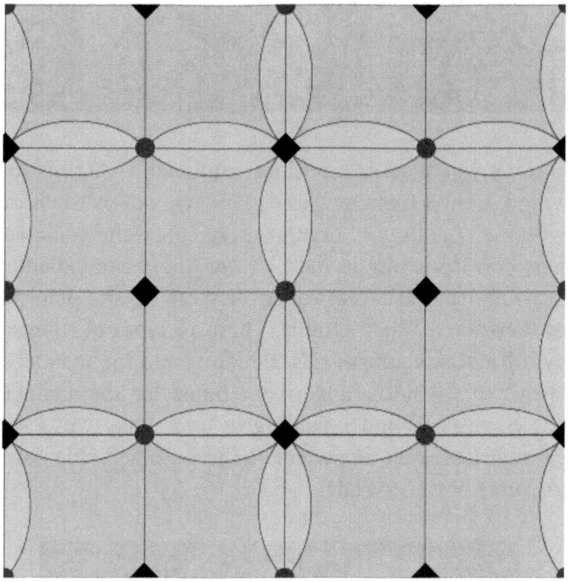

If we try to cancel the rotations of 180°, transforming their center in centers of rotations of 90°, automatically new rotations of 180° appear (see figure in next page).

Once one student told me that she really finally understood this lemma not by reading it in a book, but by looking at the tiled floor of her kitchen. The laboratory "M.C. Escher: mathematics in art" tries to do exactly this: use images, possibly beautiful, fascinating images like the ones of Escher, to arouse mathematical curiosity in young people.

The laboratory was held in both 2005/2006 and 2006/2007, involving more or less 200 high school students, of different ages (14–19) and aptitudes; there were groups of very motivated and clever students as well as of very young students who were not particularly interested in math. But the subject is very ductile and can be approached at various levels. The students in each class or group worked on their

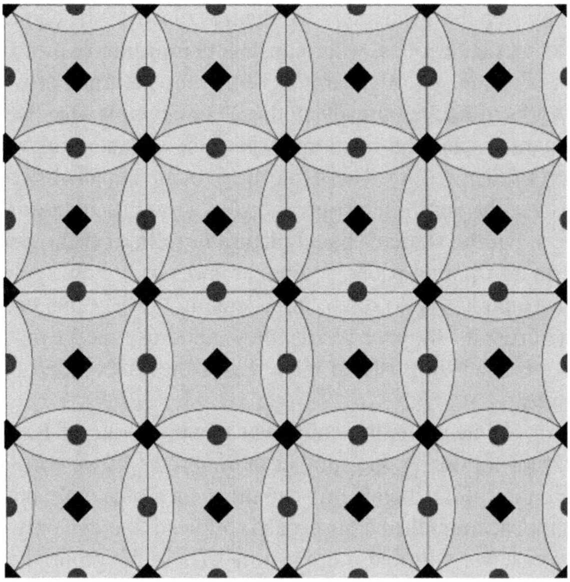

own, overseen by a teacher and an older student (usually an university or a PhD student).

The students involved in the laboratory were invited to first carefully observe some of Escher's works on the regular division of the plane and then to find the geometry lying behind them. For example, they were invited to find the translation lattice: one or more fundamental domains, that is, the possible shape of a tile; which rigid motions are symmetries for the tiling; what are the relations among those rigid motions; what happens taking or not taking the colors into account, or adding new colors, and so on. During the planning stage of the laboratory, in the first meeting the same kind of exercises were proposed to grown-up people, namely, the teachers involved in the laboratory; we all noticed that young people, once they understood the game, were much quicker in decoding images than adults, and this is clearly due to the revolution that computers and audiovisual methods in general have brought in the children's development.

Isometries of the plane are always included in scholastic programs, so many of the participants knew something about them. The teacher of the younger ones, i.e., students in the first year of high school, seized the opportunity of introducing isometries in a very intuitive way.

Successively, the students were asked to produce new patterns on their own. Different instruments, according to the age of the students concerned, were proposed, from pencil, scissors, and glue to different packages available on the net.

Some step-by-step exercises were then proposed to the older and more motivated students, these usually being students in the last or second to last year of high school, and with a penchant for math. The idea was to make them find by themselves the algebraic instruments needed for a deeper mathematical understanding of Escher's works. So step by step these exercises led them to discover the equation of a general isometry and of particular ones, what happens composing two of them, and so on until the notion of group and of generators of a group naturally arose, and permitted revisiting the works of Escher already studied. For example, they were asked to find a system of generators and the relations among those generators for the symmetry group of a given Escher's tiling. These questions treated in an abstract way and with more generality can be very interesting and also very difficult from the mathematical point of view, but the students had a picture in front of them, and reproductions of this picture on transparent paper, so that, to understand how symmetries worked, they could, for example, try to rotate, translate, and reflect this copy until it overlapped with the original. In other words, they could use their eyes and their hands to help their comprehension, and in many cases they succeeded in giving correct answers brilliantly.

Another point of interest is the color. For example, one of Escher's works has blue and pink crabs following one another in long rows. If we consider the drawing alone, forgetting the colors, a pink crab can move on a blue crab; but if we decide to take the colors into account then a pink crab is allowed to move only on another pink one. In the first case we will find more symmetries in the group than in the second one, and the structure itself of the group can change, or not, according to the cases. Older students were asked to understand what happens varying the colors in some of the pictures studied. Since the mathematical approach to color would have been too complicated for the younger ones, an "artistic" one has been used with them; they produced (with a lot of enthusiasm!) a lot of variants of a given tiling changing the colors so that it remained a tiling, i.e., taking care of the periodicity. This again was done with various instruments, on paper with crayons and paint brushes or on the computer; at the final meeting one group of students wore T-shirts on which they had printed their work!

Naturally, various difficulties arose in the course of this experience. For example, there were some students absolutely determined not to get involved; they were interested neither in mathematics nor in art, nor in general in anything proposed by the teacher; but luckily there were very few of them, and on the whole the students' reactions were very positive. As I said above, there were students attending a non-scientifically oriented high school, without any particular feeling toward mathematics; but in most cases at the beginning the aesthetic side captured them, and toward the end they were speaking with enthusiasm not only about Escher's works, but also about isometries of the plane!

I am more and more convinced that we should place, side by side to the traditional teaching of mathematics, a sort of Socratic teaching: the teacher tries to stimulate interest on a given subject, and then asks questions. Even if the student is not able to answer, the effort the student makes in trying to answer will make him/her more receptive and able to understand the real problems that the formal language of mathematics could otherwise obscure. Such a way of teaching has the evident defect that it requires a lot of time, but sometimes quality is more important than quantity!

Bibliography

Artin, M. (1997). *Algebra*. Bollati Boringhieri, Torino.
Coxeter, H. S. M. (1961). *Introduction to geometry*. John Wiley & Sons, New York.
Coxeter, H. S. M. (1985). Coloured symmetry. In *M. C. Escher: Art and science*. Proceedings on the international congress on M.C. Escher, Roma 2628 marzo 1985. Edited by H. S. M. Coxeter, M. Emmer, R. Penrose, and M. I. Tenber, North Holland 1986.
Dedò, M. (2000). *Forme: simmetria e topologia*. Zanichelli, Bologna.
Ernst, B. (1990). *Lo specchio magico di M. C. Escher*. Taschen, Köln.
Iversen, B. (1990–1991). *Lectures on crystallographic groups*. Matematisk Institut, Aarhus Universitet, Lecture Notes Series 1990/1991 No. 60.
Martin, G. E. (1982). *Transformation geometry – An introduction to symmetry*. Springer, New York.
Weyl, H. (1975). *La simmetria*. Feltrinelli, Milano.
http://web.unife.it/progetti/geometria/Escher_A/index.htm
http://www2.polito.it/didattica/polymath/htmlS/probegio/GAMEMATH/TassellaturePenrose/TassellaturePenrose.htm
http://www.mcescher.com/
http://users.erols.com/ziring/escher.htm
http://www.clarku.edu/~djoyce/wallpaper/index.html
http://matematica.uni-bocconi.it/tassellatura1/home.htm
http://www2.polito.it/didattica/polymath/htmlS/argoment/Matematicae/Maggio_05/Escher.htm
http://www.scienceu.com/geometry/articles/tiling/wallpaper.html
http://www2.spsu.edu/math/tile/index.htm
http://www.math.okstate.edu/~wolfe/border/border.html

Chapter 24
Art by Numbers

Mel Bochner, Roman Opalka, and other Philarithmics

The number, object and subject of paintings, sculptures, drawings, video, films, photographs and installations have revealed an aesthetic potential that had remained latent and unexpressed up until the first decades of the last century. For a long time, the number in figurative arts was only the result of a transitive counting, an answer to the question "How many?" Virtues, planets, apostles, ranks of angels, seasons, star signs, senses have been reproduced, personified, represented according to their number, in a correlation often tight enough to transcend into cliché (Rigon 2006). Conversely, the number has expressed measurements, relationships and proportions necessary for the shaping of forms and their conclusion, as in the much-celebrated case of the golden section. The graphic signs that embody the numbers were never given more space, in art works, than that needed to indicate a date or the coordinates of a biblical passage, with rare exceptions. Amongst these we must at least mention the allegories of *Arithmetics and Mathematics*,[1] almost invariably present in the cycles depicting the liberal arts (as was the case originally with Giacinto Brandi's

M. Bochner (✉)
New York artist represented by Peter Freeman Galery, New York, USA
e-mail: info@peterfreemaninc.com

[1] See the entries *Aritmetica* and *Mathematica* taken from the 1611 Paduan edition of Cesare Ripa's *Iconology* (respectively on pp. 30 and 328–329). "Arithmetic. A woman of handsome appearance, holding an iron hook in her right hand, a white board in her left and in the hem of her clothing the writing: Par et impar. The beauty will be a hint to the perfection of numbers, of which some Philosophers believed all things to be composed, and God, from which no other thing than perfection can proceed, made everything in number, in weight and measure, and this is the true subject of Arithmetic. The metal hook and the white board demonstrate that with those instruments we know the reason of various types of things and the things composed by the number, weight and measure of the Elements. The motto Par et impar declares what it is that gives all diversity to the accidents and all demonstrations. Arithmetic. [another definition contained in the same page]. A woman that holds in both hands a board with numbers and another one next to her feet on the ground". "Mathematics. A middle-aged woman, dressed in a white transparent veil, with wings on her head, tresses down her shoulder, with a compass in her right hand, measuring a board bearing some figures and numbers and held by a young boy to whom she is talking and teaching, with the other hand she holds a large ball representing the earth with the hours and the celestial orbits and on her dress is a frieze depicting mathematical figures, with her bare feet on a base [...]".

V. Capecchi (eds.), *Applications of Mathematics in Models, Artificial Neural Networks and Arts*, DOI 10.1007/978-90-481-8581-8_24,

oil painting now in the Whitfield Collection in London), some portraits of mathematicians and scientists, as well as very peculiar cases such as Dürer's *Melancholy II*, containing a magic square.

The number, less patently following the same fate as the word but on a similar path, knew its first emancipation from marginal note to subject with Cubist and Futurist painting, although with no immediate full autonomy or independence.

In the first and second decade of the twentieth century, avant-garde paintings – namely, the Cubist works of Pablo Picasso, Georges Braque and Juan Gris – contain numbers in ever-growing guises: excerpted from newspaper clippings, borrowed from car number plates or snippets of advertising, street numbers, telephone numbers, train timetables or sometimes built into the composition with no obvious reference to their origin. Exemplary from this viewpoint is the large 6943 standing out in *Stati d'animo: Gli Addii* (*Moods: Farewells*) by Umberto Boccioni (1911), indicating the number of the tank engine. Futurist works feature many more digits, specifically those by Gino Severini and Fortunato Depero, the latter the author, as early as the mid-1910s, of some drawings titled *Compenetrazione di numeri* (*Compenetration of Numbers*) offering elaborate graphic developments of numbers. European artists close to Futurism paid the same amount of attention to numbers, from the Portuguese Amadeo de Souza-Cardoso to the Polish Jan Hrynkowski, up to all the best exponents of the coeval and analogous Russian avant-garde, from Natalia Goncharova to Mikhail Larionov, Vladimir Majakovskij to El Lissitzky and Kazimir Malevich. The same interest was shown within the Dadaist movement, as clearly visible in many works by Kurt Schwitters, Hannah Höch, Raoul Hausmann and John Heartfield.

Giacomo Balla's *Numeri innamorati* (*Numbers in Love*), dating to the beginning of the 1920s, is one of the first examples of the liberation of the number from a more articulated and complex figurative context. Numerical figures are the uncontested protagonists of the work; they take shape and volume through a telescopic projection of the graphic sign and participate, together with the coloured planes in green, yellow, white and black, in the construction of a space markedly Constructivist in structure. Conversely, one number only dominates the famous *The Figure 5 in Gold*, an oil on carton produced by the American painter Charles Demuth in 1928 and inspired by the verses of William Carlos Williams' *The Great Figure*, where the poet lingers on the noisy and fast passage of a fire engine on the back of which a large, golden number 5 stands out: "Among the rain/and lights/I saw the Figure 5/in gold/on a red/fire truck/moving/tense/unheeded/to gong clangs/siren howls/and wheels rumbling/through the dark city" (Williams 1986, 174). The artist repeats the number three times, progressively smaller in order to convey the visual effect of the vehicle rapidly disappearing from sight. On the top left the word BILL and lower down CARLOS indicate the poets' Christian names, while the acronym WCW stands for his initials.

Although numbers appeared with a certain regularity in American painting even before this – see, for example, the work of artists such as Marsden Hartley or Stuart Davis – it was Demuth's painting that would serve as a paradigm for all those who, in the intervening years, nurtured a persistent interest in the representation of numbers. The influence exercised by *The* Figure 5 *in Gold* on Pop artists was decisive enough to be repeatedly declared, both through homage and direct quotations. The most famous take on the painting is due to Robert Indiana, who offered his own interpretation in 1963 with *The Figure 5* and *X-5*. Even before Indiana, Jasper Johns had evoked Demuth's painting in *Figure 5*, 1960, a sizable encaustic and collage piece today preserved in the Centre Georges Pompidou in Paris. The large number, like Indiana's reproduced in the same typeface as its model, loses in Johns' hands its heraldic and bright quality while acquiring pictorial qualities that, while reducing the neatness of the shape and the uniformity of the colour, soften the perception of the number as a mere, artificial abstract entity. The attraction towards numbers, shared by a vast majority of Pop artists, remained very strong for Johns and Indiana, who, over the course of the years, would continue proposing them as autonomous subjects in their compositions. Numbers, while pure pretexts for a painting for Jasper Johns, are perceived by Indiana as dominant elements in the urban landscape and rendered in an "objective" and anonymous fashion, intentionally remindful of the style of the so-called Precisionists from the 1920s and the 1930s, such as Charles Demuth and Charles Sheeler.

The phenomenon of the icastic representation of numbers was not limited to American Pop art; it was also present in analogous European movements, as proven by some famous works by Joe Tilson, Mario Schifano and Mario Ceroli. Even outside and beyond Pop art, the attraction to numbers has remained constant for artists of the most varied inclination and artistic tendency – as is the case of Pier Paolo Calzolari, Joseph Kosuth, Alighiero Boetti, Darren Almond, Micah Lexier and Charles Sandison – until becoming the main, when not exclusive, focus for some of them. Examples are Mario Merz's Fibonacci series, Hanne Darboven's body of work and, more recently, Tatsuo Miyajima's.[2]

Within this context of widely spread interest towards the number, we can identify some artists that have focused their attention not so much on the number itself but rather on the operation of counting. We refer to that intransitive counting that consists of listing the names of the numbers in their right order, potentially to infinity. "But the enactment of intransitive counting – as Mario Piazza reminds us – is not only a phonemic expression, that is to say only involving the sounds uttered (even mentally): it also includes the transcription of the letters (or figures)" (Piazza 2000, 9). The transcription of the infinite series of numbers, or the repetition of sequences, is a practice that some artists have adopted, some occasionally and some regularly, in certain cases with undertones hinting at manic obsession. Even before artists started devoting their art to the transcription of counting thus making it a piece, Aldous Huxley, in 1920, had given life to the character of Eupompus. Huxley

[2]Two recent exhibitions had as their subject the numbers in visual art. For an initial exploration on the subject, please see the respective catalogues: *Magie der Zahl in der Kunst des 20. Yahrhunderts*, exhibition catalogue (Stuttgart, Staatsgalerie, 1 February–19 May 1997), curated by Karin v. Maur, Verlag Gerd Hatje, Ostfildern 1997, *Numerica*, exhibition catalogue (Siena, Palazzo delle Papesse, 22 June 2007–6 January 2008), curated by Marco Pierini, Silvana Editoriale, Cinisello Balsamo 2007.

imagined the Alexandrine painter as the founder of a mystic–artistic sect devoted to the cult of the number, following the example of the Pythagoreans. "[Eupompus] just suddenly fell in love with numbers-head over ears, amorous of pure counting. Number seemed to him to be the sole reality, the only thing about which the mind of man could be certain. To count was the one thing worth doing, because it was the one thing you could be sure of doing right. Thus, art, that it may have any value at all, must ally itself with reality–must, that is, possess a numerical foundation. He carried the idea into practice by painting the first picture in his new style. It was a gigantic canvas, covering several hundred square feet–I have no doubt that Eupompus could have told you the exact area to an inch–and upon it was represented an illimitable ocean covered, as far as the eye could reach in every direction, with a multitude of black swans. [...] They gathered round Eupompus in a little school, calling themselves the Philarithmics. They would sit for hours in front of his great work, contemplating the swans and counting them; according to the Philarithmics, to count and to contemplate were the same thing. [...] Eupompus seems to have grown tired of painting merely numbers of objects. He wanted now to represent Number itself. And then he conceived the plan of rendering visible the fundamental ideas of life through the medium of those purely numerical terms into which, according to him, they must ultimately resolve themselves" (Huxley 1920). Some postulates of Eupompus' artistic theory seem to find an echo in researches developed almost half a century after the publication of the short story. It is astounding how Huxley introduced, albeit without being aware of it, the theme of the dissatisfaction produced by painting "numeric quantities", that is to say counting objects rather than the numbers themselves.

When Mel Bochner, in 1966, starts painting his first canvases with numeric sequences, he moves from an assumption similar to Eupompus', that is to say counting as the only thing that "one is sure one can do well". "Numbers give me the freedom to think about something else – said the artist – they have already been invented and don't belong to anyone" (Arditi 2003, 5). The certainty granted by numbers and their inevitable sequence made it possible for the artist to break free from the obligation of the "subject" in order to concentrate on painting pure and simple and on the relationship between language and space. With time, colour, which Bochner, in line with tradition, sees as the agent for the expression of emotion, has gained space within his research, without in any way downsizing the role of the "counted" numbers. These are not read exclusively proceeding from top to bottom and left to right; their reading sometimes unravels in anomalous sequences that force the eyes of the viewer to unusual journeys along the surface.

In the same year as Bochner's first paintings of numeric sequences, George Maciunas shot three very short films with numbers as their protagonists: *10 Feet*, *End After 9* and *1,000 Frames*, the last two titles being exclusively centred around intransitive counting. Both films faithfully illustrate what the titles declare, that is to say the end of the film – in the case of *End After 9* – as soon as the sequence of white numbers, starting from 1, reaches 9; in the second case, the very fast succession of 1000 frames, where the counting goes up to 1000 (although the counting is not linear: from 1 to 100 ten times, with a final result of 1000). The low resolution of the images, the unsteady camera and the tautology of the title all contribute to underline the ironic intentions of the Lithuanian artist, able to drag even cold, detached numbers into the creative chaos of Fluxus. Alighiero Boetti, too, adopted an ironic approach when he experimented with numbers for the first time in 1967.[3] *Contatore* (counter) lingers on the irrational impulse of observing the simultaneous changing of digits to tens and hundreds of thousands. Whether the attraction is purely aesthetic or whether it has to do with superstitious rites or with an unconscious (and ephemeral) desire for order, clarity and cleanliness, it is nevertheless difficult to avoid the visual appeal of such a "revolution". Boetti leaves us exactly halfway through the passage, suspending movement and catching just the instant when a number is no more and the next isn't yet. Rather than prolonging a pleasurable moment, this epoché uncovers all the vacuity and hollowness of the game.

1965/1 – ∞ is the work to which Roman Opalka has been devoting himself constantly and exclusively for over 40 years. The artist started transcribing the counting of numbers on the first canvas in the cycle, starting from one and tracing the digits with a thin brush, white against the black background. The second painting takes the counting up exactly from the last value drawn in the previous one. Opalka's monumental work carries on in the same way in the present day, the only variation being the progressive lightening of the background of the paintings, each of which, although perfectly complete in itself, is only a fragment of the project as a complex and is therefore called *Détail* (each canvas measures 196 cm × 135 cm). Later on, Opalka started taking photographic self-portraits in black and white inside his studio. The portraits, each measuring 30.5 cm × 24 cm, accompany the *Détail* paintings and complete them. The artist takes them wearing the same white shirt and the same expression, in the same white background and light conditions; they are perfectly identical, the only difference lying in the signs left by time on the artist's face. Opalka's work, a methodical transcription of the passing of time, is circumscribed within his own life and will end only with the artist's death, when the last of the painted numbers will not be followed by another one and the counting will be interrupted. This will leave the work not unfinished, but perfect. Regarding the progression of numbers applied to a life span, Opalka observed: "In the progression of my *Détails*: 1, 22, 333, 4444 belong to the beginning of the first *Détail*, 55555 is at the end of the second *Détail*. However, it took me seven years to reach 666666 after 55555. After 666666 (six time the Figure 6) I asked myself: How long will it take me to reach 7777777? I realised that, all being well, it would have taken me another thirty years to get to that 'seven times the figure seven'. Considering the hypothesis of the average life span for someone entirely devoted to this type of counting, this person would never reach 8 times the figure 8. 88888888 is the roof of a life span's space-time."[4]

---

[3]In this regard please see Bruno Corà, *Alighieroeboetti*, exhibition catalogue, Motta, Milano 2005, in particular the chapter *Numerologia, ars combinatoria*, pp. 151–157.

[4]Roman Opalka's untitled text, from which the quote is taken, is contained in *Opalka. 1965/1–∞*, Galleria Melesi, Lecco 1995, pp. unnumbered.

Jonathan Borofsky also sees the operation of counting according to the infinite progression that proceeds from the number one as a measure of one's existence, a reading of time adjusted according to a personal, intimate rhythm, inseparable from artistic practice.

As the artist recently stated: "For me, numbers are like God – They connect us all together in a way nothing else does. Like magic". Counting not only marked the dawn of his artistic activity but also deeply influenced its developments – even when he cut down on his practice or abandoned it altogether – in a journey that led Borofsky from piles of sheets of paper containing exclusively a progressive sequence of numbers (*Counting from 1 to Infinity in Progress*, 1969) to the drawings in which the number shares the space with post-surrealist representations to finish with the works signed not with the artist's name but with the last number counted that day. The artist recalls: "I began to do little 1, 2, 3; 1, 2, 3, 4; 1, 2, 3, 4, 5 writing of number sequences on paper almost as a way to pass the time and not have to think so deeply. Later, I made a decision to count from one to infinity and did write those numbers on paper. After about a year or two of doing that solely with nothing else, counting for a few hours a day as my art activity, I began to go to painting and sculpture again. I made this connection... instead of signing this painting I made today with my name, I'm going to sign it with the number I was on on this particular day when I stopped counting."[5]

Conversely, counting as the mere recording of the passing of time is at the basis of *9 Minutes* by James Riddle, one of many Fluxfilms produced by artists (mostly in 1966) and later collected by George Maciunas. Similar to Maciunas' films such as *1000 Frames*, the only protagonists of *9 Minutes* are the white numbers proceeding in a sequence. Their flow, this time, is ordered in series of 60 according to the rhythm of the passing of time; a number per second appears on the screen until reaching the first minute after 59; the sequence starts again eight times over. Real time and film time coincide perfectly, while the measuring of time becomes the only narrative plot of the work.

Although not of specific relevance to the subject of this contribution, we feel that we must at least mention in passing how in the past few decades the passing of time and its measurement in numerical terms have often been the focus of artistic investigation. Many artists – amongst whom Darren Almond, Alighiero Boetti, Charles Dreyfus, Felix Gonzalez-Torres, Joseph Kosuth, Jonathan Monk, Pablo Vargas Lugo, Ben Vautier and others – have sometimes specifically concentrated on the tool in charge of such a task, the clock.[6]

---

[5]Jonathan Borofsky interviewed by Ann Curran, published on the Carnagie Mellon Magazine (Spring 2002).

[6]Please see *Chronos. Il tempo nell'arte dall'epoca barocca all'età contemporanea*, exhibition catalogue, curated by Andrea Busto, Edizioni Marcovaldo, Caraglio 2005. We have not forgotten – we only thought it went beyond the confines of this contribution – that time can also be measured backwards, in terms of the interval separating us from a given event. In this case the time being recorded is normally extremely limited, substituting the immediate expectation of an arrival point – a zero that resolves the tension, potentially establishing a new starting point – to a perspective

Finally, Tatsuo Miyajima's research also focuses on the flowing of time, albeit not on its visual representation according to the schemes imposed by clocks or calendars. Miyajima uses hi-tech and adopts an aesthetics of numbers of undisputable modernity, the LED. The LED counters that animate his large installations as well as his smaller format works give shape to the numbers from 1 to 9, but they do so at different speeds and observe pauses of variable duration, as if each one was following its own rhythm, a tempo dictated from the inside. Even more than the veiled Pythagorean thought seemingly tangent to Miyajima's research, some of the words he has to say regarding digital numbers and their nature and potential are quite enlightening: "LED-generated digital numbers have all the digits from 0 to 9: the infinite, in every direction. All numbers can be found in LED. Digital numbers have all ten numbers contained in just one. This number has everything. This number is everything."[7] Words, once we remove the filter of time and technological distance, appear extraordinarily similar to those used by Fibonacci in the *incipit* of his *Liber Abaci*: "Novem figure Indorum he sunt 9 8 7 6 5 4 3 2 1. Cum his itaque novem figuris, et cum hoc signo 0, quod arabice zephirum appellatur, scribitur quilibet numerus".

Bibliography

Arditi, F. (2003). *Mel Bochner*. Exhibition catalogue, Roma: Il Gabbiano.
Huxley, A. (1920). *Eupompus gave Splendour to art by numbers*. In Limbo.
Piazza, M. (2000). *Intorno ai numeri. Oggetti, proprietà, finzioni utili*. Milano: Bruno Mondadori.
Rigon, F. (2006). *Arte dei numeri*. Milano: Skira.
Williams, W. C. (1986). *Sour grapes: A book of poems*. Boston: Four Seas Company, 1921 now in *Collected poems of William Carlos Williams: Vol. I 1909–1939*. New York: New Directions.

of counting towards infinity. Among the artists who interpreted the countdown with intelligence and irony and those who stand out are Guy Sherwin, with his short film on 16 mm titled *At the Academy* (1974) and Aïda Ruilova (*Countdowns* 2004), who dealt with the theme of the countdown by extracting it from the usual contexts that the collective imagination immediately places them in a film, space launches, the passage to a new year and so on.

[7] *Tatsuo Miyajima*, exhibition catalogue, curated by Achille Bonito Oliva, Electa, Milano 2004, p. 151.

Chapter 25
My Way of Playing with the Computer: Suggestions for a Personal Experience in Vector Graphics

Aldo Spizzichino

Abstract It is a widely held belief that using computers to produce graphics necessarily requires the use of sophisticated and expensive commercial software "packets." This is certainly true in the fields of advertising where hyper-realistic effects are used to emulate photography, for the visualization of scientific data, and for applications in the field of industrial production. I will show, however, that there is a possibility to follow another path, maybe technically more difficult, but probably more profitable in the sense of cultural progress. Herein I will describe designs (or experiences) realized in a Linux environment on a typical personal computer, without using proprietary software. The programs (written in Fortran 77) depend on a library of routines developed by the author and rely on the basic routines of the PGPLOT package which is freely available on the Internet.

Graphical programming is an excellent exercise for the understanding of geometric–mathematic concepts and for feeding creativity: a creativity which could take advantage of, and not be hindered by, simple programming procedures rather than using sophisticated pre-packaged inventories of effects.

If I leave you all with one main message, it is that of indicating how New Media can become the vehicle for a new form of craftsmanship and knowledge as long as it is used in a "virtuous" manner, that is, not passively.

In this post-industrial epoch of ready-made off-the-shelf products, a culture of do-it-yourself may be able to find a niche by means of new instruments, thereby rediscovering and promoting the ancient ties between art, mathematics, and science of nature.

The arrival and dissemination of computers in our society has, among other things, greatly strengthened studies and understanding in the area of the convergence between mathematics and art.

A. Spizzichino (✉)
Former researcher at INAF IASF-bo, Bologna, Italy
e-mail: aldo@computedart.org

V. Capecchi (eds.), *Applications of Mathematics in Models, Artificial Neural Networks and Arts*, DOI 10.1007/978-90-481-8581-8_25,

Having lived through the adventure of this fundamental revolution and having at my shoulders prior experience of producing graphics with traditional techniques, I found it natural since the 1980s to focus on creative activity based on the computer, exercising myself by blending geometric intuition and aesthetic sensitivity by means of the new conceptual and operative method of computer programming.

My background in physics research certainly helped in this, but probably of more influence was a certain natural inclination toward graphical expression combined with the fascination that natural shapes have always held for me.

In order to avoid ambiguity, I would immediately specify that we are not talking about frontline research, in the sense that it is not based on recent advances in mathematics or informatics; however it could be defined as a boundary under various profiles in which it exists:

In the region between art and science
Between classical and contemporary language
Between an aesthetic and a pedagogic approach

In a way it could be defined as a cutting edge (in a relative sense) from the point of view of the techniques employed and in the sense that I have always used instruments (both hardware and software) in an "improper" manner, pushing them to their limits, convinced as I am that "creativity" is the fruit of the desire to measure up to a challenge, trying to overcome the structural limits within which one works.

As an example of this attitude, I will begin by showing some works from the second half of the 1980s, created using an AppleIIe connected to a small electromechanical plotter (Figs. 25.1, 25.2, 25.3, 25.4, 25.5 and 25.6).

In those days, personal computers, as we know them today, were still a long way off, as were commercial graphics programs with their incredibly realistic, almost photographic effects.

Forms and structures, both natural and artificial, which effect aesthetic fascination and which are not excessively complex invite a modelization by means of computing.

Examples are shown in Figs. 25.1 and 25.2.

As we can see, from the first works I have experimented with a mix of regularity and random variability: an awareness which, from *De Nive Sexangula* of Kepler to today, has developed enormously.

From D'Arcy Thompson onward, we have looked at the form as an epiphenomenon of one or more developmental rules. Computer graphics is a perfect instrument with which to give body to this story.

Nature (objects or processes) may never appear to us perfectly regular, and this also influences our aesthetic standards.

Symmetry is certainly the most elementary paradigm drawing together the various forms of creative thinking and represents therefore the most obvious point of contact between art and science.

However, the classic idea of beauty has changed. Nowadays we emphasize – as Giuseppe Caglioti observes –"how a measured dose of symmetry together with elements which break the symmetry appear to be necessary for the construction of an image which is capable of seizing the unconscious mind" (Caglioti 1995).

Naturally I have also been very attracted by perfect symmetry. In particular, first independently and then encouraged by Lucio Saffaro (Spizzichino and Cavazzini 2003), I "revisited" the platonic and archimedean polyhedra, reproducing them in the "cava" manner of Leonardo.

In the 1980s there was not the abundance of sites and channels of which we avail today, and to calculate the coordinates I created an algorithm (Spizzichino 1988) which generates all the regular and semi-regular polyhedra with connectivity 3, that is, with three faces around every vertex.

I will demonstrate some examples of pieces made in those years and some more recent instances.

What I want to underline is how, through programming and automatic calculation, the possibility of a new type of experience is opened, an experience between the aesthetic and the cognitive spheres, in perfect continuity with the program first expressed several decades ago by constructivism and other independent artists.

> Artists must be involved with machines – said Bruno Munari as early as 1938 – and they must learn the language of mechanisms.... to create works of art with these same machines.

There was, for the first time since the Renaissance, a renewed interest in the fields where art and science converge, as we entered into the so-called image society.

The development of this "new" (even if, in reality, ancient) mode of communication has succeeded because it serves as a kind of Esperanto in both interpersonal

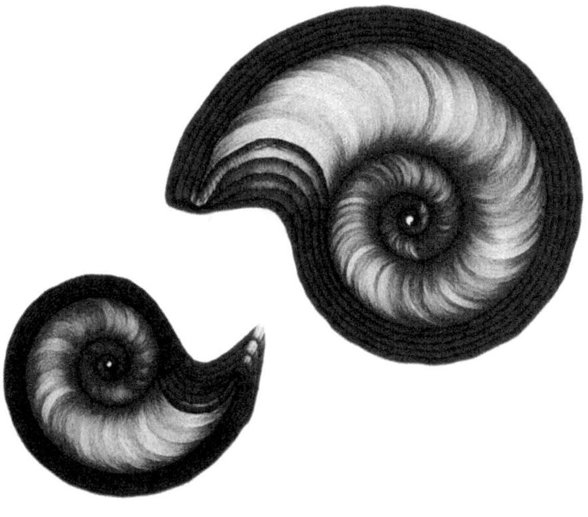

Fig. 25.1 Fossil shells (1986)

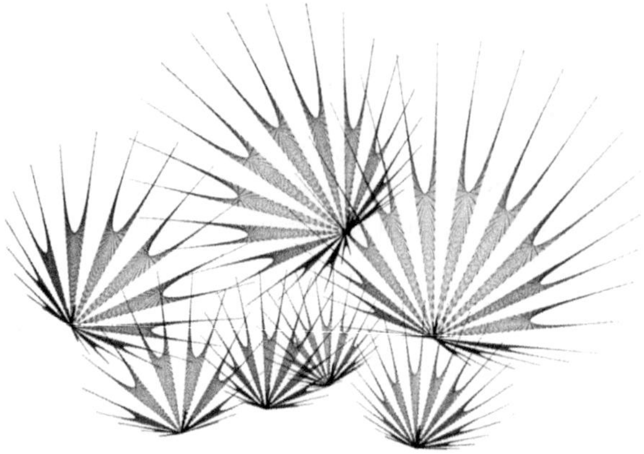

Fig. 25.2 In the desert (1986)

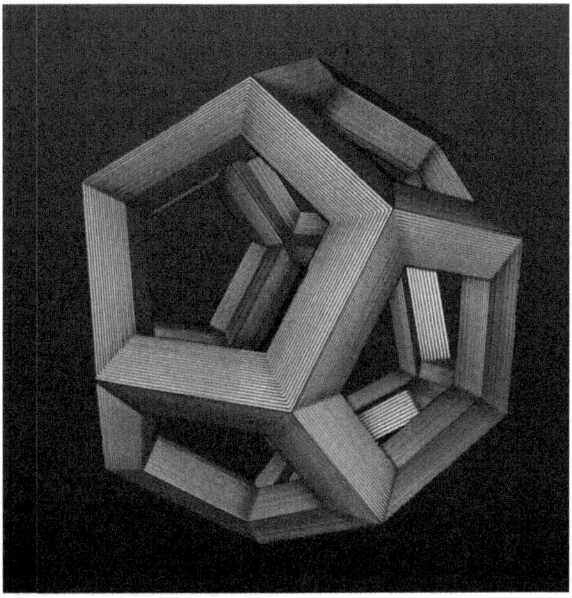

Fig. 25.3 Skeletal model of a dodecahedron (1987)

communication and that between culture and various disciplines, but also because it has its own specific characteristics (with respect to spoken or written language).

Herein, I intend to focus my attention on a particular type of graphics (technically defined as vector graphics) [G. Anceschi talked about "works whose 'visibility' is written in the form of programming code"], contiguous to the worlds of geometry and mathematics, but which has in itself rich expressive potential.

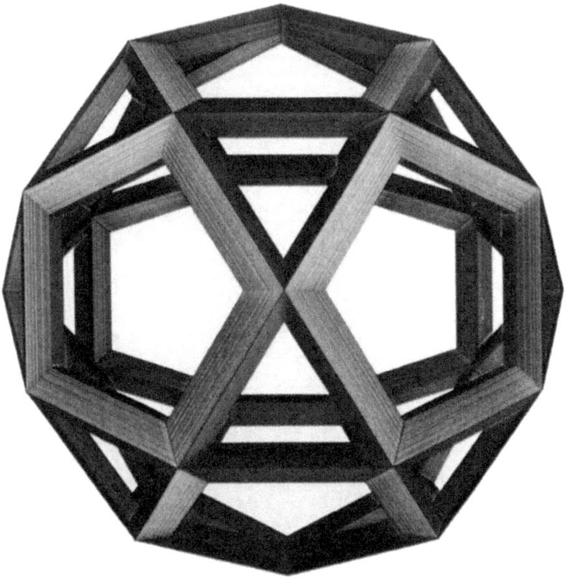

Fig. 25.4 Skeletal model of an icosidodecahedron (1987)

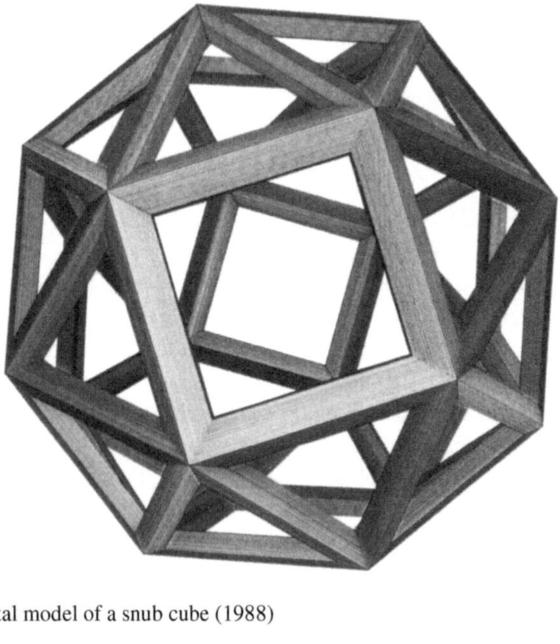

Fig. 25.5 Skeletal model of a snub cube (1988)

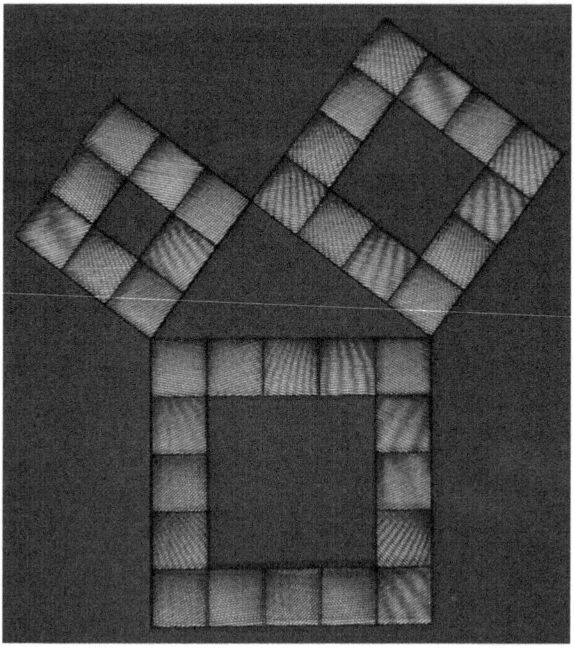

Fig. 25.6 Pitagoric mosaic (1987)

According to Jon Phillips,[1] "Whereas a bitmap/raster image is trying to describe our world in desire to the reality perceived by our vision, vectors seem to stylize reality in closer proximity to the actual concepts existing in our brain."

We will therefore see how, in a progressive augmentation of complexity, it can be considered a true and proper arena of creativity and so invests the world of art, intended not as a purely aesthetic experience but as a form of knowledge.

Naturally, this creativity, this artisanship implies an effort of personalization of graphical language, and therefore a particular attention to the constituent elements of language itself (lines, points, surfaces, etc.).

Some of the works shown here are just fragments, ideas or exercises but which are nonetheless useful in order to illustrate my personal approach to this subject.

I begin with some figures which "narrate" a mathematical property or a physical process in a visible form. The idea behind this kind of exercise is to add some visible suggestion to the cold schematic representation normally found in books, which could be of support in stimulating interest and understanding.

Figure 25.6 is based on the most famous of the Pythagorean triples (3,4,5), but also contains the sequences (1,2,3) and (2,3,4), while Fig. 25.7 is a homage to the most pervasive and intriguing number in mathematics and nature: the golden ratio φ. In the diagonal is a continued fraction representation of φ.

[1] J. Phillips: http://rejon.org/madia/writings/vector/vectorAesthetics-phillips.ps

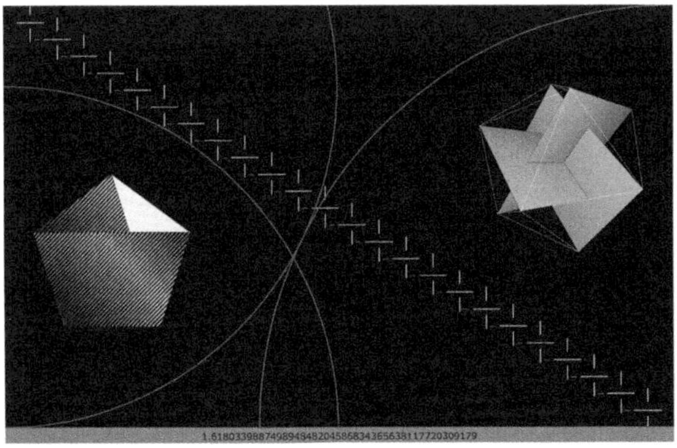

Fig. 25.7 Golden ratio (1998)

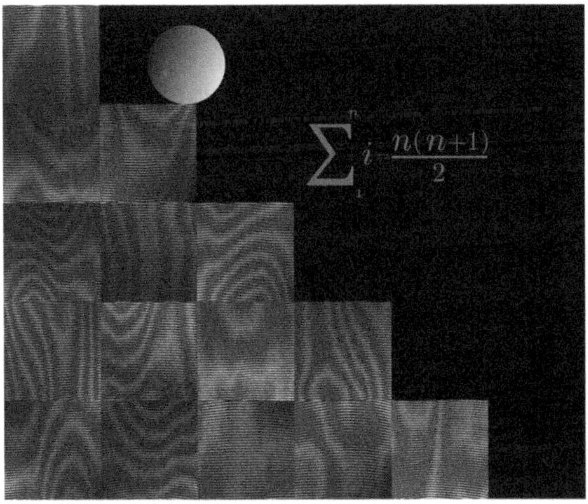

Fig. 25.8 The stair and the formula (2007)

Figure 25.8 is a geometric representation of the mathematical formula for the sum of the first n integers. Finally, Fig. 25.9 is a snapshot of a physical process – the movement of a well-known toy (*Slinky*) down a flight of steps.

Then graphic programs arrived (PhotoShop, Illustrator, etc.). I am often asked why I do not employ them.

Even though they are very useful for the requirements of today's world, these programs trick the user into a pattern of predefined options which I have always considered very annoying and not appropriate for creative activity.

In particular, these programs, operating directly on the images, that is, on the pixels, preclude a constructive approach using an algorithmic basis.

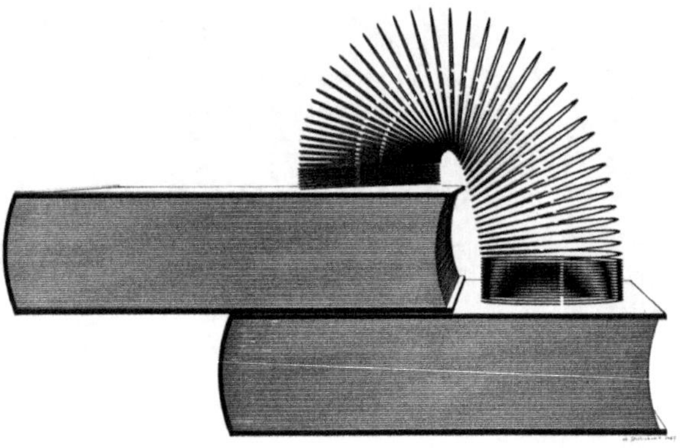

Fig. 25.9 The Slinky (1987)

However, most of the artists who work with computers have adapted so as to employ these instruments created for use in a production context, while others use robotized devices.

I, after my first experience in the 1980s with AppleIIe, have preferred not to submit to the seduction of photorealism; but as the seduction is very strong, the only manner to stay away was to use a "poor" method. Therefore I have swum against the flow by writing my programs in Fortran 77 on a PC, using, at first, the DOS operating system, thereafter Linux, and creating a personal library (still in development) of over 2500 routines.

For the basic library of graphical functions, I rely on PGPLOT, an s/w packet born in the scientific environment and freely downloadable from the Internet.

The great number of routines is equivalent to having a set of screwdrivers and various types of pliers in your toolbox which help to overcome the linguistic barrier with a medium not intended for drawing.

Here, I cannot enter into technical descriptions. The criteria which I admire are those of simplicity of use and of modularity, often counter to computational efficiency, which for my purposes is not a fundamental problem.

I continue therefore with a demonstration of a portion of my work comprising a series of images roughly grouped according to the generative algorithm employed.

25.1 Compositions of Circles

Grouped sets of tangent circles are pretty common in our everyday experience (soap foams, greasy broth, etc). In the 1970s the Italian artist Bruno Cagli used the circle as the elemental sign in a series of precious pieces of graphics. Trying to obtain similar results with a computer is an interesting and challenging exercise, affordable both with classical analytical geometry and by using complex number representation.

A couple of examples are shown in Figs. 25.10 (*Celtic necklace)* and 25.11 (*soup of circles*).

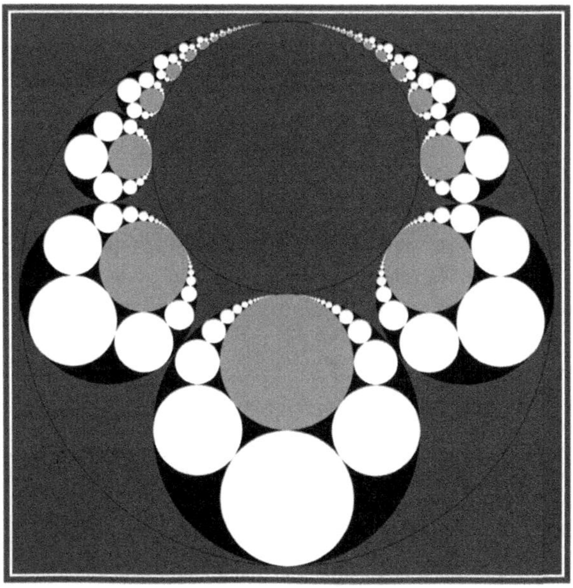

Fig. 25.10 Celtic necklace (1998)

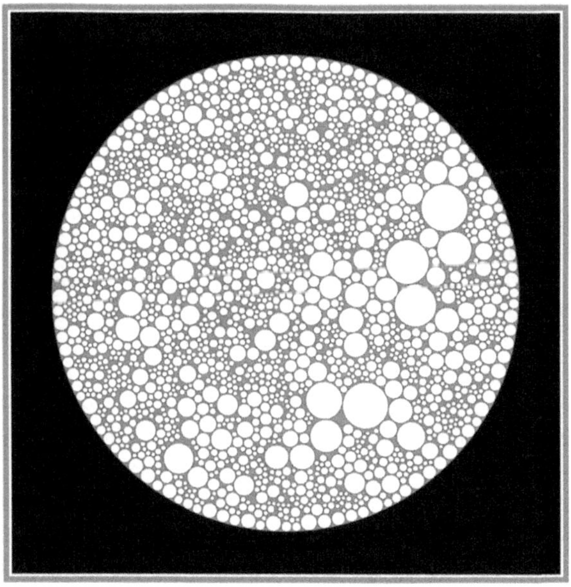

Fig. 25.11 Soup of circles (1998)

These are two different cases of osculatory packing. While the first is of *apollonian* type, the second, in which each circle needs to be in contact with at least one previous circle, deals with the so-called *tangent-1 packing* (Pickover 1990).

25.2 Complex Mapping

The following examples are based on the geometric properties of complex transformations, in which the variable w, interpreted as a point of the Euclidean plane, undergoes a transformation $w \rightarrow f(w)$, according to a process that maps the plane into itself.

The shell-like structure of Fig. 25.12 derives from a triangular heap of framed triangles through the transforming rule $w \rightarrow \exp(w)$.

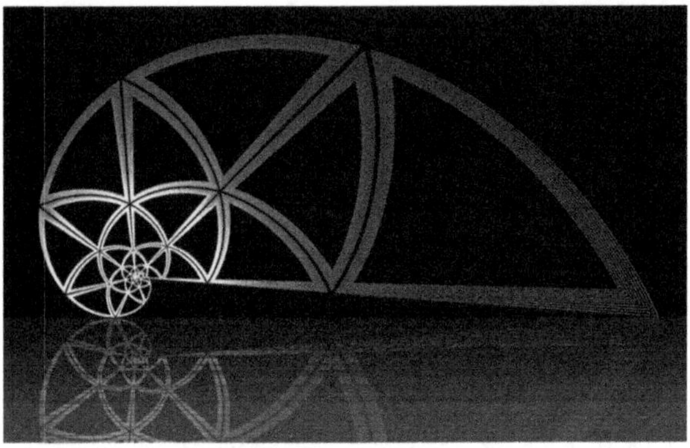

Fig. 25.12 Exponential reflection (1998)

The bunch of flowers depicted in Fig. 25.13 is generated by transforming the boundary of a number of pentagons by the rule $w \rightarrow w^6$. The transformed polygons are then randomly located inside a circle and filled with graded blue color.

The graphics titled *Math-ernity* (Fig. 25.14) derives from an elaboration of a Truchet tiling described by Pickover (1990). The generating tile is simply a square with two quarters of circle centered at two opposite corners. The square tiles are located in the tessellation regardless of their orientation. The resulting pattern is shown in the background, with just a little deformation. The central figure originates from the same pattern, where the complex transformation $w \rightarrow w^2$ is applied. The original pattern refolds in itself generating many more closed circles and intricate paths.

For a deeper insight into the subject I suggest the book *Visual Complex Analysis* by T. Needham (1997). In the Preface, the author, stressing the importance of visualization, says that it would be "patently unfair and irrational to have a law forbidding would-be music students from experiencing and understanding the subject directly through 'sonic intuition'. But in our society of mathematician we have such a law. It is not a written law..., but it says, Mathematics must not be visualized!"

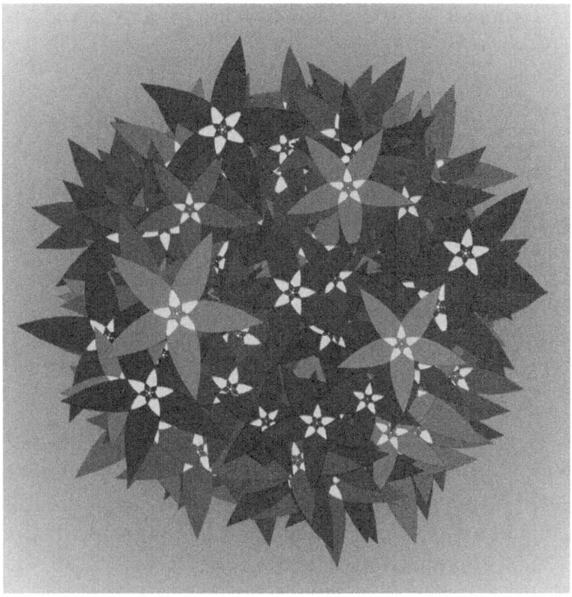

Fig. 25.13 Flowers in the complex field (2008)

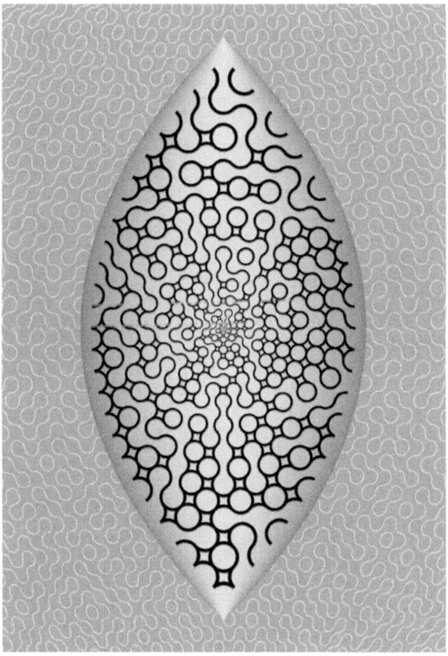

Fig. 25.14 Math-ernity (2008)

Fortunately, computer graphics is fostering a new trend in mathematical teaching.

25.3 Moiré Patterns

Moiré patterns spring up rather frequently in our everyday life, being produced by the interaction (more precisely we can say by "the logical AND") of two overlaid patterns.

In TV and computer screens, as in printing, moiré patterns are an unwanted effect, but a smart use of them is very effective, as demonstrated by kinetic artists long before the use of computers in visual arts; they add a sort of vibrating dimension to the image.

I make large use of moiré patterns, especially in the simulation of wooden objects but also in different contexts, backgrounds, etc. In my first experiences in computer art, I experimented by superposing two patterns, a set of colored lines drawn on a transparent sheet and a similar black pattern drawn on paper. It is very interesting that in this way, faint complementary colors arise.

Usually, only the simplest case of gratings of parallel lines or circles is considered in books, whereas more interesting graphic results come from the use of more general gratings.

Two overlaid spiral gratings are shown in Fig. 25.15.

Usually I generate gratings limited by two *baselines*, obtained by interpolating a randomized or a fractal line (Fig. 25.16). The intermediate lines are generated by

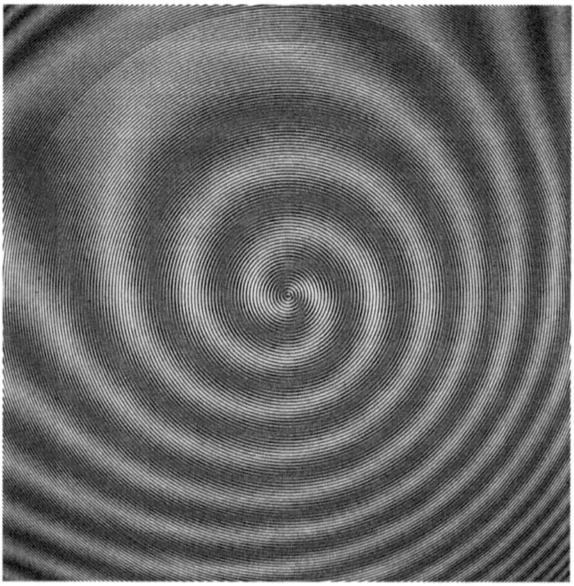

Fig. 25.15 Spiral moiré (1999)

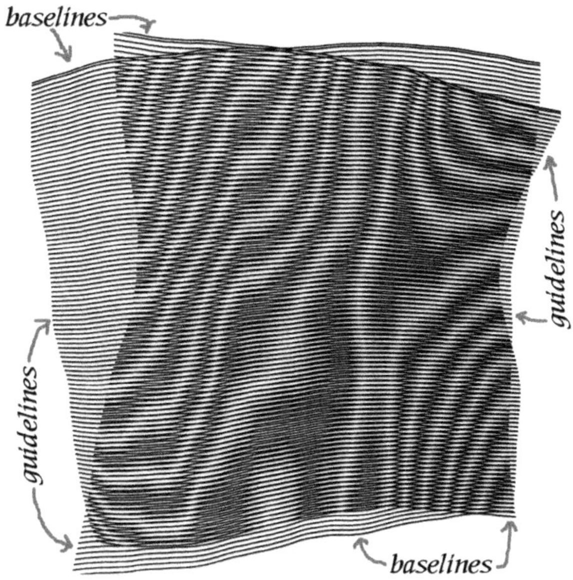

Fig. 25.16 Two overlapping layers giving rise to a moiré interference

linear morphing (I call it *blending*), with the end points of each line constrained to stay on two assigned *guidelines*. It is worth noticing that in graphics, lines have a finite width (which may be fixed or modulated), therefore in practice they are a sequence of small quadrilaterals.

Once the pattern has been obtained, it may undergo a series of operations and transformations (cutting, clipping, swelling, circular inversion, mapping on a given 2D shape or 3D surface, normal or fish-eye perspective, etc., besides the usual linear transformations).

Of particular interest for applications is the mapping of a rectangular pattern on a region derived by a rubber sheet deformation of the original.

The plumage of the bird of Fig. 25.17, as the vase in Fig. 25.18, is an example of a procedure of this type, in which each mesh of the original lattice is transformed into the corresponding mesh of the target one (irregular grid defined inside the silhouette of the bird). It is however important to notice that moiré patterns come out "spontaneously" through the wire frame representation of solid figures seen in perspective, as shown in Fig. 25.19.

25.4 Tessellations

In spite of the circumstance that the word tessellation derives from a Greek root meaning four, tessellation (or tiling) deals with the problem of covering the plane without gaps or overlaps, making use of a finite set of primary shapes having no a priori limitations in the numbers of sides.

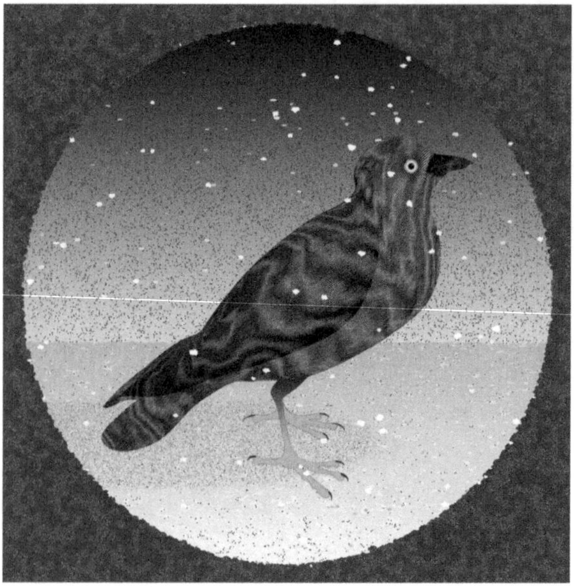

Fig. 25.17 Winter (2004)

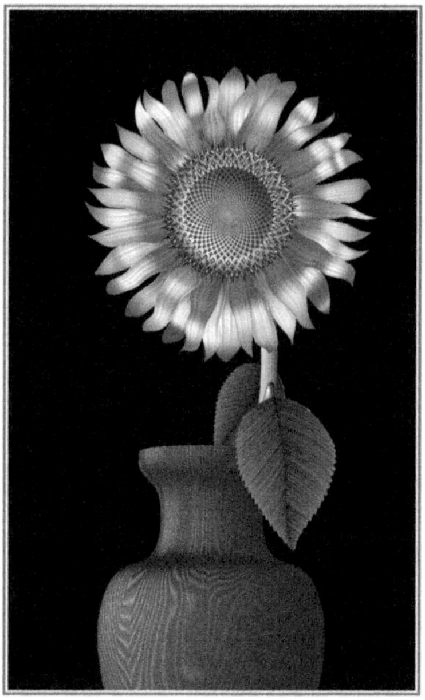

Fig. 25.18 Helianthus (2001)

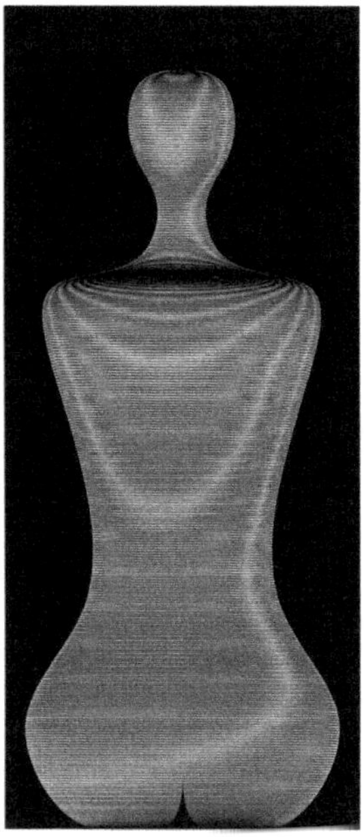

Fig. 25.19 Seating woman (2004)

The topic is so intriguing and fascinating that it has accompanied the history of civilization and still now is a subject of active research, especially regarding its extensions to higher dimensions.

I report in the present chapter four of my works inspired by or derived from tessellations.

The first has been discussed above (Fig. 25.14, Truchet tiling); the next is shown in Fig. 25.20; it has as the main subject a red ribbon toroidally wrapped, resting on a sheet of paper on which is drawn a mosaic of tiles. In this (nonperiodic) tessellation, due to M. Goldberg (Grünbaum and Shephard 1987), each tile can be subdivided into an equilateral and an isosceles-rectangular triangle. The inter-tile gaps are due to a scaling and therefore are unessential.

In the following figure (*From order to chaos*, Fig. 25.21), the prototile is a nonregular pentagon with inner angles of 40°, 140°, and 160°. Its shape is evocative of a leaf. Something is intervening to destroy the perfect order: randomness is increasing along the vertical direction.

The last figure is a spherical infinite tessellation derived from an unusual truncation of an icosahedron (Fig. 25.22). The faces of the polyhedron, before being projected on the sphere, are 12 regular pentagons plus 20 nonregular hexagons. A full description of the pattern would be too complex to be reported here; I limit myself to note that the pattern in each sector of a pentagon comes from an affine transformation of the larger sector of the hexagon, the recursive pattern of which therefore constitutes the basic element for the mosaic construction.

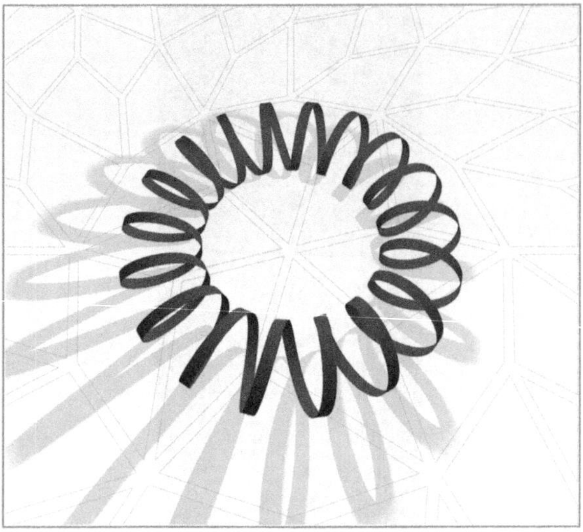

Fig. 25.20 Toroidal spring (2006)

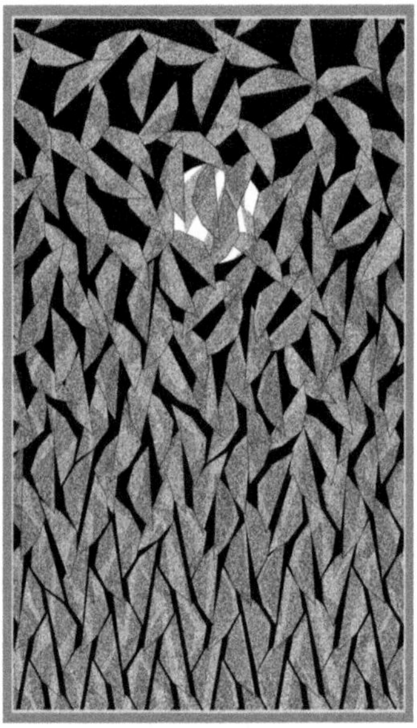

Fig. 25.21 From order to chaos (1999)

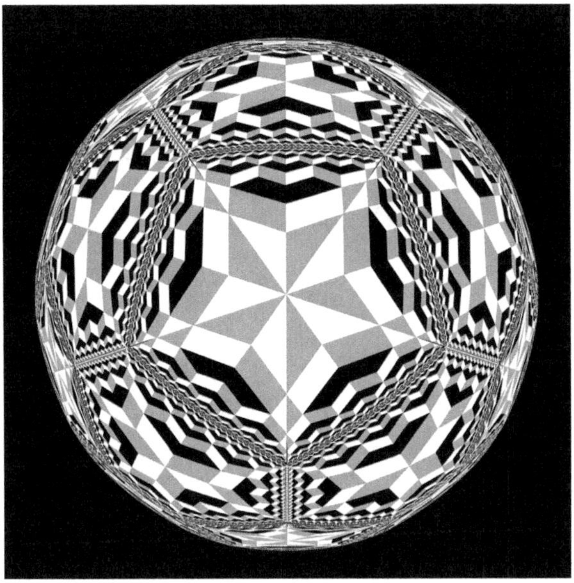

Fig. 25.22 Inlaid woodwork (2007)

A particular partition of a plane region deserves a mention at this point: the so-called Voronoi tessellation.[2] Given a distribution of points (generators), the partitioning into convex polygons is such that each polygon contains exactly one generating point and every point in a given polygon is closer to its generating point rather than to any other. The tiles of this diagram may be worked out in a variety of different ways. For instance, the *Stones under water* (Fig. 25.23) are smoothed Voronoi tiles with a slight deformation due to the refraction of the perturbed water.

25.5 Linear Fractals and Branching

After the discovery of the famous Koch's curve, at the beginning of the last century, a wealth of similar mathematical objects have been proposed and investigated. Nowadays they are incorporated in the frame of L-systems and described in terms of turtle geometry. Of particular interest for applications in graphics is a class of curves, also based on the concept of *rewriting*, which besides being self-similar, are space filling and self-avoiding. Among these I want to mention the Hilbert curve (Prusinkiewicz and Linenmayer 1990) (that I use to decorate solids, as shown later in

[2]E. W Weisstein, "Voronoi Diagram." From –MathWorld A Wolfram Web Resource http://mathworld.wolfram.com/VoronoiDiagram.html

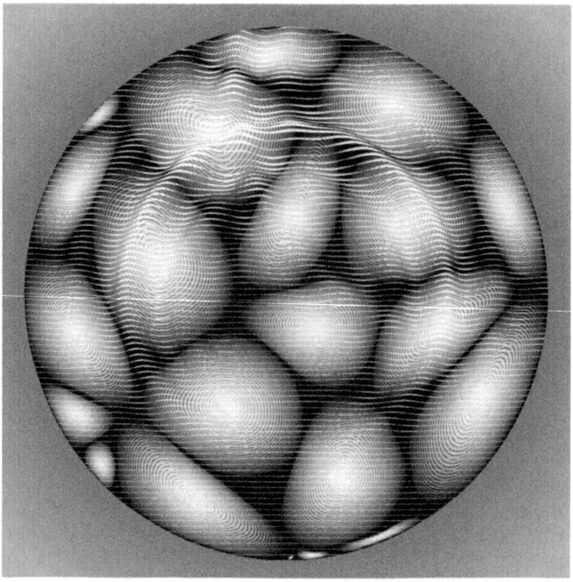

Fig. 25.23 Stones under water (2000)

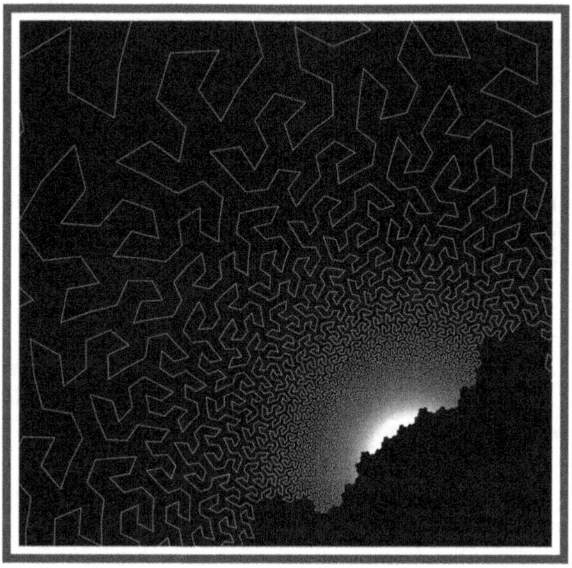

Fig. 25.24 Moolight (1999)

the chapter) and the hexagonal Gosper flake (Peitgen and Saupe 1988), which, after a suitable polar transformation, generates the *Moonlight* reproduced in Fig. 25.24.

Concepts of rewriting and self-similarity, extended in the statistical sense, are very useful in the modeling of developmental processes of biological systems and plant formation (Prusinkiewicz and Linenmayer 1990). Simple examples are given in Figs. 25.25 and 25.26. In the latter the skylines of the mountains are generated by using the midpoint displacement algorithm described in Peitgen and Saupe (1988).

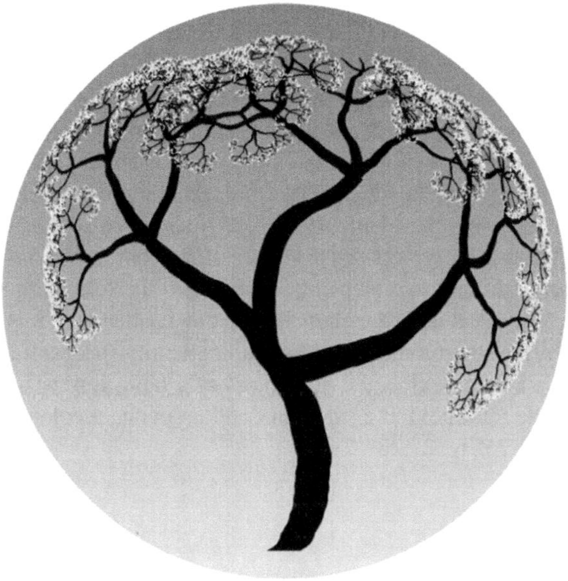

Fig. 25.25 Blooming tree (2005)

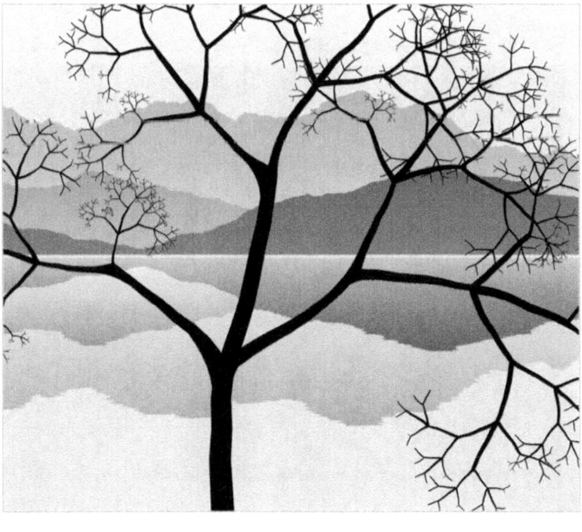

Fig. 25.26 Fractal landscape (2004)

25.6 Cellular Automata

Algorithms based on cellular automata can be very useful, especially for describing processes of evolution or growth. In Fig. 25.27 the plants which climb up the balcony have been designed using the algorithm of diffusion-limited aggregation (Peitgen and Saupe 1988); a sticky particle (a small disc) is placed at the base of the plant. A myriad of other similar particles are then one-by-one introduced at random points and each of these is then migrated linearly to be attached to the nearest pre-existing particle. As can be seen, this simple model of dendritic growth is sufficient to produce realistic branching. In the example shown, in order to create a more natural representation, the size of the discs decreases with height.

Another genetic algorithm which has interesting graphic applications is the so-called quantum foam (Pickover 1990). One takes a random binary array (e.g., 200×200) and then sets the elements outside a specified region to zero. A filter is then applied iteratively which transforms each element on the basis of the sum of the 3×3 sub-array around that element according to the following rule: if the sum is greater than 6 or equal to 4, the element is set to 1, otherwise it is set to 0. In this way a labyrinth-like structure is formed including empty spaces. If the points inside this structure are interpreted as the generators of a field, it is possible to calculate the strength of the total field at every point and associate a color to that point as a function of intensity (Fig. 25.28).

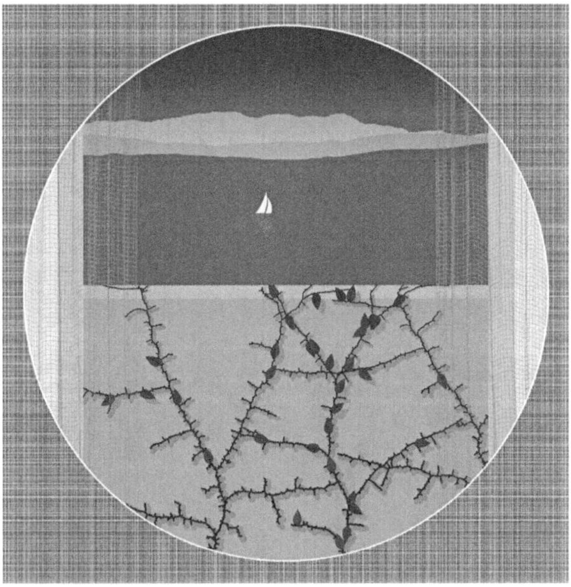

Fig. 25.27 Beyond the border (2006)

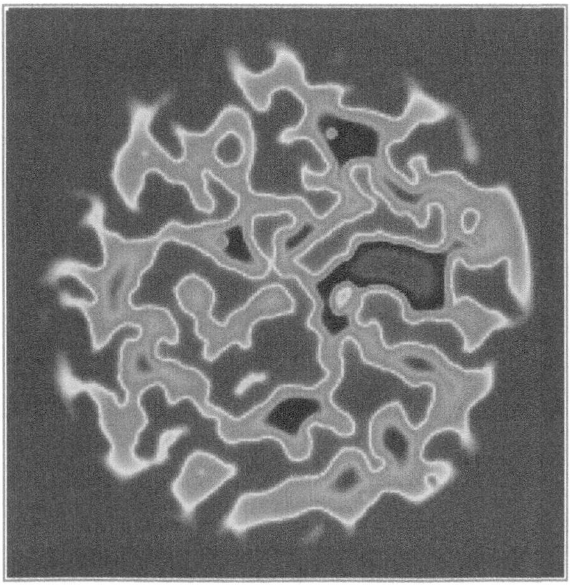

Fig. 25.28 Restless Sun (detail, 2007)

25.7 Contour Lines

As with the moiré patterns, I employ contour lines widely throughout my graphics. Depending on the situation, I may choose to use contour lines which are either defined analytically (in Fig. 25.29 the function is of the type $z=x^2-y^2+xy+g(x,y)$, where g is a Gaussian term) or by a field generated by points internal to various polygons which form the structure of the composition (e.g., the contours of the face, the eyes, the mouth, etc. of the clown in Fig. 25.30 or the two starfish in Fig. 25.31). In general the field is assumed to decrease with distance either exponentially or according to a power law. The use of contour lines is convenient in that it generates families of non-intersecting lines which create a three-dimensional effect or even evoke an interaction between objects. By linking colors to the levels, one can also obtain chromatic effects (e.g., Fig. 25.32).

25.8 Polyhedra

Regular and semi-regular polyhedra (Wenninger 1971), which have fascinated people for centuries, are a sort of a must for a computer graphics amateur. I have shown above some examples of early works created on a plotter in the 1980 s. Here are a couple of instances from my more recent experience.

Figure 25.33 represents a sticky model of the snub dodecahedron, one of the Archimedean solids. Each of the 12 pentagonal faces is surrounded by five triangular

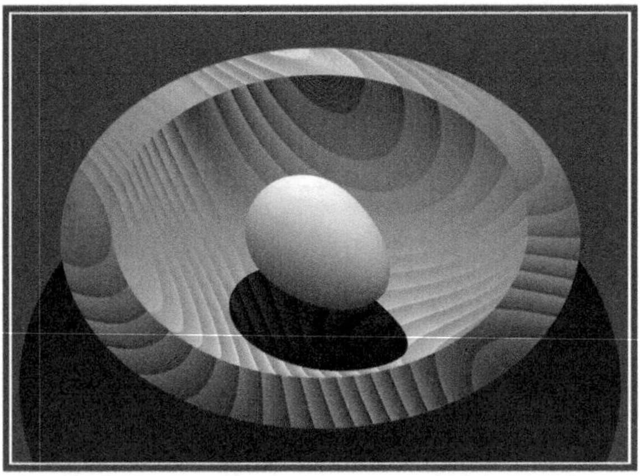

Fig. 25.29 Egg in a wooden bowl (1999)

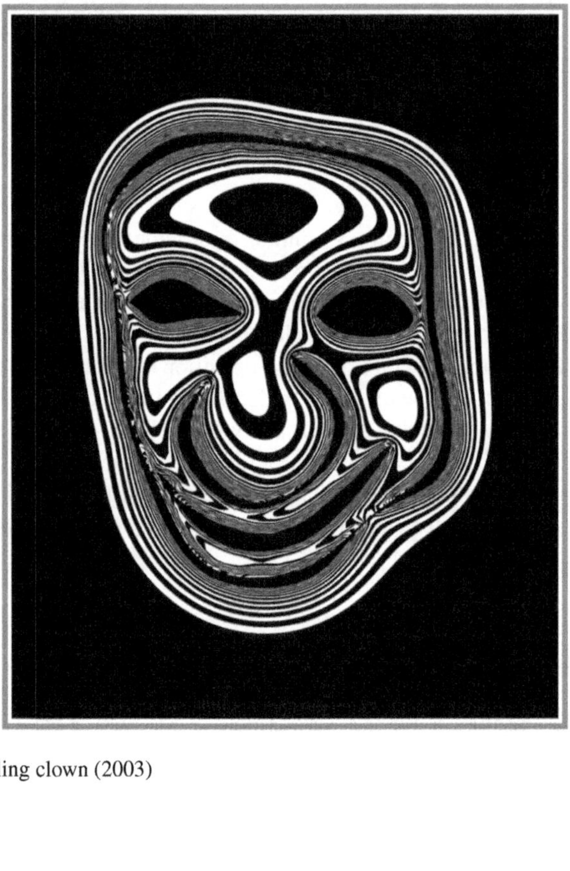

Fig. 25.30 Smiling clown (2003)

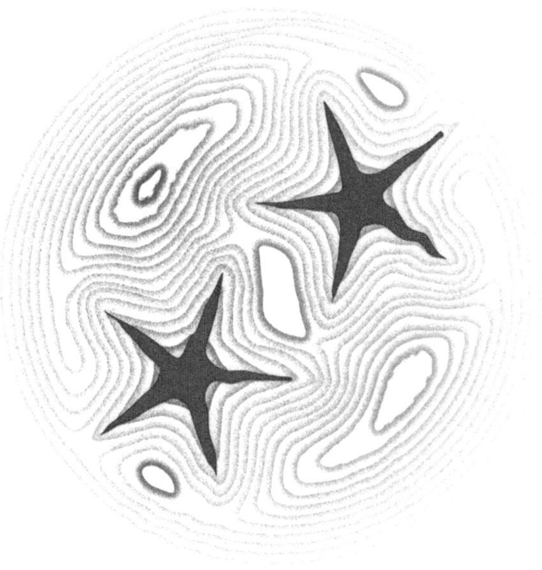

Fig. 25.31 Starfishes (2005)

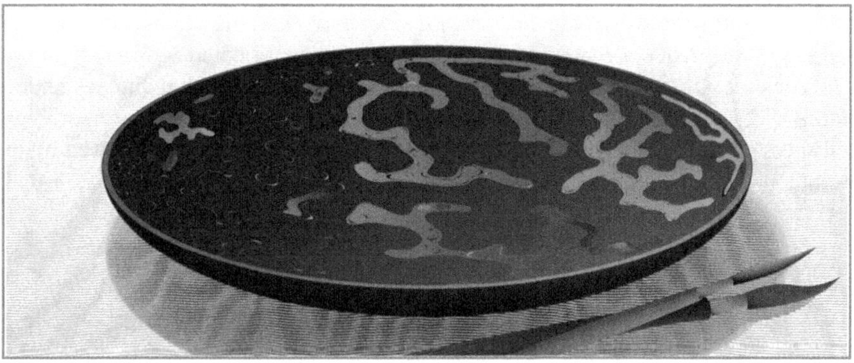

Fig. 25.32 The unfinished decoration (2008)

ones. At a first glance it is difficult to appreciate its property of being different from its mirror image, but this property stands out clearly in the framed drawing on the table, representing the same geometrical structure in a fish-eye projection taken from the center of a pentagonal face. The projection, appearing flower-like, exhibits in the central region a rotation, denoting the snub nature of the solid.

In this case, as with all convex polyhedra, for the removal of the hidden lines, it is not necessary to store all the surface elements in memory. At first the rear faces are drawn, then the front ones (with the caution that the inner facets of each stick must be drawn before the external ones).

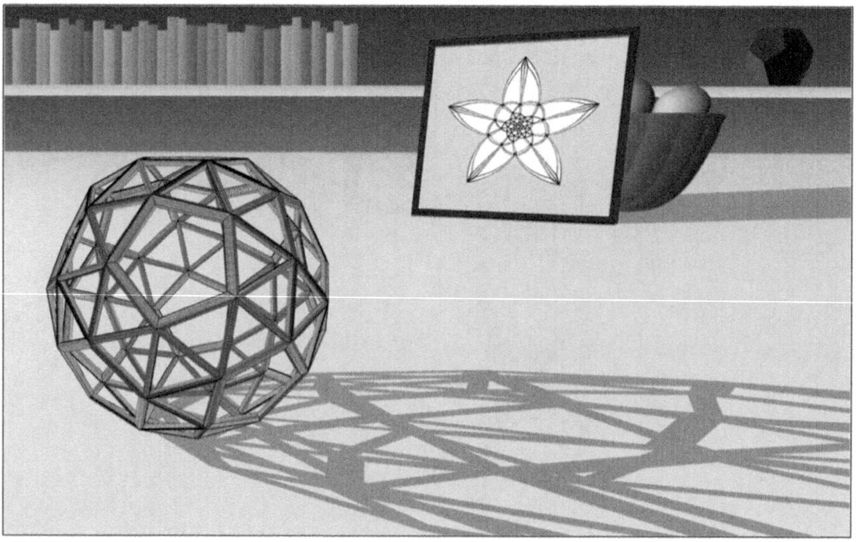

Fig. 25.33 A snub dodecahedron and its fish-eye projection (2002)

In the following work (*The library of a mathematician*, Fig. 25.34), two origami models of the great dodecahedron hang from the ceiling, oriented at different angles. The construction is similar to an origami made in paper: 20 trihedral dimples replace the faces of an icosahedron. The rendering in shaded colors is produced by polygonal spots clipped against the triangular facets, with color composition driven by the point location.

25.9 A Sample of Other 3D Figures

Computer graphics techniques are well suited for decorating solids of revolution and various mathematical surfaces with geometric motifs. In the examples shown below, a smoothed Hilbert curve is wrapped around a Möbius band (Fig. 25.35) and a terracotta vase (Fig. 25.36). To remove the hidden parts, the surface elements are plotted in decreasing order, according to their distance from the observer, while a simple model of shading is employed taking into account only the cosine of the angle between the point-like light source and the perpendicular vector to the element. The mapping of the curve is performed in the usual way of the bilinear transformation of each cell of the original grating into the new cell of the target surface.

The two *Orobori* shown in Fig. 25.37 are obtained by a tubular coating of a classical mathematical curve called a trifolium. The composition may be regarded as an exercise in using generalized cylinders, in preparation for harder tasks such as the Klein bottle. The decorating pattern is very simple, consisting of the repetition

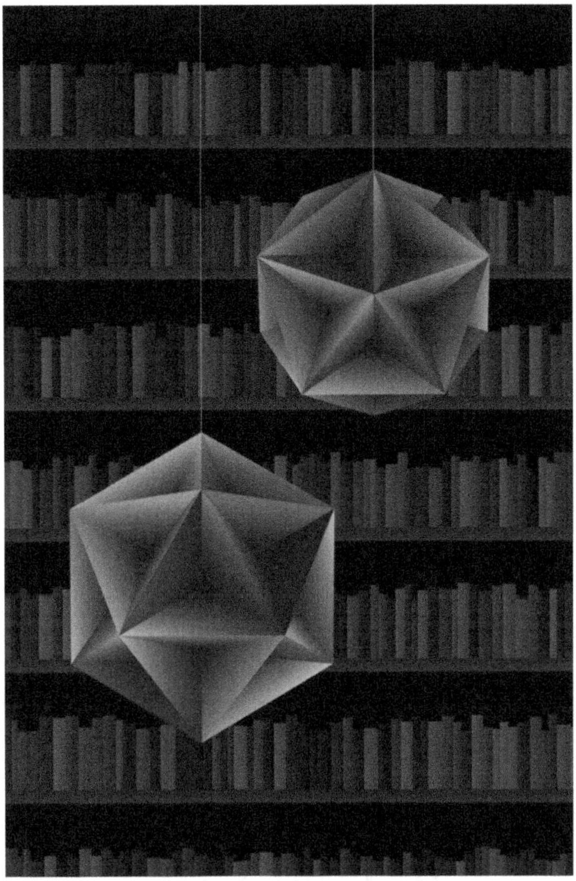

Fig. 25.34 The library of a mathematician (2006)

of a black triangle drawn inside each mesh of the grating. The white line in the background comes from an interpolated hexagonal Gosper flake.

At this point it is worth mentioning the way I followed to construct the Klein bottle shown in Fig. 25.40.

To create this figure I first define a function of one parameter $f(t)$ which has the general form of the sum of two Gaussian terms plus a constant, as shown in Fig. 25.38. This function is then sampled at equal intervals δt, creating a comb-like figure where the length of the teeth represents the radii of the local cross-section of the final bottle. The only real constraint is that the value of the function at the two end points is the same. I then define the spine of the bottle as a P-shape (as shown in Fig. 25.39) in a vertical plane. Clearly the return arm of the P must encounter the starting arm smoothly. The comb shape is then wrapped along the spine and then rotated around the spine itself through 360° at a discrete resolution. A constraint in this definition is that the maximum curvature of the spine must be such that the teeth

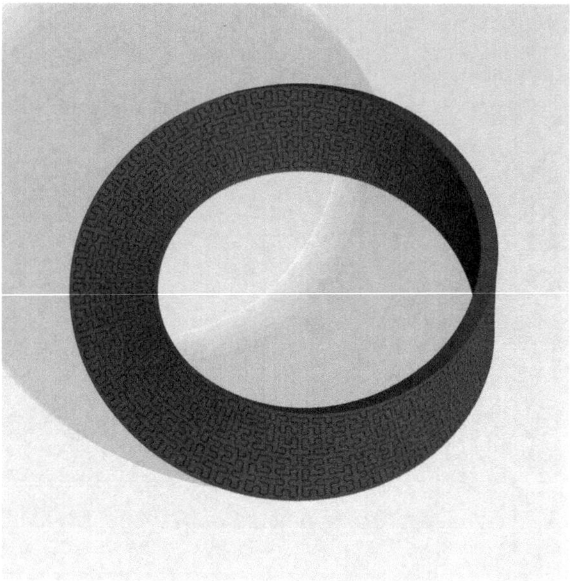

Fig. 25.35 A decorated Möbius band (2007)

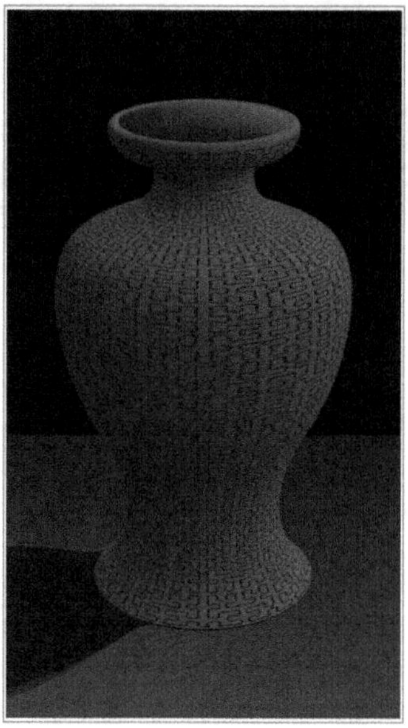

Fig. 25.36 The Hilbert's pot (2007)

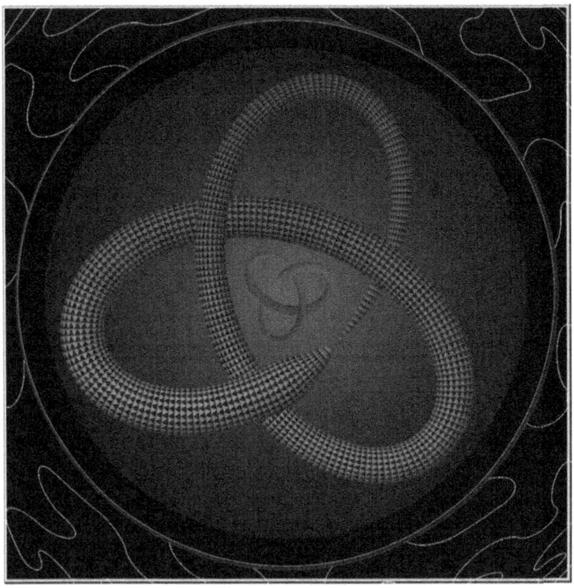

Fig. 25.37 Orobori (2006)

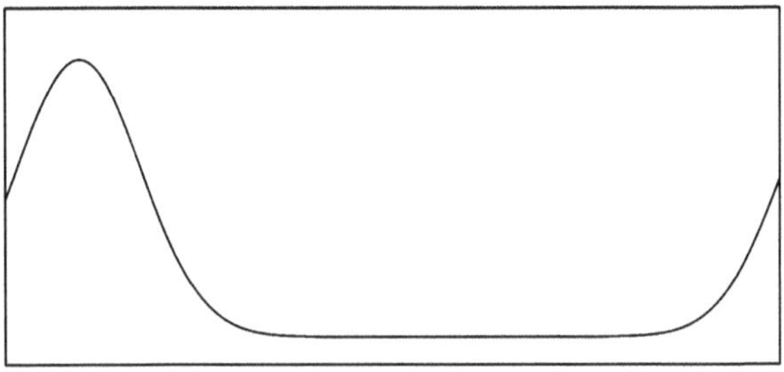

Fig. 25.38 Profile used for the construction of the Klein bottle

never intersect during the rotation. The end points of the teeth then define the surface of the Klein bottle (Fig. 25.40). Not having available any facility for transparency effects, I realized the rendering of the glass with random dots, while the casting of isophotal strips of color dots adds a suggestion of volume.

Finally, a few words about the last two works presented. In *Notturno* (Fig. 25.41), we see two mysterious figures lightly inflated by a supposed rotation, a sort of dance under the starry dome of the sky.

The volumes have been modeled by sweeping a straight segment in contact with two parallel curved polygons having convex and concave sides, respectively. A differential scaling in height produces the swelling.

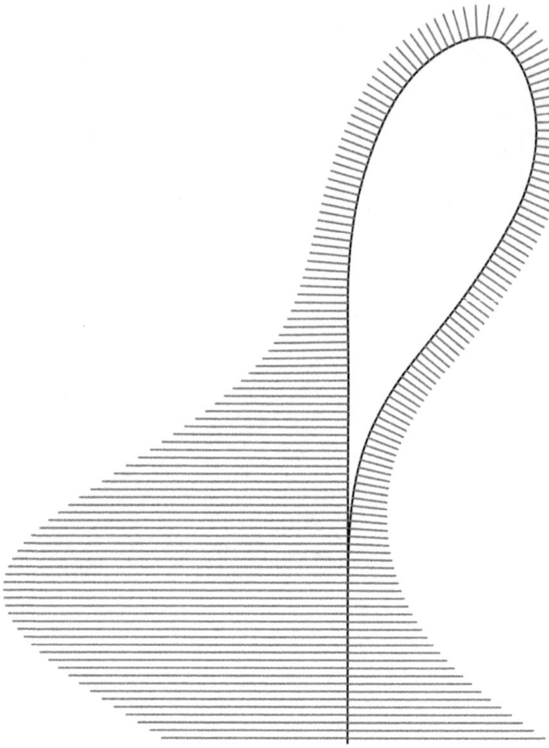

Fig. 25.39 The rotation of the rays perpendicular to the black line generates the surface

The toroidal shape shown in Fig. 25.42 represents a life belt falling from the sky in help of somebody: a metaphorical allusion to the power of rational thinking.

The sophisticated decoration consists of a curly motif on a hexagonal lattice wrapped on the torus.

The underlying mathematics is that of *hexagonal uniformly redundant arrays* (HURAs), based on the theory of cyclic difference sets (Finger and Prince 1985).

This is the only case in which I employ a slightly unusual algorithm. In general my work starts from elementary mathematics.

25.10 Final Considerations

With this presentation I hope to have demonstrated, at least in part, the multiplicity of experiences – figurative, abstract, or purely cognitive – possible through the use of computers but not based on generic pre-packaged programs: a way allowing captivating achievements.

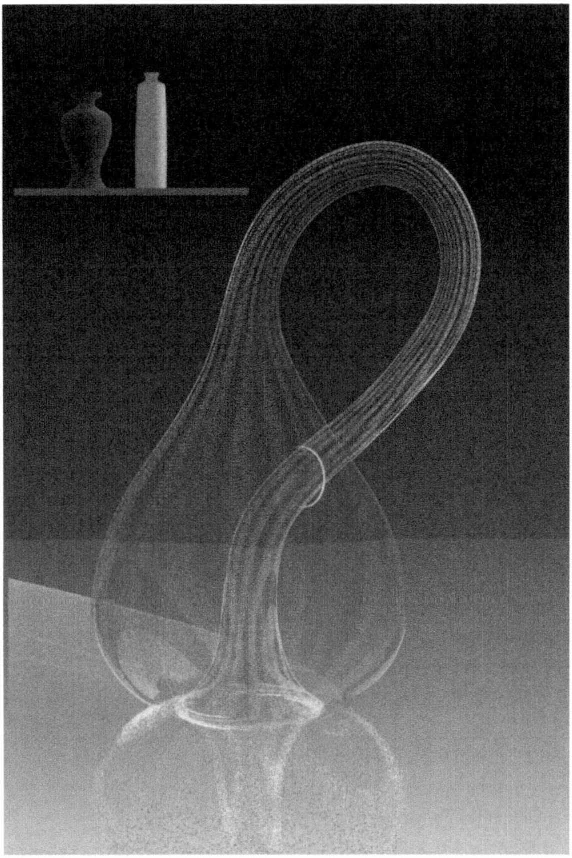

Fig. 25.40 The Klein bottle (2007)

My aim goes beyond these results, but the examples shown here seem to me to be already significant, at least at the level of method and approach; in my view *stimulation* of interest is by far more important than a perfect *simulation*.

In today's society, there is the need to give graphical form to concepts, processes, and abstract entities, but it is not certain whether the best way is that of figurative hyperbole, eye-catching, or eye-popping as it may be, as is often proposed from the American culture.

More awareness in the use of computer graphics, sustained by a conceptual architecture derived from mathematics, could liberate this graphics from its ancillary role to other disciplines to become a valuable means of connection between art and science which, 50 years after Snow's book (Snow 1959), remains a valid ideal to follow.

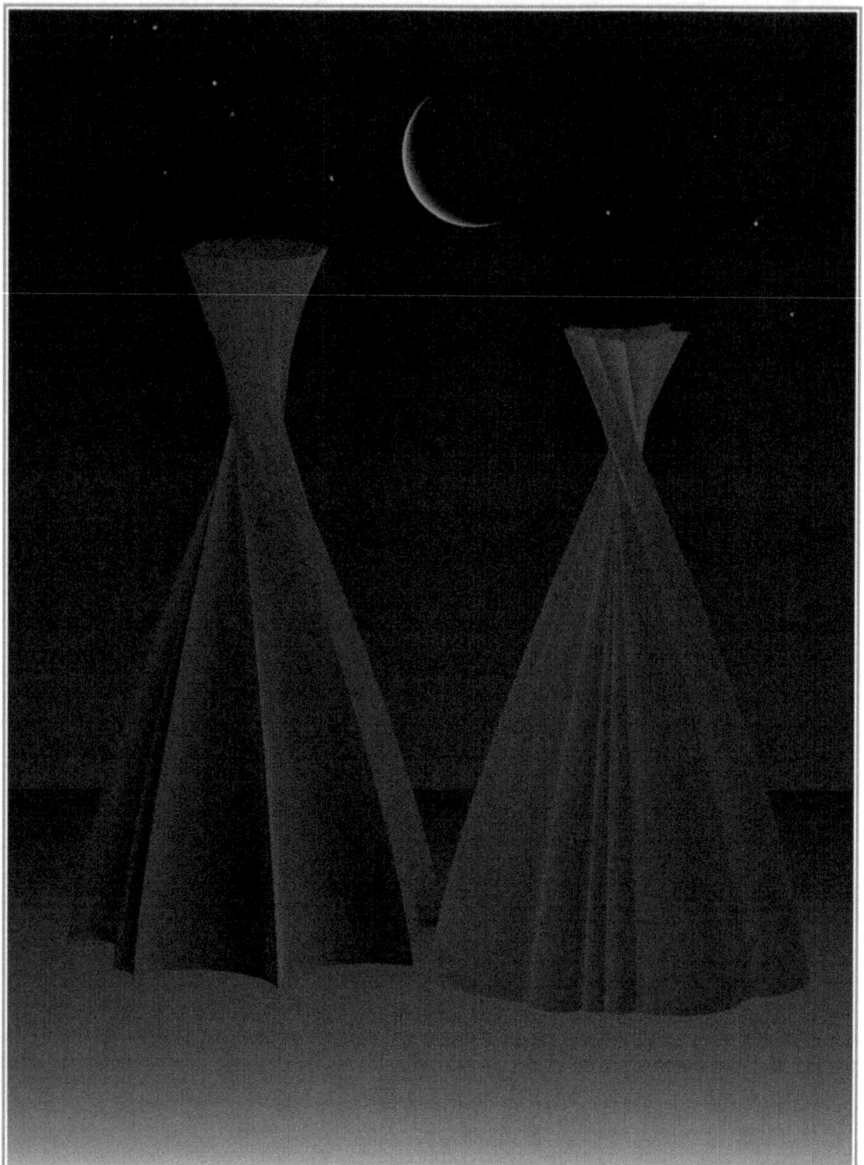

Fig. 25.41 Notturno (2006)

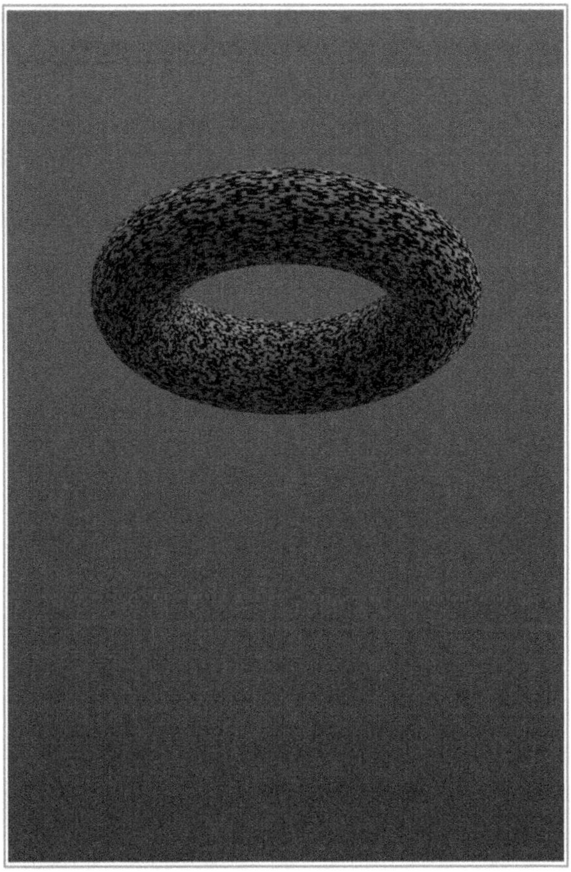

Fig. 25.42 A life belt from the sky (2008)

Bibliography

Caglioti, G. (1995). *Eidos e psiche*. Nuoro, Italy :Ilisso.
Delahaye, J. P. (1985). Nouveaux dessins géométriques et aristiques avec votre micro-ordinateur. Eyrolles.
Finger, M. H. and Prince, T. A. (1985). *Hexagonal uniformly redundant arrays for coded-aperture imaging*. 19th Intern. Cosmic Ray Conf. 3, 295–298.
Grünbaum, B. and Shephard, G. C. (1987). *Tilings and patterns*. Freeman and C.
Needham, T. (1997). *Visual complex analysis*. Oxford: Clarendon Press.
Peitgen, H. O. and Saupe, D. (Eds.) (1988). *The science of fractal image*. Springer Verlag.
Pickover, C. A. (1990). *Computers, pattern, chaos and beauty*. New York: St. Martin's Press, Inc.,
Prusinkiewicz, P. and Linenmayer, A. (1990). The algorithmic beauty of plants. Springer Verlag.
Snow, C. P. (1959). Two cultures and the scientific revolution. Cambridge: Cambridge University Press.

Spizzichino, A. (1988). An algorithm for recursive generation of a class of convex uniform polyhedra. In T. F. Banchoff et al. (Eds.), *ECM/87 Educational Computing in Mathematics* North Holland.

Spizzichino, A. and Cavazzini, E. (2003). The geometric world of Lucio Saffaro. In M. Emmer and M. Manaresi (Eds.), *Mathematics, art, technology and cinema*. Springer Verlag.

Wenninger, M. J. (1971). *Polyhedron models*. Cambridge: Cambridge University Press.

Chapter 26
Four-Dimensional Ideas

Gian M. Todesco

Abstract Living in a three-dimensional world, it is quite difficult for us to imagine a fourth geometric dimension, perpendicular to the three we already know. But a 4D geometry does not break any mathematical rule and indeed mathematicians have been studying it since the eighteenth century. Ideas referring to a 4D world have then spread beyond the math world and have inspired painters, sculptors, writers, and architects. Modern computer graphics allows us to get some more insight into this fascinating world.

Crucifixion (also known as *Corpus Hypercubus*) (Dalì 1954) was painted in 1954 by Salvador Dalì. The painting depicts the crucified Jesus floating upon a crux-shaped compound of eight cubes. This shape is the net of the *hypercube*[1]; it can be folded in a four-dimensional space to create the four-dimensional analog of the cube. Of course our mind, trained mainly with two-dimensional images of a three-dimensional world, cannot easily visualize this kind of shapes and therefore the Dalì's hypercube is a good metaphor to allude to the metaphysical and imperscrutable nature of the Christ (Kemp 1988).

We can guess that Dalì's public – educated people, probably without a specific training in math – had enough math knowledge to recognize the shape of the hypercube and therefore to understand the metaphor. More or less in the same decades, the popular culture celebrated the physicist Albert Einstein, whose relativity theory, developed between 1905 and 1915, uses four-dimensional geometry to represent the space–time structure.

In the second part of the twentieth century, four-dimensional shapes (for the most part the hypercube, also known as *tesseract*) have been used by sculptors (e.g., some

G.M. Todesco (✉)
(http://www.toonz.com/personal/todesco), Digital Video S.p.A. (http://www.toonz.com), matematita (http://www.matematita.it)

[1]Hypercube, Wikipedia, The Free Encyclopedia, <http://en.wikipedia.org/wiki/Hypercube> Hypercube, from MathWorld, Eric W. Weisstein, <http://mathworld.wolfram.com/Hypercube.html>

V. Capecchi (eds.), *Applications of Mathematics in Models, Artificial Neural Networks and Arts*, DOI 10.1007/978-90-481-8581-8_26,

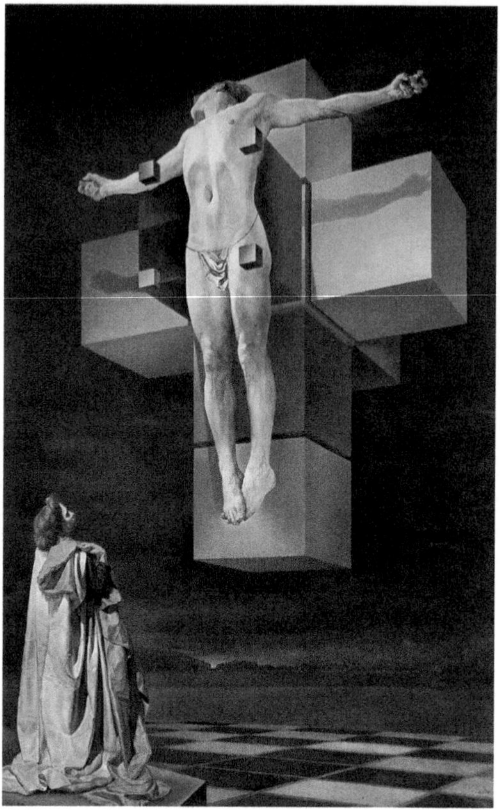

Fig. 26.1 Corpus Hypercubus, Salvador Dalí. Note: (c) 1999 Artists Rights Society (ARS), New York / VEGAP, Madrid. Probably it can be used under fair use. See http://en.wikipedia.org/wiki/Image:Dali_Crucifixion_hypercube.jpg.

metal sculptures by Attilio Pierelli), architects (e.g., the *Grande Arche* in Paris, resembling a perspective view of the tesseract), novelists (e.g., Robert Heinlein, who wrote a novel (1941) in which a house, similar to the Dalì's crux, collapses in the fourth dimension, driving his inhabitants into a very strange alien world), etc.

Apparently, the four-dimensional geometry, challenging to explore something that cannot be completely understood, fascinates not only mathematicians.

Formal study of the four-dimensional geometry started since the mid-nineteenth century. The German mathematician and astronomer A. Möbius is believed to be the first to speculate about four spatial dimensions, while the Swiss mathematician L. Schläfli determined all the regular four-dimensional polytopes (the analog of the regular polyhedra) (Robbins 1992). One of the richest sources of information about the four-dimensional world is the work of Coxeter (1973, 1991).

Probably the popular interest for the theory has been driven by the availability of images and figures. In 1880 W. Stringham wrote a paper (Stringham 1880) with some illustrations of many four-dimensional figures. In the late-twentieth century, the computer graphics made available new models. In 1966 M. Nöll and his associates at Bell Laboratories produced the first animation of a rotating hypercube and in 1978 T. Banchoff and C. Strauss produced the film *The Hypercube: Projections and Slicing*, winner of the *Prix de la Recherche Fondamentale* at the *Festival of Scientific and Technical Films* in Brussels. (Remarkably Banchoff became a friend of Salvador Dalì in 1975, after his research was mentioned in an article in the Washington Post, illustrated by a painting by Dalì.)

Today it is possible to create interactive representations of four-dimensional shapes using a simple laptop. Aim of this chapter is to show how the computer graphics can be used to push forward our capacity to visualize the four-dimensional world. We will try to explore something slightly more complex than the hypercube.

26.1 Flatland

Representing four-dimensional objects on a two-dimensional screen is a tricky task. Luckily it is not so different from representing three-dimensional objects on a piece of paper and there are a number of well-established techniques to do that. For instance, it is possible to make a projection, as in a perspective drawing. Another approach is to present many parallel sections as in the magnetic resonance imaging. Some simple shapes can be represented with a foldout.

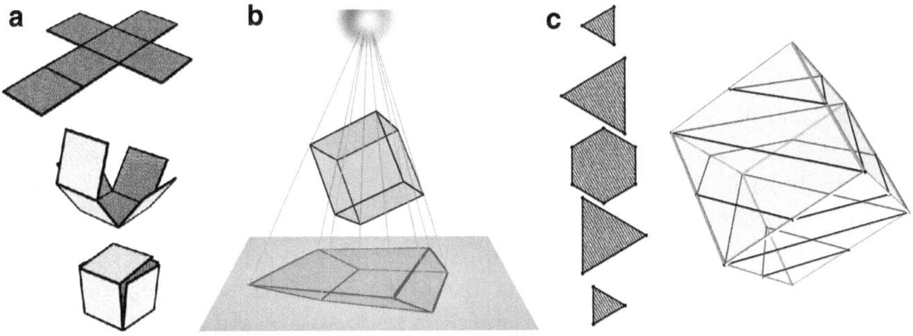

Fig. 26.2 Three different ways to represent a cube in two dimensions: **(a)** a foldout, **(b)** some sections, and **(c)** a projection

It is possible to use the same methods with four-dimensional objects using a dimensional analogy. This approach is largely used in the novel *Flatland*, written in 1884 by E.A. Abbot (2008). The main character is a square, living in a flat, two-dimensional world. One night, the Square has a dream about visiting a one-dimensional world (*Lineland*). In the dream, he tries to convince the Lineland monarch of a second dimension but finds essentially impossible to make him see outside of his eternally straight line. Of course the Square himself is absolutely unable to imagine the third dimension and therefore is completely mystified when a Sphere crosses his house, appearing to his two-dimensional eyes as a point, suddenly enlarging in a perfect circle. After a while, the Square starts to accept the existence of the Sphere, living in a three-dimensional world: *Spaceland*. In fact the Square's understanding of the matter is so deep that he postulates the existence of a fourth (and a fifth, a sixth, etc.) spatial dimension. The Sphere refuses to accept this advanced concept and abandons the Square.

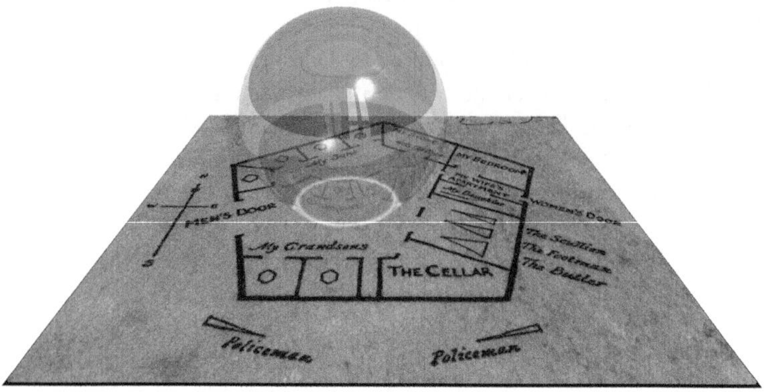

Fig. 26.3 The Sphere crosses Flatland, appearing in the Square's house

In this context, the fourth dimension is a purely spatial dimension, perfectly analogous to the three that we are already familiar with. In other words, we are not referring to the space–time, in which the fourth dimension is quite different from the other three. Let us consider the sequence: point, segment, square, and cube. Each item can be obtained from the previous one sliding it along a difference direction. Each direction is perpendicular to the others. We cannot image a fourth direction perpendicular to the other three, but its existence does not violate any geometrical rule. Therefore it is possible to think that it exists (as a mathematical object), albeit we cannot visualize it.

To get a better understanding of this subject, it is useful to follow Abbot's example using the power of the analogy; we will examine a solid shape from the point of view of a *flatlander*. We shall focus on the difficulties of the two-dimensional being trying to grasp three-dimensional features. Eventually we will consider an analog shape in four dimensions and this will guide our mind to deduce its four-dimensional properties from three-dimensional clues.

26.2 The Sphere

Let us start our exploration with the surface of a simple sphere (after all, the Sphere in Flatland does introduce higher dimensions). The sphere surface, which is a two-dimensional entity, is relatively easy to understand for a flatlander. Indeed, Flatland could be placed on a very big sphere and, locally, no one would be aware of the difference with a purely flat surface. Actually the almost spherical shape of our own world has been erroneously considered flat for long time. In a small region of the sphere the flatlander could not detect anything strange. It is its global structure that is definitely different from the plane. To investigate this global structure, let us draw a number of parallel circles on the sphere surface. All the circles are concentric, but they have two common centers, not just one. Let call those two centers *North Pole* and *South Pole*. An inhabitant of the surface, living near the South Pole, would see a sequence of concentric circles around the pole, each containing the other. Traveling from south to north, he or she would cross the circles, which would become bigger and bigger (as expected). Suddenly a strange phenomenon would happen. After crossing the equator, the circles would start become smaller and smaller and eventually the last circle would degenerate in a single point: the North Pole. This is very difficult to understand for our explorator, who cannot leave the sphere surface and see it from the space, as we do.

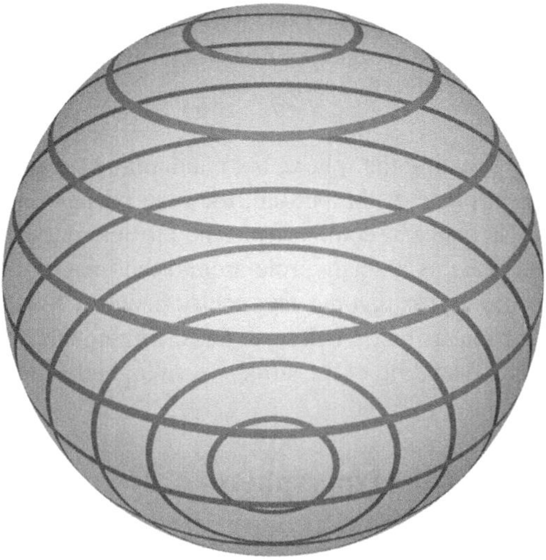

Fig. 26.4 The sphere with a number of parallels

To get an intuitive understanding of this strange phenomenon, our two-dimensional explorer could draw a planar map of the surface. There are many ways to do that; for instance, two disjoined disks can be used to represent the north and the south hemispheres. Of course a two-dimensional being can hardly imagine how to "glue" the two disks, joining the boundaries, because this process requires a third dimension. Nevertheless the two maps together provide a good representation of the whole spherical world. Unfortunately the strange behavior of the parallels happens just across the equator: the common limit between the two maps. Therefore this representation is not very useful to investigate the phenomenon.

A better choice is to use a stereographic projection. The sphere is placed above a plane, touching it at the South Pole. The projection source is located at the North Pole. Each point on the sphere surface, except the North Pole, has a projected image somewhere on the plane. This kind of projection preserves angles and therefore shapes, e.g., circles remain circles (they can possibly become straight lines, which could be considered circles with infinite radius).

In our new map the parallels appear as a sequence of concentric circles, each bigger than the previous one. A small parallel near the North Pole would appear as an enormous circle, containing the images of all the other parallels closer to the South Pole.

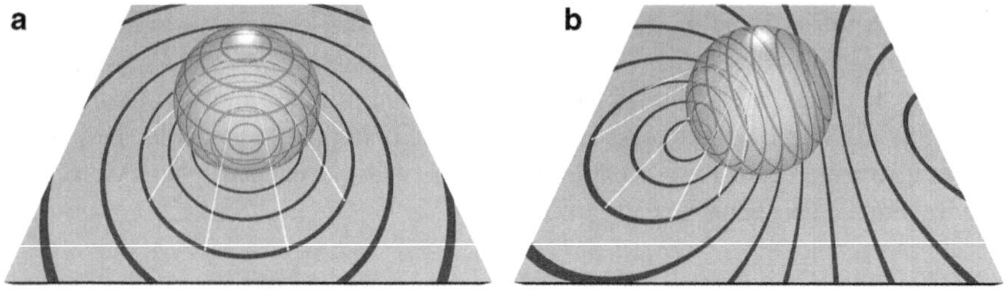

Fig. 26.5 Stereographic projections of the parallels on the sphere surface: (a) from the North Pole and (b) rotating the sphere

Rotating the sphere, but maintaining the projection source at the top and the tangent plane at the bottom, the map changes dramatically. The image of the North Pole appears, coming from the far horizon. The small parallel near the North Pole appears as a small circle around the image of the North Pole. The sphere rotation makes clear that the asymmetry between North Pole and South Pole is a mere projection artifact. Looking at this changing map, the flatlander can develop an intuitive understanding of the strange parallel behavior.

26.3 The Hypersphere

Now we can start to explore the four-dimensional analog of the sphere: the *hypersphere*[2] also known as *glome*.[3] The hyper-surface of the hypersphere would be a three-dimensional space, bended in a direction we cannot visualize. If the hypersphere were big enough, the curvature of the hyper-surface would be small and not noticeable. The "parallels" of the hypersphere would be a sequence of concentric spheres, each containing the others. Also in this case, the parallels have two different centers: the North Pole and the South Pole. Of course, we (three-dimensional being) cannot imagine a sphere with two different centers. We have to use the analogy with the circular parallels of the three-dimensional sphere we have just examined in the previous paragraph.

Traveling from the South Pole toward the North Pole, we cross bigger and bigger spheres, but behind the "equator" the spheres become smaller and smaller. The very last sphere degenerates in a single point: the North Pole of the hypersphere.

---

[2]The word *hypersphere* can in general describe any higher-dimensional analog of the sphere (i.e., spheres in four, five, six, etc. dimensions).

[3]*3-sphere, Wikipedia, The Free Encyclopedia. <http://en.wikipedia.org/w/index.php?title=3-sphere&oldid=208966785> Hypersphere*, from Math World, *Eric W. Weisstein*, *<http://mathworld.wolfram.com/Hypersphere.html>*

We can represent the hypersphere using two balls, filled with concentric spheres. The boundaries of the two balls are identified, i.e., the two balls should be considered "glued" along their surfaces. The North and the South Poles of the hypersphere are the centers of those two balls.

It is also possible to use a stereographic projection: the two poles are both visible in the same image. The spherical parallels are distributed in the space between the two poles. The curvature of the spheres changes in such a way that those closer to a pole contain it.

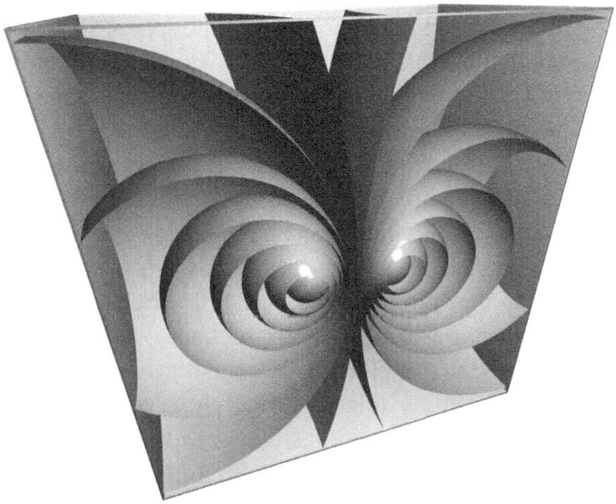

Fig. 26.6 Stereographic projection of the spherical parallels on the hypersphere

The structure of the hypersphere (a sequence of concentric spheres, limited in opposite directions by two different poles) resembles very closely a well-known literary image: the Dante Alighieri's Heaven (Egginton 1999, Osserman 1996). In his journey across the heaven, Dante crosses a number of spheres whose center is the earth center. Eventually Dante crosses the last sphere and realizes that its center is a very bright point representing God. In other words, all the celestial spheres and the spheres of the angels have two opposite centers: the center of the earth (where Lucifer lives) and God. This cosmological description is difficult to understand completely and that is very appropriate for such a metaphysical subject. The geometrical structure of the hypersphere fits surprisingly well the Dante's description. In fact, Dante pictured the universe as two balls: the first is the "Primum Mobile," which has the earth in its center and contains all the "skies." The other is the "Empyrean," which contains the angels and God at the center. The surfaces of the two balls are "glued" together; the Empyrean is surrounding the visible universe, although it has a different center. This is exactly the hypersphere structure we have just described. Of course Dante had no clues about high-dimensional geometry which has been studied five centuries after the publication of the *Divina Commedia*, but apparently artists and scientists, living in the same universe and sharing the same "ideosphere," can speculate – each with his or her own tools – on similar ideas, sometimes creating very similar models.

26.4 Tiling and Polyhedra

As we have already noticed, a small part of a spherical surface is quite similar to a flat plane. It is possible to draw geometric figures on it and to measure distances, angles, etc. Indeed the first four Euclid's postulates are valid on the sphere, while the fifth is wrong. The geometry of the sphere surface is non-Euclidean. One consequence of the fifth postulate is the existence of similar, but noncongruent figures and indeed such figures do not exist on the sphere. For instance, two spherical squares of different sizes do have different angles. The square angles are never 90° and therefore it is not possible to place four squares around a vertex without overlaps. This is an important difference between the flat and the spherical geometries. The whole plane can be tiled using squares, while the sphere cannot. On the other side, a spherical square whose size has been carefully selected (in rapport to the sphere radius) has 120° angles and therefore three of those squares can be placed around a vertex without overlaps. In fact six of those squares can tile the sphere completely. Of course this tiling – six squares, three around each vertex – is closely related to the cube; it can be obtained by "inflating" a cube inscribed in the sphere until the faces touch the sphere surface. There is a correspondence between the regular tilings of the sphere and the regular polyhedra in the space.

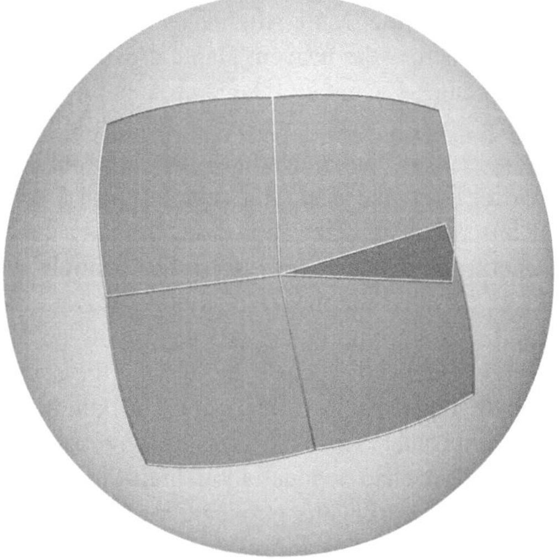

Fig. 26.7 It is not possible to place four squares around a vertex on the surface of the sphere

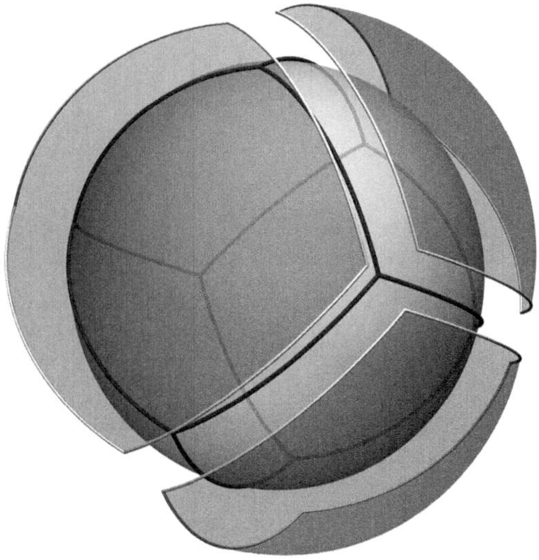

Fig. 26.8 A tiling of the sphere made of six squares, three around each vertex

To create a representation of the spherical tilings that can be understood by a Flatland inhabitant, we use again the stereographic projection. Let us take a regular dodecahedron, which is a convex polyhedron made of 12 regular pentagons, "inflated" in order to obtain a sphere tiling. The stereographic projection of this tiling is a set of 12 curvilinear pentagons, meeting – three at each vertex – at 120° angles and covering the whole plane. The faces closer to the projection source are more distorted and enlarged. In fact when the projection source is well inside a face (not touching any edge), the image of that face extends around the figure up to the horizon and only the other 11 pentagons are visible.

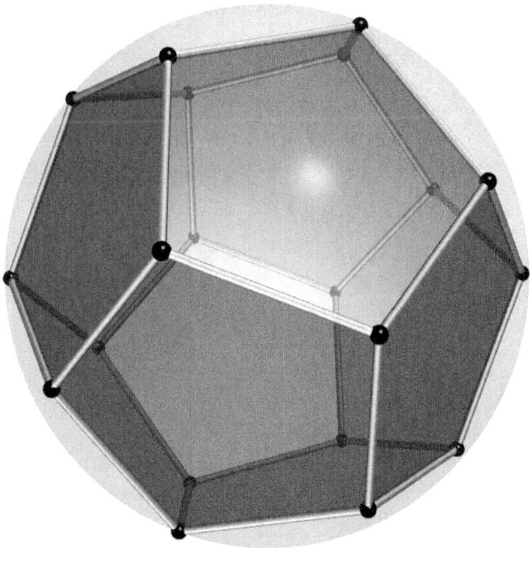

Fig. 26.9 A dodecahedron inscribed in a sphere

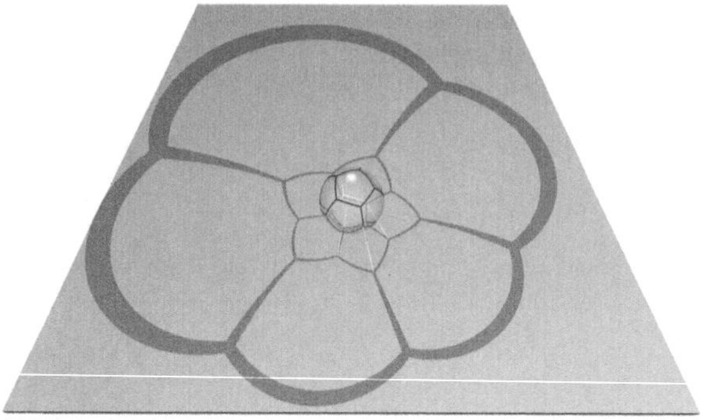

Fig. 26.10 The stereographic projection of the "inflated" dodecahedron

Rotating the sphere changes the map; the small faces, almost not distorted, become larger and larger and eventually they spread toward the horizon, while the distorted, far faces become smaller and regular.

26.5 The 120-cell or Hyperdodecahedron

Following the approach we have already used, we consider the stereographic projection of the hypersphere. Instead of showing the projection of the spherical parallels, we start with the image of a single curvilinear dodecahedron, "drawn" on the hypersurface of the hypersphere. We add another dodecahedron with a face in common with the first one. Then a third is attached to the second through the opposite face. The small tower of three dodecahedra is slightly bent because of the curvature of the hypersphere. Indeed other dodecahedra added to the tower take place along a circular path. The size of the dodecahedra is carefully selected such that exactly 10 dodecahedra fit in a circular shape; the tenth touches the ninth, but also the first.

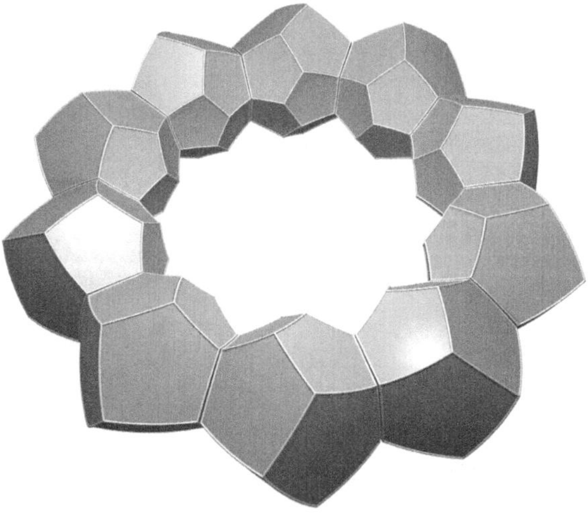

Fig. 26.11 Stereographic projection of ten 10 dodecahedra on the hyper-surface of the hypersphere

It is possible to add another chain of 10 dodecahedra, each touching two consecutive dodecahedra of the first chain. This second chain wraps around the first one: the two chains are linked. For symmetry reason, it is possible to add four more chains around the first one. All the dodecahedra touch each other with no overlaps or leaks. To summarize, we have placed six chains of 10 dodecahedra each for a total of 60 dodecahedra. They cover exactly half of the hyper-surface of the hypersphere. The shape of this part is identical to the rest of the hypersphere. Therefore we can add other 60 dodecahedra covering the whole hypersphere. The 120 dodecahedra are the hyper-faces of the four-dimensional analog of the dodecahedron.

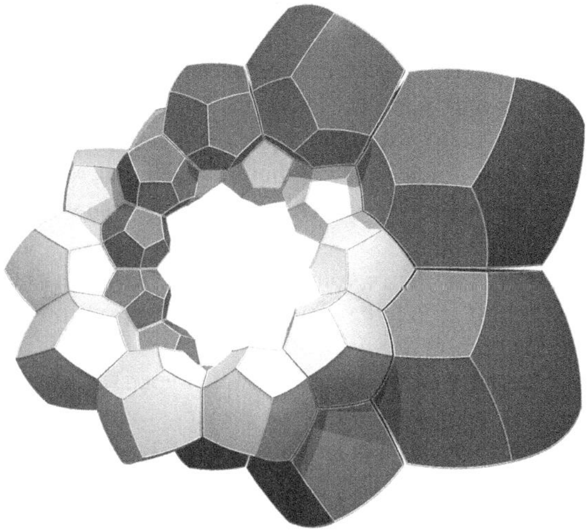

Fig. 26.12 A second chain of dodecahedra linked to the first one

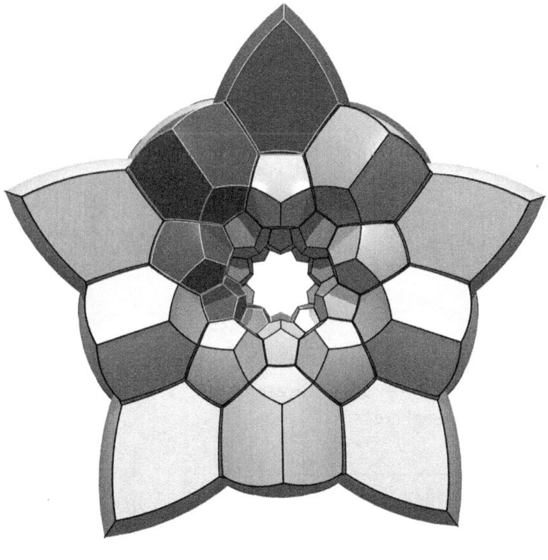

Fig. 26.13 60 dodecahedra coevering half of the hyper-surface of the hypersphere

It is a polychoron (polychora are the analog of polyhedra in four dimensions) called 120-cell (or *hecatonicosachoron* or *hyperdodecahedron*).[4]

26.6 Tori

The shape made of the first 60 dodecahedra of the 120-cell is topologically equivalent to a solid torus (it can be deformed, without cutting or gluing, into a solid resembling a doughnut). Also the rest of the 120-cell is equivalent to a solid torus. The two tori are linked as two rings in a chain, and their surfaces are completely "glued" together (as in the case of the two balls, it is quite difficult for us to imagine how they are glued).

The stereographic images of the two parts are quite different. As usual the difference is only a projection artifact and rotating the hypersphere the shapes swap and it is possible to see their equivalence.

We have just realized that the hypersphere can be split not only in two balls but also in two solid tori. This is something new and peculiar of the four-dimensional world.

Moreover if we consider the first chain of 10 dodecahedra, we realize that it is also equivalent to a solid torus. This torus is completely contained in the torus made of the first 60 dodecahedra.

Indeed we can cover the whole hyper-surface of the hypersphere with a sequence of tori, each containing the previous one. Therefore the hypersphere has toroidal parallels beside spherical ones.

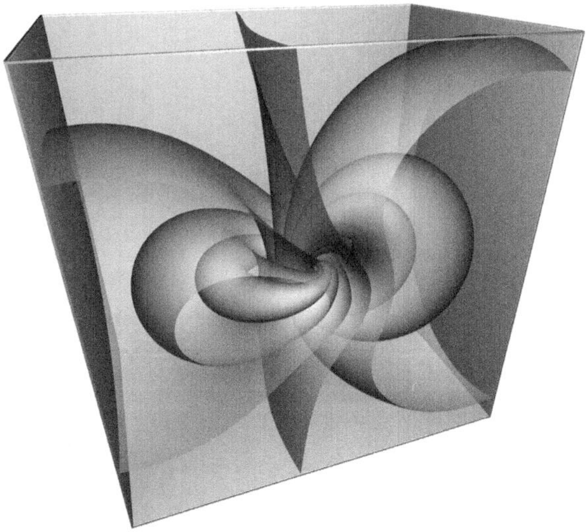

Fig. 26.14 The toroidal parallels on the hyper-surface of the hypersphere

[4]120-cell, *Wikipedia, The Free Encyclopedia*, *<http://en.wikipedia.org/wiki/120-cell>*120-cell, from MathWorld, *Eric W. Weisstein*, *<http://mathworld.wolfram.com/120-Cell.html>*

The image of the two tori linked together is strong and evocative and has been used by artists. For instance, J. Robinson created in 1979 *Bonds of Friendship*, a bronze sculpture made of two large tori linked together. According to the author this sculpture "[...] can symbolise the 'Bonds' between Mathematics and the Visual Art."[5]

Bibliography

Abbot, E. A. (2008). *Flatland: A romance of many dimensions. Oxford world's classics*. Oxford: Oxford University Press. [Full text is available on the web: <*http://www.gutenberg.org/etext/97*>]

Coxeter, H. S. M. (1973). *Regular polytopes*. New York: Dover.

Coxeter, H. S. M. (1991). *Regular complex polytopes*. Cambridge: Cambridge University Press.

Dalì, S. (1954). *Crucifixion (Corpus Hypercubus). oil on canvas 194.5 × 124 cm*. New York: Metropolitan Museum of Art.

Egginton, W. (April 1999). On Dante, Hyperspheres, and the curvature of the medieval cosmos. *J. Hist. Ideas* 60,(2), 195–216.

Heinlein, R. (1941). —And he built a crooked house. In *Astounding Science Fiction*.

Kemp, M. (1988). Dalì's dimensions. *Nature* 391(27), doi:10.1038/34063

Robbins, T. (1992). *Computers, art & the 4th dimension*. A Bulfinch Press Book, ISBN: 0-8212-1909-X.

Robinson, J. (1979). *Bonds of friendship. Polished bronze 5 ft × 3 ft*, Circular Quay, Sydney Cove, NSW, Australia.

Stringham, W. (1880). Regular figures in n-dimensional space. *Am. J. Math* 2(1 Mar), 1–14.

Osserman, R. (1996). *Poetry of the universe*. New York: Anchor Books/Doubleday.

[5]Bonds of Friendship, *J. Robinson*, <*http://www.bradshawfoundation.com/jr/bonds_of_friendship.php*>

Chapter 27
From Art to Mathematics in the Paintings of Theo van Doesburg

Paola Vighi and Igino Aschieri

Abstract The aim of this chapter is to show how present, use or find some mathematical concepts, starting from an artistic production. In particular, we chose Arithmetic Composition I (1930), painted from Theo van Doesburg: we propose to read it with mathematical eyes. In our path we touch the concepts of ratio, geometrical progression, gnomon, perimeter and area, symmetry and so on. We wish that our suggestion can promote the need and the opportunity of mathematical instruments for investigating more in depth, in any context.

27.1 Introduction

This chapter is inspired by pictures by the Dutch artist Theo van Doesburg (1883–1931), one of the founders of the De Stijl group. The aim of this group was to renew the arts, beginning with painting. The artist's own description of his ideas is significant:

> The evolution of painting is nothing but an intellectual search for the truth by means of a visual culture. [...] We are painters who think and measure. [...] Most painters work like pastry-cooks and milliners. In contrast we use mathematical data (whether Euclidean or not) and science, that is to say, intellectual means. [...] We reject artistic handwriting. If one cannot draw a circle by hand, one may use a compass. All instruments which were created by the intellect due to a need for perfection are recommended. (van Doesburg 1930/1974, 181–182).

The chapter makes an in-depth examination of a van Doesburg's painting, it focuses on the "hidden" mathematics and on use of mathematical concepts for interpret the painting.

P. Vighi (✉)
Local Research Unit of Didactics of Mathematics; Mathematics Department, University of Parma, Parma, Italy
e-mail: paola.vighi@unipr.it

V. Capecchi (eds.), *Applications of Mathematics in Models, Artificial Neural Networks and Arts*, DOI 10.1007/978-90-481-8581-8_27,

27.2 Mathematics and Art

The so-called separation between cultures often leads us to consider mathematics and art as separate and even opposing. But the study of a work of art can be enriched and completed if technical aspects are examined. It is also important to know about the historical period in which it has been created. "Human creations, both artistic and scientific, have their own specificity, but at the same time they are linked in multiple relationships: both types constitute development of thought dating from the same period. There have been times in which the relationship was more close (during the Renaissance for instance, 'mathematical rules' were used to organize figurative space); at other times the ties were present, but less obvious" (Speranza and Vighi 1997). In our schools nowadays there is often a lack of integration between artistic and scientific culture, although "Art is inseparable from science and surely also from philosophy, history, literature, music, so the science finds in artistic expression [...] a concrete visualization of the transformations that it produces in human thought and in civilization" (Lazzotti 1986, 24). Returning to mathematics, it is important to restore its educational and formative role. We can use it to guide the students to go beyond contents of lessons and put them in touch with the external world, to help them transfer their own knowledge, to understand the usefulness of in-depth study of mathematics and refining mathematical concepts and instruments.

27.3 From a Painting to Mathematics

We start by observing van Doesburg's painting *Arithmetic Composition I* (1930). It is part of a sequence of paintings in which the square is the main element (Fig. 27.1).

A preliminary look at the picture shows four black squares, all "tilted", in a squared canvas. They are homothetic figures. The centre of homothety is one vertex of the canvas. The right lines that connect the corresponding points of the tilted squares pass through this point. A question arises in the mind of the viewer: why the title uses the adjective "arithmetic" when the picture, at least initially, seems to be based on geometrical concepts? This question has been answered from a mathematical point of view by Marion Walter: "I focused first on the horizontal squares because they are so obviously in geometric progression. I let the outside square length 1 unit, and then the side lengths of successive horizontal squares (starting with the largest) are: 1, 1/2, 1/4, 1/8 squares units.

If, instead of sides, I focus on the *areas* of these squares, I obtain areas of: 1, 1/4, 1/16, 1/64 square units. Though the artist, for his own reasons, stopped after four squares, we can theoretically continue the pattern obtaining two geometrical sequences" (Walter 2001). We do not know why van Doesburg chose this title, but the question raises didactically opportune points for discussion with students. Subsequently, we can ask questions such as "What is the relationship between the

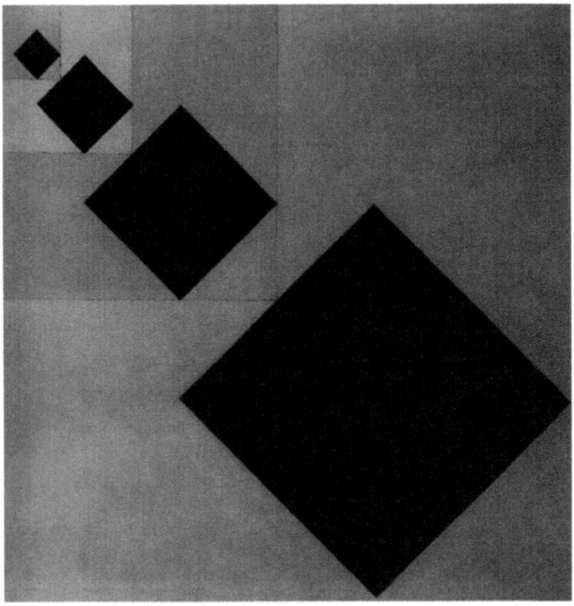

Fig. 27.1 *Arithmetic Composition I*

measurements of the sides of the black squares? And between their areas?" We can next introduce *geometrical sequences*. The discussion could also be enriched by making reference to Plato's dialogue between Socrates and the servant, based on the fact that if the sides of two squares are in the ratio of 1:2, then their areas are in the ratio 1:4. From the didactical point of view, this is an important and difficult concept. We can also use van Doesburg's sketch *Study for Forme Universelle II* (Fig. 27.2) as useful material for calculating perimeters and areas.

Here we can see that the black squares are drawn on squared paper, but the background of the other tilted squares changes and it becomes "smaller" if we go from right to left and from low to high. The sides of the background's squares are halved and halved and so on. This sketch provides the opportunity to speak about *units of measurement* and their change. Each black square occupies 32 squares of the paper on which it is drawn, but the surface occupied is different! We again meet the ratio 1:2 between the sides and, as a consequence, the ratio 1:4 between the areas.

In other words, from a didactical point of view, the painting can furnish a first approach to idea of "similitude". In effect, homothety is a particular similitude.

27.4 The Gnomon

Now let us observe the first painting again more closely (Fig. 27.1). Our eyes see in the background other squares, "straight" and overlapping, in light colours (Fig. 27.3). More precisely, to the left of the canvas there is a grey square, and the

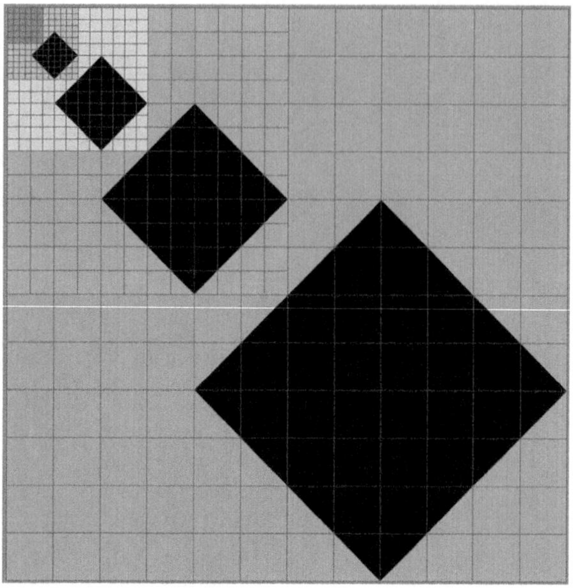

Fig. 27.2 *Study for Forme Universelle II* reproduction

Fig. 27.3 Background squares in *Arithmetic Composition I*

other shapes in the background recall the Euclidean *gnomon*. The word "gnomon" had different meanings in Greece. The first was an astronomic meaning: the time's measures were based on the use of a stick planted in earth; the stick and its shadow produce a shape named gnomon. In Euclid's "*Elements*", Definition 2 of

Book II is "And in any parallelogrammic area let any one whatever of the parallelograms about its diameter with the two complements be called a gnomon" (http://aleph0.clarku.edu/~djoyce/java/).

So a *gnomon* is a figure obtained by removing a parallelogram from a larger similar parallelogram. A gnomon is "L" shaped. In Fig. 27.4, we have a gnomon cutting from the parallelogram ABCD the smaller parallelogram with BE as diagonal. The previous figure suggests also another important Euclidean theorem, named "The gnomon theorem": "In any parallelogram the complements of the parallelograms about the diagonal equal one another." On this proposition was based a fundamental method of Greek mathematics, the "area's applications method".

The gnomon has a relevant role in Greek mathematics. After the "crisis of incommensurables", the mathematicians choose to pass from numbers to geometry and they developed a method for the treatment of algebraic problems, named "geometric algebra" from the historian Paul Tannery. In other words, the resolution of algebraic problems and of particular equations is carried out by means of geometric constructions. It could be very interesting and suitable to study this method in our schools. They allow to go in depth in some concepts and also to see them from another point of view.

On the other hand, if we opportunely add a gnomon to a parallelogram, we obtain a similar parallelogram. The idea of increase in size while maintaining shape is present also in the "figural" numbers of Pythagoras (Fig. 27.5). We find again the similitude of shapes.

The discovery of the "invariance in the variation" was an important aspect of Pythagoras' philosophy. Also biology has used the gnomon in order to study laws of increase to spiral (Thompson 1992). The role of gnomon in mathematics went very beyond the geometrical aspect, involving the number, let only technical algorithmic: "This technique of increase (or decrease) of spatial shapes as instrument of generation of numbers ended to represent not only an initial moment, but the same

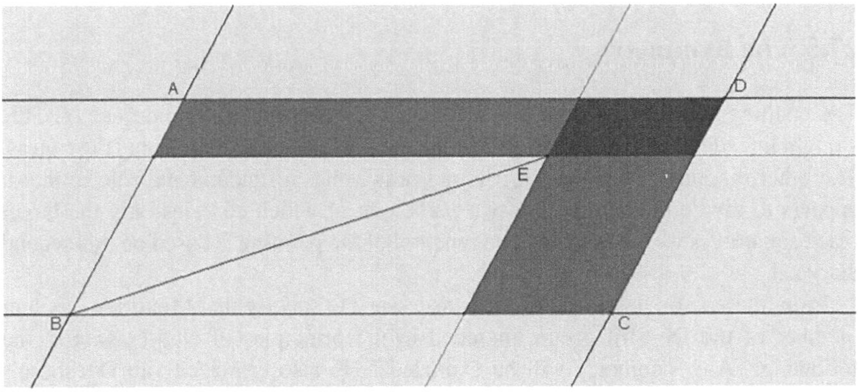

Fig. 27.4 Gnomon construction

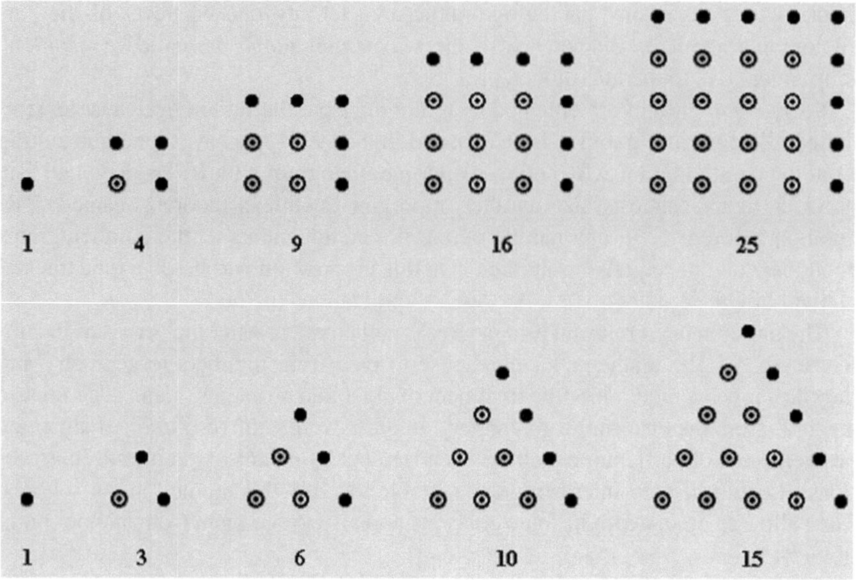

Fig. 27.5 Pythagoras *Figural numbers*

key of a way to conceive the number and the measure in the Occident" (Zellini 1999).

Heron of Alexandria (75 d.C.) applies the same technique to other geometric figures, for example, to an isosceles triangle with two angles of 72°. Tracing the bisector of one of these angles we obtain two isosceles triangles. One of these is the gnomon of ABC, since it is similar to it (Fig. 27.6). The procedure can be continued to the infinite! In this way we can also communicate the ideas of recursiveness and of fractal.

27.5 The Symmetry

The painting *Arithmetic Composition I* (Fig. 27.1) presents a symmetrical axis, the straight line identified from one of the diagonals of the square that demits the canvas. The other diagonal, even though it is not drawn, has a fundamental role in that it appears to divide the canvas into two parts, one of which contains only the larger black square. As we will see, the construction of the painting is based on this second diagonal.

From the artistic point of view, it is necessary to specify that Mondrian, another member of the De Stijl group, included in the principles of Neo-Plasticism the following: "Any symmetry will be excluded." He also criticized van Doesburg's decision to use the diagonal, and in fact even broke off relations with him. Pimm (2001) compares the problem of use of the diagonal in Neo-Plasticism with the

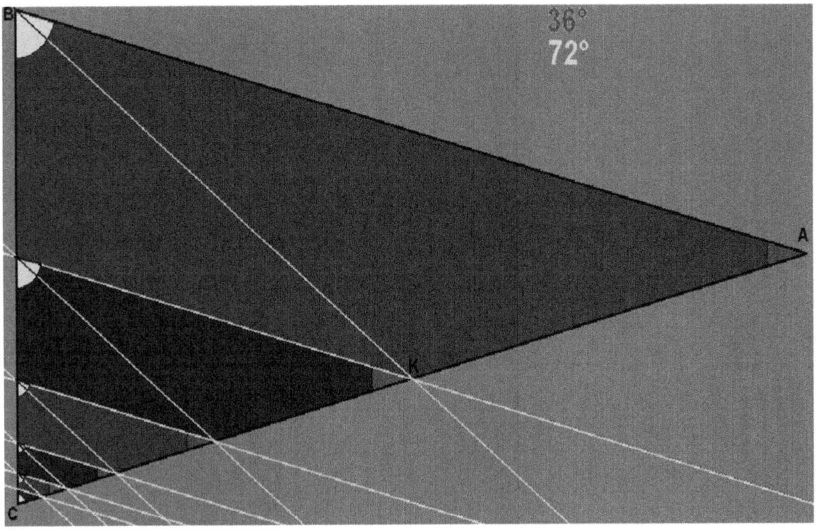

Fig. 27.6 Recursive construction

use of the procedure of "neusis" or "sliding" in Ancient Greek mathematics: "Is it of the same order as those ancient Greek mathematicians who would allow *neusis* constructions and those who would not?" (Pimm 2001, 33). In Ancient Greek mathematics, the only acceptable constructions were those executed with rule and compass and those made with neusis were not acceptable.

We now discuss a further aspect of the painting.

The square of the canvas, ABCD, contains two squares AGFE and HIJK (Fig. 27.7), the first "straight" and the second "tilted", which have F as common point. Some questions arise: Are the squares AGFE and HIJK isometric or not? Is the segment HI on the diagonal line BD? Is it possible that the answer is "yes" for both questions?

We develop the answer with "synthetic geometry"s' arguments.

Wc chosc (Fig. 27.8) to put IH on the diagonal line BD and to take the point F as the medium point of BD and, as a consequence, of IH. So, according to theorem named in Italy "Tale's theorem",[1] G is the medium point of AB and E is the medium point of AD. There are many isometric segments: AE, ED, AG, GB, AG, EF, GB. The triangles EDF and GFB are rectangular and isosceles. Triangles DHK and BIJ are rectangular, isosceles and congruent too: $DH \cong HK$ and $BI \cong IJ$, but also $HK \cong IH \cong IJ$ because they are sides of a square, then $BI \cong IH \cong HD$ for the transitive property of equal. Lastly we find that IH is one-third of BD, while AE half of AD.

[1] If we cut some parallel straight lines with two lines, equal segments correspond to equal segments etc.

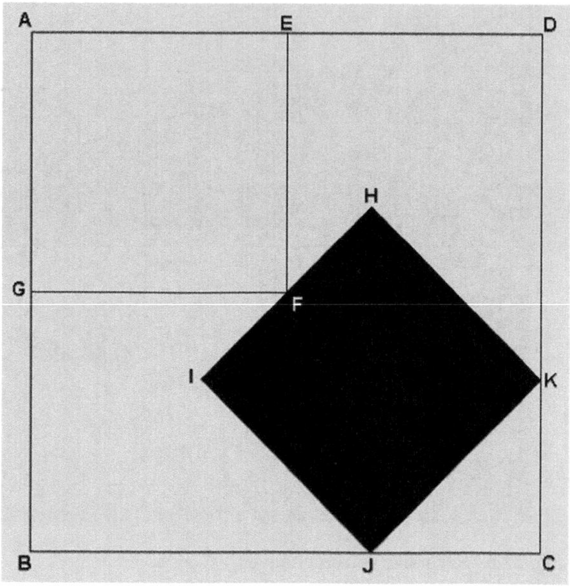

Fig. 27.7 Comparison between squares AGFE and IJKH

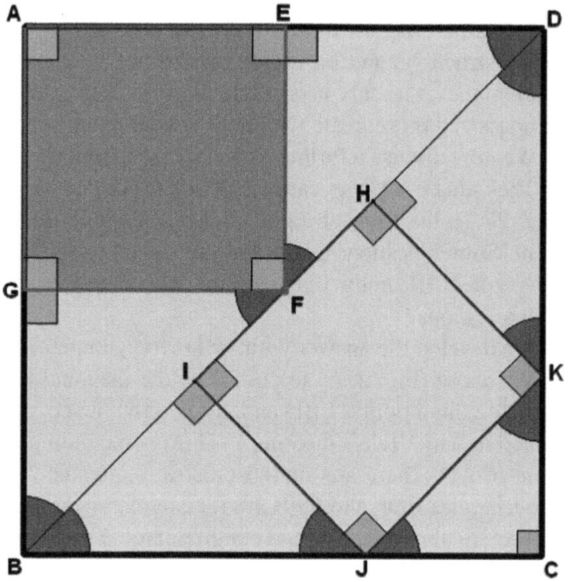

Fig. 27.8 Geometrical analysis

If we indicate with 1 the length of each side of the canvas, we obtain the following measurements wrote in Fig. 27.9.

Therefore the squares **A** and **B** are not equal. If we want equal squares, we must exit from the diagonal line! (Fig. 27.10) (IH segment not lying on diagonal).

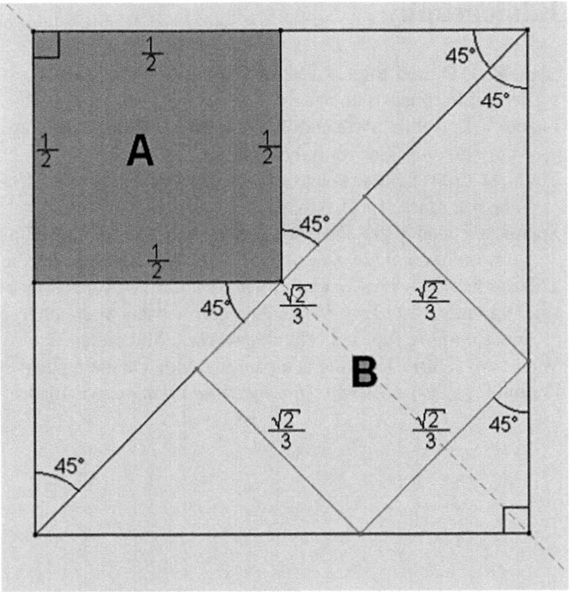

Fig. 27.9 Quantitative analysis

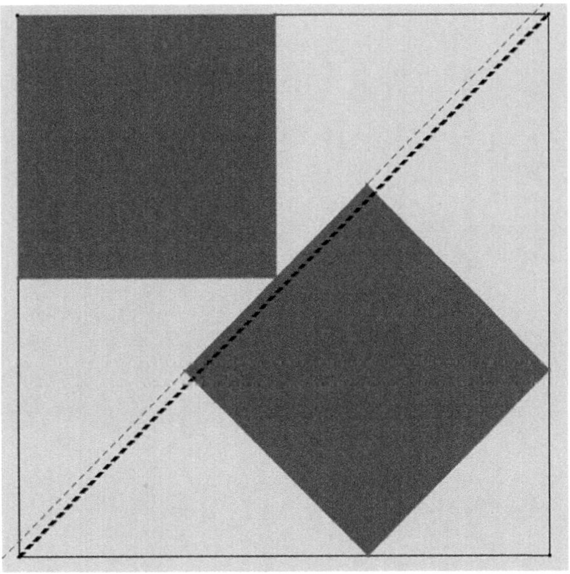

Fig. 27.10 Relationship between squares and diagonal

Another problem arise: how is it possible to draw a "tilted" square inscribed in a triangle? For this, we suggest to read the Walter's explanations (Walter 2001).

Bibliography

Bedient, J. D. and Bunt, L. N. H. (1976). *The historical roots of elementary mathematics*. New Jersey: Prentice-Hall.
Lazotti F. L. (1986). Arte and Scienza: riflessioni teoriche e prospettive didattiche. In *Quaderni di Villa Falconieri*, no. 8, Italy: Frascati.
Pimm, D. (2001). Some notes on Theo van Doesburg (1883–1931) and his Arithmetic Composition I. *Learn. Math.* 21(2), 31–36.
Speranza, F. and Vighi, P. (1997). Spazio dell'arte, spazio della matematica. In *Arte e Matematica: un sorprendente binomio*. Italy: Vasto Atti Convegno Mathesis.
Thompson, D. W. (1992). *On growth and form*. Dover reprint of 1942 2nd edn. (1st edn., 1917).
van Doesburg, T. (1974). Comments on the basis of concrete painting. In Banlieu, J. (Ed.), *Theo van Doesburg* (pp. 181–182). New York: Macmillan.
Walter, M. (2001). Looking at a painting with a mathematical eyes. *Learn. math.* 21(2) 26–30.
Zellini, P. (1999). *Gnomon. Una indagine sul numero*. Milano: Adelphi.

ERRATUM

Erratum to: Art by Numbers

Marco Pierini
Direttore della Galleria civica di Modena

V. Capecchi (eds.), *Applications of Mathematics in Models, Artificial Neural Networks and Arts*,
DOI 10.1007/978-90-481-8581-8_24, © Springer Science+Business Media B.V. 2010

DOI 10.1007/978-90-481-8581-8_28

The contributing author of chapter 24 (Art by Numbers) has mistakenly been interpreted in the chapter opening page as well as the table of contents. The correct contributing author of this chapter is **Marco Pierini**.

The online version of the original chapter can be found at
http://dx.doi.org/10.1007/978-90-481-8581-8_24

Author Index

V. Capecchi (eds.), *Applications of Mathematics in Models, Artificial Neural Networks and Arts*, DOI 10.1007/978-90-481-8581-8,

GPSR Compliance

The European Union's (EU) General Product Safety Regulation (GPSR) is a set of rules that requires consumer products to be safe and our obligations to ensure this.

If you have any concerns about our products, you can contact us on ProductSafety@springernature.com

In case Publisher is established outside the EU, the EU authorized representative is:

Springer Nature Customer Service Center GmbH
Europaplatz 3
69115 Heidelberg, Germany

Batch number: 10584520

Printed by Printforce, the Netherlands